Practical Pediatric Urology

Prasad Godbole • Duncan T. Wilcox
Martin A. Koyle
Editors

Practical Pediatric Urology

An Evidence-Based Approach

Springer

Editors
Prasad Godbole
Department of Paediatric Surgery
Sheffield Children's Foundation Trust
Sheffield
UK

Duncan T. Wilcox
Division of Urology
University of Colorado Division of Urology
Aurora, CO
USA

Martin A. Koyle
Department of Surgery and IHPME
University of Toronto Paediatric Urology
The Hospital for Sick Children
Toronto, ON
Canada

ISBN 978-3-030-54019-7 ISBN 978-3-030-54020-3 (eBook)
https://doi.org/10.1007/978-3-030-54020-3

This Springer imprint is published by the registered company Springer Nature Switzerland AG
The registered company address is: Gewerbestrasse 11, 6330 Cham, Switzerland

Foreword

Paediatric Urology is one of the youngest surgical specialties and much of its development has occurred during the era of evidence based medicine. By promoting clinical and experimental research in Pediatric Urology, specialist societies such as the Society for Pediatric Urology and European Society for Paediatric Urology have played valuable roles in ensuring that the new specialty has been built on firm scientific foundations. The establishment of the Journal of Pediatric Urology in 2005 was another influential landmark in Pediatric Urology's development as an evidence based specialty.

Opportunities to attain the levels of evidence achieved in other areas of medical research are inevitably more limited in a small volume surgical specialty such as Pediatric Urology. With certain exceptions (such as the RIVUR, PRIVENT and Swedish Reflux trials) it has proved very difficult to design and conduct prospective randomised controlled trials with the statistical power required to meet the highest levels of evidence based medicine. However, to some extent this deficiency is now being addressed by systemic reviews and meta analyses of case—controlled clinical studies. Other obstacles to high quality research include the difficulty in attracting funding and the length of time before long term outcomes can be reliably evaluated in adolescence or adulthood. Against this challenging background the editors and contributors have set themselves a daunting task in seeking to define the scientific evidence underpinning best practice in clinical Pediatric Urology.

The opening chapter sets the scene by providing an authoritative account of the history and development of evidence based medicine. This is followed by chapters on the development of evidence based guidelines, antibiotic usage and the role of effective pain management: important topics which rarely feature in standard Pediatric Urology textbooks. For the most part, Pediatric Urologists are practical clinicians for whom evidence based medicine exists primarily to assist them in caring for their young patients to the highest standards. With this in mind, most of this excellent book is devoted to enabling Pediatric Urologists to adopt an evidence based approach to the management of a wide range of practical problems encountered in their day to day clinical practice. This book will undoubtedly serve as a valuable resource for trainees—particularly those preparing for examinations. In addition it will provide established Pediatric Urologists with an opportunity to appraise their own specialist practice and decision—making in the context of the latest published evidence. The editors and contributors have distilled a wealth of valuable and clinically relevant evidence into this textbook and are to be commended on their achievement.

David F. M. Thomas
Emeritus Consultant Paediatric Urologist
Leeds Teaching Hospitals & Professor of Paediatric Surgery
University of Leeds
Leeds, England

Preface

The world of pediatric urology is progressing at a rapid pace. With the advances in pharmaceuticals, technologies and greater understanding of disease process, treatment decisions can be based on evidence as opposed to anecdotal experience. Furthermore increasing patient/parental awareness of pediatric urological conditions mandate that the Pediatric Urologist discuss the various treatment options with the patient and family to enable a shared decision making approach.

With this background, we are delighted to introduce this book 'Practical Pediatric Urology—An Evidence Based Approach'. The book is predominantly in a question and answer scenario based format to enable higher order thinking and decision making process. Wherever evidence is available, this has been cited in the discussion. A small minority of chapters are descriptive in nature where the scenario based format would not have been suitable.

This book would be of use to all Pediatric Urologists, Adult Urologists practising Pediatric Urology, Pediatric Urology and Pediatric Surgery trainees as well as Trainers. The book can also be used as a self assessment tool for preparation of Board exams.

We would like to thank the outstanding and timely contributions from the authors. A special thanks to Ms Madona Samuel, project coordinator for her periodic prompting to ensure our consistent focus on the project and to Melissa Morton Executive Editor at Springer for giving us the opportunity to publish this important book.

Finally it goes without saying that we are grateful to our families for their patience and support throughout this process.

Sheffield, UK — Prasad Godbole
Aurora, CO — Duncan T. Wilcox
Toronto, ON, Canada — Martin A. Koyle

Contents

The Evolution of Evidence Based Clinical Medicine

1

Paul Dimitri

Learning Objective

- To understand the rationale and need for evidence based medicine for clinical practice
- To recognise the hierarchies and systems designed to support the evaluation and classification of clinical evidence
- To understand the challenges and controversies with current systems used in evidence based medicine

1.1 Introduction

Evidence Based Medicine (EBM) proposed by David Sackett over a quarter of a century ago is the integration of the best research evidence with clinical expertise and patient values defined as 'the conscientious, explicit and judicious use of current best evidence in making decisions about the care of individual patients' supported by 'integrating individual clinical expertise with the best available external clinical evidence from systematic research' [1]. The concept of EBM was initiated in 1981 when a group of clinical epidemiologists at McMaster University (Hamilton, Ontario, Canada), led by David Sackett, published the first of a series of articles in the Canadian Medical Association Journal based upon 'critical appraisal' providing a framework for clinicians to use when appraising medical literature [1]. Subsequent to this in 1985, Sackett and co-workers published 'Clinical Epidemiology: a Basic Science for Clinical Medicine' based upon the critical appraisal of research

P. Dimitri (✉)
Sheffield Children's NHS Foundation Trust, Sheffield, UK

Sheffield Hallam University, Sheffield, UK

University of Sheffield, Sheffield, UK
e-mail: Paul.Dimitri@nhs.net

P. Godbole et al. (eds.), *Practical Pediatric Urology*,
https://doi.org/10.1007/978-3-030-54020-3_1

providing the foundations that have gone on to support the principles of EBM [2]. Whilst David Sackett is considered the father of EBM, it was not until nearly a decade after the first principles of EBM were published that the term 'evidence based medicine' was coined by Gordon Guyatt, the Program Director of Internal Medicine and Professor of Epidemiology, Biostatistics, and Medicine at McMaster University [3]. Sackett believed that the truth of medicine could only be identified through randomised-controlled trials which eliminated the bias of clinical opinion when conducted appropriately. Furthermore, Sackett distinguished the difference between EBM and critical appraisal by defining the three principles of EBM (a) consideration of the patient's expectations; (b) clinical skills; and (c) the best evidence available [4]. Thus whilst EBM is founded on robust clinical research evidence, there is a recognition that practitioners have clinical expertise reflected in effective and efficient diagnosis and incorporates the individual patients' predicaments, rights, and preferences. In 1994 Sackett moved to Oxford, United Kingdom where he worked as a clinician and Director of the Centre for Evidence-Based Medicine. From here Sackett lectured widely across the UK and Europe on EBM. He would begin his visits by doing a round on patients admitted the previous night with young physicians and showing evidence based medicine in action. Junior doctors learned how to challenge senior opinions encapsulated in expert based medicine through evidence based medicine [5]. Based upon the growing support and recognised need for EBM, in 1993 Iain Chalmers co-founded the Cochrane Centre which has evolved to become an internationally renowned centre for the generation of EBM. Thus the foundations of EBM had been laid to pave the way for an revolution in interventional medical care, robust in quality, but subsequently open to challenge from critics that believed that EBM had developed into an overly rigid system limited by generalisation.

1.2 The Evolution of Evidence Based Medicine

Over the subsequent decade the popularity and recognition for EBM grew exponentially. In 1992, only two article titles included the term EBM; within 5 years, more than 1000 articles had used the term EBM [6]. A survey in 2004 identified 24 dedicated textbooks, nine academic journals, four computer programs, and 62 internet portals all dedicated to the teaching and development of EBM [7]. Evidence based medicine derives its roots from clinical epidemiology. Epidemiology and its methods of quantification, surveillance, and control have been traced back to social processes in eighteenth and nineteenth-century Europe. Toward the middle of the twentieth century doctors began to apply these tools to the evaluation of clinical treatment of individual patients [6]. The new field of clinical epidemiology was established in 1938 by John R Paul. In 1928, Paul joined the faculty of the Yale School of Medicine as a Professor of Internal Medicine and subsequently held the Position of Professor of Preventive Medicine from 1940 until his retirement. Paul established the Yale Poliomyelitis Study Unit in 1931 together with James D. Trask. It was through this work that the concept of 'clinical epidemiology' was established in which the path of disease outbreaks in small communities was directly studied. The concepts of clinical epidemiology were furthered by Alvan Feinstein, Professor of Medicine and Epidemiology at Yale University School of Medicine from 1969. Feinstein introduced the use of statistical research methods into the quantification of clinical practices and study of the medical decision-making process. In 1967 Feinstein challenged the traditional process of clinical decision making based upon belief and experience in his publication 'Clinical Judgement' [8], followed shortly by Archie Cochrane's publication 'Effectiveness and Efficiency' describing the lack of controlled trials supporting many practices that had previously been assumed to be effective [9]. In 1968, The McMaster University was established in Canada. The new medical school introduced an integrative curriculum called 'problem-based learning' combining the study of basic sciences and clinical medicine using clinical problems in a tutorship system. The McMaster Medical School established the world's first department of clinical epidemiology and biostatistics, which was directed by David Sackett. The process of problem-based learning led by Sackett was fundamental to the curriculum; Alvan Feinstein was invited as a visiting Professor for the first 2 years of the programme to combine clinical epidemiology with the process of problem-based learning. Thus a new approach to clinical epidemiology arose combining the methods problem-based learning curriculum, practical clinical problem solving and the analysis of medical decision making. In 1978 they developed a series of short courses at McMaster University based upon the use of clinical problems as the platform for enquiry and discussion. This approach was described in the Departmental Clinical Epidemiology and Biostatistics Annual report 1979; 'these courses consider the critical assessment of clinical information pertaining to the selection and interpretation of diagnostic tests, the study of etiology and causation, the interpretation of investigation of the clinical course and natural history of human disease, the assessment of therapeutic claims and the interpretation of studies of the quality of clinical care'. The approach adopted in these courses demonstrated that what we now know as EBM was practiced prior to its formal introduction into the medical literature. These courses were the catalyst for the landmark series of publications in the Canadian Medical Association Journal in 1981 [2] describing the methodological approaches to critical appraisal, culminating in Guyatt's publication in 1992 in JAMA (Journal of the American Medical Association) popularising the term 'Evidence Based Medicine' [10]. Guyatt stated 'a new paradigm for medical practice is emerging. Evidence-based medicine de-emphasises intuition, unsystematic clinical experience, and pathophysiologic rationale as sufficient grounds for clinical decision making and stresses the examination of evidence from clinical research', thus challenging past medical knowledge, established medical literature and practice formed by consensus and expertise based upon knowledge derived from clinical research, epidemiology, statistics and bioinformatics. However, to ensure the that the principles of EBM carried credibility and authority from consensus, this and other subsequent publications were written by an anonymous Evidence-Based Medicine Working Group to ensure the greatest impact. JAMA under the editorial authority of Drummond Rennie became one of the first and principle proponents of EBM; of 22 articles on EBM published in the first 3 years, 12 were published by JAMA with a further 32 published over the proceeding 8 years [6]. The terminology 'evidence-based' had been previously used by David Eddy in the study of population policies from 1987 and subsequently published in 1990 in JAMA, describing evidence-based guidelines and policies stating that policy must be consistent with and supported by evidence [11, 12].

EBM is an approach to medical practice intended to optimise decision-making by emphasising the use of evidence from well-designed research rather than the beliefs of practitioners. The process of EBM adopts an epistemological and pragmatic approach dictating that the strongest recommendations in clinical practice are founded on robust clinical research approaches that include meta-analyses, systematic reviews, and randomised controlled trials. Conversely, recommendations founded upon less robust research approaches (albeit well-recognised) such as the case-control study result in clinical recommendations that are regarded as less robust. Whilst the original framework of EBM was designed to improve the decision making process by clinicians for individual or groups of patients, the principles of EBM have extended towards establishing guidelines, health service administration and policy known as evidence based policy and evidence based practice. More recently there has been a recognition that clinical 'interpretation' of research and clinical 'judgement' may also influence decisions on individual patients or small groups of patients whereas policies applied to large populations need to be founded on a robust evidence base that demonstrates effectiveness. Thus a modified definition of EBM embodies these two approaches—evidence-based medicine is a set of principles and methods intended to ensure that to the greatest extent possible, medical decisions, guidelines, and other types of policies are based on and consistent with good evidence of effectiveness and benefit [13]. Following the implementation of the National Institute of Clinical Evidence (NICE) in the UK in 1999, there was a recognition that evidence should be classified according on rigour of its experimental design, and the strength of a recommendation should depend on the strength of the evidence.

1.3 A Methodological Approach to Evidence Based Medicine

1.3.1 Reviewing the Evidence

Fundamental to the process of defining an evidence-base, is the 'systematic review' which was established to evaluate the available and combined evidence in order to provide a robust and balanced approach. There are a number of programmes established to conduct and present systematic reviews. The Cochrane Collaboration established in 1993 was founded on 10 principles to provide the most robust evidence; collaboration, enthusiasm, avoiding duplication, minimising bias, keeping up to date, relevance, promoting access, quality, continuity and world wide participation [14]. The founders of the Cochrane Collaboration, Iain Chalmers, Tom Chalmers and Murray Enkin attributed the name to Archie Cochrane who had conducted his first trial whilst imprisoned during World War II defining the principles of the randomised-control trial. Through later work Cochrane demonstrated the value of epidemiological studies and the threat of bias [15]. Cochrane's most influential mark on healthcare was his 1971 publication, 'Effectiveness and Efficiency' strongly criticising the lack of reliable evidence behind many of the commonly accepted healthcare interventions at the time, highlighting the need for evidence in medicine [9]. His call for a collection of systematic reviews led to the creation of The Cochrane Collaboration. The framework for the Cochrane Collaboration came from preceding work by Iain Chalmers and Enkin through their development of the Oxford Database of Perinatal Trials [16]. Through their work in this field, Chalmers and Enkin uncovered practices that were unsupported by evidence and in some cases dangerous, thus acting as a catalyst for adopting the same approach to establish and evidence base across all medical specialities.

The Cochrane Collaboration has grown into a global independent network of researchers, professionals, patients, carers and people interested in health from 130 countries with a vision to 'to improve health by promoting the production, understanding and use of high quality research evidence by patients, healthcare professionals and those who organise and fund our healthcare services' (uk.cochrane.org). The Cochrane Library now provides a comprehensive resource of medical evidence for clinicians and researchers across the globe. The aim of the Cochrane Library is to prepare, maintain, and promote the accessibility of systematic reviews of the effects of healthcare interventions. It contains four databases: the Cochrane Database of Systematic Reviews (CDSR), the Database of Abstracts of Reviews of Effectiveness (DARE), the Cochrane Controlled Trials Register (CCTR), and the Cochrane Review Methodology Database (CRMD) [17].

1.3.2 Categorising the Quality of Evidence

The utilisation of EBM in different healthcare settings is underpinned by the quality of evidence available. Different aspects of EBM including evidence-based policy and evidence-based practice require a certain quality of evidence to inform practice. Evidence ranges from meta-analyses, systemic review and appropriately powered blinded randomised-control trials, to expert consensus opinion and case reports; the inclusion of expert consensus is controversial as it is not felt to represent empirical evidence. Categorising EBM is derived from the freedom from bias inherent in the process by which the evidence was derived. There are many examples derived from organisations that categorise EBM according to the quality of evidence. In 1989 Sackett provided a pragmatic classification of evidence quality based upon trial design using antithrombotic agents as described in Table 1.1 [18].

An adapted approach to the earlier classifications is the well-established 'Evidence Pyramid' (Fig. 1.1) which divides the evidence level pragmatically into study level data and subject level data based upon trial design. The pyramid prioritises randomised control trials due to the ability to provide high levels of internal validity supporting causal inferences and minimising bias due to selection,

Table 1.1 1989 classification of evidence based upon trial design

Level	Type of evidence
I	Large RCTs with clear cut results
II	Small RCTs with unclear results
III	Cohort and case-control studies
IV	Historical cohort or case-control studies
V	Case series, studies with no controls

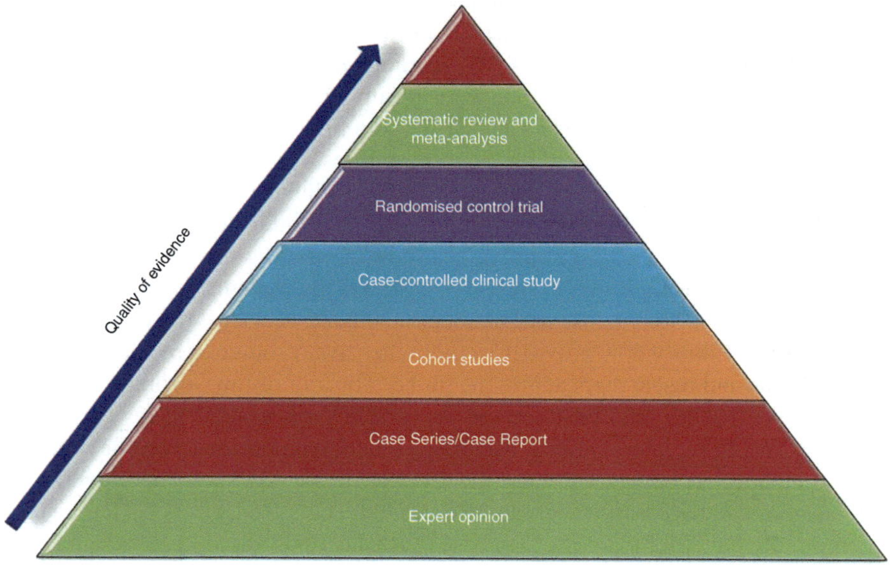

Fig. 1.1 Pyramid of evidence

measurement and confounding. As randomised control trials proliferated the use of systematic review and meta-analyses were established as means of reviewing the outputs of multiple trials.

Early evidence hierarchies were initially developed primarily to help clinicians appraise the quality of evidence for therapeutic effects. The Oxford Centre for Evidence Based Medicine (CEBM) is a not-for-profit organisation dedicated to the practice, teaching and dissemination of high quality evidence based medicine to improve healthcare in everyday clinical practice. Recognising the need to expand the evidence hierarchy to consider evidence related to the area it is being applied to, the Oxford CEBM released the first iteration of their guidelines in 2000 based upon evidence relating to prognosis, diagnosis, treatment benefits, treatment harms, economic decision analysis and screening; these levels were revised in 2011 (Table 1.2).

The type of evidence required is determined by the area in which the question is being asked. Thus evidence for treatment, and prognosis will be depend on studies that use relevant methodologies. For example, a randomised control trial may not be used to determine prognosis and so the highest level of evidence (type 1) may be based upon a systematic review of cohort studies. This is because prognosis may be determined by the impact of not providing introducing an intervention compared to the use of an intervention. Thus well powered prospective cohort analyses or systematic reviews would provide the best evidence (Table 1.2). The Oxford CEBM state '*The levels are not intended to provide you with a definitive judgment about the quality of evidence. There will inevitably be cases where 'lower level' evidence—say from an observational study with a dramatic effect—will provide stronger evidence than a 'higher level' study—say a systematic review of few studies leading to an inconclusive result*'. Moreover, the Oxford CEBM website states that the levels have not been established to provide a recommendation and will not determine whether the correct question is being answered. The following questions need to be considered to determine a recommendations [19].

1. Do you have good reason to believe that your patient is sufficiently similar to the patients in the studies you have examined? Information about the size of the

Table 1.2 Oxford Centre for evidence-based medicine 2011 levels of evidence [19]

Question	Step 1 (Level 1[a])	Step 2 (Level 2[a])	Step 3 (Level 3[a])	Step 4 (Level 4[a])	Step 5 (Level 5)
How common is the problem?	Local and current random sample surveys (or censuses)	Systematic review of surveys that allow matching to local circumstances[b]	Local non-random sample[b]	Case-series[b]	n/a
Is this diagnostic or monitoring test accurate? (Diagnosis)	Systematic review of cross sectional studies with consistently applied reference standard and blinding	Individual cross sectional studies with consistently applied reference standard and blinding	Non-consecutive studies, or studies without consistently applied reference standards[b]	Case-control studies, or "poor or non-independent" reference standard[b]	Mechanism-based reasoning
What will happen if we do not add a therapy? (Prognosis)	Systematic review of inception cohort studies	Inception cohort studies	Cohort study or control arm of randomized trial[a]	Case-series or case-control studies, or poor quality prognostic cohort study[b]	n/a
Does this intervention help? (Treatment Benefits)	Systematic review of randomized trials or *n*-of-1 trials	Randomised trial or observational study with dramatic effect	Non-randomized controlled cohort/follow-up study[b]	Case-series, case-control studies, or historically controlled studies[b]	Mechanism-based reasoning

(continued)

Table 1.2 (continued)

Question	Step 1 (Level 1[a])	Step 2 (Level 2[a])	Step 3 (Level 3[a])	Step 4 (Level 4[a])	Step 5 (Level 5)
What are the COMMON harms? (Treatment Harms)	Systematic review of randomized trials, systematic review of nested case-control studies, *n*-of-1 trial with the patient you are raising the question about, or observational study with dramatic effect	Individual randomized trial or (exceptionally) observational study with dramatic effect	Non-randomized controlled cohort/ follow-up study (post-marketing surveillance) provided there are sufficient numbers to rule out a common harm. (For long-term harms the duration of follow-up must be sufficient)[b]	Case-series, case-control, or historically controlled studies[b]	Mechanism-based reasoning
What are the RARE harms? (Treatment Harms)	Systematic review of randomized trials or *n*-of-1 trial	Randomized trial or (exceptionally) observational study with dramatic effect			
Is this (early detection) test worthwhile? (Screening)	Systematic review of randomized trials	Randomized trial	Non-randomized controlled cohort/ follow-up study[b]	Case-series, case-control, or historically controlled studies[b]	Mechanism-based reasoning

[a]Level may be graded down on the basis of study quality, imprecision, indirectness (study PICO), because of inconsistency between studies, or because the absolute effect size is very small; Level may be graded up of here is a large or very effect size

[b]As always, a systematic review is generally better than an individual study

variance of the treatment effects is often helpful here: the larger the variance the greater concern that the treatment might not be useful for an individual.

2. Does the treatment have a clinically relevant benefit that outweighs the harms? It is important to review which outcomes are improved, as a statistically significant difference (e.g. systolic blood pressure falling by 1 mmHg) may be clinically irrelevant in a specific case. Moreover, any benefit must outweigh the harms. Such decisions will inevitably involve patients' value judgments, so discussion with the patient about their views and circumstances is vital

3. Is another treatment better? Another therapy could be 'better' with respect to both the desired beneficial and adverse events, or another therapy may simply have a different benefit/harm profile (but be perceived to be more favourable by some people). A systematic review might suggest that surgery is the best treatment for back pain, but if exercise therapy is useful, this might be a more acceptable to the patient than risking surgery as a first option.
4. Are the patient's values and circumstances compatible with the treatment? If a patient's religious beliefs prevent them from agreeing to blood transfusions, knowledge about the benefits and harms of blood transfusions is of no interest to them. Such decisions pervade medical practice, including oncology, where sharing decision making in terms of the dose of radiation for men opting for radiotherapy for prostate cancer is routine

Other frameworks and tools exist for the assessment of evidence. The PRISMA statement is a checklist and flow diagram to help systematic review and meta-analyses authors assess and report on the benefits and harms of a healthcare intervention. The Scottish Intercollegiate Guidelines Network (SIGN) Methodology provides checklists to appraise studies and develop guidelines for healthcare interventions. The CONsolidated Standards of Reporting Trials (CONSORT) is an evidence-based tool to help researchers, editors and readers assess the quality of the reports of trials and the PEDro scale considers two aspects of trial quality, namely internal validity of the trial and the value of the statistical information.

1.3.3 Grading

Another approach to the evaluation of clinical evidence was proposed in 2000, by the Grading of Recommendations Assessment, Development and Evaluation (GRADE) working group providing a transparent and reproducible framework for assessment [20–22]. It is the most widely adopted tool for grading the quality of evidence and for making recommendations, with over 100 organisations worldwide officially endorsing GRADE. It requires users of GRADE assessing the quality of evidence, usually as part of a systematic review, to consider the impact of different factors based upon their confidence in the results. A stepwise process is employed by which the assessors determine the clinical question, the applicable population and the relevant outcome measures. Systemic reviews are scored accordingly:

- Risk of bias: Is a judgement made on the basis of the chance that bias in included studies has influenced the estimate of effect?
- Imprecision: Is a judgement made on the basis of the chance that the observed estimate of effect could change completely?
- Indirectness: Is a judgement made on the basis of the differences in characteristics of how the study was conducted and how the results are actually going to be applied?

- Inconsistency: Is a judgement made on the basis of the variability of results across the included studies?
- Publication bias: Is a judgement made on the basis of the question whether all the research evidence has been taken to account?

Objective tools may be used to assess each of the domains. For example, tools exist for assessing the risk of bias in randomised and non-randomised trials [23–25]. The GRADE approach to rating imprecision focuses on the 95% confidence interval around the best estimate of the absolute effect. Thus, certainty is lower if the clinical decision is likely to be different if the true effect was at the upper versus the lower end of the confidence interval. Indirectness is dictated by the population studied assessing whether the population studied is different from those for whom the recommendation applies or the outcomes studied are different for those which are required.

The GRADE system also provides a framework for assessing observational studies but conversely utilises a positive approach to assessing the quality of the evidence.

- Large effect: This is when methodologically strong studies show that the observed effect is so large that the probability of it changing completely is less likely.
- Plausible confounding would change the effect: This is when despite the presence of a possible confounding factor which is expected to reduce the observed effect, the effect estimate is still significant
- Dose response gradient: This is when the intervention used becomes more effective with increasing dose.

Following the assessment of the quality of evidence derived from systemic reviews and other methodological approaches, the GRADE system moves to a second stage relating to the strength of recommendation (certainty) which will act to inform guidelines, policy and may also act as a determinant for further research [26].

- High Quality Evidence: The authors are very confident that the estimate that is presented lies very close to the true value.
- Moderate Quality Evidence: The authors are confident that the presented estimate lies close to the true value, but it is also possible that it may be substantially different.
- Low Quality Evidence: The authors are not confident in the effect estimate and the true value may be substantially different.
- Very low quality Evidence: The authors do not have any confidence in the estimate and it is likely that the true value is substantially different from it.

Evidence-based medicine approaches also objectively evaluate the quality of clinical research by critically assessing techniques reported by researchers in their publications. Consideration is given to trial design by which high-quality studies

Table 1.3 Cochrane's table of evidence to guide evaluations of the internal and external validity—(efficacy, effectiveness and cost-effectiveness) of medical intervention [9, 19]

Type of evidence	Question	Description
Efficacy	Can it work?	Extent to which an intervention does more good than harm under ideal circumstances
Effectiveness	Does it work in practice?	Extent to which an intervention does more good than harm under usual circumstances
Cost-effectiveness	Is it worth it?	The effect of an intervention in relation to the resources

have clearly defined eligibility criteria and have minimal missing data. Some studies may only be applicable to narrowly defined patient populations and may not be generalisable in other clinical contexts. Studies also have to be sufficiently powered to ensure that the number of patients studied is sufficient to determine a difference between interventions and also need to run over a sufficient period of time to ensure sustainable change. Randomised placebo controlled trials are considered the gold standard in this respect providing they are sufficiently powered and have minimised missing data points.

As early as 1972, Cochrane proposed a simple framework for evaluating medical care that could be applied to treatment and policy in current-day medical practice [9]. The questions posed test the internal and external validity of an intervention (Table 1.3).

The fundamental importance in this approach lies in the extent to which the process focusses on the external validity accounting for the application of an intervention in clinical practice and the resulting financial impact.

1.4 Challenges to Evidence Based Medicine

Evidence Based Medicine has clearly revolutionised the practice of medicine, the choice of investigations and treatments and has challenged therapies which had previously been built on limited evidence and opinion, but had gone unchallenged due to the hierarchical constraints of the medical profession. However, there has been criticism about inherent weaknesses of EBM. Some have suggested there is an over-reliance on data gathering that ignores experience and clinical acumen, and data which may not have formed part of the clinical trial process, and does not adequately account for personalised medicine and the individual holistic needs of the patient. Thus, EBM does not seek to extend to more recent advances in stratified medicine. Others have argued that the hierarchical approach to EBM places the findings from basic science at a much lower level thus belittling the importance of basic science in providing a means of understanding pathophysiological mechanisms, providing a framework and justification for clinical interventions and an explanation for inter-patient variability [27, 28]. Furthermore, EBM has been regarded as overly generalisable, considering the treatment effect to large populations, but not accounting for the severity of a disease, whereby a treatment may offer significant effect to those who are seriously affected compared to little or no impact for those who are mildly affected by the same condition. Thus within analyses, sub-stratification of patient cohorts may overcome this issue. Although a doyenne of EBM, Feinstein also argued that some of the greatest medical discoveries, for example the discovery of insulin and its use in diabetic ketoacidoisis have come about from single trials and would not stand up to the rigours of evidence based medicine [29]. Feinstein argued that there was too much emphasis placed upon the randomised-control trial and the process simply tests one treatment against another, with additional acumen needed to treat a patient in relation to presentation and severity of symptoms. Thus there is a concern that practice that does not conform to EBM is marginalised as a consequence. EBM is also restricted in its use for the defined patient population and does not consider alternative patient groups using the same therapies and interventions. Evidence defined by the RCT should also be challenged by observational and cohort studies in which supported treatments may lead to adverse effects in certain patient populations. Meta-analyses often include highly heterogeneous studies and ascribe conflicting results to random variability, whereas different outcomes may reflect different patient populations, enrolment and protocol characteristics [30]. Richardson and Doster proposed three dimensions in the process of evidence-based decision making: baseline risk of poor outcomes from an index disorder without treatment, responsiveness to the treatment option and vulnerability to the adverse effects of treatment; whereas EBM is focused on the potential therapeutic benefits it does not usually account for the patient inter-variability in the latter two dimensions [31].

The GRADE approach described earlier attempts to overcome some of these challenges by defining a system that provides a 'quality control' for evidence such that powerful observational studies for example may be upgraded due to the dramatic observed effect. The use of meta-analyses and systematic reviews as a gold standard are also scrutinised by GRADE for their inherent weaknesses. Heterogeneity (clinical, methodological or statistical) has been recognised as an inherent limitation of meta-analyses [32]. Different methodological and statistical approaches used in systematic reviews can also lead to different outcomes [33]. To this extent some have suggested that the approach to the evidence based pyramid should be adapted to incorporate a more rational approach to the assessment of evidence and with the use of systematic reviews at all levels of the evidence pyramid to determine the quality of the evidence [34]. Others have argued that the rigidity of the randomised-control trial has allowed an exploitation through selective reporting, exaggeration of benefits and the misinterpretation of evidence [35, 36]. Greenhalgh and colleagues state that through '*overpowering trials to ensure that small differences will be statistically significant, setting inclusion criteria to select those most likely to respond to treatment, manipulating the dose of both intervention and control drugs, using surrogate endpoints, and selectively publishing positive studies, industry may manage to publish its outputs as unbiassed in high-ranking peer-reviewed journal*s' [37]. Fundamentally and most importantly, whilst Sackett believed that the predicament of the patient formed part of the process of EBM, the rigidity of the system has resulted in a paradigm shift away from this principle. Some believe that EBM provides an oversimplified and reductionistic view of treatment, failing to interpret the motivation of the patient, the value of clinical interaction, co-morbidities, poly-pharmacy, expectations, environment and other confounding and influential variables and demand a return to 'real evidence based medicine' [37]. Others recognise that published evidence should also be presented in a way that is readable and usable for patients and professionals [38].

1.5 Conclusion

Since the foundations of evidence based medicine were introduced by David Sackett and colleagues in 1981 and the concept defined a decade later by Gordon Guyatt, EBM has provided a revolutionary framework defining medical interventions that challenged conventions of opinion-based medical practices based upon experience and position. Medical guidelines, policy and practice were founded by the evidence defined by research with frameworks subsequently applied that provided a means of defining the quality of the research and a system (GRADE) that assessed the quality of the research output and the ability to apply the evidence to clinical practice. Well established organisations now exist to systematically assess research evidence to provide an evidence-based resource for clinicians and researchers. Despite the recognised impact of evidence based-medicine, in the rapidly advancing era of personalised and stratified medicine, and the established role that basic science research plays in understanding the pathophysiology of disease and the impact of therapeutic intervention, the value of EBM has been questioned. In current day medical practice, many now recognise the need to balance the value of EBM with other methodological approaches to define future healthcare and interventions for patients.

References

1. Sackett DL, Rosenberg WM, Gray JA, Haynes RB, Richardson WS. Evidence based medicine: what it is and what it isn't. BMJ. 1996;312(7023):71–2.
2. Sackett DL, Haynes RB, Guyatt GH, Tugwell P. Clinical epidemiology: a basic science for clinical medicine. 2nd ed. Boston: Little Brown; 1991.
3. Guyatt G. Evidence-based medicine. Ann Intern Med. 1991;14(Supp 2):A-16.
4. Sackett D. How to read clinical journals: I. why to read them and how to start reading them critically. Can Med Assoc J. 1981;124(5):555–8.
5. Smith R, Rennie D. Evidence based medicine—an oral history. BMJ. 2014;348(21):g371.
6. Zimerman A. Evidence-based medicine: a short history of a modern medical movement. American Medical Association Journal of Ethics. 2013;15(1):71–6.
7. Haynes B. Advances in evidence-based information resources for clinical practice. ACP J Club. 2000;132(1):A11–4.
8. Feinstein AR. Clinical Judgement. Baltimore, MD: Williams & Wilkins; 1967.
9. Cochrane AL. Effectiveness and efficiency: random reflections on health services. London: Nuffield Provincial Hospitals Trust; 1972.

10. Evidence-Based Medicine Working Group. Evidence-based medicine. A new approach to teaching the practice of medicine. JAMA. 1992;268(17):2420–5.
11. Eddy DM. Practice Policies: Guidelines for Methods. JAMA. 1990;263(13):1839–41.
12. Eddy DM. Guidelines for policy statements. JAMA. 1990;263(16):2239–43.
13. Eddy DM. Evidence-based medicine: a unified approach. Health Aff. 2005;24(1):9–17.
14. Sur RL, Dahm P. History of evidence-based medicine. Indian J Urol. 2011;4:487–9.
15. Cochrane AL, Cox JG, Jarman TF. Pulmonary tuberculosis in the Rhondda Fach; an interim report of a survey of a mining community. Br Med J. 1952;2:843–53.
16. Chalmers I, Enkin M, Keirse MJ, editors. Effective Care in Pregnancy and Childbirth. New York, NY: Oxford University Press; 1989.
17. Dawes M. EBM Volume 5 July/August 2000 103. https://ebm.bmj.com/content/5/4/102.
18. Sackett DL. Rules of evidence and clinical recommendations on the use of antithrombotic agents. Chest. 1989;95:2S–4S.
19. OCEBM Table of Evidence Working Group: Howick J, Chalmers I (James Lind Library), Glasziou P, Greenhalgh T, Heneghan C, Liberati A, Moschetti I, Phillips B, Thornton H, Goddard O, Hodgkinson M. The Oxford 2011 levels of evidence. Oxford Centre for Evidence-Based Medicine. http://www.cebm.net/index.aspx?o=5653.
20. Schünemann H, Brożek J, Oxman A, editors. GRADE handbook for grading quality of evidence and strength of recommendation (Version 3.2 ed.); 2009.
21. Guyatt GH, Oxman AD, Vist GE, Kunz R, Falck-Ytter Y, Alonso-Coello P, et al. GRADE: an emerging consensus on rating quality of evidence and strength of recommendations. BMJ (Clinical research ed). 2008;336(7650):924–6.
22. Guyatt G, Oxman AD, Akl EA, Kunz R, Vist G, Brozek J, et al. GRADE guidelines: 1. Introduction-GRADE evidence profiles and summary of findings tables. J Clin Epidemiol. 2011;64(4):383–94.
23. Higgins JP, Altman DG, Gøtzsche PC, Jüni P, Moher D, Oxman AD, et al. The Cochrane Collaboration's tool for assessing risk of bias in randomised trials. BMJ (Clinical research ed). 2011;343:d5928.
24. Wells G, Shea B, O'connell D, Peterson J, Welch V, Losos M, et al. The Newcastle-Ottawa scale (NOS) for assessing the quality of nonrandomised studies in meta-analyses. Ottawa: Ottawa Hospital Research Institute; 2011. Oxford. Asp; 2011
25. Sterne JA, Hernan MA, Reeves BC, Savovic J, Berkman ND, Viswanathan M, et al. ROBINS-I: a tool for assessing risk of bias in non-randomised studies of interventions. BMJ (Clinical research ed). 2016;355:i4919.
26. Guyatt GH, Oxman AD, Kunz R, Falck-Ytter Y, Vist GE, Liberati A, et al. Going from evidence to recommendations. BMJ (Clinical research ed). 2008;336(7652):1049–51.
27. La Caze A. The role of basic science in evidence-based medicine. Biology & Philosophy. 2011;26(1):81–98.
28. Timmermans S, Berg M. The gold standard: the challenge of evidence-based medicine and standardization in health care. Philadelphia: Temple University Press; 2003.
29. Feinstein AR, Massa RD. Problems of 'evidence' in 'evidence-based medicine'. Am J Med. 1997;103:529–35.
30. Fava GA, Guidi J, Rafanelli C, Sonino N. The clinical inadequacy of evidence-based medicine and the need for a conceptual framework based on clinical judgment. Psychother Psychosom. 2015;84(1):1–3.
31. Richardson WS, Doster LM. Comorbidity and multimorbidity need to be placed in the context of a framework of risk, responsiveness, and vulnerability. J Clin Epidemiol. 2014;67:244–6.
32. Berlin JA, Golub RM. Meta-analysis as evidence: building a better pyramid. JAMA. 2014;312:603–5.
33. Dechartres A, Altman DG, Trinquart L, et al. Association between analytic strategy and estimates of treatment outcomes in meta-analyses. JAMA. 2014;312:623–30.
34. Murad MH, Asi N, Alsawas M, Alahdab F. New evidence pyramid. Evid Based Med. 2016 Aug;21(4):125–7.

35. James J. Reviving Cochrane's contribution to evidence-based medicine: bridging the gap between evidence of efficacy and evidence of effectiveness and cost-effectiveness. Eur J Clin Investig. 2017;47(9):617–21.
36. Ioannidis JP. Why most published research findings are false. PLoS Med. 2005;2:e124.
37. Greenhalgh T, Howick J, Maskrey N. Evidence based medicine: a movement in crisis? BMJ. 2014;348:g3725.
38. Lavis JN, Davies HT, Gruen RL, Walshe K, Farquhar CM. Working within and beyond the Cochrane collaboration to make systematic reviews more useful to healthcare managers and policy makers. Healthcare Policy. 2006;1:21–33.

Clinical Practice Guidelines: Choosing Wisely

2

Prasad Godbole

Learning Objectives
- To understand the process of developing guidelines
- To understand the process of critically reviewing guidelines
- To understand how/which guidelines should be implemented

2.1 Introduction

As Paediatric Urologists or in fact as clinicians in any discipline, we come across a vast array of guidelines from which to choose. The ultimate aim of clinical guidelines is to offer the clinicians an evidence based patient focused resource to improve patient outcomes, maintain patient safety and provide the most cost effective treatments. Guidelines can be found nationally, regionally or locally. Most local guidelines are adopted from existing guidelines but tailored for local use. With the vast array of guidelines available it can be a daunting task to determine which guidelines to choose from for patient management as not all guidelines are consistent and may differ widely in their content and recommendations. This chapter will focus on how guidelines are developed and how end users—the clinicians can determine which guidelines have been developed in a robust fashion to use with the highest level of evidence.

2.1.1 Clinical Guideline Development

There are several key steps when developing guidelines. These are:

1. Identify an area in which to develop the guidelines

P. Godbole (✉)
Department of Paediatric Surgery, Sheffield Children's NHS Foundation Trust, Sheffield, UK
e-mail: p.godbole@nhs.net

P. Godbole et al. (eds.), *Practical Pediatric Urology*,
https://doi.org/10.1007/978-3-030-54020-3_2

2. Establish a core guideline developmental group
3. Agree on guideline appraisal process
4. Assess existing guidelines for quality and clinical content
5. Decision to adopt or adapt guideline
6. External peer review of the guideline
7. Endorsement and ratification at local level
8. Local adoption
9. Periodic Review of the guideline

2.2 Identifying an Area in Which to Develop Guidelines

The key consideration is to develop a guideline for areas which may be prevalent in the local population or which will have improved outcomes for a maximum number of patients. This could be areas such as urinary tract infections in children, congenital obstructive uropathies, urinary tract calculi, nocturnal enuresis to name a few.

2.3 Establish a Core Guideline Developmental Group

Once an area has been established, all stakeholders including patients/carers should be involved in the guideline development process. For urinary tract infections this may include pediatricians, Paediatric urologists, general practitioners, nursing staff, microbiologists, parents of infants and young children and older children. In essence any stakeholder who may provide a clinical service for or who may benefit from the area that the guideline is designed for should be included.

2.4 Agree on a Guideline Appraisal Process

How can one determine whether a guideline is sufficiently rigorously developed to adopt? The guideline development group therefore needs to agree on how the guidelines will be appraised. The AGREE instrument is one such appraisal methodology and is shown below

2.5 Assessing Existing Guidelines

The initial chapters on Evidence Based Medicine already highlights the levels of evidence and the hierarchy of evidence. As clinical guidelines are outcome focused and are aimed to be cost effective, the following levels of evidence and their implication for clinical decision making may be used to assess existing guidelines. A strategy to retrieve guidelines has to be agreed eg. Search terms, language/s, databases etc.

Levels of evidence for therapeutic studies

Level	Type of evidence
1A	Systematic review (with homogeneity) of RCTs
1B	Individual RCT (with narrow confidence intervals)
1C	All or none study
2A	Systematic review (with homogeneity) of cohort studies
2B	Individual Cohort study (including low quality RCT, e.g. <80% follow-up)
2C	"Outcomes" research; Ecological studies
3A	Systematic review (with homogeneity) of case-control studies
3B	Individual Case-control study
4	Case series (and poor quality cohort and case-control study
5	Expert opinion without explicit critical appraisal or based on physiology bench research or "first principles"

[a]From the Centre for Evidence-Based Medicine, http://www.cebm.net

Grade practice recommendations

Grade	Descriptor	Qualifying evidence	Implications for practice
A	Strong recommendation	Level I evidence or consistent findings from multiple studies of levels II, III, or IV	Clinicians should follow a strong recommendation unless a clear and compelling rationale for an alternative approach is present
B	Recommendation	Levels II, III, or IV evidence and findings are generally consistent	Generally, clinicians should follow a recommendation but should remain alert to new information and sensitive to patient preferences
C	Option	Levels II, III, or IV evidence, but findings are inconsistent	Clinicians should be flexible in their decision-making regarding appropriate practice, although they may set bounds on alternatives; patient preference should have a substantial influencing role
D	Option	Level V evidence:little or no systematic empirical evidence	Clinicians should consider all options in their decision making and be alert to new published evidence that clarifies the balance of benefit versus harm; patient preference should have a substantial influencing role

From the American Society of Plastic Surgeons. Evidence-based clinical practice guidelines. Available at: http://www.plasticsurgery.org/Medical_Professionals/Health_Policy_and_Advocacy/Health_Policy_Resources/Evidence-based_GuidelinesPractice_Parameters/Description_and_Development_of_Evidence-

While the agree criteria may be used to determine the quality of the guideline, a quick screening process that has been advocated is to determine the rigor of development (number 7 of the AGREE criteria). Furthermore, the guideline should be current. The content of the guideline also must be considered. Where more than one guideline is being considered, a comparison between guidelines, recommendations and levels of evidence may result in evolution of a guideline incorporating recommendations from more than one guideline.

2.6 Decision to Adapt or Adopt a Guideline

Once the process above is completed, a decision must be made by the guideline development group as to the robustness of the guideline for local use. The guideline may be used un modified or may need to be adapted for local use but maintaining the key principles within the guideline.

2.7 External Peer Review

If a decision is made to adopt a guideline, the guideline should be sent to a specialist in that field for peer review of the applicability of the guideline for local use. In some instances when local guidelines are being developed without reference to national/international guidelines, the peer reviewer may be a senior clinician within the speciality. For example a guideline on the management of Transanal irrigation or on insertion of catheters may be developed by specialist urology nurses and reviewed by a Paediatric Urologist.

2.7.1 Endorsement and Ratification at Local Level

Once peer reviewed, the guideline has to pass through a formal process of ratification usually via a committee that approves the guideline for local use. In the authors' institution, this is the Clinical Audit and Effectiveness Committee. Guidelines for approval are sent out in advance of the meeting and discussed in the meeting prior to approval.

2.8 Local Adoption

Once approved, the guidelines are adopted for local use. Guidelines are reviewed at periodic intervals of 2–3 years with updates.

2.9 Conformity to Guideline Adherence

While the process above describes best practice in developing guidelines and how to determine which guidelines are robust, getting clinicians to adhere to the guidelines can be a different matter. In the past, surgical training was more paternalistic in that the 'doctor was always right' and training was more experience based rather than evidence based. In such scenarios, changing mindset of individuals can be a daunting task. So imagine a scenario where a guideline is developed in a robust fashion using the AGREE tool and the surgeon does not adhere to the guideline. How can that be reversed?

In many organisations and indeed nationally there are specific standards that need to be met in terms of guideline adherence. In England for example the National Institute for Health and Clinical Excellence (NICE) publishes monthly requests for information regarding guidelines adherence and new technology appraisals. Individual organisations are expected to provide a baseline assessment of adherence to the guideline (Urinary tract infection is a good example) or provide deviation statements with rationale for the deviation from the guideline. These baseline assessments are required to be updated every 2 years. In many instances individual organisations may face a financial penalty for not providing these reports. As a result at local level, organisations have mechanisms in place led by clinicians to ensure this information is collected in a prompt manner.

Guidelines are developed to ensure standardised care and best possible clinical outcomes. Hence audit of outcomes are also important in ensuring adherence to guidelines. If outcomes are poorer than expected than a review of the guideline or adherence to the same by clinicians should be triggered.

2.10 Conclusion

It is important for clinicians to understand the process of guideline development. Wherever possible guidelines that are developed using the highest level of evidence should be considered for local use. These guidelines may be tailored for local use and must be reviewed periodically to incorporate any new evidence that may be available. Regulatory oversight and audit of outcomes are useful tools to ensure guidelines are being followed.

Appendix: Domains of AGREE II Appraisal Instrument

Scope and purpose
1. The overall objective(s) of the guideline is (are) specifically described
2. The health question(s) covered by the guideline is (are) specifically described
3. The population (patients and public) to whom the guideline is meant to apply is specifically described
Stakeholder involvement
4. The guideline development group includes individuals from all the relevant professional groups
5. The views and preferences of the target population (patients, public, etc.) have been sought
6. The target users of the guideline are clearly defined

Rigor of development
7. Systematic methods were used to search for evidence
8. The criteria for selecting the evidence are clearly described
9. The strengths and limitations of the body of evidence are clearly described
10. The methods for formulating the recommendations are clearly described
11. The health benefits, side effects, and risks have been considered in formulating the recommendations
12. There is an explicit link between the recommendations and the supporting evidence
13. The guideline has been externally reviewed by experts before its publication
14. A procedure for updating the guideline is provided
Clarity of presentation
15. The recommendations are specific and unambiguous
16. The different options for management of the condition or health issue are clearly presented
17. Key recommendations are easily identifiable
Applicability
18. The guideline describes facilitators and barriers to its application
19. The guideline provides advice and/or tools on how the recommendations can be put into practice
20. The potential resource implications of applying the recommendations have been considered
21. The guideline presents monitoring and/or auditing criteria
Editorial independence
22. The views of the funding body have not influenced the content of the guideline
23. Competing interests of guideline development group members have been recorded and addressed

AGREE appraisal of guidelines research and evaluation

Antibiotic Stewardship in Pediatric Urology: Editorial Comment

3

Prasad Godbole, Duncan T. Wilcox, and Martin A. Koyle

Learning Objectives
- To understand the principles of use of antimicrobials in Pediatric Urology
- To identify key causes of bacterial resistance to antimicrobials
- Appropriate prescribing in Pediatric Urology

3.1 Introduction

There is no doubting the fact that antibiotics are the mainstay in the treatment of bacterial infections. Since the advent of antibiotics beginning with use of Penicillin in the 1940's, mankind has been plagued with the problem of bacterial resistance. This has perpetuated a cycle of isolating the causative pathogenesis of bacterial resistance and finding ways of circumventing it and developing a new antibiotic. Often there is a significant delay between the development of resistance and the introduction of a new antibiotic. Organisms are becoming increasingly resistant to newer antibiotics and in some cases this has prompted a media frenzy of the 'superbug'.

This phenomenon of bacterial resistance is encountered frequently in pediatric urological practice. Improper use of antibiotics, excessive use of antibiotics remains

P. Godbole (✉)
Department of Paediatric Surgery, Sheffield Children's NHS Foundation Trust, Sheffield, UK
e-mail: p.godbole@nhs.net

D. T. Wilcox
Division of Urology, University of Colorado, Aurora, CO, USA
e-mail: duncan.wilcox@childrenscolorado.org

M. A. Koyle
Department of Surgery and IHPME, University of Toronto Paediatric Urology,
The Hospital for Sick Children, Toronto, ON, Canada
e-mail: Martin.Koyle@SickKids.ca

P. Godbole et al. (eds.), *Practical Pediatric Urology*,
https://doi.org/10.1007/978-3-030-54020-3_3

common despite campaigns urging a reduction in the prescribing of antibiotics for pediatric urological conditions. In some instances this is also driven by patients or their families. Antibiotic prophylaxis for insignificant isolated hydronephrosis, low grade ureterovesical reflux without febrile UTI's, or antibiotic treatment for bacteriuria in a child doing clean intermittent catheterization without symptoms is still being practiced globally. We are all guilty of such practices and this includes general practitioners, family physicians, pediatricians and pediatric urologists.

Appropriate teaching and knowledge sharing to both the medical fraternity as well as the patients and their families is required to reduce the incidence of bacterial resistance in pediatric urology. We will look at a few examples where there is inappropriate use or overuse of antibiotics in pediatric urology contrary to available evidence and patient factors contributing to this.

3.2 Antenatal Hydronephrosis

One of the practices certainly common in the UK is to put children with antenatal diagnosis of hydronephrosis on antibiotic prophylaxis from birth irrespective of the severity of the antenatal hydronephrosis and whether associated with ureterovesical reflux or not. Evidence suggests that newborns with high grade hydronephrosis may benefit from antibiotic prophylaxis compared to low grade in reducing the risk of febrile UTI's. If associated reflux, the incidence of febrile UTI's appears to be higher than without reflux. There seems to be little difference in the incidence of febrile UTI in newborns with low grade hydronephrosis. Hence one should avoid the use of antibiotic prophylaxis in newborns with isolated low grade hydronephrosis.

3.3 Vesicoureteral Reflux

There appears to be differing practices in antibiotic prophylaxis in children with vesico ureteral reflux. Some clinicians put all children with reflux on antibiotic prophylaxis for varying periods of time. There is very little evidence in support of putting all children on prophylaxis. A number of studies have demonstrated no benefit of antibiotic prophylaxis in low grade (I–III) reflux in preventing recurrent febrile urinary tract infections. The Swedish Reflux Study has demonstrated some benefit of antibiotic prophylaxis in dilating reflux (Grade IV–V) in girls between 1 and 2 years of age but not in boys in preventing recurrent febrile UTI's.

3.4 Compliance

There is a direct relationship between development of resistance to antibiotics and compliance to the antibiotic regime. It has been shown by a review of a large pharmacy database that up to 60% of children being treated for vesicoureteral reflux are not compliant with the antibiotic schedule suggesting the need for increased patient/clinician contact and counselling.

3.5 Choice of Antibiotics

Most hospitals have their own antibiotic regime for the urinary tract. In the UK, the first line treatment for simple uncomplicated lower urinary tract infection is Trimethoprim with Nitrofurantoin reserved for recurrent or resistant UTI's. Cephalosporins should be avoided as first line therapy for prophylaxis due to their association with antibiotic resistance. The National Institute for Health and Care Excellence (UK) has reviewed and published guidelines for managing urinary tract infections in children updated in February 2019 to reduce misuse of antibiotics and it is essential that similar guidelines are available internationally.

3.6 Conclusion

Bacterial resistance to antibiotics in Pediatric Urology is here to stay. However the natural evolution of this resistance can be slowed by appropriate use of antibiotics based on evidence. Teaching of clinicians as well as counselling of parents is important in reducing the risk of bacterial resistance.

Suggested Further Reading

1. Edlin RS, Copp HL. Antibiotic resistance in pediatric urology. Ther Adv Urol. 2014;6(2):54–61.
2. Wong NC, Koyle MA, Braga LH. Continuous antibiotic prophylaxis in the setting of prenatal hydronephrosis and vesicoureteral reflux. Can Urol Assoc J. 2017;11(1–2 Suppl1):S20–4.
3. Shuangmei Tong MB, Pan J, Lu S, Tang J. Patient compliance with antimicrobial drugs: a Chinese survey. Am J Infect Control. 2018;46:e25–9.
4. Lee T, Park JM. Vesicoureteral reflux and continuous prophylactic antibiotics. Investig Clin Urol. 2017;58(Suppl 1):S32–7.
5. Brandström P, Esbjörner E, Herthelius M, Swerkersson S, Jodal U, Hansson S. The Swedish reflux trial in children: III. Urinary tract infection pattern. J Urol. 2010;184(1):286–91.

Pain Management in Paediatric Urology

4

Judith Morgan

Learning Objectives

- Understand the need for good pain management and tailor the appropriate treatment to the type of surgery
- Assess pain in children using the age appropriate tools
- Use multimodal analgesia effectively in children to enable good recovery
- Use regional anaesthesia blocks where possible and select the most appropriate block for the type and location of surgery

4.1 Introduction

Effective pain management is essential for the successful recovery from surgery. Not only is it important for the child's comfort and wellbeing, it improves recovery, allowing early mobilisation and discharge from hospital. A successful plan must be appropriate for the child's age and size. That includes method of pain assessment, the drug choice and dosage, the staff skill mix, whether suitable for regional analgesia and if a day case or inpatient. The majority of paediatric urology surgery is done as a day case and suitable for some form of peripheral or regional anaesthesia block as part of a multimodal approach to analgesia.

The sensation of pain produces a biological and emotional response. Physiological changes in response to pain include sympathetic stimulation which can increase the heart rate and blood pressure, alter blood flow to the damaged tissue, and stimulate nausea and vomiting amongst other things. Emotional and behavioral responses alter the perception of pain and result in restlessness, insomnia, mood changes, and can modulate the pain pathway to a significant degree. Understanding the source of the painful stimulus, the pathway it travels and the effects on the child can better

J. Morgan (✉)
Sheffield Children's NHS Foundation Trust, Sheffield, UK
e-mail: Judith.morgan3@nhs.net

P. Godbole et al. (eds.), *Practical Pediatric Urology*,
https://doi.org/10.1007/978-3-030-54020-3_4

direct the treatment. This is so important not only to enable a faster recovery and return to full mobility, but also to prevent adaptive changes in the neurons and long term abnormal pain perception. The tissue trauma caused by surgery stimulates the peripheral nociceptors producing substances that pass information to the brain via nerves through the dorsal horn of the spinal cord. At each level of the pathway, different analgesics can act to inhibit or modify this transmission in different ways and form the basis of multimodal pain relief.

4.2 Assessment of Pain

There are many aspects to assessing and therefore managing pain in children. Validated scoring tools are widely used and should be age appropriate and where possible, self-reporting rather than staff interpretation. Dedicated pain teams and regular assessment have improved safety and efficacy. Consideration should be given to other influences around the time if surgery such as fear and anxiety, particularly separation from parents which should be avoided, hunger and thirst which should be minimised, and the effect of a hospital environment which should be made as child friendly as possible.

The very young and those with learning disabilities require a pain assessment tool based on physiological and behavioral changes such as facial expression, leg movement, activity level, crying and consolability (FLACC score). Older children require some cognitive ability to understand and relate their level of pain to a score and then compare it at regular intervals after intervention and treatment. From the age of 4 years, many children are able use an adapted 'smiley faces' scale with pictures of faces from smiling to crying to describe their pain. A linear visual analogue score such as simple numerical scale 1–10 is more suitable from the age of 7 years, 1 being mild discomfort and 10 being the worst pain ever felt.

Staff in recovery, on the ward, and in dedicated pain teams should regularly assess pain scores with children using an age appropriate system and use it to guide treatment.

4.3 Analgesia

4.3.1 Paracetamol (Acetaminophen)

The most commonly used simple non opioid analgesic for mild to moderate pain relief.

It acts both in the periphery by inhibiting prostaglandin synthesis, and centrally on the hypothalamus and descending serotonergic pathways.

It is analgesic and anti pyretic but does not produce the anti inflammatory effects seen in non-steroidal anti-inflammatory drugs (NSAIDS).

Routes of administration are oral, intravenous and rectal.

Oral administration is the commonest, easiest and possibly safest route. It has rapid absorption and very good bioavailability. It is best given preoperatively and then regularly post-operatively to be most effective.

IV administration is increasingly used for intra and post-operative administration where oral is unsuitable. It has the greatest central potency and fastest uptake with analgesic effects within 10–15 min and peak effect within 1 h.

Care is needed with intravenous administration to prevent significant overdose problems when calculating weight based dose and volumes in children. The preparation comes as 10 mg/ml and therefore can lead to mistakes with calculating volume in milliliters and doses in milligrams with a ten-fold drug calculation error. There have been numerous national safety warnings issued following such high numbers of inadvertent drug overdoses [1, 2]. The IV preparations should only be administered for a short course and converted to oral preparations when possible.

Rectal administration is less suitable with a highly variable bioavailability, slower onset and is often unacceptable to the patient or parent (Table 4.1).

4.3.2 Non-Steroidal Anti-Inflammatory Drugs (NSAIDS)

They are effective for mild to moderate pain. They work well alone but give better analgesia in combination with paracetamol. NSAIDS have opiate-sparing effects and reduce the requirement for opiate analgesia when used in combination for more major surgery.

Like paracetamol they inhibit production of prostaglandins mainly in the peripheral tissues to produce analgesia, but also have more of an anti inflammatory action.

Ibuprofen can be used down to 1 month of age and only comes in an oral preparation, but other formulations such as diclofenac sodium are limited in children to 6 month of age and over, given via the oral and rectal route with good bioavailability, and intravenously for children over the age of 2 years.

Caution is needed in children with renal impairment and they may not be suitable for some urological surgery. A history of gastro intestinal bleeding or ulceration, coagulation disorders and brittle asthma or those known to be sensitive to NSAIDS, may also prevent administration and need to be considered.

Table 4.1 Paracetamol dose ranges

Neonates	ORAL	10–15 mg/kg 6 h	Max 60 mg/kg/24 h
	IV	10 mg/kg 6 h	Max 40 mg/kg/24 h
	PR	Up to 20 mg/kg load 10–15 mg/kg 6 h	Max 60 mg/kg/24 h
1 month–18 years	ORAL	15–20 mg/kg 4–6 h	Max 90 mg/kg/24 h
	IV	15 mg/kg 6 h	Max 60 mg/kg/24 h
	PR	Up to 40 mg/kg load 20 mg/kg 6 h	Max 90 mg/kg/24 h

4.3.3 Opioids

Opioid analgesics are the main choice for effective control of moderate to severe pain. These range from codeine, tramadol and oxycodone, to fentanyl, morphine and diamorphine.

They all have dose dependent side effects of nausea and vomiting, respiratory depression, sedation, itching, as well as causing constipation and urinary retention. All patients should be monitored for side effects and treated appropriately.

Moderate pain is well managed with codeine medicines, however they are metabolised to their active component, morphine, to varying degrees.

Since 2015 safety reviews have issued warnings that no child under the age of 12 years should be prescribed codeine medicines due to the risk of respiratory depression and death [3, 4]. Some children are genetically predisposed to excessive metabolism of codeine into its active metabolite, morphine, resulting in dangerously high plasma levels (ultra or rapid metabolisers).

As an alternative in the younger patient, oral morphine liquid on a PRN basis, has been used to achieve a more predictable and therefore safer analgesia level, suitable for use for more moderate daycare surgery as part of a multi modal plan.

Tramadol is a synthetic codeine analogue with dual effects. It has both opioid analgesic effects and enhances the inhibitory pain pathways via serotonin and noradrenaline. It has less effect on sedation and provides another useful analgesic for moderate pain.

Morphine is by far the commonest opioid used in hospital particularly as intravenous infusions, patient controlled analgesia (IV-PCA) or nurse controlled analgesia (NCA) systems. To use a patient controlled system, the child needs to be old enough to realise that pushing a button will help take away the pain, and this may be possible from the age of 5 years. Fentanyl can be used intravenously in PCA systems where morphine is not suitable or causes dose-related side effects. Fentanyl also comes as transdermal patches in a range of doses useful in providing a background reservoir of analgesia where there is no IV access (Table 4.2).

4.3.4 Local Anaesthetics

Bupivicaine, levobupivicaine (chirocaine) and ropivicaine are all longer acting amide local anaesthetic drugs used for prolonged analgesia in local blocks.

Table 4.2 Doses for commonly used opioid

Drug	Route	Dose
Codeine (>12 years)	Oral	1 mg/kg
Tramadol (>12 years)	Oral/IV	1–2 mg/kg 4–6 h
Oxycodone (>1 month)	Oral	0.2 mg/kg 4–6 h
Fentanyl	IV	1 mcg/kg
Morphine	Oral/IV	0.05–0.2 mg/kg 4–6 h

Levobupivicaine is the single enantiomer of bupivicaine and has the same effect and dosage but a safer profile with lower cardiac and neurotoxicity. It is more suitable in neonates and infants where there is a greater risk of local anaesthetic toxicity due to less protein binding of the drugs. Concentrations of 0.125–0.25% are adequate for successful blockade. Maximum dose for bupivacaine is 2.5 mg/kg but often volumes required for many regional blocks may be up to 1–1.25 ml/kg without seeing problems of toxicity.

The use of some form of local anaesthetic used as wound infiltration, nerve blockade or regional anaesthesia is suitable for almost all types of urology surgery in children. Performed under general anaesthesia, they are particularly useful for daycase procedures.

An audit of regional blockade for daycase urology surgery in 2017 looked at post-operative pain management and showed that with a LA regional block, fewer than 5% of patients had any moderate pain score in recovery (an accepted target standard) unlike those who received only local infiltration, where the pain scores were significantly higher [5].

4.4 Types of Blocks Performed

4.4.1 Penile Block

Dorsal penile nerve block (DPNB) is easily performed either using landmark or ultra sound guidance. This deposits local anaesthesia into the sub pubic space either side of the midline suspensory ligament, where run the dorsal nerves of the penis, lateral to the vessels. The needle is advanced until a pop is felt through Scarpa's fascia and a dose of 1 ml plus 0.1 ml/kg to a maximum 5 mls is injected each side. It should be combined with a small subcutaneous injection of local at the base of the ventral surface to cover an area of skin on the frenulum [6]. The local solution must not contain epinephrine. Complications include haematoma. Simple ring block does not provide as good post operative pain relief as penile block [7].

4.4.2 Caudal Block

Caudal anaesthesia is one of the most frequently used blocks in children as it is safe, reliable, easy to perform, and provides prolonged analgesia with few side-effects. The caudal epidural space is reached via injection through the sacrococcygeal ligament. It contains the cauda equina and epidural venous plexus. The extent of the block into the lumbar epidural space is dependant on age and weight for the volume of local anaesthetic injected as suggested by Armitage [8, 9].

It is most suitable for surgery below the umbilicus and best tolerated in the younger patients. Higher blocks can be achieved using larger volumes or via a catheter threaded into the caudal space. The lowest concentration possible should be used to minimise motor blockade of the lower limbs, as children can become very upset if they cannot feel and move their legs properly.

Onset of block with bupivacaine is within 10–15 min after administration and although a single shot last 4–6 h, the level of block starts receding within 2 h. Block duration can be extend by addition of variety of substances, however there are concerns over neurotoxicity particularly in the very young. Adrenaline, narcotics, alpha agonists (clonidine and dexmetatomidine), tramadol and ketamine are just some used.

A RCT in 2017 by Kannojia et al. found 1 mcg/kg of dexmetatomidine added to caudal bupivicaine for urogenital surgery, improved analgesia and increased the length of block with minimal side effects, compared with either fentanyl or bupivacaine alone [10] Another RCT looked at the addition of 0.1 mg/kg dexamethasone to ropivicaine for orchidopexy surgery in 80 children and found significantly improved analgesia up to 48 h post operatively [11]. A meta-analysis of ketamine use in caudal also showed prolonged analgesia [12]. Better analgesia with more prolonged block and local anaesthesia sparing effects has also been shown using the addition of clonidine [13].

4.4.3 Ilio Inguinal Block

The ilioinguinal and iliohypogastric nerves originate from T12 and L1 of the lumbar plexus and they run between external, internal oblique and transversus abdominis (with some variation). Injection is placed into the abdominal wall via landmark or ultra sound, just medial to the anterior superior iliac spine (ASIS), to deposit local between the layers of internal oblique and transverses abdominis in a dose of 0.5 ml/kg of levobupivicaine. The spread of this block can be complicated by a femoral nerve block in 10% of cases resulting in weak hip flexion and care needs to be taken in ambulant children prior to discharge [14].

4.4.4 Transversus Abdominus Plane (TAP) Block

This is suitable for infra umbilical surgery and can be performed either uni- or bilateral. Local anaesthesia is deposited in the layer between internal oblique and transverses abdomens muscles, where the sensory nerves from T6-L1 lie. It is performed with either landmark or ultra sound guidance, between the costal margin and iliac crest in the mid axillary line.

4.4.5 Paravertebral Blocks

These are a good alternative for a unilateral block for more major unilateral upper abdominal renal surgery as an alternative to epidurals and with catheter insertion can provide more prolonged post operative analgesia. However they are technically more difficult to perform as less frequently placed and therefore the guarantee of efficacy is less assured. They require similar monitoring of effect post operatively as epidurals although more peripheral, for safety and familiarity reasons.

4.4.6 Epidural Block

These can be placed in the caudal, lumbar or thoracic region depending on the dermatome level required. They are placed under general anaesthesia by an experienced paediatric anaesthetist—In the very young patient, plain local anesthesia infusions provide good analgesia. The addition of fentanyl may reduce dose requirement of local but increase side effects of sedation and pruritus [15] A dilute concentration of 0.1% bupivacaine with 1–2 mcgs/ml of fentanyl is commonly used and infusions can successfully be used for usually no longer than 72 h post operatively and then should be reviewed regarding risks of infection and effectiveness. Close observations are needed not only for adequacy of block spread therefore analgesia but also looking for side effects including hypotension, urinary retention, pruritus or respiratory depression with opioids.

A really good alternative if a particular block is not suitable is to place a catheter in the tissue layers and run a continuous local anaesthesia wound infusion [32, 33].

4.5 Types of Surgery

4.5.1 Cystoscopy

Often performed as a daycare procedure and although of short duration, can be very stimulating. Paracetamol given preoperatively allows time for it to work as the procedure time is too short. Intravenous is an alternative in theatre as well as short acting opioid such as IV fentanyl.

Simple analgesics, paracetamol and ibuprofen are suitable for postoperative analgesia.

Cystoscopy to perform incision of posterior urethral valves is more invasive and can result in significant pain intra and post operatively. This is often performed in babies and caudal provides good analgesia with paracetamol administration prior to the block wearing off. Caution with NSAIDS depending on the renal function in these patients. Paracetamol provides adequate post operative pain relief.

4.5.2 Circumcision

A daycare procedure suitable for caudal, ring block, dorsal penile or pudendal nerve block depending on the age and size of the patient. Cochrane review found little difference in outcomes with any method but small studies made evidence limited [16].

Caudal block using bupivicaine 0.5–1 ml/kg may provide better analgesia in the first 6 h postoperatively but prolong time to walking [17–19]. Postoperative analgesia is provided with simple analgesics such as regular paracetamol and NSAIDS. Oral morphine in low dose can be given on a PRN basis if required. Opioids may be required intra operatively depending on the regional block [20].

4.5.3 Orchidopexy

For simple inguinal orchidopexy, an ilioinguinal block with local anaesthetic is suitable for unilateral surgery, but if bilateral, then a caudal may be more appropriate, depending on the patient's age. Some local anaesthetic infiltration is needed in the scrotum in addition to an ilioinguinal block. Laparoscopic surgery for intra abdominal testes will require opioid analgesia and local infiltration of the port sites, unless in the very young child where a caudal may be appropriate. Post operative analgesia includes regular paracetamol and NSAIDs, with the addition of oral morphine on a PRN basis. Orchidopexy does induce significant nausea and vomiting and so prophylactic antiemetics are helpful.

The use, wherever possible, of regional local anaesthesia reduces the need for morphine and therefore reduces the incidence of post operative nausea and vomiting; a common cause of unexpected admission after daycare surgery [21].

4.5.4 Hypospadias Repair

The choice of anaesthesia and analgesia depends to some degree on the severity of hypospadias, proximal or distal meatus and whether one stage or two stage procedure with or without foreskin or buccal mucosal graft. Suitable regional anaesthesia includes penile, pudendal or caudal block, alongside regular paracetamol and NSAIDs.

Recent reports have suggested an increased association of urogenital fistula amongst post operative complications associated with the use of caudal analgesia for hypospadias repair. A suggestion that venous engorgement due to caudal placement may be responsible for suture failure has been published [22]. In one study, Kim et al. did a retrospective notes review of 342 patients undergoing urethroplasty and found those receiving a caudal had a 2:1 odds ratio of developing complications [23] Taicher et al. looked at 395 single stage repairs, receiving either caudal or penile block, and excluding all other confounding factors, found a 13 fold increase risk of complications in the caudal group [24].

However a retrospective review of over 500 patients published in 2017 found hypospadias severity and not type of regional anaesthesia to be the only risk factor in post operative complications [25] Caudal anaesthesia has a higher success rate with easier landmarks to achieve a successful block [26] and is also sited away from the tissues layers of the operative field.

Comparison of other blocks has shown no difference in analgesia between pudendal and caudal block in one study [27] however another double blind RCT of 84 children found better pain scores and longer analgesia in the pudendal group compared with the caudal group [28] There is a question of familiarity and skill mix however with pudendal blocks, which are not commonly performed and not as simple to perform as a caudal for the majority of anaesthetists.

4.5.5 Pyeloplasty

Performed either laparoscopically or via an open incision in the subcostal region, this surgery is suitable for either a caudal epidural block in the very young or ultra sound guided TAP block for regional analgesia. Equally effective if not superior analgesia has been shown with opiates and local infiltration of the surgical field [29].

4.5.6 Nephrectomy

Unilateral renal surgery is suitable for a one sided paravertebral block as an alternative to epidural. They do require specialist skill to perform as are technically challenging with significant risks of pleural or epidural puncture. The level of injection is at T9 for the kidney and can be landmark or ultra sound guided. The majority of these more major procedures are best managed with an opiate infusion of some kind post operatively, unless an epidural catheter or equivalent infusion of local anaesthesia is used.

4.6 Ureteric Reimplantation

Pain results not only from the incision wound but also from bladder spasms post operatively. Open is more commonly performed and an epidural works well but if not then local infiltration or block of the incision and an opiate infusion is suitable, including if surgery is performed laparoscopically. Paracetamol and ibuprofen given regularly should be enough a few days after surgery.

4.7 Repair of Bladder Extrophy

This congenital abnormality is as a result of failure of the midline structures to fuse, leaving an exposed abdominal bladder and splayed pelvis. Anaesthesia and analgesia depend on the severity of the condition as there is a considerable spectrum of disease with few specialist centres performing the repair. Due to the extensive surgery, pelvic osteotomies and use of external fixators, most would choose to site an epidural to continue post operatively, as long as any congenital spinal abnormalities have been excluded, including tunnelled caudal epidural in neonates. The younger patient may also be adequately analgesed with NCA opiate infusion and some centres have shown them to be equally effective [30] Good analgesia is essential in these cases for recovery from such extensive surgery, to assist in healing, ensure the abdomen is relaxed and therefore reduce the risk of wound dehiscence [31].

4.8 Summary

- Multi modal analgesia should be used for optimal pain relief
- Pain assessment tools should be age appropriate and used regularly to guide analgesia
- Most surgery is suitable for some form of regional block with local anaesthesia and provides excellent pain relief, allows improved mobility and improves recovery.

References

1. MHRA Drug Safety Advice. Intravenous paracetamol (Perfalgan): risk of accidental overdose, especially in infants and neonates. Drug Saf Updat. 2010;3(12):2–3.
2. Safe Anaesthesia Liason Group. Intravenous paracetamol; 2013.
3. Codeine for analgesia: restricted use in children because of reports of morphine toxicity—GOV.UK [Internet]. [cited 2018 Aug 20]. https://www.gov.uk/drug-safety-update/codeine-for-analgesia-restricted-use-in-children-because-of-reports-of-morphine-toxicity.
4. Research C for DE and. Drug Safety and Availability—FDA Drug Safety Communication: FDA restricts use of prescription codeine pain and cough medicines and tramadol pain medicines in children; recommends against use in breastfeeding women. [cited 2018 Aug 20]. http://wayback.archive-it.org/7993/20170722032956/https://www.fda.gov/Drugs/DrugSafety/ucm549679.htm.
5. Paschou V, Garcia-Verdugo Peralta O. Day case paediatric urological surgery-regional blockade reduces postoperative pain and is opiate sparing. Reg Anesth Pain Med. 2017;42(5). (conference abstract).
6. Long RM, McCartan D, Cullen I, Harmon D, Flood HD. A preliminary study of the sensory distribution of the penile dorsal and ventral nerves: implications for effective penile block for circumcision. BJU Int [Internet]. 2010 Jun [cited 2018 Jul 29];105(11):1576–8. http://doi.wiley.com/10.1111/j.1464-410X.2009.09044.x.
7. Holder K, Peutrell J, Weir P. Regional anaesthesia for circumcision. Subcutaneous ring block of the penis and subpubic penile block compared. Eur J Anaesthesiol. 1997;14:495–8.
8. Armitage E. Caudal block in children. Anaesthesia. 1979;34:396–9.
9. Dalens BJ. Regional anesthesia in infants, children, and adolescents [Internet]. Waverly Europe; 1995 [cited 2018 Aug 16]. p. 550. https://books.google.co.uk/books?id=dI5sAAAAMAAJ&vq=%22Pediatric+Regional+Anesthesia%22&source=gbs_citations_module_r&cad=2.
10. Kannojia U, Meena R, Paswan A, Meena K, Prakash S, Loha S. Comparison of caudal dexmedetomidine and fentanyl combined with bupivacaine in pediatric patients undergoing urogenital surgery. Pain Intensive Care. 2017;21(2):204–11.

11. Kim EM, Lee JR, Koo BN, Im YJ, Oh HJ, Lee JH. Analgesic efficacy of caudal dexamethasone combined with ropivacaine in children undergoing orchiopexy. Br J Anaesth [Internet]. 2014 May [cited 2018 Aug 7];112(5):885–91. http://linkinghub.elsevier.com/retrieve/pii/S0007091217308395.
12. Schnabel A, Poepping DM, Kranke P, Zahn PK, Pogatzki-Zahn EM. Efficacy and adverse effects of ketamine as an additive for paediatric caudal anaesthesia: a quantitative systematic review of randomized controlled trials. Br J Anaesth [Internet]. 2011 Oct [cited 2018 Aug 7];107(4):601–11. https://linkinghub.elsevier.com/retrieve/pii/S0007091217330441.
13. Disma N, Frawley G, Mameli L, Pistorio A, Alberighi ODC, Montobbio G, et al. Effect of epidural clonidine on minimum local anesthetic concentration (ED50) of levobupivacaine for caudal block in children. Pediatr Anesth [Internet]. 2011 Feb 1 [cited 2018 Aug 7];21(2):128–35. http://doi.wiley.com/10.1111/j.1460-9592.2010.03478.x.
14. Leng SA. Transient femoral nerve palsy after ilioinguinal nerve block. Anaesth Intensive Care [Internet]. 1997 Feb [cited 2018 Aug 7];25(1):92. http://www.ncbi.nlm.nih.gov/pubmed/9075530.
15. Research Society of Anaesthesiology Clinical Pharmacology., Sharma K, Raghavendran T. Journal of anaesthesiology, clinical pharmacology. [Internet]. Vol. 24, Journal of Anaesthesiology Clinical Pharmacology. Research Society of Anaesthesiology Clinical Pharmacology; 1985 [cited 2018 Aug 7]. 25. http://www.joacp.org/article.asp?issn=0970-9185;year=2008;volume=24;issue=1;spage=25;epage=29;aulast=Bhardwaj;type=0.
16. Cyna AM, Middleton P. Caudal epidural block versus other methods of postoperative pain relief for circumcision in boys. Cochrane Database Syst Rev [Internet]. 2008 Oct 8 [cited 2018 Aug 7];(4). http://doi.wiley.com/10.1002/14651858.CD003005.pub2.
17. Margetts L, Carr A, McFadyen G, Lambert A. A comparison of caudal bupivacaine and ketamine with penile block for paediatric circumcision. Eur J Anaesthesiol [Internet]. 2008 Dec [cited 2018 Aug 7];25(12):1009–13. https://insights.ovid.com/crossref?an=00003643-200812000-00008.
18. Kazak Bengisun Z, Ekmekci P, Haliloğlu AH. Levobupivacaine for postoperative pain management in circumcision: caudal blocks or dorsal penile nerve block. Agri [Internet]. 2012 [cited 2018 Aug 7];24(4):180–6. http://www.ncbi.nlm.nih.gov/pubmed/23364781.
19. Kaya Z, Süren M, Arici S, Karaman S, Tapar H, Erdemir F. Prospective, randomized, double-blinded comparison of the effects of caudally administered levobupivacaine 0.25% and bupivacaine 0.25% on pain and motor block in children undergoing circumcision surgery. Eur Rev Med Pharmacol Sci [Internet]. 2012 Dec [cited 2018 Aug 7];16(14):2014–20. http://www.ncbi.nlm.nih.gov/pubmed/23242731.
20. Sandeman D, Reiner D, Dilley A, Bennett M, Kelly K. A retrospective analysis of three different regional anaesthetic techniques for male circumcision. Pediatr Anesth. 2009;19(August 2007):554–5.
21. Al-Zaben KR, Qudaisat IY, Abu-Halaweh SA, Zuabi WS, Al-Momani HM, Albsoul NM, et al. Comparison of ilioinguinal/iliohypogastric nerve blocks and intravenous morphine for control of post-orchidopexy pain in pediatric ambulatory surgery. Middle East J Anaesthesiol [Internet]. 2014 Feb [cited 2018 Aug 7];22(4):393–8. http://www.ncbi.nlm.nih.gov/pubmed/25007693.
22. Kundra P, Yuvaraj K, Agrawal K, Krishnappa S, Kumar LT. Surgical outcome in children undergoing hypospadias repair under caudal epidural vs penile block. Pediatr Anesth [Internet]. 2012 Jul [cited 2018 Aug 7];22(7):707–12. http://www.ncbi.nlm.nih.gov/pubmed/21957982.
23. Kim MH, Im YJ, Kil HK, Han SW, Joe YE, Lee JH. Impact of caudal block on postoperative complications in children undergoing tubularised incised plate urethroplasty for hypospadias repair: a retrospective cohort study. Anaesthesia. 2016;71(7):773–8.
24. Taicher BM, Routh JC, Eck JB, Ross SS, Wiener JS, Ross AK. The association between caudal anesthesia and increased risk of postoperative surgical complications in boys undergoing hypospadias repair. Veyckemans F, editor. Pediatr Anesth [Internet]. 2017 Jul 1 [cited 2018 Aug 7];27(7):688–94. http://doi.wiley.com/10.1111/pan.13119.

25. Braga LH, Jegatheeswaran K, McGrath M, Easterbrook B, Rickard M, DeMaria J, et al. Cause and Effect versus Confounding—Is There a True Association between Caudal Blocks and Tubularized Incised Plate Repair Complications? J Urol [Internet]. 2017 Mar [cited 2018 Aug 7];197(3):845–51. http://www.ncbi.nlm.nih.gov/pubmed/27794432
26. Azerfarin R, Amiri M, Seyedhejazi M, Kazemi F. Comparing caudal and penile nerve blockade using bupivacaine in hypospadias repair surgeries in children. African J Paediatr Surg [Internet]. 2011;8(3):294. http://www.afrjpaedsurg.org/text.asp?2011/8/3/294/91673
27. Hecht S, Piñeda J, Bayne A. Ultrasound-guided Pudendal Block Is a Viable Alternative to Caudal Block for Hypospadias Surgery: A Single-Surgeon Pilot Study. Urology [Internet]. 2018 Mar [cited 2018 Aug 7];113:192–6. http://www.ncbi.nlm.nih.gov/pubmed/29155191.
28. Kendigelen P, Tutuncu AC, Emre S, Altindas F, Kaya G. Pudendal Versus Caudal Block in Children Undergoing Hypospadias Surgery. Reg Anesth Pain Med [Internet]. 2016 [cited 2018 Aug 7];41(5):610–5. http://www.ncbi.nlm.nih.gov/pubmed/27501015.
29. Lorenzo AJ, Lynch J, Matava C, El-Beheiry H, Hayes J. Ultrasound Guided Transversus Abdominis Plane vs Surgeon Administered Intraoperative Regional Field Infiltration with Bupivacaine for Early Postoperative Pain Control in Children Undergoing Open Pyeloplasty. J Urol [Internet]. 2014 Jul [cited 2018 Aug 7];192(1):207–13. http://www.ncbi.nlm.nih.gov/pubmed/24518763.
30. Kost-Byerly S, Jackson E V, Yaster M, Kozlowski LJ, Mathews RI, Gearhart JP. Perioperative anesthetic and analgesic management of newborn bladder exstrophy repair. J Pediatr Urol [Internet]. 2008 Aug [cited 2018 Aug 7];4(4):280–5. http://linkinghub.elsevier.com/retrieve/pii/S1477513108002131.
31. Sekhri C, Georgiou M, Thomas M. Bladder Exstrophy repair: analgesia and wound dehiscence. Reg Anaesth pain Med. 2008;33(5):e230.
32. Hidas G, Kelly MS, Watts B, Kain ZN, Khoury AE, Application of continuous incisional infusion of local anesthetic after major pediatric urological surgery: Prospective randomized controlled trial. J Pediatr Surg. 2015:50(3);481–4.
33. Chalmers DJ, Bielsky A, Wild TT, Siparsky GL, Wilcox DT, Continuous local anesthetic infusion for children with spina bifida undergoing major reconstruction of the lower urinary tract. J Pediatr Urol. 2015:11 (2);72.e1-72.e5.

Antenatal Urology

5

Martin Kaefer

Learning Objectives
Upon reading the chapter the reader should be able to:

1. Describe the prenatal sonographic presentation, postnatal evaluation and treatment of multicystic dysplastic kidney (MCDK).
2. Delineate the differential diagnosis of a prenatally identified upper pole renal cyst and describe the postnatal methods for determining the etiology.
3. Provide an algorithm for how to differentiate between the various etiologies of prenatally identified bilateral hydronephrosis with a distended bladder in a male fetus.
4. List the six criteria that must be met prior to proceeding with placement of a vesicoamniotic shunt in a fetus with suspected posterior urethral valves.
5. Outline the four most likely differential diagnosis of a fetus found to have an anterior abdominal mass on prenatal sonogram.
6. Describe the differential diagnosis for a female fetus with bladder distension and bilateral hydronephrosis.

5.1 Scenario 1

The department of maternal fetal medicine contacts you to discuss the care of a 22-year-old G1P0 female carrying a 26-week-old male fetus with apparent hydronephrosis.

Question 1: What further information do you wish to have regarding the fetal sonogram?

M. Kaefer (✉)
Division of Pediatric Urology, Indiana University School of Medicine, Indianapolis, IN, USA
e-mail: mkaefer@iupui.edu

P. Godbole et al. (eds.), *Practical Pediatric Urology*,
https://doi.org/10.1007/978-3-030-54020-3_5

5.2 Answer 1

1) General: Gender, presence of other anatomical abnormalities involving non-genitourinary systems. Amniotic fluid volume.
2) Renal: Laterality, size of the renal pelvis, calyceal dilation, location of the kidney, presence of a hydroureter, condition of contralateral kidney, evidence of duplication, echogenicity of renal parenchyma, presence of cysts.
3) Bladder: Relative fullness of bladder, bladder wall thickness, presence or absence of ureterocele or distended ureter posterior to the bladder.

5.3 Question 2

What are the two most likely diagnoses in a patient with apparent hydronephrosis?

5.4 Answer 2

Antenatal hydronephrosis is identified in 1–3% of all pregnancies and is one of the most common birth anomalies detected on prenatal sonography [1]. The majority of fetuses with a renal anterior posterior diameter (APD) of <10 will not have significant pathology. In patients that have areas of dilation >10 mm, it is likely that a significant problem may exist with the involved kidney. Since we are not yet aware of the specific degree of hydronephrosis or renal architecture in this case, the two most likely diagnoses would be.

1. Ureteropelvic junction obstruction (UPJO): When identified in utero, the most common cause of UPJ is intrinsic narrowing of the ureter. Although far less common, intrinsic occlusion may also occur due to high insertion of the ureter on to the renal pelvis or the presence of a fibroepithelial polyp. External compression from a lower pole crossing blood vessel is typically identified later in life.
2. Multicystic Dysplastic Kidney (MCDK)—The finding of multiple non-communicating cysts, minimal or absent renal parenchyma, and the absence of a central large cyst support a diagnosis of MCDK. Many believe that MCDK has a similar etiology to that of UPJO with the obstruction occurring far earlier in embryologic life and hence resulting in more significant renal dysplasia.

Following delivery, the following sonographic picture is obtained (Image 5.1).

5.5 Question 3

How would you confirm the diagnosis? What would be your recommended treatment for this entity?

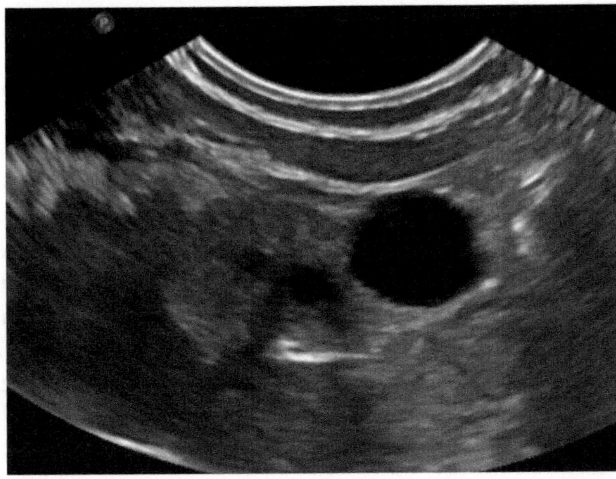

Image 5.1 Renal ultrasound of a newborn child with MCDK. Large polar cyst within a small 2.5 cm kidney. Solid elements are hyperechoic and lack coritomedullary differentiation. These are both consistent with dysplastic parenchyma

5.6 Answer 3

Real-time sonographic imaging of the kidneys to demonstrate the absence of a central large cyst and lack of communication between the peripheral cystic structures is highly suggestive of the diagnosis of MCDK. The presence of minimal, often severely echogenic parenchyma without corticomedullary differentiation is typical. Doppler ultrasonography of the renal vasculature pulse pattern has also been reported to help make the distinction between MCDK and a severe UPJO.

The diagnosis may be confirmed by the absence of renal function on a DMSA scan.

The majority of MCDKs will involute over time and require no intervention. Serial ultrasounds are used to follow this process. Ultimately, very few of these kidneys will need to be removed. Increasing size, hypertension and compression of neighboring structures leading to such symptoms as poor feeding may lead one to consider nephrectomy.

5.7 Scenario 2

A 32-week EGA female fetus is found to have a cyst that appears to involve the upper pole of the left kidney.

5.8 Question 1

What is the differential diagnosis? What further sonographic information would help you to ascertain the etiology of this cyst like structure?

5.9 Answer 1

1. Obstructed upper moiety of a duplex kidney. This is the most likely etiology of an upper pole renal "cyst".
2. Simple Cyst
3. Fetal Adrenal Hemorrhage

Sonographic features that will help establish the diagnosis of an obstructed upper pole moiety include the presence of a hydroureter along with the presence of a ureterocele or impression of a distended ectopic ureter pushing in on the posterior bladder wall (so called pseudoureterocele). Simple cysts are very uncommon in the fetus and fetal adrenal hemorrhage may resolve during the course of the pregnancy.

5.10 Question 2

A distended ureter is identified on the subsequent prenatal sonogram. What investigations would you consider in the postnatal period?

5.11 Answer 2

1. Renal Bladder Ultrasound: A postnatal ultrasound will provide excellent definition of renal and bladder architecture. For unilateral renal pathology in a patient who is voiding spontaneously and otherwise stable it is best obtained a few days after delivery. An ultrasound obtained during the first 48–72 h of life will often underestimate the degree of hydronephrosis due to a relative state of dehydration in the immediate postnatal period.
2. Voiding Cystourethrogram (VCUG): A VCUG should be performed to evaluate for bladder contour, associated reflux into the lower pole of the duplex system and identify a ureterocele or diverticulum (which can be due to an everting ureterocele). The study should be performed with a non-balloon catheter so that the balloon itself does not give a false impression of there being a mass or ureterocele.
3. MAG-3 renal scan: Functional Scintigraphy should be performed to evaluate both function and drainage of each kidney and of the upper pole relative to the lower pole. If possible, it is best to wait until the child has reached 1 month of age before obtaining this test. Prior to this time the kidney is in a state of transition and may not concentrate the radionuclide sufficiently to provide the most accurate assessment of relative function and drainage.

5.12 Question 3

What are the various forms of treatment you could offer the family of this child after reviewing the following Images 5.2, 5.3, and 5.4?

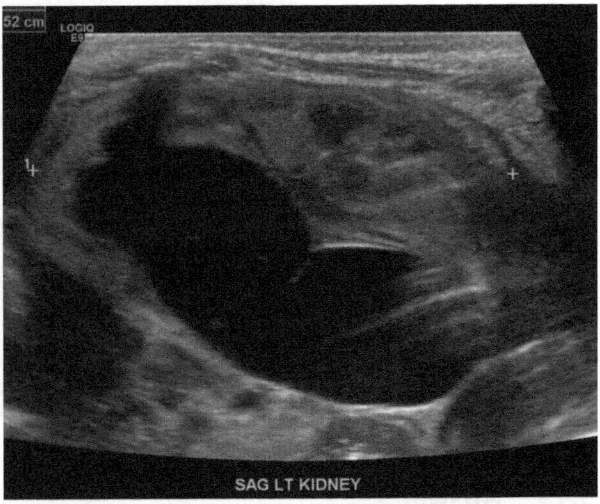

Image 5.2 Renal ultrasound of a duplex left kidney with markedly dilated upper pole and ureter. Small rim of upper pole parenchyma is noted

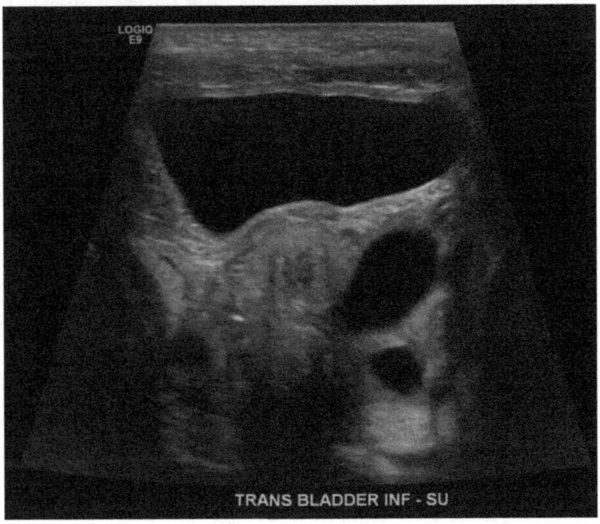

Image 5.3 Bladder ultrasound with posterior distended left ureter consistent with the presence of a left upper pole ectopic ureter

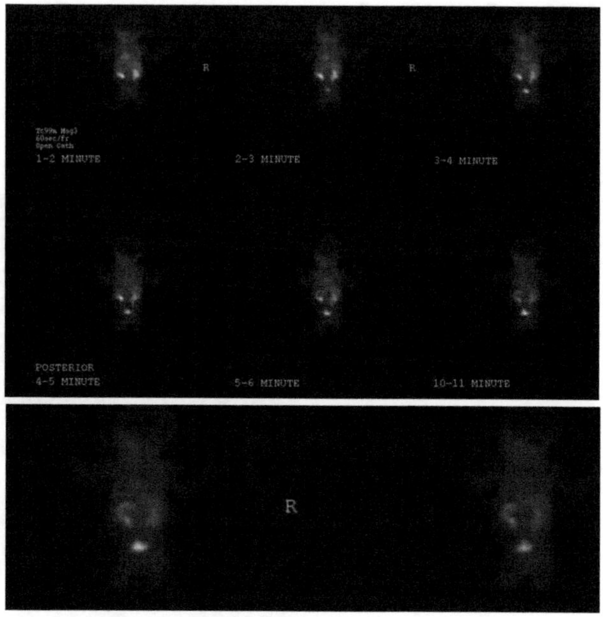

Image 5.4 MAG-3 renal scan demonstrating a left duplex kidney with delayed transit time through upper pole suggestive of obstruction. Reasonable upper pole function is observed

5.13 Answer 3

1) Observation: In that the upper pole has reasonable function on the MAG-3 renal scan, one option would be to observe the neonate until they are older and then perform a duplex ureteral reimplantation with upper pole ureteral tapering. Although some surgeons have advocated for immediate repair, the relative size of the ureter compared to the bladder may make this a challenging operation in the neonatal setting.
2) Upper to lower pole ureteroureterostomy: In the absence of lower pole vesicoureteral reflux, anastomosis of the upper pole system to the lower pole system is a good option. Surgeons continue to debate whether this is best performed at the renal level or distally near the bladder. Proponents of the former cite concerns regarding possible yo-yo reflux and continued stasis when a low ureteroureterostomy is performed.
3) Cutaneous ureterostomy or refluxing ureteral reimplantation [3]: A temporary diversion from the site of obstruction may be utilized in the neonatal setting if there is concern regarding potential for loss of function. Subsequent ureteral reimplantation after the bladder has had chance to grow is then typically undertaken after 9 months of age.

5.14 Scenario 3

A 20-week gestational age boy is found to have bilateral hydroureteronephrosis with a distended bladder and normal amniotic fluid volume.

5.15 Question 1

Why is the initial prenatal sonogram typically obtained at this time? What is the differential diagnosis and what associated findings are typical of each of these diagnosis?

5.16 Answer 1

After 16 weeks gestational age, amniotic fluid production shifts from a primarily placental transudate to fetal urine. By 20–22 weeks the overwhelming majority of amniotic fluid is fetal urine, allowing for proper assessment of hydronephrosis, bladder filling and amniotic fluid volume. The differential diagnosis includes:

1. Posterior Urethral Valves (PUV): The diagnosis of PUV should immediately be entertained when presented with this sonographic picture. The incidence is approximately 1.5 per 10,000 male births. A wide spectrum of sequelae can be appreciated depending on the degree of outlet obstruction.
2. Bilateral High Grade VUR: High-grade bilateral reflux may result in chronic distension of the bladder even in the absence of outlet obstruction. A helpful adjunct for differentiating between this nonobstructive form of bladder distension and posterior urethral valves is the degree of renal echogenicity. Patients with increased renal echogenicity and cysts are far more likely to have an obstructive etiology [2].
3. Prune Belly Syndrome: Marked hydroureteronephrosis and bladder distension are typical of the prune belly syndrome. The associated abdominal wall laxity typical of this condition can aid in identifying these very rare cases. In the later part of the third trimester, the finding of bilateral undescended testis and the presence of a megalourethra may also support this diagnosis.

5.17 Question 2

Two weeks later the amniotic fluid index (AFI) is noted to be <3. The following fetal MRI is obtained. Describe what is seen on these images (Image 5.5).

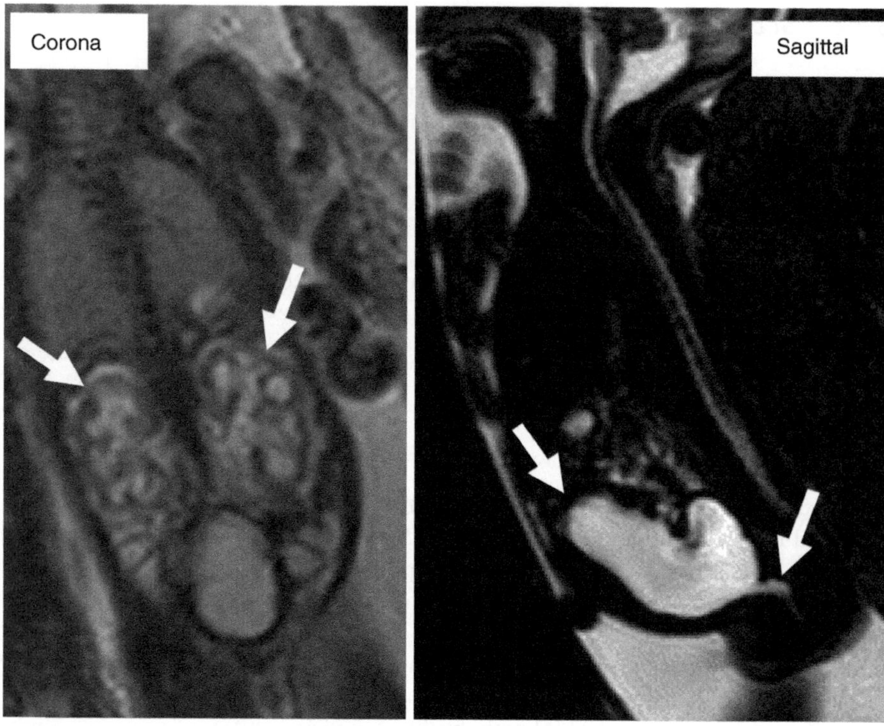

Image 5.5 Fetal MRI findings consistent with posterior urethral valves. *Left*: Coronal image demonstrates bilateral severe hydroureteronephrosis with thinned renal parenchyma. *Right*: Sagittal image demonstrates irregular bladder contour (*upper arrow*) with distended posterior urethra (*lower arrow*). (Images Courtesy of Dr. Brandon Brown, Department of Pediatric Radiology, Indiana University School of Medicine)

5.18 Answer 2

These images demonstrate bilateral severe hydroureteronephrosis with thinned renal parenchyma. Posterior urethral dilation is seen on the right hand image supporting posterior urethral valves as the most likely diagnosis.

5.19 Question 3

What measures must be taken prior to offering the family intervention in the form of a vesicoamniotic shunt?

5.20 Answer 3

In addition to demonstrating evidence of bladder outlet obstruction and oligohydramnios, the following criteria should be met prior to proceeding with placement of a vesicoamniotic shunt.

1. Gestational age less than 25 weeks
2. Normal karyotype by amniocentesis
3. Singleton pregnancy
4. Non-cystic kidneys
5. Favorable urinary indices. Analysis of fetal urine electrolytes is the most widely accepted indicator of salvageable renal function [4]. When Na < 100 mg/dl, Cl < 110 mg/dl and osmolality <210 mOsm/dl renal function appears to be salvageable with in utero intervention. Serial bladder sampling over 3 days appears to have greater predictive value than a single sampling.
6. Informed consent after discussion of risks. Potential complications include initiation of premature labor and intraperitoneal shunt placement. In the case of the very large bladder, the shunt may become dislodged after the bladder decompresses.

5.21 Question 4

A vesicoamniotic shunt is placed and the child is delivered at term. A VCUG is performed and confirms the diagnosis of posterior urethral valves with high-grade right-sided reflux into a dysplastic appearing kidney. What advice can you provide the family regarding long term renal and bladder function?

5.22 Answer 4

1. The nadir creatinine value is the most cited indicator of long-term renal function. A value less than 0.8 mg/dl appears to indicate a minimal risk of developing end-stage renal failure. The value at 1 year of life appears to be a more accurate predictive tool than a value obtained at 1 month. Although it was once felt that presence of high-grade reflux into a dysplastic kidney would help preserve contralateral renal function, this so called VURD syndrome (Vesicoureteral Reflux and Dysplasia) does not appear to provide a reliable benefit to the contralateral unit.
2. Bladder function may often remain impaired after the valves have been resected. Impairment can exist in a spectrum ranging from hypercontractile to relatively atonic. Detrusor hyperreflexia is most common in infancy. This often evolves into improved compliance in childhood and subsequent hypotonia in adolescence. Each of these forms of bladder dysfunction can have an occult onset and thus the management of these children requires constant monitoring.

5.23 Scenario 4

A 32-week G3P2 female presents for prenatal assessment and is found to be carrying a 24-week EGA fetus. The child is noted to have an anterior abdominal wall mass.

5.24 Question 1

What is the differential diagnosis?

5.25 Answer 1

1. Omphalocele (exomphalos): Incidence of 2–2.5/10,000. The omphalocele sac protrudes through the umbilicus as a result of failure of normal return of abdominal contents into abdomen during the 9th week of prenatal development. This condition is associated with severe malformations such as cardiac abnormalities and neural tube defects. Approximately 30% of infants have associated congenital anomalies.
2. Gastroschisis: Incidence 4/10,000. Abdominal contents protrude next to umbilicus with no membrane covering the abdominal contents. There are no common associated congenital anomalies in this condition.
3. Bladder exstrophy: Incidence of 1/50,000. The abdominal "mass", which is made up of the two everting bladder halves, does not protrude to the same degree as with the other three diagnosis.
4. Cloacal exstrophy: Incidence of 1/200,000–1/400,000. The abdominal mass consists of a midline hindgut that protrudes between two bladder halves.

5.26 Question 2

The maternal fetal medicine team comments that they do not see a distinct bladder? How do you counsel the family?

5.27 Answer 2

The parents should be informed that inability to visualize the bladder on one imaging study does not necessarily indicate the absence of an intact bladder. Patient observation of the fetal pelvis for the absence of bladder feeling is critical in making the diagnosis.

Assuming that a bladder is not visualized after a prolonged attempt to do so, then the most likely diagnosis is some form of bladder exstrophy. A fetal MRI may help with the diagnosis. Additional findings consistent with classic bladder exstrophy include normal kidneys in the orthotopic location, low umbilical cord insertion, abnormal diastasis of the symphysis, an anteriorly displaced anus, and normal

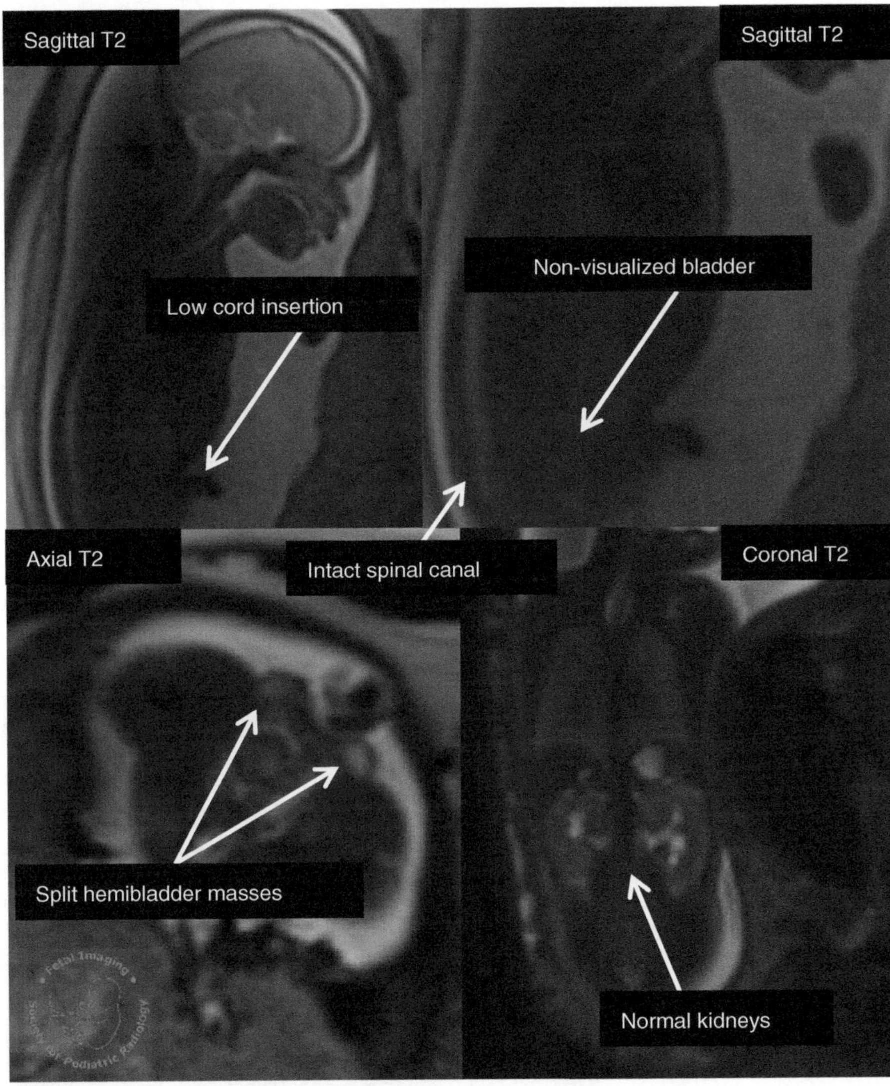

Image 5.6 Fetal MRI findings consistent with classic bladder exstrophy. *Upper left*: Sagittal image showing low umbilical cord insertion. *Upper Left*: Sagittal image showing non visualized badder. *Lower Left*: Axial image demonstrating split hemi-bladder masses. *Lower Right*: Coronal image demonstrating normal kidneys. (Images Courtesy of Dr. Brandon Brown, Department of Pediatric Radiology, Indiana University School of Medicine)

vertebrae and spinal cord [5]. An example of this (not representing the patient at hand) is shown below (Image 5.6).

Question 3: The following week an MRI of the patient you have been asked to consult on is obtained The MRI image and immediate postoperative picture of the child are shown (Image 5.7 and 5.8).

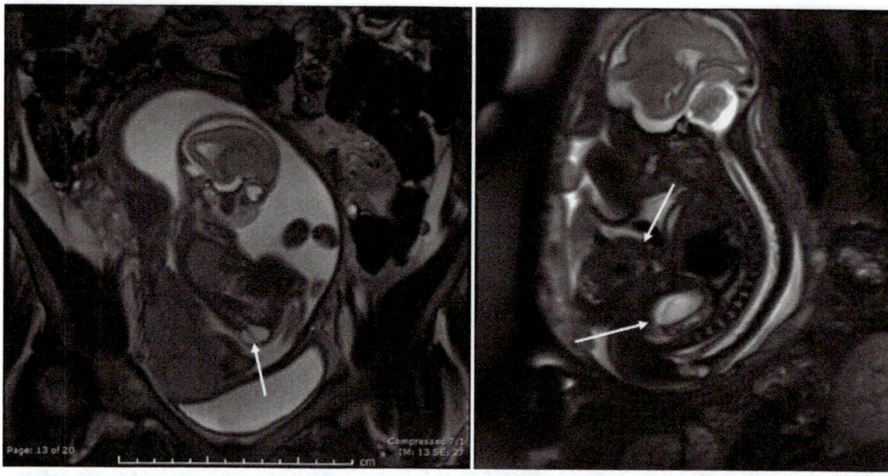

Image 5.7 Fetal MRI findings consistent with Cloacal Exstrophy. *Left*: Sagittal image demonstrating myelomeningocele (*arrow*). *Right*: Sagittal image demonstrating absence of anterior abdominal wall (*upper arrow*) and low lying stomach (*lower arrow*) with absence of bladder. (Images Courtesy of Dr. Brandon Brown, Department of Pediatric Radiology, Indiana University School of Medicine)

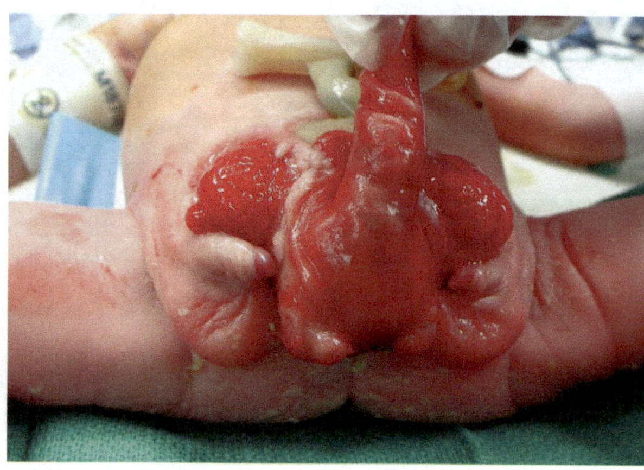

Image 5.8 Postnatal picture of cloacal exstrophy. Note the central ileum prolapsing through the cecal plate, two laterally displaced bladder halves and two widely separated halves of the penis

5.27.1 Prenatal MRI of Cloacal Exstrophy

Describe what is seen on both the fetal MRI and the newborn photo. Describe what other organ systems can be affected in this condition and what initial management steps are recommended for the proper care of these children.

5.28 Answer 3

The fetal MRI demonstrates findings consistent with cloacal exstrophy. The classic “elephant trunk” configuration of the prolapsing ileum is appreciated. One can also appreciate the lumbosacral spine abnormalities and myelomeningocele that are present in the majority of these neonates. Abnormal number or location of kidneys, cardiac abnormalities and limb abnormalities can also be seen in these infants.

The post-delivery picture shows the classic cecal plate in the midline with the ileum prolapsing through the ileocecal valve. The two hemi-bladders and widely separated penile corpora can also be appreciated. Initial management includes separating the prolapsed hindgut from between the two bladder halves, tubularizing the cecum and bringing the intestine out as a colostomy. Although immediate closure of the bladder has been typically performed in the past, it is now common to simply approximate the two bladder halves during the initial operation. Subsequent closure of the bladder is aided by pelvic osteotomies.

5.29 Scenario 5

A 24-year-old G3P2 female presents for prenatal assessment. At 32 weeks estimated gestational age bilateral hydroureteronephrosis and a somewhat distended bladder are noted. Maternal cell-free DNA screening is negative for the presence of a Y-chromosome. Amniotic fluid volume is normal.

5.30 Question 1

What is the differential diagnosis?

5.31 Answer 1

Maternal cell-free DNA is highly effective in predicting the gender of a fetus. This technology is based on polymerase chain reaction amplification of 200 base pair fragments of DNA that are passed from the baby across the placental circulation to the mother. The assumption in this case is that the child is a genetic female and therefore that the common form of bladder outlet obstruction noted in a boy (i.e. posterior urethral valves) is not in the differential diagnosis. In females the most common forms of fetal bladder outlet obstruction are

a. Ureterocele: A cecoureterocele that projects in to the bladder neck can result not only in obstruction of the ipsilateral kidney, but also in bladder outlet obstruction with subsequent bladder distension. A ureterocele will typically be appreciated on prenatal sonography.

b. Hydrometrocolpos: Distension of the fetal vagina can result in the bladder outlet obstruction. With persistent cloaca, the rectum, vagina(s) and urethra all come together proximal to the perineum and exit as a common channel. When this occurs, voided urine can fill the vagina(s) to such a great degree that they create a posterior mass effect on the bladder neck, effectively creating bladder outlet obstruction. Obstruction of the bladder neck from a distended vagina can also occur in patients with a common urogenital sinus (with or without underlying congenital adrenal hyperplasia). In cases of vaginal filling from voided urine the patient may also demonstrate ascites due to urine passing out the fallopian tubes in to the peritoneal cavity. Finally, hydrometrocolpos can be seen in association with transverse vaginal septum, intact hymen or Herlyn-Werner-Wunderlich Syndrome [5, 6].

Other causes of bilateral hydroureteronephrosis in a female include bilateral UVJ obstruction such as might occur in bilateral single system ectopic ureters. However, in such cases one would not anticipate bladder distension.

5.32 Question 2

The ultrasound findings prompt a fetal MRI. The results are shown. Describe the findings (Images 5.8 and 5.9).

5.33 Answer 2

The first set of images demonstrates bilateral hydroureteronephrosis with an anterior displaced bladder. The fluid collection posterior to the bladder represents the fluid filled vagina and uterus. The second set of images shows the distended vagina, hydronephrotic kidneys and urinary ascites in the axial plane (left arrow), while the sagittal picture demonstrates retained meconium (right arrow) secondary to imperforate anus in this patient with a diagnosis of cloaca.

5.34 Question 3

What possible management options once the patient has been delivered?

5.35 Answer 3

Upon delivery the child will require a diverting colostomy. Treatment of vaginal distension (and as a result bladder obstruction) can be achieved through intermittent catheterization of the common sinus. When effective catheterization cannot be performed the child may require the creation of a vesicostomy and possible vaginostomy.

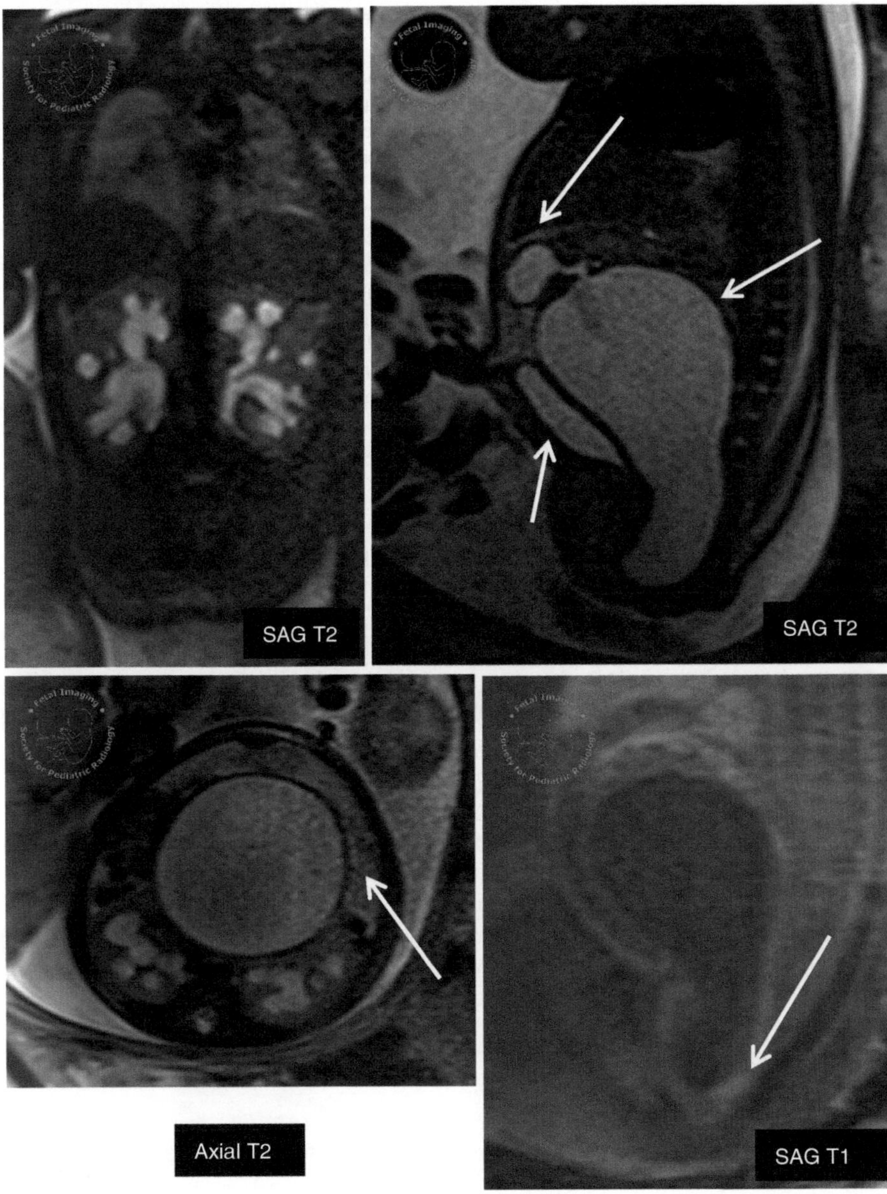

Image 5.9 Fetal MRI findings consistent with cloaca. *Upper left*: Coronal image demonstrating bilateral hydronephrosis. *Upper right*: Sagittal image demonstrating anterior displaced bladder with posterior fluid collection representing distended vagina. *Top arrow* pointing to a small intraluminal uterine fluid collection. *Bottom left*: Axial image demonstrating fluid filled vagina and posteriorly positioned hydronephrotic kidneys. *Bottom right*: Sagittal image demonstrating meconium (*right arrow*) secondary to imperforate anus. (Images Courtesy of Dr. Brandon Brown, Department of Pediatric Radiology, Indiana University School of Medicine)

References

1. Fernbach SK, Maizels M, Conway JJ. Ultrasound grading of hydronephrosis: introduction to the system used by the society for fetal urology. Pediatr Radiol. 1993;2396:478–80.
2. Kaefer M, Peters CA, Retik AB, et al. Increased renal echogenicity: a sonographic sign for differentiating between obstructive and nonobstructive etiologies of in utero bladder distension. J Urol. 1997;158:1026–9.
3. Glick PL, Harrison MR, Golbus MS, et al. Management of the fetus with congenital hydronephrosis II: prognostic criteria and selection for treatment. J Pediatr Surg. 1985;20:376–87.
4. Kaefer M, Misseri R, Frank E, Rhee A, Lee SD. Refluxing ureteral reimplantation: a logical method for managing neonatal UVJ obstruction. J Pediatr Urol. 2014;10(5):824–30.
5. Gearhart JP, Ben-Chaim J, Jeffs RD, Sanders RC. Criteria for the prenatal diagnosis of classic bladder exstrophy. Obstet Gynecol. 1995; 85(6):961–4.
6. Kaefer M. Management of Abnormalities of the genitalia in girls. In: Wein AJ, Kavoussi LR, Partin AW, Peters CA, editors. Campbell's urology. 11th ed. Philadelphia, PA: W.B Saunders; 2016.
7. Celayir AC, Kurt G, Sahin C, Cici I. Spectrum of etiologies causing hydrometrocolpos. J Neonatal Surg. 2013;2(1):5–8.

6 Office Paediatric Urology

Joana Dos Santos, Mandy Rickard, Armando J. Lorenzo, and Martin A. Koyle

Learning Objectives

- Provide a practical approach for the management of common paediatric urology conditions often seen by primary care physicians and pediatricians in the office
- Describe an itemized overview along with pertinent history and physical examination
- Demonstrate key points and provide recommendations on when to refer to specialists

6.1 Introduction

In this Chapter we will address some common paediatric urology concerns and conditions often by primary care physicians and pediatricians. We will provide an itemized overview along with pertinent history and physical examination key points, recommendations on when to refer to specialists and management of these conditions.

6.2 Undescended Testicles

Undescended testicles (UDT) or cryptorchidism is a relatively common congenital condition affecting 1–5% of full term boys. It is characterized by the inability to palpate one or both testes in their correct scrotal position [1]. The incidence at birth

J. D. Santos (✉) · M. Rickard · A. J. Lorenzo
Division of Urology, The Hospital for Sick Children, Toronto, ON, Canada
e-mail: joana.dossantos@sickkids.ca

M. A. Koyle
Department of Surgery and IHPME, University of Toronto Paediatric Urology, The Hospital for Sick Children, Toronto, ON, Canada

P. Godbole et al. (eds.), *Practical Pediatric Urology*,
https://doi.org/10.1007/978-3-030-54020-3_6

is impacted by gestational age, being more common in pre-term boys. Other known risk factors include multiple births, family history, low birth weight and associated genetic syndromes [2]. There have been some reports of maternal and paternal characteristics as well as certain environmental exposures playing a role in the development of UDT, however these associations are relatively weak and based on observational studies [3]. Spontaneous descent can be seen in the first 3–6 months of life (appropriately adjusting gestational age in pre-term infants). After this period, if the testes are not in their normal anatomical position, referral to a surgical specialist should be initiated. As recommended in the American Urological Association (AUA) and Canadian Urological Association (CUA)guidelines, cryptorchidism should be surgically corrected by 18 months of age, therefore timely referral is important [1, 4]. Routine testicular examination should be carried out at every well child visit by primary care providers, especially in light of the fact that 1.5% of prepubertal boys may develop an "ascending testis" where the gonad is initially present in the scrotum but subsequently retracts into the inguinal canal [1].

A true UDT is either non-palpable or detected outside of the scrotum. During examination it may not be gently maneuvered into the scrotum at all, or immediately retracts once manipulated into the scrotum. Non-palpable testes may be gonads that are in the inguinal region, groin or scrotumbut are difficult to detect on physical exam, may be intraabdominal, or be absent. Palpable testes that can be brought into the scrotum and remain there once the cremasteric reflex has been fatigued are considered retractile and a normal findings that does not require surgical correction. In the event of bilateral non-palpable testes (NPT) in a newborn, karyotyping and hormonal testing is recommended before discharge to rule out congenital adrenal hyperplasia.

Routine imaging for UDT is not indicated. Many reports have demonstrated that ultrasound (US) is not a reliable test for this condition, and is in fact less accurate than physical examination followed by selective surgical exploration. Further, US for UDT is expensive, causes confusion for referring providers, and may result in a delay in referral, assessment and surgical intervention for these children [5]. The most important aspect of diagnosis of UDT is the physical examination carried out during the clinical assessment.

6.3 History and Physical Examination

In the assessment of an infant with UDT, birth history, family history and other risk factors identified above should be obtained. For older patients, parents should be asked if they have ever noted to the testes to be visible and descended, even if only intermittently, during activities such as bathing.

During physical examination, it is helpful to remember the physiologic response of the testes to changes in temperature and the cremasteric reflex. Examining the testes in an uncooperative anxious child may be very challenging, as such, it is important provide a safe, calm environment, and to simply observe before palpating. There is useful information that can be obtained by simple visual assessment of

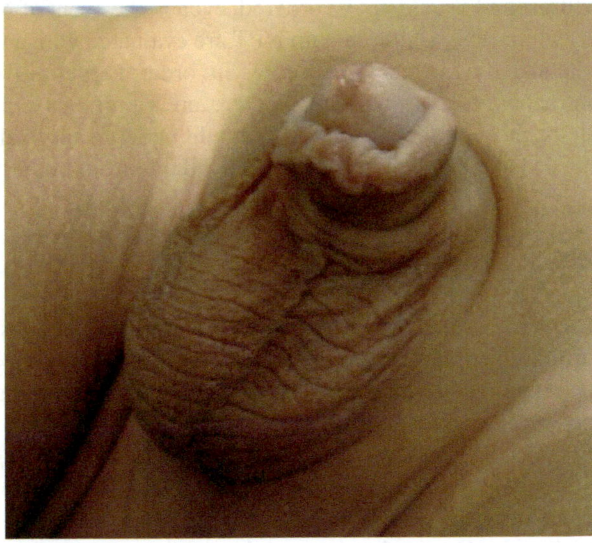

Fig. 6.1 Undescended testicle and underdeveloped scrotum

this patient population. First, pay attention to the fullness of the scrotum while the child is initially exposed, the testes may be visible and descended before the child is handled. Next, assess for symmetry of the scrotum. Typically, in the event of unilateral UDT, the ipsilateral hemi-scrotum appears smaller and underdeveloped when compared to the contralateral side (Fig. 6.1). Finally, noting a prominent genital fat pad allows for recognition of a more challenging physical examination as the type of anatomy generally makes palpation of testes more difficult.

During palpation of the testes, clinicians develop individual techniques over time that are modified based on experience. Some clinicians prefer the child supine and in a frog leg position, while others prefer a squatting or "catchers" position. Examination should be carried out while standing on the same side of the child as the test is being palpated for, while the testis is tracked along the natural path of descent. It may be necessary to apply gentle pressure/traction in in inguinal region, and at times the testes become visible in the scrotum upon doing so. Finally, in the event that the testes cannot be palpated, it may be helpful to attempt to palpate them with the assistance of lubricant or hand soap. This technique will usually allow for identification of a palpable testis in the inguinal canal that cannot be brought into the scrotum by minimizing friction and direct visualization of a "pop" in the location of the testis.

6.4 Summary

If testes are undescended, whether palpable or nonpalpable, by 6 months of age a prompt referral to a surgical specialist should be initiated, in order to have adequate time to further assess and plan for a potential surgical intervention (if required).

Ultrasound should not be ordered, even in the event of NPT, due to the poor sensitivity of this test. Children with NPT are evaluated with an examination under anesthesia and diagnostic laparascopy in order to definitively rule in or rule out an intraabdominal testis. Unless there are significant comorbidities or contraindications, most children with UDT should undergo surgical correction by 18 months of age. Management algorithms are available from both the AUA and the CUA.

6.5 Hernia/Hydrocele

Inguinal herniais one of the most common surgical issues presenting to paediatric urology and surgery clinics. It is diagnosed in approximately 0.8–4% of children [6]. Inguinal hernia occurs due to a patent processus vaginalis that fails to obliterate postnatally and is more common in boys. Spontaneous resolution may occur in the first year of life, becoming less likely with increasing age. Classical presentation of a hernia is painless swelling of the scrotum in boys, or labial folds in girls. If the contents or the patient processus vaginalis is only fluid, it is called a communicating hydrocele. Once other intra-abdominal structures (i.e. bowel, omentum) enter the canal, it is labelled as a hernia. The groin, scrotal or labial swelling is noted in the absence of pain, erythema and discoloration, and a report of regular fluctuation in size is often given. Hernias may be unilateral or bilateral with a small risk of contralateral occurrence after unilateral surgical correction. Risk factors for inguinal hernia are preterm birth, low birth weight and often present simultaneously with UDT.

Imaging is not routinely indicated for this condition and the diagnosis is made based on history and physical examination. US may be selectively used to confirm presence of a patent processus vaginalis, to rule out alternative diagnoses (such as a testicular tumor or para-testicular mass), visualization of the testis and demonstration of blood flow, and the presence of Mullerian structures in girls [7]. In the event of a persistent hydrocele/hernia in infants older than 6 months of age a referral should be initiated for timely assessment and surgical planning. Inguinal hernias are repaired electively either laparoscopically or through a small inguinal incision—depending on the age of the child—with ligation of the processus vaginalis. Surgical intervention is required due to the small but serious risk of incarceration, however infants are typically observed for 1–2 years to allow for spontaneous resolution [8]. There are some exceptions, more notably premature children with large inguinal hernias and children with prior incarceration. In these, surgical correction is expedited.

6.6 History and Physical Examination

A thorough history is important in the decision-making process. Often times a physical examination may be negative, which makes an accurate and detailed history necessary for diagnosis. The child (or parents) should be asked about duration of the

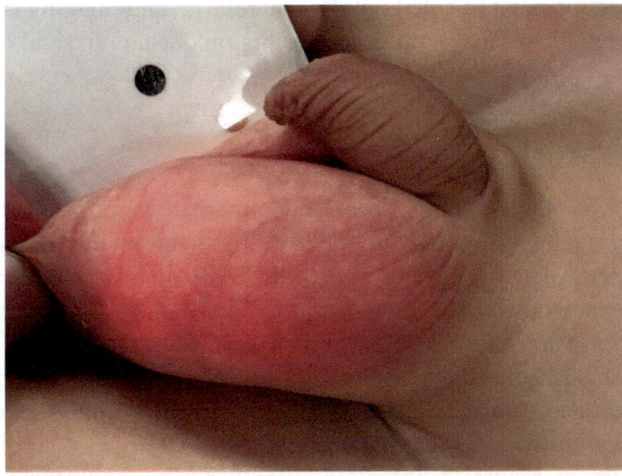

Fig. 6.2 Hydrocele with transillumination

presumed hernia, and the presence of fluctuation, which is one of the most important finding to note. This will help distinguish between a communicating hydrocele (surgical problem) vs. a non-communicating hydrocele which should improve without surgery. It is also important to determine the presence of pain associated with the hernia as well as any discoloration or bulging in the groin. Timing of when the hernia was noticed is important for older children as it may coincide with a history of viral illness or trauma [8].

There may be instances when physical examination is positive for an obvious fluid collection or mass in the scrotum/labial fold that is suggestive of a hernia. There may be opportunity to confirm communication if it is reducible and the fluid or other contents can be pushed back into abdomen. There is some controversy surrounding the so-call "silk glove sign" in boys with hernia. It is thought to be elicited by gently rolling the cord structures across the pubic bone and feeling the hernia sac gliding on itself. This finding is felt to be suggestive of a patent processes vaginalis but it's not diagnostic [9]. For boys, it is important to document if the ipsilateral testicle is normal and descended into the scrotum, as a large hydrocele may mask an associated UDT. As well, transillumination can be performed to confirm the presence of fluid in the scrotum (Fig. 6.2) and help rule out an acute scrotum or underlying testicular pathology [10].

6.7 Summary

Hernias and communicating hydroceles represent a common surgical condition seen in paediatric surgery clinics, amenable to conservative management in the first 1–2 years of life. Elective repair is encouraged due to the risk of incarceration and a history of fluctuation is considered a surgical indication. Importantly, in the event of scrotal pain, erythema, discoloration, swelling or an unwell appearing child, immediate referral to an emergency department should occur as incarceration or testicular torsion must be ruled out. Urgent referral and imaging is also indicated for suspicion of testicular mass or testicular torsion during physical examination.

6.8 Phimosis

Physiologic phimosis is a developmentally appropriate finding in infants and prepubertal boys and refers to the inability to retract the foreskin due to congenital attachment of the inner prepuce to the glans penis. In North America there has been a somewhat recent trend towards not routinely circumcising children, resulting in confusion about the correct management of foreskin in infants and young boys [11]. At birth, the inner prepuce is adherent to the glans and should not be forcefully retracted, with gradual release expected over time. During this period, children may present with some ballooning of the foreskin with voiding, deviation of the urinary stream, recurrent 'infections' or other vague symptoms related to the penis. Parents and patients should be reassured that resolution will occur naturally with slow release of the preputial adhesions through the accumulation of smegma and with reflex erections. Children with physiologic phimosis do not have an indication for circumcision solely based on this diagnosis and should be encouraged to manage the issue conservatively should the family choose to do so.

In contrast, pathologic phimosis occurs when the prepuce is unable to be retracted due to a buildup of scar tissue. This reaction may occur as a result of chronic inflammatory processes such as balanitis xerotica obliterans (BXO or lichen sclerosis), repeated episodes of infections (balanitis/balanoposthitis) or poor healing after previous forced retraction. Children with pathologic phimosis may have progressive difficulty with voiding including significant ballooning, a weak stream, and dribbling or spraying with voiding, which may lead to urinary retention. Pathologic phimosis does not spontaneously improve and is an indication for circumcision in this population of children.

6.9 History and Physical Examination

In the assessment of a child with phimosis, age, duration of phimosis and presence of urinary symptoms are important to consider.

6.9.1 Physiologic Phimosis

6.9.1.1 History

Boys with physiologic phimosis typically have not been able to have their foreskin retracted. Many are asymptomatic with respect to both urinary symptoms and lower urinary tract complains (often misdiagnosed as "infections") and are being brought for assessment due to parental concerns about the skin being tight and uneasiness about the time frame when the skin should be retracted. Those with symptoms may also report ballooning with micturition but are able to void easily with minimal effort and resistance. If 'infections' are reported, they usually are reported as redness/irritation, dysuria and 'discharge' which is usually a mixture of entrapped urine and smegma that emanates through the foreskin opening and is mistaken as exudate or pus. Most of these infections are managed with topical treatments, are not usually associated with fever, and do not require systemic antibiotics. Rarely, some children may develop balanitis/balanoposthitis and may be treated with oral antibiotics. In some patients, recurrent episodes may lead to pathologic phimosis [12]. Other children, particularly infants with underlying urinary tract conditions may develop urinary tract infections (UTI) as a result of phimosis. In this instance a circumcision may be indicated.

6.9.1.2 Physical Examination

Physical examination of a boy with physiologic phimosis is relatively unremarkable. With any examination it is important to note the presence of bilaterally descended testes. On inspection, the foreskin should appear elastic and supple without erythema or obvious scarring (Fig. 6.3). The opening may be pinpoint, or the meatus may be visible through a small opening. The skin should never be retracted past the point of skin placed on tension or discomfort. When examining the foreskin, if it is ever retracted past the glans, it is important that it is always reduced back over the glans to prevent paraphimosis.

6.9.1.3 Management

For asymptomatic physiologic phimosis, no treatment is required as this condition will improve spontaneously with age. These children do not need routine

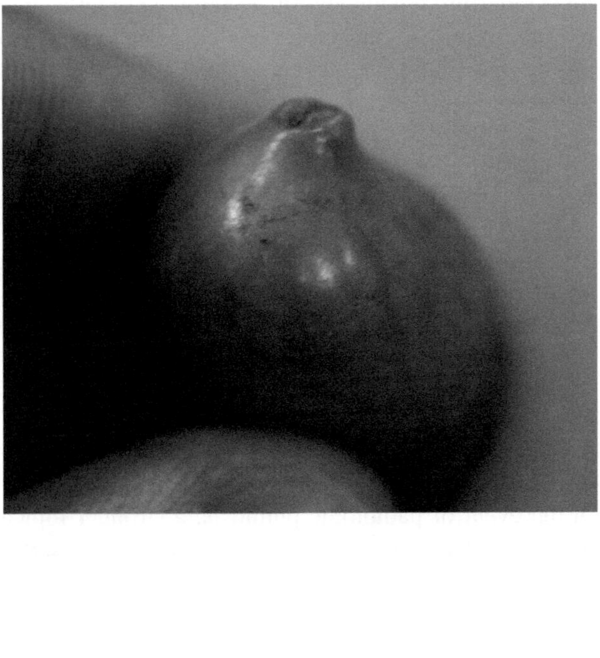

Fig. 6.3 Physiologic phimosis

assessment by a paediatric urologist and can be managed by their primary care provider. Parents should be encouraged to work on gentle stretching of the skin with diaper changes and baths to stimulate slow separation of adhesion between the foreskin and glans from an early age. Older boys should be encouraged to retract he foreskin each time they void and during baths or showers. Intermittent ballooning also does not require treatment if in the absence of other symptoms. In the event of recurrent episodes of erythema or edema, parents may be encouraged to apply an over the counter antibiotic ointment and Epsom salts in the bath which should help to alleviate those symptoms. Finally, to expedite the separation of the physiologic adhesions, application of a topical steroid—such as a 0.05–0.1% betamethasone—once or twice per day for 6 weeks will help facilitate this. It is beneficial to demonstrate to the patient or parent the most effective method of application of this cream to ensure success. Parents should be counselled that with cessation of the cream, the skin may become tight again. Elective circumcision may be performed for this condition however, it should be explained to the family that there is no medical reason for doing so.

6.10 Pathologic Phimosis

6.10.1 History

The history of a child with pathologic phimosis may differ from the physiologic counterpart. Most children with pathologic phimosis are older, as this condition is rare in infants and toddlers. There may be a report of a previous ability to retract the skin which has since disappeared. This condition may occur after development of scar tissue after forceful retraction. There may also be a history of recurrent infections requiring treatment with systemic antibiotics with or without fever. Children may also report voiding issues, including ballooning. However, unlike children with physiologic phimosis, this may also occur with a weak stream or dribbling, straining to void and dysuria.

6.10.2 Physical Examination

The primary finding to note on an examination of these children is the presence of white, fibrotic scar tissue on the tip of the foreskin with a small or pinpoint opening. When attempting to retract, the skin is not pliable or elastic and no stretching occurs (Fig. 6.4).

6.10.3 Management

In the event of pathologic phimosis, a stronger topical steroid such as clobetasol may be indicated in an attempt to manage it conservatively, however the reported

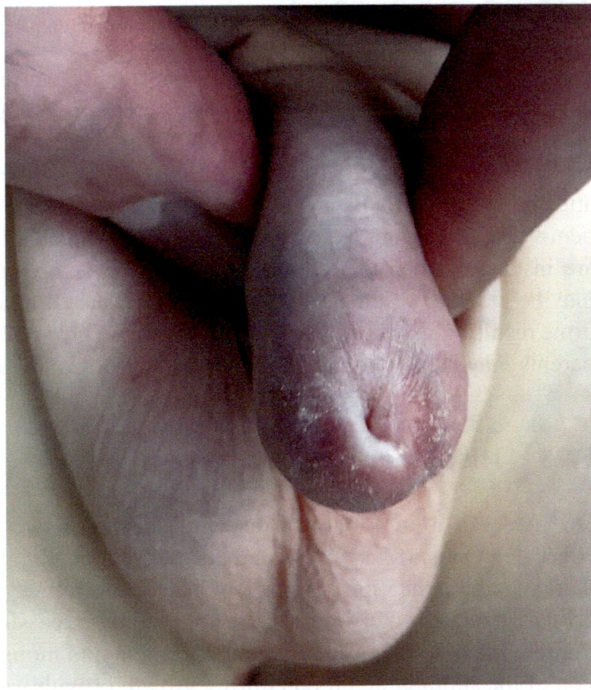

Fig. 6.4 Pathologic phimosis/BXO

success rates are low [11]. In many instances circumcision is the required management option.

6.11 Summary

Physiologic phimosis is a developmentally normal finding for many boys and does not require assessment in a paediatric urology clinic or treatment other than conservative measures. It will improve with age, however in the event of bothersome symptoms it can be managed with topical steroids. Pathologic phimosis occurs in older children and is the result of accumulation of scar tissue on the tip of the foreskin. This condition does not spontaneously improve and may require a circumcision for management. A referral to paediatric urologist is indicated in the event of scarring of the preputial ring, recurrent episodes of balanitis, genital lichen sclerosis (also known as balanitis xerotica obliterans), UTIs or failure of topical steroids.

6.12 Concealed Penis

A concealed penis is a congenital abnormality caused by numerous anatomical defects including deficient penile skin, scrotal webbing and prominent suprapubic fat pad [13]. This condition is most common in infancy and may also become apparent during adolescence. Typically, children with a concealed penis are asymptomatic and concerns focus primarily on cosmesis. Parents often express distress about penis size, sometimes exacerbated by previous misdiagnosis as "micropenis". There are instances when this condition may cause symptoms and surgical intervention may be indicated. Some children may experience difficulty voiding and trapping of urine resulting in significant ballooning and recurrent balanitis [14]. In severe cases, parents may have to manually express the urine after each void.

6.13 History and Physical Examination

On history it is important to determine the presence of symptoms related to the concealed penis. If the patient had been experiencing infections or difficulty voiding there may be indication for surgical intervention. If asymptomatic and concerns are primarily related to cosmesis, parents should be reassured that many children have improvement with conservative management and monitoring, typically with reduction of the suprapubic fat pad during growth or with weight loss [15].

During physical examination, retract ability of the foreskin should be assessed as a tight phimotic ring contributes to urine entrapment. This can be further suspected in the presence of erythema, local irritation and expression of urine when the penis is palpated. Location of the penoscrotal angle and presence of suprapubic fat should also be considered.

6.14 Summary

Concealed penis is a congenital condition causing the penis to be hidden and not extending outside the body. This may cause distress for some families due to the cosmetic appearance and cause voiding symptoms and other complaints for others. Some children will experience natural improvement with growth and development while others may require surgical intervention. This condition is a contraindication for newborn circumcision and any necessary surgical intervention should occur with a paediatric urologist and optimally deferred until the child has passed the infancy period. Children with this condition should be referred to a paediatric urologist for assessment and monitoring.

6.15 Routine Newborn Circumcision Contraindications

While routine newborn circumcision has become a controversial topic, many parents choose to have their boys circumcised. Because of this persistent demand, practitioners still offer this procedure in their office, and assessment and recognition of potential contraindications is important. Unrecognized contraindications may result in poor cosmetic result, parental distress and anxiety and possible complications requiring assessment by a paediatric urologist.

6.15.1 Hypospadias

Hypospadias is a congenital defect of the penis occurring in approximately 1 in 300 infant boys [16]. It is characterized by an abnormal position of the urethral meatus on the ventral aspect of the penis, ventral curvature and skin deficiency, and dorsal hooded foreskin. Boys with hypospadias may have varying degrees of severity with all or some of these characteristics, which may not always be obvious on routine exam. Hypospadias is a reconstructive surgical condition and the prepuce is used for the urethral reconstruction. Therefore, a missed hypospadiac penis that is circumcised may make the hypospadias repair technically challenging and potentially risk a less favorable outcomes. If there is any suspicion of hypospadias the circumcision should not be completed until the patient is assessed by a paediatric urologist.

6.15.2 Webbed or Buried Penis

A webbed or buried penis occurs when the penoscrotal angle is obscured by skin webbing resulting in a shorter than normal shaft skin and foreskin. This may be accompanied by a prominent suprapubic fat pad. When a circumcision is performed in this setting the penis tends to entrap into the surrounding tissue resulting in the formation of adhesions. Parental anxiety worsens as the penis is not visible protruding outside the body. Surgical intervention in the form of concealed or buried penis repair may be required for these boys if parents wish to have them circumcised, otherwise it is recommended to leave them intact.

6.15.3 Penile Curvature/Torque

Curvature of the penis may occur in unison with hypospadias or on its own and may be due to ventral skin tethering of penis and scrotum or from intrinsic corporal disproportion. Penile torque occurs when there is torsion of the penis within its longitudinal axis, in contrast to ventral curvature where the longitudinal axis is deviated. It may range from mild to a complete 180° and is reported in up to 20% of infant males [17]. A handy assessment tool for determining the presence of torque is to use the midline raphe on the ventral aspect as a guide as it should line up with the midline of the scrotum and proceed in a straight line along the ventral side of the penis.

In the event of either of these conditions it is recommended to have the infant assessed by a paediatric urologist before proceeding with circumcision.

6.16 Circumcision Complications

Careful and accurate assessment prior to performing a newborn circumcision and disclosure during consent is important due to the possibility of post-procedure complications. In this section, we will review the most common circumcision complications.

6.16.1 Preputial Adhesions

Preputial adhesions form during the healing period after a circumcision when the penis retracts into the surrounding tissue and superficial adhesions form between the glans and the circumcision wound edges. They may be more prone to occur when there is a prominent suprapubic fat pad, pre-procedure concealed penis or penoscrotal webbing. Parents can try to prevent these from forming during the initial healing period and afterwards by ensuring that they expose the glans and corona by regularly applying pressure on the fat pad during diaper changes followed by generous application of petroleum jelly. In some cases, regardless of parental diligence, adhesions will form which will need to be addressed. Adhesions can be taken down in the clinic by applying a topical anesthetic and manually separating them, bearing in mind that there is a strong likelihood of reforming during the first few days of healing. For some boys, if left untreated the adhesions will eventually become skin bridges which require surgical intervention.

6.16.2 Buried/Trapped Penis

If a circumcision is performed on a child with penoscrotal webbing (identifiable by a suboptimal penoscrotal angle) or a concealed penis they could develop an acquired buried or trapped penis. This occurs when the penis "disappears" after a circumcision and is completely concealed only visible with pressure applied to the fat pad to expose the glans. These boys may also develop a cicatrix, which is a fibrotic ring which prevents the penis from being exposed. A cicatrix may benefit from application of a topical steroid. In some cases, management may require re-operation.

6.16.3 Meatal Stenosis

Meatal stenosis is a long-term complication of circumcision that occurs in approximately 2.8–11% of cases [11]. It is thought to occur due to chronic irritation of the exposed meatus leading to scar tissue formation, ammoniacal meatitis, and/or ischemia due to division of the frenular artery [11]. It is usually noted several years after the procedure and results in a thin urinary stream that is deviated upwards, making it difficult to direct. In many instances this is self-limiting and improves with age, however in some circumstances it requires intervention in the form of meatotomy. Topical steroids may be helpful in relieving symptoms.

6.17 Bladder and Bowel Dysfunction

Bladder and bowel dysfunction (BBD) is an umbrella term used to describe a series of symptoms related to the lower urinary tract (LUTS) with or without constipation [18]. BBD is one of the most common referrals to paediatric urology clinics and can be a source of distress to parents and clinicians. In the majority of children, there is no anatomical explanation of the symptoms and they occur secondary to voiding habits and the presence of constipation. Children may present with urinary incontinence, frequency, urgency, infrequent voiding, dysuria, recurrent urinary tract infection and constipation, however the fundamental management of these complaints is the same and requires education and behaviour modification with pharmacologic intervention when appropriate.

6.18 History and Physical Examination

A detailed history about duration of symptoms as well as requesting completed voiding diaries from the child is important and it is common to note the onset of LUTS to coincide with the child starting school. Voiding diaries provide an accurate measure of how often the child is voiding, volumes of urine output, fluid intake, degree of incontinence and assessment of constipation. Timing of incontinence (prevoid vs. post-void) should also be determined and differentiated as each may provide evidence as to which interventions and further testing may be required for each child. Age of toilet training and any periods of dryness are important to note as girls with complaints of constant dampness despite acceptable voiding habits should be assessed with an ultrasound for the purpose of ruling out a duplex kidney with ectopic ureter. An inability of achieve toilet training with complaints of lifelong LUTS ad constipation could also be indicative of neurogenic bladder as well as if the symptoms appeared suddenly after a growth spurt which may occur in those children with tethered cord. Characteristics about the stream should be ascertained as interrupted stream with start-stop patterns may be suggestive of dysfunctional voiding and a thin or weak stream in boys could be evidence of meatal stenosis and resulting high post void residual.

Investigations such as ultrasound and laboratory tests are not normally indicated for BBD patients. US may be done in those with UTIs or for a need to assess for high post void residuals. Further testing such as renal scans and VCUG should be left for specialists to order and interpret. Urine specimens should only be obtained for symptoms consistent with suspicion of UTI such as fever and dysuria. Routine screening for UTI or testing urine on the basis of foul smelling urine is not recommended. Culture and sensitivity is not indicated in the event of a negative urinalysis, especially in the absence of distinct symptoms.

During the physical examination, an abdominal assessment for constipation should be completed. It is important to perform a complete assessment of the genitalia for both genders. In boys circumcision status should be assessed and for those not circumcised phimosis could cause pooling of urine with local irritation which may mimic LUTS. In females, the urethral meatus and vaginal orifice should be clearly visible with no evidence of labial fusion or vulvovaginitis. Labial adhesions often contribute to post-void dribbling and recurrent UTIs and tend to be recurrent until puberty. Vulvovaginitis may be present and contribute to LUTS in girls that may be mistaken for signs of UTI. A neurological examination should be completed, paying attention to the presence of any dimples or abnormalities in the lower back, sacral area as well as any features of the lower extremities suggestive of neurological deficits.

6.19 Management

The pediatrician or family physician's office is an ideal setting for the implementation of management strategies for this condition that can be initiated prior to or while waiting for the child to be assessed by paediatric urology specialists. The management of BBD consists primarily of behaviour modification strategies with pharmacologic additions when appropriate. There are several examples of how these strategies are best delivered including individual clinic visits, group sessions, videos and inpatient delivery [19–21]. Regardless of the delivery modality, initially families should be encouraged to purchase a vibrating watch for their child to assist them with timed voiding. Children are required to void every 2 h during waking hours whether they feel the need to void or not. In addition, they should be encouraged to double or triple void when necessary. Adequate fluid intake is important and a minimum of 4–6 cups of water per day is recommended. Finally, aggressive monitoring and management of constipation is imperative and in fact, bladder strategies may be less effective if constipation is present and persistent. Medications such as anticholinergic therapy and prophylactic antibiotics may be indicated in some instances, but their use should be assessed and initiated by a specialist for challenging or refractory cases.

6.20 Summary

In summary, bladder and bowel dysfunction is a common reason for referral to paediatric urology clinics and typically presents in the absence of any anatomical abnormality. A thorough history and physical examination is important to support the diagnosis as most families are hesitant to accept that the concerns will most

Table 6.1 Causes of ANH (adapted from Nguyen et al. J Ped Urol 2010 6 [3] 212–231. Copyright Elsevier)

Etiology of antenatal hydronephrosis	Incidence
Transient hydronephrosis	41–88%
UPJ obstruction	10–30%
VUR	10–20%
UVJ obstruction/megaureters	5–10%
Multicystic dysplastic kidney	4–6%
PUV/ urethral atresia	1–2%
Ureterocele/ectopic ureter/duplex system	5–7%
Others: prune belly syndrome, cystic kidney disease, congenital ureteric stricture, megalourethra	Uncommon

likely be addressed by behaviour modifications. The majority of children with BBD will improve by implementation of bladder retraining strategies and aggressive management of constipation. Those have persistent symptoms despite these strategies should be referred to a paediatric urology clinic or community paediatrician who has studied the management of this condition.

6.21 Antenatal Hydronephrosis

Antenatal hydronephrosis (ANH), defined as the dilation of the renal pelvicalyceal system, is the most common fetal anatomical abnormality affecting 1–5% pregnancies [22–25]. A variety of congenital abnormalities of the kidneys and urinary tract (CAKUT) can present with ANH (Table 6.1). Transient idiopathic hydronephrosis, ureteropelvic obstruction (UPJ), and vesicoureteral reflux (VUR) are the most common etiologies, occurring in up to 88, 30, and 20% of ANH cases, respectively (Table 6.1). The vast majority of cases are known to be transient and will resolve or remain stable overtime [26]. However, the primary goal for the postnatal management of children with ANH is the early identification of obstructive cases who would benefit of surgical intervention, aiming to prevent deterioration of renal function. During pre and postnatal evaluation of ANH, several factors such as cause, severity and whether ANH is unilateral or bilateral are considered for the decisions about additional assessment and potential intervention.

6.22 Epidemiology

Seventy five percent of ANH cases are unilateral; mostly on the left side, and it occurs more frequently in males in a 2:1 ratio [22–25]. Over the past 20 years, with significant advancements in prenatal hydronephrosis screening, the most common presentation of ANH is of asymptomatic neonates. Palpable flank mass in newborns or worsening hydronephrosis in serial ultrasounds are also often seen. Even in congenital cases, symptoms can manifest at any time in life. In older children, UPJ obstruction must be ruled out in the presence of intermittent acute flank or abdominal pain, nausea or vomiting, and more rarely hematuria, after fluid intake, known as Dietl's crisis [27]. Increased risk of febrile UTI is also described in patients with ANH [28–32].

6.23 History and Physical Examination

Prenatal history must include the presence or absence of oligohydramnios, associated anatomical abnormalities, spinal defects, ultrasound findings, APD measurements when available, gestational age and delivery history. Specifically ask about family history of hydronephrosis and other congenital abnormalities of the kidneys and the urinary tract. For the postnatal history it is important to inquire about birth weight, postnatal resuscitation and care, weight gain, number of wet diapers, history of confirmed or suspected UTIs and circumcision status. A thorough physical examination must include weight, height and blood pressure measurement, abdominal exam looking for palpable kidneys or bladder, genitalia inspection, and circumcision status. Back exam may reveal midline or nearby dimples, hair tuft, clefts, skin-discoloration or tags that are often associated with an underlying spinal cord abnormality.

6.24 Diagnosis

6.24.1 Antenatal Diagnosis

There is lack of consensus for the definition of ANH in the literature. The Society for Fetal Urology (SFU) defines ANH as the measurement of anteroposterior diameter of the renal pelvis diameter (APD) greater than 4 mm on prenatal ultrasound at second trimester and/or >7 mm at third trimester [28], while the Canadian Urological Association (CUA) defines hydronephrosis as APD $\geq$ 7 mm at second trimester and/or $\geq$9 mm at third trimester [29].

6.24.2 Postnatal Diagnosis

Renal ultrasound is the noninvasive instrument of choice for monitoring hydronephrosis postnatally. The Society for Fetal Urology (SFU) grading system [28, 30]

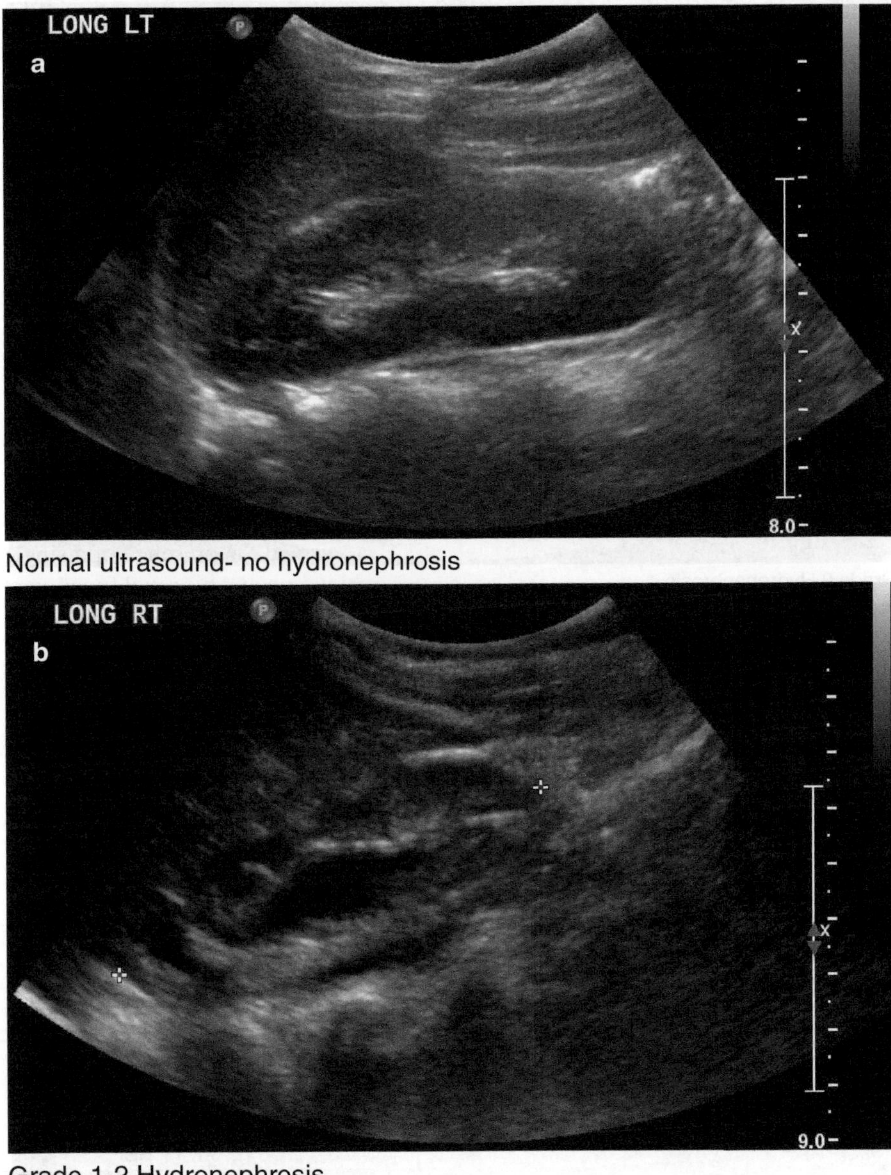

Fig. 6.5 SFU grades of hydronephrosis (**a**) Normal ultrasound- no hydronephrosis. (**b**) Grade 1–2 hydronephrosis. (**c**) Grade 3 hydronephrosis. (**d**) Grade 4 hydronephrosis

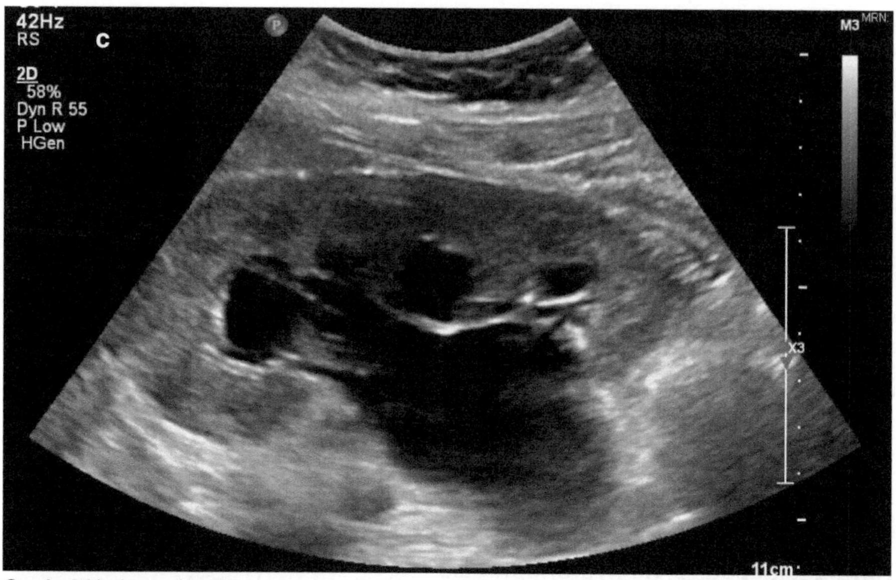

Grade 3 Hydronephrosis

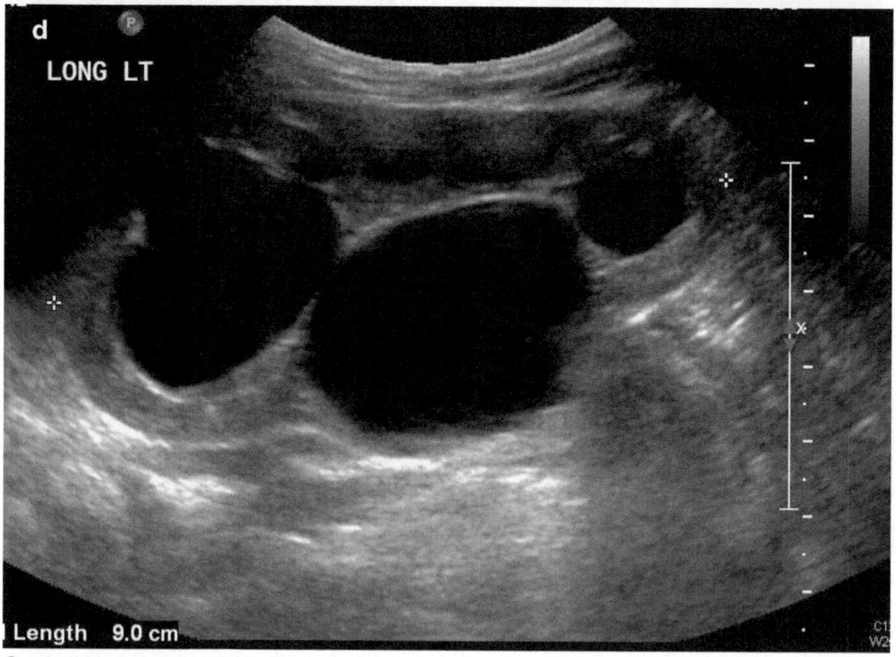

Grade 4 Hydronephrosis

Fig. 6.5 (continued)

and the measurement of the APD are the two most common standardized systems for evaluating hydronephrosis [22, 31]. Briefly, the SFU grading system provides a qualitative assessment of hydronephrosis based on the degree of pelvicaliectasis and the presence of cortical thinning (Fig. 6.5), while APD is a quantitative assessment of the degree of pelviectasis with the measurement of the greatest diameter of the renal pelvis on ultrasound images acquired in transverse plane. Previous studies have shown high interobserver variability for the SFU grading likely due to the subjective evaluation of nonquantitative features mentioned above [25, 28]. Similarly to prenatal diagnosis, several cut-off measurements have been proposed for the APD classification postnatally [32]. Regardless of the grading system of choice, trends in serial ultrasounds are still the cornerstone of the postnatal management of ANH.

6.25 Investigations and Management

6.25.1 Based on Current Literature and Expert Opinion [22–25, 28–32] We Recommend the Above

Ultrasound:

- All children with isolated ANH (third trimester prenatal RPD ≥7 mm in most centres) and/or any urinary tract abnormalities (ureteral dilatation, abnormal bladder) should have a postnatal renal ultrasound (Level 3 evidence; Grade C recommendation);
- Ideally, the first postnatal ultrasound should not be done in the first 48–72 h given the expected lower urine output during this period. Exception for this recommendation apply to cases of bilateral severe hydronephrosis or hydronephrosis in a solitary kidney, for which the postnatal ultrasound must be obtained before hospital discharge. The remaining should have an ultrasound between 4 and 30 days;
- The interval between postnatal serial ultrasounds will vary depending on the severity of hydronephrosis and clinical judgement.

Voiding cystourethrogram (VCUG):

- Any child with suspected bladder outlet obstruction (i.e. posterior urethral valves) should have a VCUG before discharge from the hospital;
- Other absolute indications of VCUG: severe bilateral hydronephrosis, suspected infravesical obstruction, hydroureter, duplex kidney, abnormal echogenicity or abnormal bladder.

Diuretic nuclear scan

- Diuretic nuclear scan (MAG3 or DTPA) should be done at 4–6 weeks of age for unexplained grade 3–4 hydronephrosis or worsening hydronephrosis in serial ultrasounds ((Level 4 evidence; Grade D recommendation). Nuclear scan results may be equivocal in infants [33].

Continuous antibiotic prophylaxis (CAP)

- The use of CAP in the neonatal period is controversial. Both the AUA and CPS suggest potential benefit in the presence of SFU grades 3 and 4 hydronephrosis, hydroureter or bladder abnormalities.
- Females and uncircumcised boys may benefit more CAP than circumcised males. (Level 3 evidence; Grade C recommendation).

6.26 Surgical Indications

Approximately 1/3 of children with UPJ will need surgery [32]. Indications for intervention: worsening hydronephrosis on serial ultrasounds, symptoms, impairment of renal function (<40% function on nuclear scan), stones, infection, hypertension. The goals of treatment are preservation or improvement of renal function and relief of symptoms. Pyeloplasty, which can be open, laparoscopic or robotic, is the surgical modality of choice which involves the removal of obstructed segment and reanastomosis of ureter to renal pelvis. The ureter is reanastomosed above the vessel if there is an aberrant vessel (Fig. 6.6). Other options of treatment are endopyelotomy (endoscopic incision of the obstructed proximal ureter), stents insertion (double J, nephrostomy), angiopexy, endoscopic removal of a fibroepithelial polyp, among others.

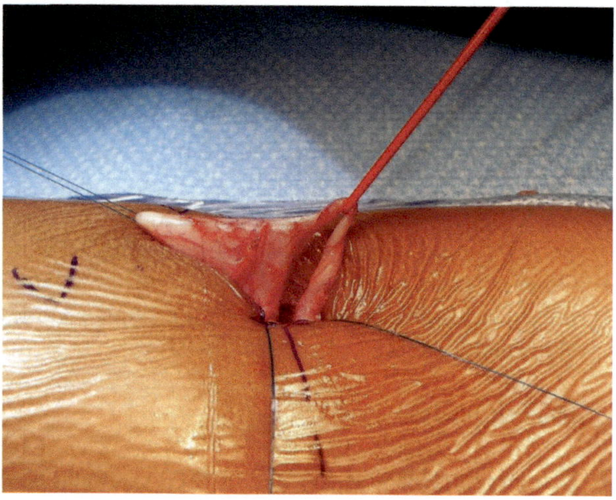

Fig. 6.6 UPJO. Dilated pelvis and narrowed UPJ is noted during open pyeloplasty

6.27 Summary

ANH is the most common fetal anatomical abnormality affecting 1–5% pregnancies. Most cases are transient and will resolve or remain stable overtime. However, the primary goal for the postnatal management is the early identification of obstructive cases who would benefit of surgical intervention, ultimately aiming to prevent deterioration of renal function. Serial ultrasounds associated with diuretic renography are still the main tools used to guide surgical indication for obstructive cases. The use of CAP in the neonatal period is controversial, however, its use must be considered for females and uncircumcised boys with grade 3–4 hydronephrosis. We recommend caution and case by case consideration for CAP in the presence of recurrent UTIs.

6.28 Vesicoureteral Reflux and Urinary Tract Infection

Vesicoureteral reflux (VUR), defined as the retrograde flow of urine from the bladder into the upper urinary tracts, can be primary or secondary. Primary VUR is usually due to malfunction of the ureterovesical junction (UVJ) anti-reflux mechanisms, while secondary VUR is associated with high bladder pressures secondary to functional or anatomical bladder outlet obstruction. This chapter will focus on the office management of primary VUR and its relationship with urinary tract infection (UTI).

The management of primary vesicoureteral reflux (VUR) in children has evolved significantly over the past 30 years, however in 2018, VUR is still one of the most controversial topics in Pediatric Urology. Dramatic progress occurred in the understanding of the relationship between VUR and urinary tract infections resulting in a shift from surgery for all to conservative management with or without antibiotic prophylaxis in most cases.

Approximately 30–45% of children who present with a febrile UTI or pyelonephritis have underlying VUR [34] however, the natural history of this condition is to

Table 6.2 International classification of vesicoureteral reflux and 5 year resolution rates after presentation

Grade	Appearance on VCUG	Resolution by 5 year After Presentation
I	Contrast in ureter, not reaching renal pelvis, no ureteral dilatation	90%
II	Contrast up to pelvis, no ureteral dilatation	80%
III	Contrast up to pelvis, mild dilatation of ureter and pelvis, slight/no blunting of calyces	60%
IV	Moderate dilatation of ureter and pelvicalyceal system, mild tortuosity and blunting of calyces	30%
V	Significant dilatation and tortuosity of ureter, severe dilatation of pelvis, significant blunting of calyces	Rarely

resolve overtime with resolution rates varying according to the grade of reflux (Table 6.2). VUR-related short term concerns are the morbidity of pyelonephritis and urosepsis, while potential lifelong implications of recurrent febrile UTIs are renal scarring, proteinuria, hypertension and progressive renal impairment [34–36]. Surgical repair is left for children with recurrent febrile UTIs despite CAP, progressive renal scarring, or early signs of renal deterioration (proteinuria, abnormal creatinine or hypertension).

Recently, the clinical significance of VUR and the use of continuous antibiotic prophylaxis (CAP) to prevent UTIs and renal scarring have been questioned based on results of large randomized controlled trials, like the RIVUR and PREVENT studies [37]. Consequently, the importance of diagnosing VUR in first place, the role of diagnostic imaging and treatment recommendations have been reassessed. As a result, the Canadian Pediatric Society no longer recommends CAP for otherwise healthy children with grades 1–3 VUR [35]. Moreover, concerns with an increasing risk for antibiotic resistance may soon deny the benefits of prophylaxis even in cases of grade 4 or 5 VUR. Ultimately, the role of severe VUR in the development of renal scarring and kidney failure is unclear [34].

6.29 Initial Diagnosis and Evaluation of a Child with VUR

6.29.1 History and Physical Examination

On history it is important to inquire about antenatal history, prenatal ultrasound findings, postnatal hospitalizations, previous UTIs, unexplained fevers, and failure to thrive. In toilet trained children, daily fluid intake, voiding, and stooling patterns must be obtained in addition to dietary history to rule out BBD. On physical examination, palpable fecal mass in the abdomen suggest constipation. The child with VUR should undergo careful general medical evaluation including measurement of height, weight, blood pressure, serum creatinine, and urinalysis for proteinuria if bilateral renal abnormalities are found. If proteinuria is seen in the urinalysis, two first morning samples obtained in two different occasions are recommended to rule out orthostatic proteinuria. Finally, if first morning samples are positive, protein quantification in the urine is warranted (protein/creatinine ratio for non-toilet trained and 24 h urine protein measurement for toilet trained children).

In the event VUR is diagnosed in an asymptomatic child, we recommend CAP for grades 4 or 5 VUR during the first year of life and a referral should be made to the pediatric urologist or pediatric nephrologist. There is currently no evidence CAP would be beneficial beyond the age of 12 months. Such recommendations are also supported by both the American Urological Association (AUA) and CPS [35, 36], but are mostly based on expert opinion.

6.30 Investigations

With the advancement of prenatal ultrasounds, VUR is commonly diagnosed in asymptomatic, otherwise healthy children with antenatal hydronephrosis (ANH). Indications to perform voiding cystourethrogram (VCUG) postnatally in children with ANH have been previously discussed in the Antenatal Hydronephrosis section of this chapter.

For children presenting with a UTI, both the American Academy of Pediatrics (AAP) and the CPS recommend that a renal and bladder ultrasound should be done following the first appropriately confirmed febrile urinary tract infection in children between 2- and 24-months [38, 39] and VCUG is recommended following the second confirmed febrile UTI or if urinary tract abnormalities are seen on the ultrasound. Newborns with a febrile UTI should be investigated with a baseline ultrasound and VCUG must be considered in the presence of hydronephrosis, hydroureters and/or abnormal bladder on ultrasound, especially in boys with bilateral hydronephrosis or a trabeculated bladder to rule out posterior urethral valves. Index of suspicion for BBD is high for children who onset of UTIs occurs around the toilet training phase. In this scenario, a baseline ultrasound should be considered to check upper tracts status, but BBD treatment is critical and must precede ordering a VCUG if the ultrasound is normal.

6.31 Circumcision

Boys with high grade VUR or lower grades with recurrent UTIs may benefit from circumcision in the first year of life, with a number needed to treat (NNT) of 4–6 to prevent 1 UTI [40].

6.32 Continuous Antibiotic Prophylaxis

CAP use should be carefully individualized and considered for high grade VUR in the first year of life, recurrent febrile UTIs regardless of VUR grade, or in the presence of complex urological anomalies. Short term CAP (approximately 3 months) may be considered for toilet-trained children with recurrent febrile UTIs in the context of BBD while working on bladder and bowel habits. Combined data from two longitudinal studies (RIVUR and CUTIE trials) showed that toilet-trained children with both BBD and VUR are at higher risk of developing recurrent UTIs than children with isolated VUR or children with isolated BBD and, therefore may benefit from CAP [41].

Table 6.3 Differential diagnosis of hematuria

Upper Tract
• Glomerular: PSGN, IgA nephropathy, Thin membrane disease, Lupus nephritis, systemic vasculitis, Alport syndrome, HUS, shunt nephritis, Granulomatosis with polyangiitis, MPGN/C3G
• Tubulointerstitial:
– Infection
– Tumors
– Nephrotoxins
– Stones, nephrocalcinosis, hypercalciuria
– Renal cystic diseases
Lower Tract
• Infection
• Calculi
• Trauma
• Obstruction
• Urethrorrhagia
• Vulvovaginitis
Vascular
• Renal vein or artery thrombosis
• Vascular malformation (hemangioma, arteriovenous malformation)
• Coagulopathy, thrombocytopenia
• Sickle cell disease/trait

6.32.1 Hematuria

Hematuria, which can be either macro ormicroscopic, is usually a cause of significant distress for patients, caregivers and health care providers. Macroscopic hematuria, or the presence of blood in the urine visible to the naked eye, is uncommon in children with an estimated incidence of 1.3 per 1000 [42]. Most frequent causes are: benign urethrorrhagia (19%), trauma (14%) and UTIs (4%) [43]. Microscopic hematuria, defined as the presence of >3–5 RBCs/high-power field in spun urine, is usually identified during routine urinalysis or urine dipstick. Microhematuriais more frequently seen than macrohematuriawith an estimated prevalence of 1.5% in children and adolescents [42, 43]. Children with microscopic hematuria are more often referred to the pediatric nephrologist rather than the urologist. The most common causes of isolated microscopic hematuria in children are idiopathic hypercalciuria, glomerulopathies and nutcracker syndrome [44]. Although most cases of macro or microscopic hematuria are benign (Table 6.3), the challenge for clinicians in face of macro or microscopic hematuria is to differentiate benign conditions from serious underlying diseases, avoiding unnecessary stress to families and extra health care costs, while not missing potentially morbid yet treatable pathologies. It is important to keep in mind not all that resembles hematuria is blood. Common causes of "dark urine", but not true hematuria include pigments such as haemoglobin, myoglobin, bilirubin, beets, blackberries, and urates, and medications such as rifampin, nitrofurantoin, methyldopa, levodopa, and metronidazole.

6.33 History and Physical Examination

Initially it is important to characterize the patterns of hematuria, especially if blood is seen in the beginning or only at the end of micturition (terminal hematuria) or mixed with urine. Terminal painless hematuria suggests urethrorrhagia. The presence of clots suggests post-renaletiology and associated symptoms, such as abdominal pain, flank pain, dysuria, frequency or urgency must raise the level of suspicion of UTI or urolithiasis. Additionally, it is crucial to inquire about constitutional symptoms, commonly seen in malignancies. Other sites of bleeding, such as gingival, GI or skin, may reveal possible underlying coagulopathy. Recent trauma, menses, fever, strenuous exercise, or bladder catheterization may be associated with transient hematuria. A sore throat or skin infection within the past 7–30 days makes the diagnosis of post infectious glomerulonephritis (PSGN) very likely. Drugs and toxins can potentially cause either hematuria or hemoglobinuria. A thorough family history must include questions about hematuria, renal stones, glomerular or renal cystic diseases, renal transplant or dialysis, hearing loss, hypertension, hemophilia and other bleeding disorders and, sickle cell trait. Although hematuria rarely causes significant anemia, physical examination must include heart rate and blood pressure measurement, assessment of pallor, skin inspection for ecchymosis or petechiae, and palpable lymph nodes. Abdominal examination may reveal palpable masses, hepatosplenomegaly, or flank pain. Ultimately, meatal stenosis in boys and signs of vulvovaginitis, trauma or foreign body in girls may be seen during genital inspection of children with hematuria.

6.34 Investigations

Macroscopic hematuria: The presence of macroscopic hematuria prompts a baseline ultrasound to rule out renal or bladder masses, stones and anatomical abnormalities. Further imaging, such as KUB X-ray, CT or MRI must be individualized according to the case. Ultimately, cystoscopy is recommended for cases of persistent macroscopic hematuria to rule out urinary tract vascular malformations, bladder or more rarely, ureteral masses. Routine imaging, laboratory, and cystoscopy are unnecessary for evaluating urethrorrhagia. However, when cystoscopy is done, it reveals inflammation of the bulbar urethra.

Persistent microscopic hematuria: Persistent microscopic hematuria (on three urinalysis or urine dipsticks) should prompt further investigations.

Laboratory studies:

Recommended serum tests include CBC, urea, creatinine, electrolytes, calcium, C3, C4; and urine studies: culture, creatinine, albumin, calcium (for protein/creatinine and calcium creatinine ratios).

Imaging studies: Renal and bladder ultrasound.

The following scenarios warrant additional studies and referral to the nephrologist. If recent sore throat or skin infection, please order ASO titres. If features of lupus, ANA and anti-dsDNA are recommended; and renal biopsy may be required. If persistent, asymptomatic, isolated hematuria, consider screening other family members as workup of thin basement membrane disease and a referral to the nephrologist is warranted.

Management:

Management must be individualized depending on the cause of hematuria. For more details, please refer to specific chapters. We would like, however, to highlight the management of urethrorrhagia which is a common cause of painless terminal hematuria in prepubertal boys, with only 33% of boys presenting dysuria [44]. Benign urethrorrhagia is often associated with Bladder and Bowel Dysfunction (BBD) [44]. It is a benign condition that resolves spontaneously in 90% of boys. We recommend watchful waiting and treatment of underlying BBD. Refractory cases may benefit from short course of alpha blockers (i.e tamsulosin) and biofeedback.

6.35 Summary

Hematuria is a cause of significant distress for patients, caregivers and health care providers. Differently than adults, malignancy is a rare cause of micro or macroscopic hematuria in children. Although most cases are benign, the challenge for clinicians in face of hematuria is to differentiate benign conditions from serious underlying diseases, avoiding unnecessary stress to families and extra health care costs, while not missing potentially morbid yet treatable pathologies.

References

1. Braga LH, Lorenzo AJ, Romao RLP. Canadian Urological Association-pediatric urologists of Canada (CUA-PUC) guideline for the diagnosis, management, and follow up of cryptorchidism. Can Urol Assoc J. 2017;11(7):E251–60.
2. Gurney JK, McGlynn KA, Stanley J, Merriman T, Signal V, Shaw C, et al. Risk factors for cryptorchidism. Nat Rev Urol. 2017;14(9):534–48.
3. Brouwers MM, de Bruijne LM, de Gier RPE, Zielhuis GA, Feitz WFJ, Roeleveld N. Risk factors for undescended testis. J Pediatr Urol England. 2012;8(1):59–66.
4. Kolon TF, Herndon CDA, Baker LA, Baskin LS, Baxter CG, Cheng EY, et al. American Urological Association (AUA) guidelines: Evaluation and treatment of cryptorchidism: American urological association cryptorchidism. 2014;(April):1–38. https://www.auanet.org/guidelines/cryptorchidism-guideline.
5. Kanaroglou N, To T, Zhu J, Braga LHP, Wehbi E, Hajiha M, et al. Inappropriate use of ultrasound in Management of Pediatric Cryptorchidism. Pediatrics. 2015;136(3):479 LP–486.

6. Chang S-J, Chen JY-C, Hsu C-K, Chuang F-C, Yang SS-D. The incidence of inguinal hernia and associated risk factors of incarceration in pediatric inguinal hernia: a nation-wide longitudinal population-based study. Hernia. 2016;20(4):559–63.
7. Bandarkar AN, Adeyiga AO, Reynolds D, Cielma T, Safdar N, Shalaby-Rana E. Inguinolabial hernia containing ovary, fallopian tube and uterus in female children. Adv Pediatr Res. 2017;4:3.
8. Christensen T, Cartwright PC, Devries C, Snow BW. New onset of hydroceles in boys over 1 year of age. Int J Urol. 2006;13(11):1425–7.
9. Luo C-C, Chao H-C. Prevention of unnecessary contralateral exploration using the silk glove sign (SGS) in pediatric patients with unilateral inguinal hernia. Eur J Pediatr. 2007;166(7):667–9.
10. Kogen Barry EE. Hydrocele. Br Med J. 2017;BMJ Best Practices. https://bestpractice.bmj.com/topics/en-gb/1104.
11. Dave S, Afshar K, Braga LH, Anderson P. CUAJ—Guideline Dave et al Guideline: Foreskin care and neonatal circumcision CUA guideline on the care of the normal foreskin and neonatal circumcision in Canadian infants. 2017;12(2).
12. McGregor TB, Pike JG, Leonard MP. Pathologic and physiologic phimosis: approach to the phimotic foreskin. Can Fam physician. College of Family Physicians of Canada; 2007;53(3):445–8.
13. Metcalfe PD, Rink RC. The concealed penis: management and outcomes. Curr Opin Urol. 2005;15(4):268–72.
14. Wang T, Chen HW. Contemporary review of buried penis repair. J Genit Syst Disord. 2017;6(1):2016–8.
15. Hadidi AT. Buried penis: classification surgical approach. J Pediatr Surg. 2014;49(2):374–9.
16. Marrocco G, Grammatico P, Vallasciani S, Gulia C, Zangari A, Marrocco F, et al. Environmental, parental and gestational factors that influence the occurrence of hypospadias in male patients. J Pediatr Urol. 2015;11(1):12–9.
17. Eroglu E, Gundogdu G. Isolated penile torsion in newborns. Can Urol Assoc J Can Med Assoc. 2015;9(11–12):E805–7.
18. Yang S, Chua ME, Bauer S, Wright A, Brandström P, Hoebeke P, et al. Diagnosis and management of bladder bowel dysfunction in children with urinary tract infections: a position statement from the international Children's continence society. Pediatr Nephrol. 2017;33(12):2207–19.
19. Braga LH, Rickard M, Farrokhyar F, Jegatheeswaran K, Brownrigg N, Li C, et al. Bladder training video versus standard Urotherapy for bladder and bowel dysfunction: a non-inferiority randomized controlled trial. J Urol. 2017;197(3):877–84.
20. Dos Santos J, Lopes RI, Koyle MA. Bladder and bowel dysfunction in children: an update on the diagnosis and treatment of a common, but underdiagnosed pediatric problem. Can Urol Assoc J Can Med Assoc. 2017;11(1–2Suppl1):S64–72.
21. Brownrigg N, Pemberton J, Jegatheeswaran K, DeMaria J, Braga LH. A pilot randomized controlled trial evaluating the effectiveness of group vs individual urotherapy in decreasing symptoms associated with bladder-bowel dysfunction. J Urol United States. 2015;193(4):1347–52.
22. Sidhu G, Beyene J, Rosenblum ND. Outcome of isolated antenatal hydronephrosis: a systematic review and meta-analysis. Pediatr Nephrol. 2006;21(2):218–24.
23. Mallik M, Watson AR. Antenatally detected urinary tract abnormalities: more detection but less action. Pediatr Nephrol. 2008;23(6):897–904.
24. Timberlake MD, Herndon CDA. Mild to moderate postnatal hydronephrosis—grading systems and management. Nat Rev Urol. Nature Publishing Group, a division of Macmillan Publishers Limited. All Rights Reserved. 2013;10:649.
25. Davenport MT, Merguerian PA, Koyle M. Antenatally diagnosed hydronephrosis: current postnatal management. Pediatr Surg Int. 2013;29(3):207–14.
26. Rickard M, Lorenzo AJ, Braga LH, Munoz C. Parenchyma-to-hydronephrosis area ratio is a promising outcome measure to quantify upper tract changes in infants with high-grade prenatal Hydronephrosis. Urology. Elsevier Inc. 2016;104:166–71.
27. Alagiri MPS. Dietl's crisis: an under-recognized clinical entity in the pediatric population. Int Braz J Urol. 2006;32(4):451–3.

28. Nguyen HT, Benson CB, Bromley B, Campbell JB, Chow J, Coleman B, et al. Multidisciplinary consensus on the classification of prenatal and postnatal urinary tract dilation (UTD classification system). J Pediatr Urol Elsevier Ltd. 2014;10(6):982–98.
29. Capolicchio JP, Braga LH, Szymanski KM. Canadian Urological Association/pediatric urologists of Canada guideline on the investigation and management of antenatally detected hydronephrosis. Can Urol Assoc J. 2018:85–92.
30. Fernbach SK, Maizels M, Conway JJ. Ultrasound grading of hydronephrosis: introduction to the system used by the society for fetal urology. Pediatr Radiol. 1993;23(6):478–80.
31. Cheng A, Phan V, Geary MR. Outcome of isolated antenatal Hydronephrosis. Arch Pediatr Adolesc Med. 2004;158(1):38–40.
32. Dos Santos J, Parekh RS, Piscione TD, Hassouna T, Figueroa V, Gonima P, et al. A new grading system for the management of antenatal Hydronephrosis. Clin J Am Soc Nephrol. 2015;10(10):1783 LP–1790.
33. Radulovic M, Pucar D, Jaukovic L, Sisic M, Krstic ZAB. Diuretic 99mTc DTPA renography in assessment of renal function and drainage in infants with antenatally detected hydronephrosis. Vojn Pregl. 2015;72(12):1080–4.
34. Garcia-Roig M KA. Urinary tract infection in the setting of vesicoureteral reflux. F1000Research. 2016;5(F1000 Fa(1552).
35. Robinson J, Finlay J, Lang M, Bortolussi R. Canadian pediatric society, community pediatrics committee ID and IC. Prophylactic antibiotics for children with recurrent urinary tract infections. Pediatr Child Heal. 2015;20(1):45–7.
36. Peters CA, Skoog SJ, Arant BS, Copp HL, Elder JS, Hudson RG, et al. Summary of the AUA guideline on Management of Primary Vesicoureteral Reflux in children. J Urol Elsevier Inc. 2010;184(3):1134–44.
37. Mathews R, Mattoo TK. The role of antimicrobial prophylaxis in the Management of Children with Vesicoureteral Reflux — the RIVUR study outcomes. Adv Chronic Kidney Dis Elsevier Ltd. 2015;22(4):325–30.
38. AAP. Urinary tract infection: clinical practice guideline for the diagnosis and Management of the Initial UTI in febrile infants and children 2 to 24 months. Pediatrics. 2011;128(3):595–610.
39. Robinson JL, Finlay JC, Lang ME, Bortolussi R. Urinary tract infection in infants and children : diagnosis and management. Paediatr Child Health. 2014;19(6):1–7.
40. Ellison JS, Dy GW, Fu BC, Holt SK, Gore JL, Merguerian PA. Neonatal circumcision and urinary tract infections in infants with Hydronephrosis. Pediatrics. 2018;142(1):e20173703.
41. Shaikh N, Hoberman A, Keren R, Gotman N, Docimo SG, Mathews R, et al. Recurrent urinary tract infections in children with bladder and bowel dysfunction. Pediatrics. 2016;137(1):e20152982.
42. Ingelfinger JR, Davis AE, Grupe WE. Frequency and etiology of gross hematuria in a general pediatric setting. Pediatrics. 1977;59(4):557 LP–561.
43. Greenfield SP, Williot P, Kaplan D. Gross hematuria in children: a ten-year review. Urology Elsevier. 2007;69(1):166–9.
44. Feld LG, Waz WR, Luis MP, Joseph DB. HEMATURIA: an integrated medical and surgical approach. Pediatr Clin N Am. 1997;44(5):1191–210.

Neonatal Urological Emergencies

7

Martin Kaefer

Learning Objectives
Upon reading the chapter the reader should be able to:

1. Describe the presentation, evaluation and treatment of renal vein thrombosis in the newborn.
2. Provide a cogent algorithm for the evaluation and treatment of the male infant presenting with bladder distension and elevated serum creatinine—with specific attention to the short and long term renal and bladder characteristics of children with posterior urethral valves.
3. Discuss the differential diagnosis of a newborn presenting with a swollen hemi-scrotum with particular attention to the management of neonatal testicular torsion.
4. List the five most common etiologies of an intra-labial mass in a newborn girl.
5. Describe the various treatment options for newborn UVJ obstruction.

7.1 Scenario 1

A 7-day-old infant girl with a palpable abdominal mass is noted to have gross hematuria. A urinalysis and CBC with platelets demonstrate the following:

- Proteins ++
- Ketones –
- Blood: +++
- Leucocytes: –
- Nitrites: –

M. Kaefer (✉)
Division of Pediatric Urology, Indiana University School of Medicine, Indianapolis, IN, USA
e-mail: mkaefer@iupui.edu

P. Godbole et al. (eds.), *Practical Pediatric Urology*,
https://doi.org/10.1007/978-3-030-54020-3_7

- Hgb: 7.8 g/dl
- WBC: 4.5 k/ml
- Platelets: 50 k/ml

The baby was born at an estimated gestational age of 37 weeks to a diabetic mother by prolonged vaginal delivery.

7.2 Question 1

What does the combination of physical findings, urinalysis and hematologic results suggest?

7.3 Answer 1

The presence of gross hematuria with anemia and thrombocytopenia in the neonate strongly suggest a diagnosis of renal vein thrombosis. Predisposing factors include dehydration, sepsis, polycythemia, maternal diabetes, traumatic delivery and indwelling umbilical catheters [1]. Approximately 20% of infants with gross hematuria are found to have renal vein thrombosis. The thrombosis is typically peripheral and does not often propagate centrally. Physical signs include a palpable mass and hypertension. Oliguria may occur in bilateral cases. Although Wilms Tumor may be considered in the older child with a palpable mass and gross hematuria, malignant renal lesions associated with gross hematuria are exceedingly uncommon in the neonatal period.

7.4 Question 2

What additional testing would be recommended to confirm diagnosis?

7.5 Answer 2

1. Color doppler renal ultrasound: Renal sonography is the modality of choice for making the diagnosis of renal vein thrombosis. Renal enlargement with loss of corticomedullary differentiation associated with reduced or absent flow through the renal vein are the most common findings. Branching hyperechoic vessels and clot in the vena cava may also be noted in select cases.
2. Serum Electrolytes. Acute renal dysfunction can be seen in renal vein thrombosis. Bilateral cases can result in oliguria. The resultant alterations in renal function can be seen in an elevation of serum creatinine and significant alterations in electrolyte homeostasis.
3. Evaluation of coagulation factors. Nearly 50% of neonates with RVT are found to have prothrombotic abnormalities and hence should be screened [2]. Studies

have shown that factor V mutations and elevated lipoprotein A are more commonly identified in patients with neonatal renal vein thrombosis when compared to controls.

7.6 Question 3

What would be your subsequent management plan?

7.7 Answer 3

1. Management is directed at reversing the factors that predispose to renal vein thrombosis. Fluid resuscitation and correction of electrolyte imbalances form the cornerstone of treatment. Management of hypertension is also important.
2. If an umbilical venous catheter is present, it should be removed so that it can no longer serve as a nidus for further clot propagation.
3. Management with anticoagulants remains controversial but may include the use of heparin or fibrinolytic therapy with streptokinase in specific situations. While treatment with heparin has been shown to be of benefit in reducing renal functional abnormalities, treatment with anticoagulants can be associated with significant complications. Twenty percent of cases of neonatal renal vein thrombosis are bilateral and may benefit from more aggressive therapy to prevent end stage renal dysfunction.

7.8 Scenario 2

A 2-month old boy presents with failure to thrive and abdominal distension. Urine analysis demonstrates no sign of infection. Serum creatinine is 2.4 mg/dl. Renal Bladder Ultrasound is shown below (Images 7.1, 7.2, and 7.3).

7.9 Thickened Bladder on Ultrasound

7.9.1 Question 1

What does your initial evaluation suggest is the diagnosis?

7.9.2 Answer 1

Posterior urethral valves is the most likely diagnosis. Sonographic findings of a thick walled bladder with bilateral hydroureteronephrosis in a male should be considered posterior urethral valves until proven otherwise. Although most patients will be identified prenatally, the occasional patient with posterior urethral valves may

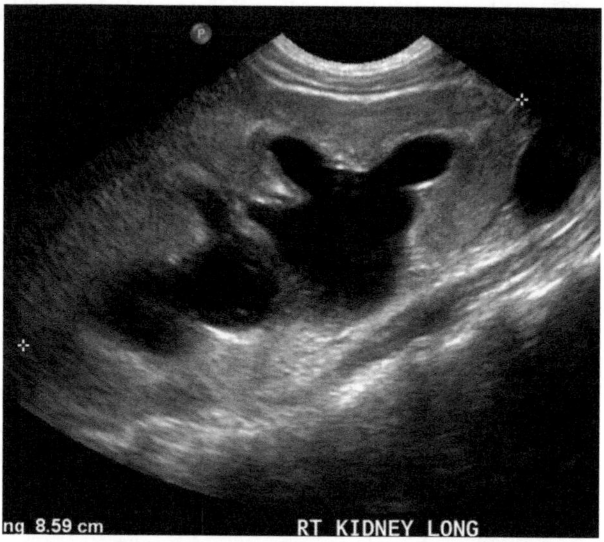

Image 7.1 Renal ultrasound demonstrating high grade right hydronephrosis with hydroureter

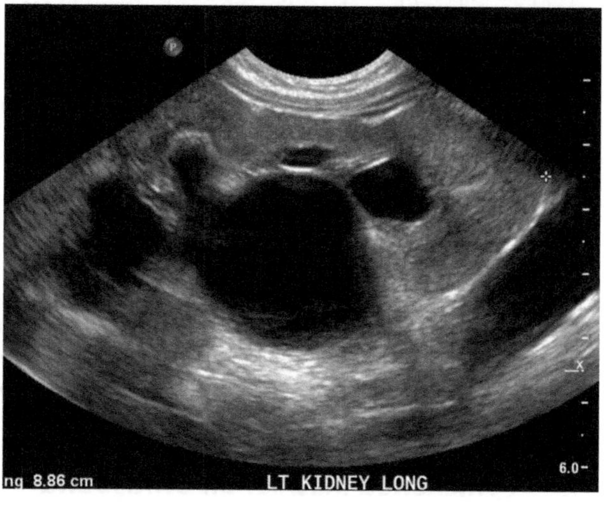

Image 7.2 Renal ultrasound demonstrating high grade left hydronephrosis with hydroureter

escape detection and present in this fashion. Long-term prognosis hinges on the creatinine level that is achieved after the obstruction has been relieved.

7.9.3 Question 2

What investigations would you consider?

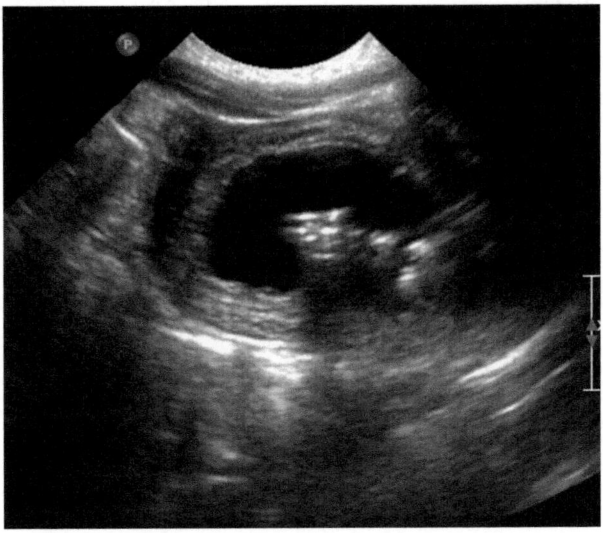

Image 7.3 Bladder ultrasound demonstrating thick wall and inflamed mucosa

7.9.4 Answer 2

1. Immediate placement of a urethral catheter with close attention to fluid and electrolyte status is paramount in the early management of these children. Post-obstructive diuresis with subsequent vascular collapse may occur in this setting unless close attention is paid to fluid shifts and electrolyte disturbances.
2. Voiding cystourethrogram to confirm diagnosis followed by close monitoring of serum creatinine until a nadir value is reached.
3. Surgical relief of obstruction with transurethral resection of valves after nadir creatinine has been reached. If serum creatinine does not drop to a suitable level with catheter placement then supravesical diversion in the form of a vesicostomy or ureterostomy may be considered.

7.9.5 Question 3

After initial evaluation and successful treatment with transurethral resection of valves, what advice would you give to the family?

7.9.6 Answer 3

1. Close follow up with radiographic imaging and monitoring of serum creatinine is critical to the long-term outcome of the child.
2. Vesicoureteral reflux, which is present in 50% of children at the time of diagnosis, has a 50% chance of spontaneous resolution.

3. Circumcision may reduce the risk of future urinary tract infections.
4. Despite successful valve resection, many children with posterior urethral valves have persistent bladder dysfunction and may require additional medical intervention in the form of anticholinergics and intermittent catheterization to optimize the patient's continence and renal status [3].

7.10 Scenario 3

A 1-day-old otherwise healthy boy is noted to have a swollen left hemi-scrotum. The child is afebrile.

7.11 Question 1

What is the differential diagnosis?

7.12 Answer 1

1. Neonatal testicular torsion
2. Hydrocele or Inguinal Hernia
3. Epididymitis
4. Testicular tumor

7.13 Question 2

Scrotal ultrasound reveals a left testicle with heterogeneous echotexture, yet the radiologist states that there is blood flow noted (peripherally). The contralateral hemi-scrotum is remarkable for a testicle of homogenous echotexture with a large hydrocele. How do you interpret the ultrasound findings?

7.14 Answer 2

The findings are most consistent with testicular torsion of greater than 24 h duration with subsequent necrosis. A rim of blood flow along the capsule can be misleading and is not the same as demonstrable blood flow within the testicular parenchyma with a clear Doppler signal. In the absence of the later finding, testicular torsion should be considered the most likely diagnosis. Although tumors are distinctly rare, the finding of heterogeneous echotexture should lead one to include this in the differential diagnosis.

7.15 Question 3

What are your recommendations for treatment?

7.16 Answer 3

It is important to explain to the family prior to the procedure that the chance of viability is very low and that the primary reason for exploration is to secure the diagnosis and perform pre-emptive contralateral septopexy.

1. Exploration of the left side via an inguinal incision (in case this represents a rare case of tumor). If torsion is identified and testicle appears viable then ipsilateral three point septopexy with permanent suture is performed. The testicle is removed if it appears necrotic and nonviable.
2. Contralateral scrotal exploration with septopexy.
3. The contralateral hydrocele is likely a reaction to the inflammatory process involving the left testicle. It may also represent a true communicating hydrocele. Due to the fact that the majority of communicating hydroceles will spontaneously improve we advocate simple drainage of the hydrocele. Contralateral inguinal exploration should not be undertaken due to risk of damaging the contralateral vasculature in a patient with a solitary testicle [4].

7.17 Question 3

How do you counsel the parents regarding future management?

7.18 Answer 3

1. If contralateral swelling is noted in the future then immediate presentation to the emergency department is indicated. Inform the family that contralateral hernia could develop and that if it did, surgical correction would be required.
2. Fertility with one testicle should be roughly equivalent to that of a child with two. Assisted reproduction is unlikely to be required.
3. Placement of a testicular prosthesis can be considered in the future. Waiting until the child has progressed through puberty is advised in order to properly judge the appropriate size of prosthesis to place (once the final size of the viable testicle is reached).

7.19 Scenario 4

A 2-day-old otherwise healthy girl is noted to have an intralabial mass. The abdomen is distended and the child is fussy but afebrile. External appearance is shown below (Image 7.4).

7.20 Question 1

What is the differential diagnosis of an intralabial mass in a newborn girl and what is the most likely diagnosis based on this image?

7.21 Answer 1

Differential diagnosis [5]:

1) Periurethral cyst. Typically white in appearance. Incision and drainage is curative.

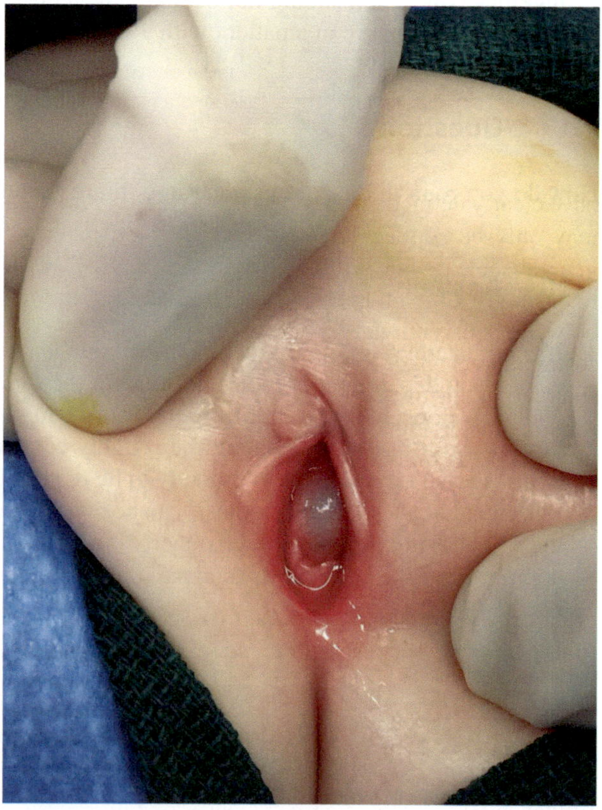

Image 7.4 Intralabial Cyst

2) Imperforate hymen with resultant hydrocolpos. A posteriorly placed whitish intralabial bulge typically associated with a palpable abdominal mass. Management is incision and drainage.
3) Prolapsed ectopic ureterocele. Typically clear to bluish in appearance. May take on a black appearance if necrotic. Most commonly noted to emerge from the posterior aspect of the urethral meatus.
4) Urethral prolapse: uncommon in newborns.
5) Vaginal Rhabdomyosacroma: grape like appearance, rare in newborns.

The appearance of this intralabial mass is most consistent with a prolapsed ureterocele in that it emanates from the posterior aspect of the urethra.

7.22 Question 2

Images from a renal bladder ultrasound are shown below. Describe what you see (Images 7.5, 7.6, 7.7, and 7.8).

7.23 Answer 2

The renal ultrasound shows a duplex left kidney with a large hydronephrotic upper pole with significant cortical thinning. The bladder view shows a ureterocele with extension into the intralabial location. The collapsed vagina and uterus are noted posterior to the bladder.

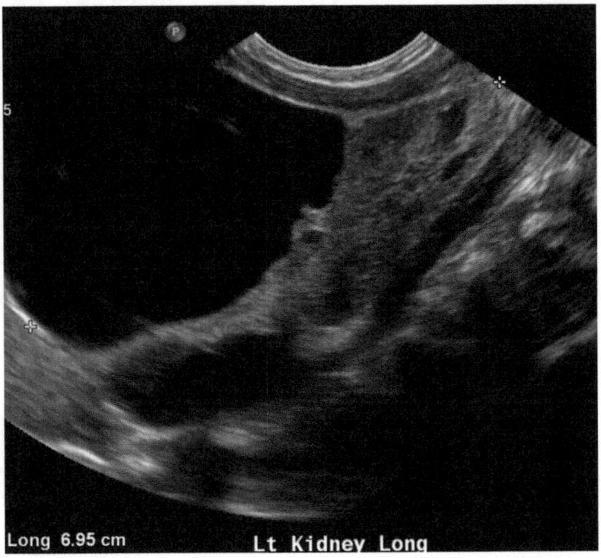

Image 7.5 Renal ultrasound of left duplex kidney with massive upper pole hydronephrosis

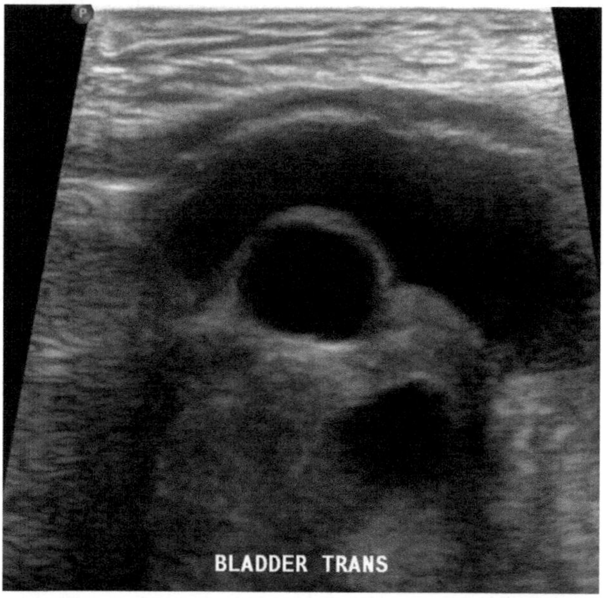

Image 7.6 Bladder ultrasound demonstrating a left intravesical ureterocele

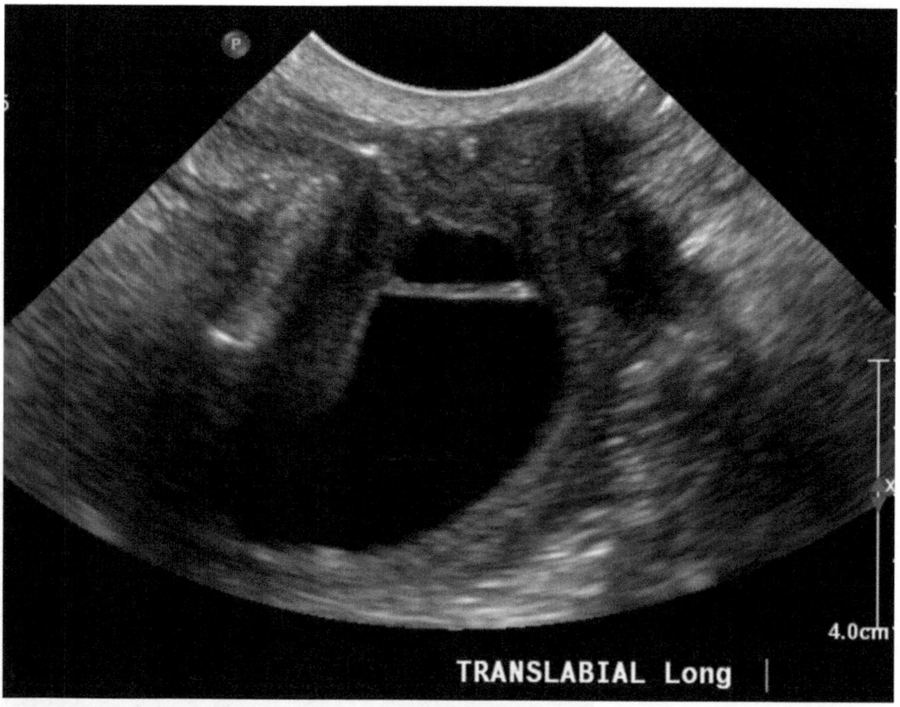

Image 7.7 Translabial ultrasound demonstrating ureterocele extending through urethra down to the level of the perineum.

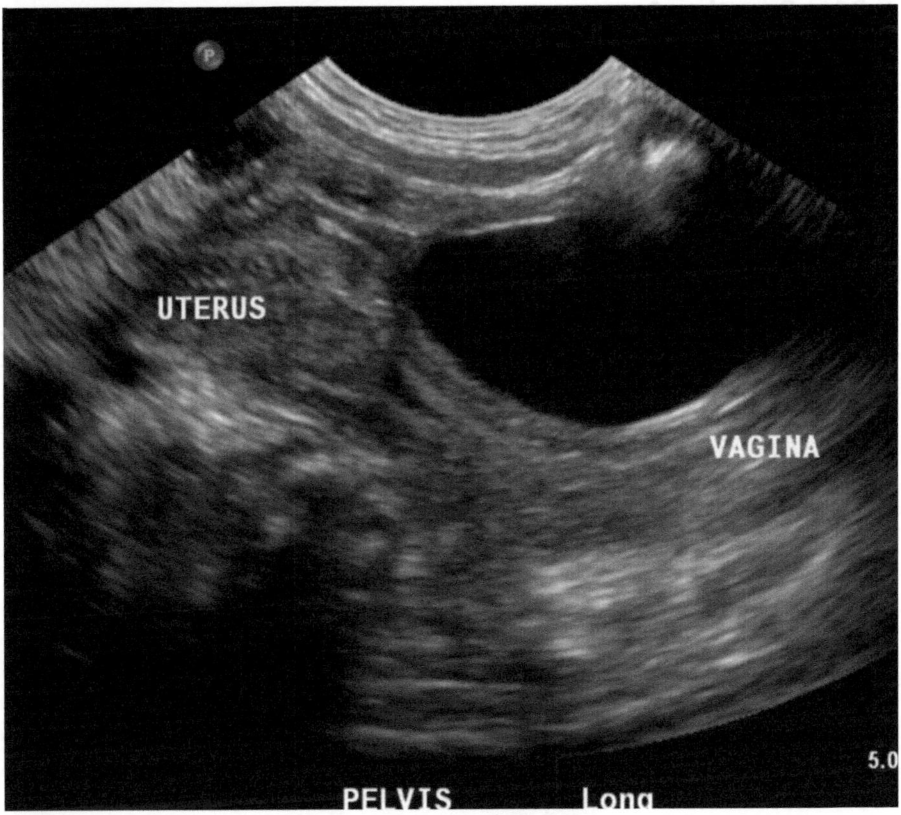

Image 7.8 Abdominal ultrasound demonstrating collapsed vagina and uterus posterior to the fluid filled bladder

7.24 Question 3

What is the treatment for this condition.

7.25 Answer 3

1) Incision of ureterocele. This can be undertaken at the bedside and should be made in a vertical orientation.
2) Prophylactic antibiotics should be provided.
3) Catheter drainage and repeat renal ultrasound to demonstrate upper tract decompression.

7.26 Question 4

Two days following incision of the ureterocele the catheter is removed. The child subsequently has poor urine output and appears to be grunting when voiding. A VCUG is obtained. What does this demonstrate (Image 7.9)?

7.27 Answer 4

The VCUG demonstrates obstruction at the bladder neck and right-sided vesicoureteral reflux. The obstruction can be explained by an anterior valve like filling of the distal part of the incised uretrerocele (see below). Treatment consists of endoscopic vertical incision of the residual distal lip. If this is not feasible then a vesicostomy may be required as a temporizing maneuverer until the patient is old enough to proceed with formal open ureterocele excision and ureteral reimplantation (Image 7.10).

Distal lip of incised ureterocele filling with urine as child voids—Effectively creating bladder outlet obstruction.

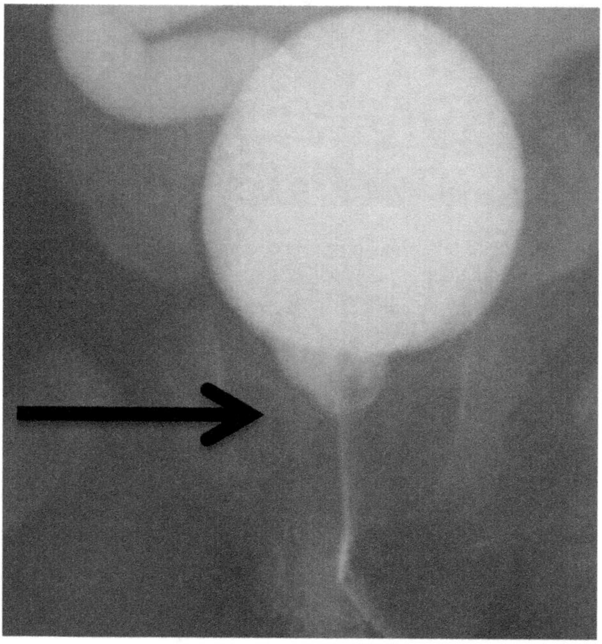

Image 7.9 Voiding Cystourethrogram demonstrating right sided vesicoureteral reflux and distal valve like filling of the distal end of the incised cecoureterocele

Image 7.10 Graphic description of fluid filling the distal segment of an incised cecoureterocele and thereby causing urethral obstruction

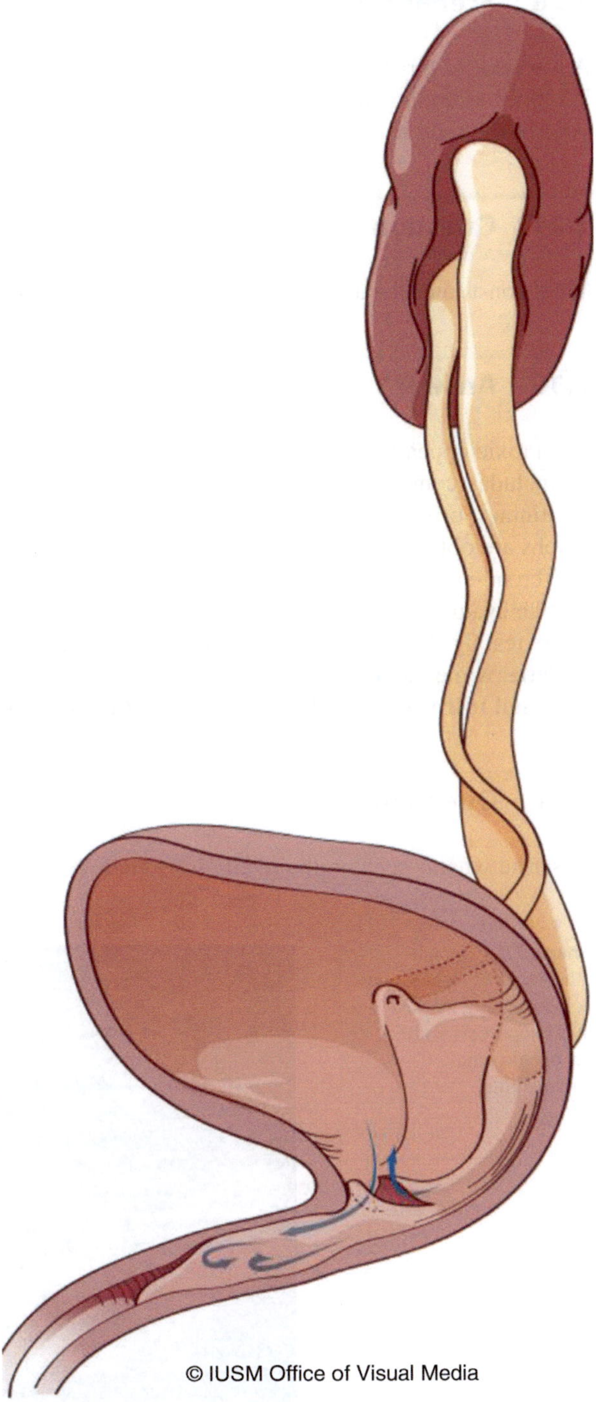

7.28 Scenario 5

A 6-week-old girl presents to an outside emergency room with hypoxia and a pH of 7.1. She has undergone initial resuscitation and has subsequently been transferred to your hospital by helicopter.

7.29 Question 1

What constitutes the appropriate work up for neonatal sepsis.

7.30 Answer 1

For a toxic appearing child under 60 days of age who presents with fever the work up includes complete blood count, basic metabolic panel (serum electrolytes and creatinine), urine analysis, blood culture, urine culture and spinal tap. Chest radiographs are obtained for children in respiratory distress/hypoxia. Fluid resuscitation and broad-spectrum antibiotics such as vancomycin and ceftriaxone are utilized. Further evaluation is dictated based on physical signs and symptoms as well as laboratory testing. This child was found to have a urinalysis that was positive for nitrites, bacteria, white blood cells and red blood cells.

Renal ultrasound findings are shown below (Images 7.11, 7.12, and 7.13).

7.31 Question 2

Describe what is seen on the renal ultrasound. What is the most likely diagnosis?

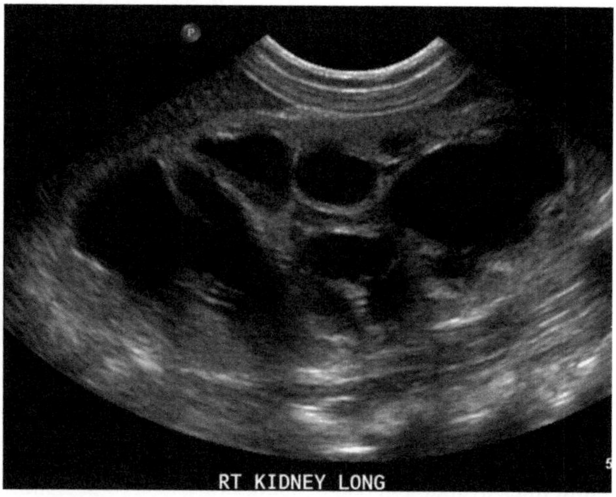

Image 7.11 Renal ultrasound of right kidney demonstrating marked hydronephrosis with echogenic renal parenchyma

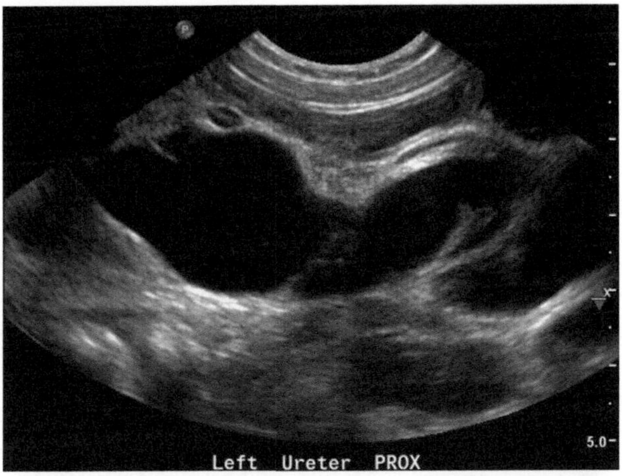

Image 7.12 Renal ultrasound of left fossa demonstrating hydronephorosis with marked dissension of proximal ureter

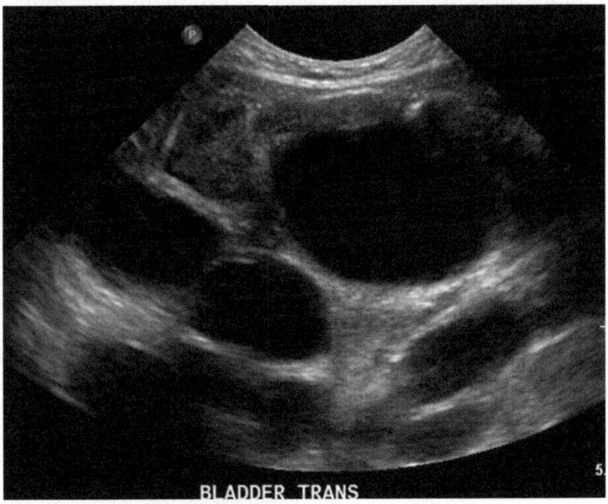

Image 7.13 Bladder ultrasound demonstrating normal bladder wall thickness and bilateral distally distended ureters

7.32 Answer 2

The renal ultrasound scan shows two large hydronephrotic kidneys with significant cortical thinning and debris within the collecting system. Marked ureteral dilatation is present extending down to the level of the bladder. This suggests that there are infected obstructed systems—bilateral UVJ obstruction with pyonephrosis. A component of vesicoureteral reflux could also be present (but in this case was shown not to be present on later VCUG).

7.33 Question 3

What are the potential options for initial management?

7.34 Answer 3

After initial resuscitation with catheter drainage, upper tract decompression is the critical step in management. This could theoretically take the form of internal stents, but the challenge of successfully placing these in tortuous ureters in this critically ill patient would preclude their use [6]. The placement of bilateral percutaneous nephrostomy tubes provides the most rapid and reliable method of clearing infection. Subsequent functional imaging with a MAG-3 renogram with the nephrostomy tubes clamped and antegrade nephrostograms are then utilized to obtain an adequate measure of function and drainage.

Question 4: The patient's subsequent imaging demonstrates bilateral UVJ obstruction. Creatinine has fallen from an initial value of 3.8–0.8 mg/dl and function is distributed equally between the two kidneys. What surgical options should be presented to the family (Image 7.14)?

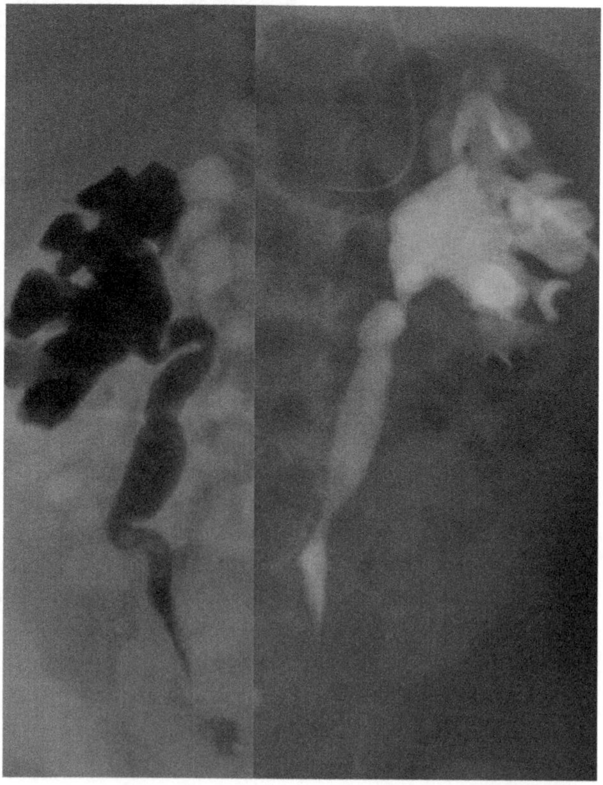

Image 7.14 Bilateral nephrostograms demonstrating bilateral distal ureteral obstruction

7.35 Answer 4

Bilateral cutaneous ureterostomies has been the classic choice for treatment in cases of bilateral ureterovesical junction obstruction in neonates. Additional options that can be used to maintain bladder cycling include placement of JJ stents (either antegrade or retrograde) or to perform bilateral temporary refluxing reimplants [6, 7]. This patient underwent the later procedure and at 18 months underwent definitive nonrefluxing bilateral ureteral reimplantation.

References

1. Brandao LR, Simpson EA, Lau KK. Neonatal renal vein thrombosis. Semin Fetal Neonatal Med. 2011;16(6):323–8.
2. Kosch A, Kuwertz-Broeking E, Heller C, Kurnik K, Schobess R. U. Renal venous thrombosis in neonates: prothrombotic risk factors and long-term follow-up. Blood. 2004;104:1356–60.
3. Peters C, Bauer SB. Evaluation and management of urinary incontinence after surgery for posterior urethral valves. Urol Clin N Am. 1990;17(2):379–87.
4. Kaefer M. Management of Abnormalities of the genitalia in girls. In: Wein AJ, Kavoussi LR, Partin AW, Peters CA, editors. Campbell's urology. 11th ed. Philadelphia, PA: W.B Saunders; 2016.
5. Kaefer M, Agarwal D, Misseri R, Whittam B, Hubert K, Rink R, Cain M. Treatment of contralateral hydrocele in neonatal testicular-torsion: is less more? J Pediatr Urol. 2016;12(5):306e1–4.
6. Farugia MK, Hitchock R, Radford A, Burki T, Robb A, Murphy F. British Association of Pediatric Urologists consensus statement on the management of the primary obstructive megaureter. J Pediatr Urol. 2014;10(1):26–33.
7. Kaefer M, Misseri R, Frank E, Rhee A, Lee SD. Refluxing ureteral reimplantation: a logical method for managing neonatal UVJ obstruction. J Pediatr Urol. 2014;10(5):824–30.

Urinary Tract Infection in Infants and Children

8

Prasad Godbole

Learning Objectives
At the end of the chapter, the reader will be able to:

- Prioritize and judiciously use appropriate imaging modalities for the diagnosis and evaluation of various pediatric urinary tract infection scenarios.
- Understand the role of antimicrobials and their appropriate use in paediatric urinary tract infections.

8.1 Scenario 1

A 4 month old baby girl presents to the emergency department with a high fever, vomiting and very smelly cloudy urine. A midstream sample urinalysis demonstrates the following:

- Proteins –
- Ketones +
- Blood: ++
- Leucocytes: ++
- Nitrites: ++

The baby has been previously fit and well with no significant antenatal history.

P. Godbole (✉)
Department of Paediatric Surgery, Sheffield Children's NHS Foundation Trust, Sheffield, UK
e-mail: p.godbole@nhs.net

P. Godbole et al. (eds.), *Practical Pediatric Urology*,
https://doi.org/10.1007/978-3-030-54020-3_8

8.2 Question 1

What does the urinalysis suggest?

8.3 Answer 1

The presence of leucocytes and nitrites on a dipstick urinalysis in the context of the history would strongly suggest a urinary tract infection. The systemic symptoms would in keeping with an upper urinary tract (pyelonephritic) type UTI. The test of leukocyte esterase detects the presence of this enzyme that is released from white blood cells (WBCs) in urine. Therefore, positive leukocyte esterase is comparable to pyuria (WBC $\geq$ 5/HPF or approximately 25 WBCs/μl) by microscopy using centrifuged urine, with a sensitivity of about 79% and specificity of 87%. Nitrites are produced by bacterial conversion of nitrates that are normally present in the urine. Most gram-negative bacteria that are cultured in urinary infections are capable of producing positive results of nitrite test. The combination of both leukocyte esterase and nitrite tests is highly sensitive and specific. A recent study shows dipstick may be an adequate screening test for UTI with a negative predictive value of 98.7%. Adding microscopy increases the negative predictive value to 99.2%.

8.4 Question 2

What would be your recommended initial treatment plan?

8.5 Answer 2

1. As this 4 month old is systemically unwell, the initial approach would be to resuscitate as appropriate depending on the clinical picture
2. Urine should be sent for culture
3. Baseline full blood count, urea and electrolytes, C Reactive protein and blood culture should be obtained before commencing on intravenous antibiotics or oral antibiotics depending on the clinical picture. The NICE guidance recommends commencing either oral/parenteral cephalexin or co-amoxiclav in the first instance. If the culture results show a resistant organism, the antibiotic must be changed based on sensitivities.
4. Had the UTI been lower urinary tract in nature, oral antibiotics in the form of Trimethoprim (first line) or Nitrofurantoin (second line) should be considered.

8.6 Question 3

What would be your subsequent management plan?

8.7 Answer 3

A renal ultrasound is required either during the acute infection or within 6 weeks of the acute infection based on the following criteria:

- During the acute infection in all children with atypical infection, indicated by:
  - Poor urine flow.
  - Abdominal or bladder mass.
  - Raised creatinine.
  - Sepsis.
  - Failure to respond to treatment with suitable antibiotics within 48 h.
  - Infection with non-*E. coli* organisms.
- During the acute infection in children aged under 6 months with recurrent UTI.
- Within 6 weeks for children aged 6 months and over with recurrent UTI.
- Within 6 weeks, for all children younger than 6 months of age with first-time UTI that responds to treatment.

8.8 Scenario 2

A 7 year old girl is referred to you with recurrent episodes of dysuria, frequency and proven lower urinary tract infections. She remains systemically well during these episodes.

8.9 Question 1

What history would you consider in this girl?

8.10 Answer 1

1. A careful history of voiding habits and bowel habits. Symptoms of lower urinary tract dysfunction should be elucidated. Such as urgency, incontinence, holding manouevres
2. A voiding diary and fluid intake chart and stooling chart
3. Detailed clinical examination including neurological examination and spinal examination

8.11 Question 2

What investigations would you consider?

8.12 Answer 2

1. As this girl has had recurrent UTI's, a renal ultrasound scan should be obtained looking at the upper tracts, bladder pre and post micturition volume and rectal diameter.
2. If there is evidence of scarring on the renal ultrasound, a DMSA scan should be done after at least a minimum of 3 months following the last UTI
3. If there is evidence of ureteric dilatation that resolves postmicturition (suggesting ureterovesical reflux), a VCUG may be considered if there is intention to treat the reflux.
4. If there is suggestion of lower urinary tract dysfunction or dysfunctional elimination, uroflowmetry with or without EMG studies may be considered.

8.13 Question 3

If her investigations are normal, what advice would you give to the family?

8.14 Answer 3

1. Advice regarding timed and regular voiding, adequate fluid intake and avoiding bladder irritants such as caffeinated and carbonated drinks, blackcurrant should be given
2. Control of constipation with stool softeners may be necessary
3. A short duration of antibiotic prophylaxis may be considered to break the cycle and allow time without UTI for the urotherapy program to be effective

8.15 Scenario 3

A 6 month old boy presents with a febrile illness, vomiting and a palpable mass in the left loin. His US scan is shown (Fig. 8.1)

8.16 Question 1

What is the most likely diagnosis?

8.17 Answer 1

The renal ultrasound scan shows a large hydronephrotic left kidney with significant cortical thinning and debris within the collecting system. The bladder view does not show any ureteric dilatation behind the bladder. This suggests an infected obstructed system on the left—a left pyonephrosis.

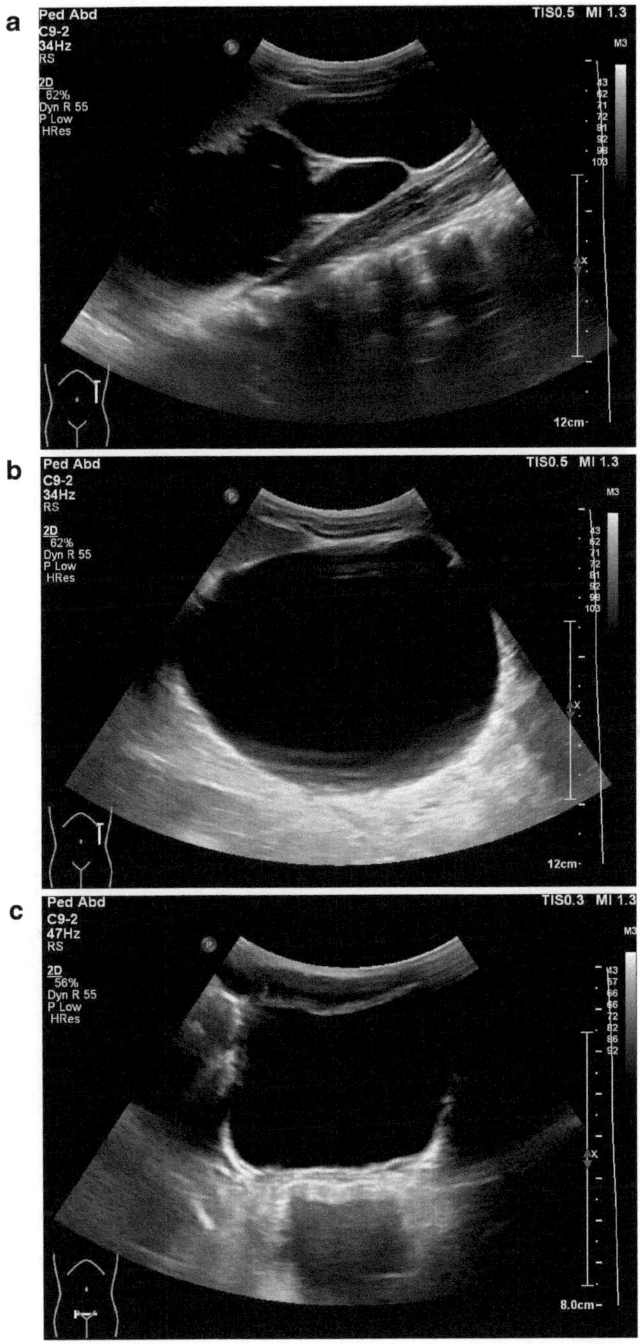

Fig. 8.1 (**a**) Ultrasound scan showing a grossly hydronephrotic kidney with corcial thinning. (**b**) Ultrasound scan of the same kidney with a massively dilated renal pelvis. (**c**) Ultrasound scan of the bladder with no dilated ureters behind the bladder

8.18 Question 2

What would be your initial management and subsequent management?

8.19 Answer 1

1. The child needs to be treated as sepsis. He requires full resuscitation, IV cannulation, baseline bloods for CBC, U&E, CRP, blood and urine culture
2. He requires commencing on a broad spectrum intravenous antibiotic such as Co-Amoxiclav
3. The infected left system needs to be drained either internally (JJ stent) or externally via a percutaneous nephrostomy and the infected urine sent for culture. In this case the boy had a percutaneous left nephrostomy.
4. He should then have some functional imaging (MAG3 renogram) with the nephrostomy clamped or a DMSA scan with an antegrade nephrostogram.

His subsequent imaging is shown (Figs. 8.2 and 8.3)

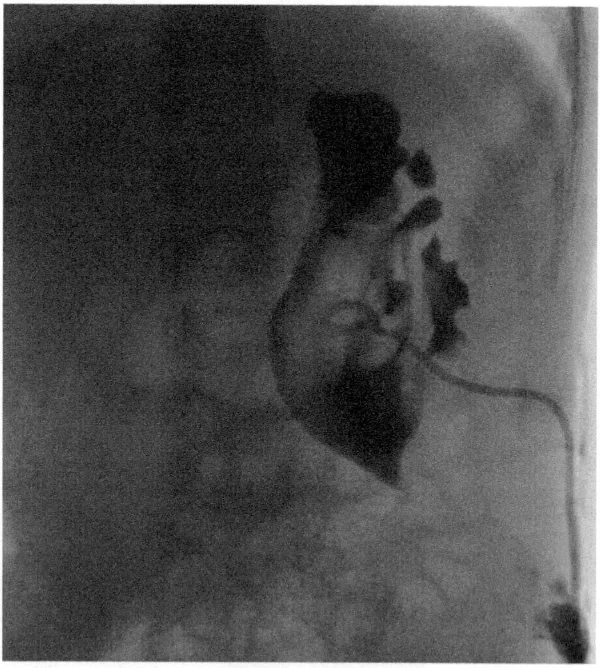

Fig. 8.2 Image of an antegrade study via the nephrostomy showing a dilated renal pelvis and no flow of contract across the pelvi ureteric junction

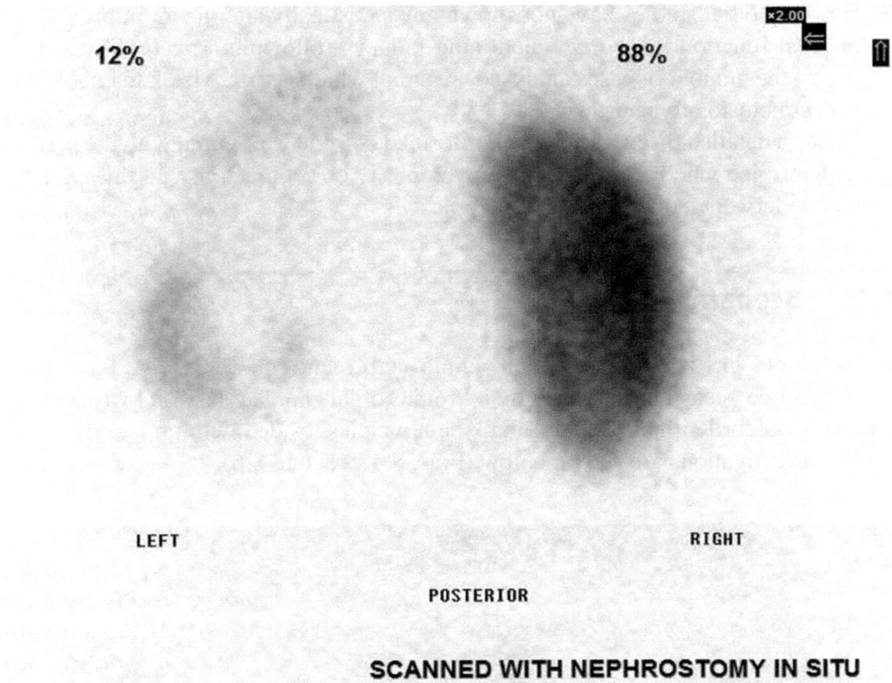

Fig. 8.3 DMSA scan showing 12% function of the left kidney

8.20 Question 3

What are the treatment options and why?

8.21 Answer 3

1. The treatment options are either a left nephrectomy or a left pyeloplasty as the left renal function is 12% and there is no drainage across the left UPJ on the antegrade study.
2. Traditionally a nephrectomy has been advocated in kidneys where the split renal function is less than 10%. However several studies have demonstrated an improvement in SRF and drainage following a pyeloplasty even for poorly functioning kidneys at 6 and 12 months after pyeloplasty.

3. However other studies have not shown any statistically significant improvement in renal function in poorly functioning kidneys following a pyeloplasty. In all series, the number of cases analysed are small which is a drawback to enable any firm conclusion to be drawn.
4. Hence a detailed discussion for full informed consent is required with the parents to determine whether to undergo a pyeloplasty or nephrectomy. In this case the boy underwent a dismembered pyeloplasty.

8.22 Scenario 4

A 6 year old girl is referred to your clinic with recurrent UTI's. She has grown *E. coli* on two occasions and recently a Proteus organism. Her last UTI was accompanied by a febrile illness and left flank pain which subsided with oral antibiotics.

Her investigations are shown below (Figs. 8.4, 8.5, and 8.6).

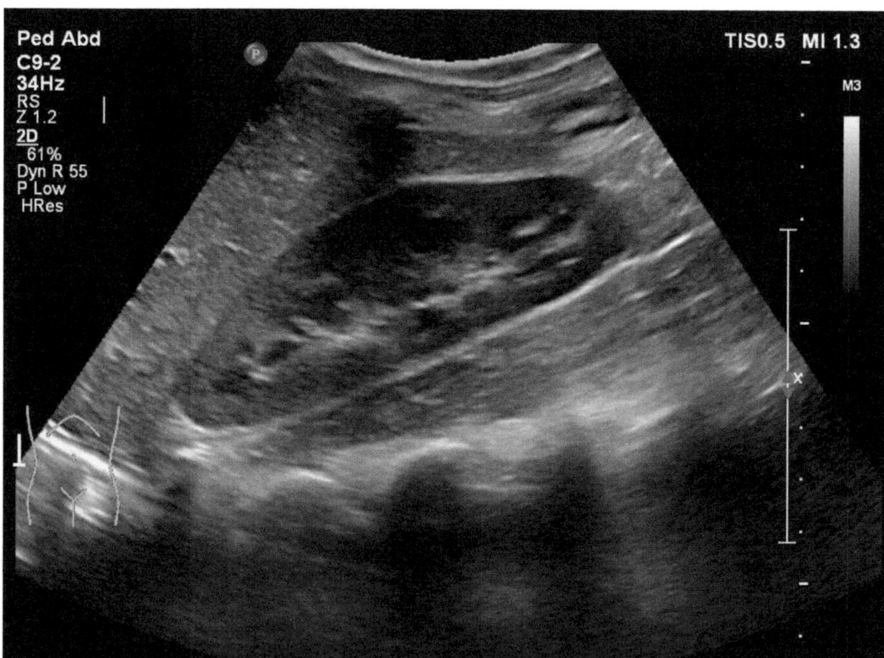

Fig. 8.4 Ultrasound scan showing normal right kidney

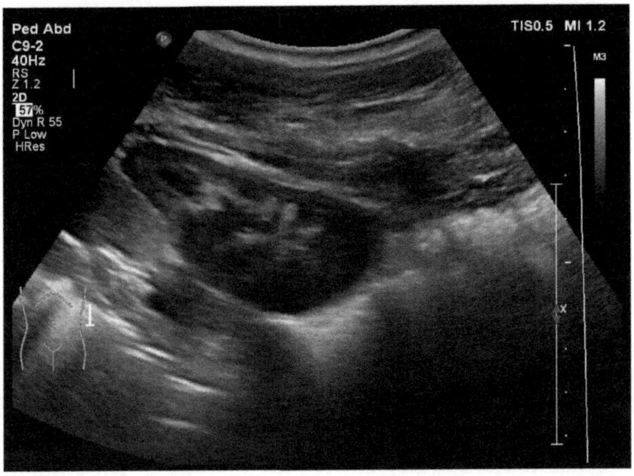

Fig. 8.5 Ultrasound scan showing irregular outline of the left kidney suggestive of scarring

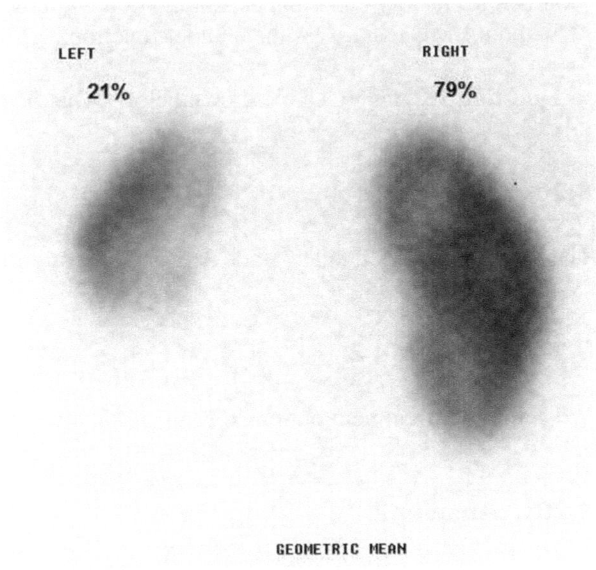

Fig. 8.6 DMSA scan confirms scarring of left kidney with reduced function

8.23 Question 1

a. What does this show?
b. What other investigation might you consider and why?

8.24 Answer 1a

The renal ultrasound shows a normal right kidney which is non dilated. The left kidney shows no pelvicalyceal dilatation but demonstrates cortical irregularity suggestive of renal scarring. The DMSA scan confirms scarring of the left kidney with reduced function.

8.25 Answer 1b

1. Combination of a scarred kidney and dilated ureter behind the bladder could suggest ureterovesical reflux. After discussion with the family, if correction of the reflux (if any) is considered then a VCUG should be obtained with the catheter inserted urethrally under play therapy or Entonox analgesia.
2. The other option would be to consider if this girl has dysfunctional elimination. A careful history and clinical examination combined with uroflowmetry with or without EMG can assess the bladder function.

Question 1c. Her VCUG is shown below- what does this show (Fig. 8.7)?

8.26 Answer 1c

The VCUG shows left sided grade 3 vesicoureteral reflux.

8.27 Question 2

What are your treatment options for this girl and why?

8.28 Answer 2

1. Most of this girls UTI's have been lower urinary tract in origin. Hence a detailed history of voiding habits and bowel habits should be taken. Standard urotherapy with timed and regular voiding, adequate fluid intake, double voiding and managing any bladder dysfunction with anticholinergics and antibiotic prophylaxis may be considered as an option in the first instance. Where standard urotherapy fails and LUTS persist a video urodynamic investigation would be useful.
2. The other option would be endoscopic correction of the reflux. It is suggested that reflux with LUTD will resolve faster after LUTD correction and that patients with LUTD are at higher risk for developing UTIs and renal scarring. Alternatively, it is possible that LUTD is secondary to VUR and that treatment of

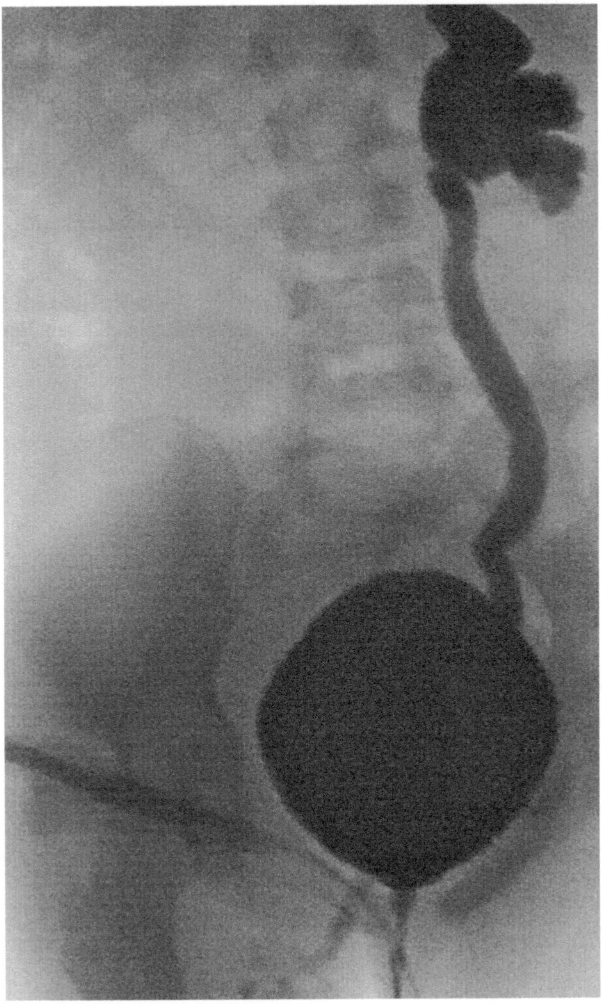

Fig. 8.7 VCUG showing left sided dilating uretero vesical reflux

VUR will therefore result in correction of LUTD. Or, it may be that there is a high coprevalence, but the treatment of one condition does not correct the other. In recent literature, no data support any of these hypotheses.

Suggested Further Reading

1. Glissmeyer EW, Korgenski EK, Wilkes J, Schunk JE, Sheng X, Blaschke AJ, et al. Dipstick screening for urinary tract infection in febrile infants. Pediatrics. 2014;133:e1121–7.
2. Williams GJ, Macaskill P, Chan SF, Turner RM, Hodson E, Craig JC. Absolute and relative accuracy of rapid urine tests for urinary tract infection in children: a meta-analysis. Lancet Infect Dis. 2010;10:240–50.

3. Urinary tracy infection—children: National institute for Health and Care Excellence (NICE). https://cks.nice.org.uk/urinary-tract-infection-children#!scenarioRecommendation.
4. Cooper CS and Nepple KG. Etiology and clinical features of bladder dysfunction in children. https://www.uptodate.com/contents/etiology-and-clinical-features-of-bladder-dysfunction-in-children.
5. Abdelaziz AY, Shaker H, Aly H, Aldaqados H, Hussein EM. Early outcome of pediatric pyeloplasty in kidneys with split renal function less than 10%: a prospective study of 25 cases. Afr J Urol. 2018;24(4):324–30.
6. Ekberli G, Tiryaki HT. Is differential renal function improved after Pyeloplasty? Evaluation of 13 cases with low differential renal function. Turkish J Pediatr Dis/Türkiye Çocuk Hast Derg. 2018;1:36–8.
7. Tekgu S, Riedmiller H, Hoebeke P, Koc˘vara R, Nijman RJM, Radmayr C, Stein R, Dogan HS. EAU guidelines on Vesicoureteral reflux in children. Eur Urol. 2012;62:534–42.

Upper Urinary Tract Obstruction

9

UPJO, Megaureter, Ureterocele

Mike O'Brien

Learning Objectives
After reading the chapter, the reader should

1. Be able to appropriately investigate obstructive uropathies of the upper urinary tract
2. Understand the rationale for conservative versus surgical management for the various pathologies and indications for surgical intervention
3. Be able to appropriately follow up patients with or without surgical intervention for upper urinary tract obstructive pathologies.

9.1 Case 1

Two-week old male presenting with a history of bilateral hydronephrosis that was diagnosed antenatally on ultrasonagraphy (US) at the 22-week gestation scan. The transverse Antero-Posterior dimensions (APDs) at the level of the renal hilum were reported as 18 mm on the right and 22 mm on the left. Repeat scanning in the 34th week of the pregnancy showed persistent bilateral renal pelvis dilatation, with calyceal dilatation. There was no mention of bladder appearances or evidence of dilated ureters and amniotic fluid volumes were reported as normal. The patient was born at term and immediately started on prophylactic antibiotics.

Question 1. What Would Be Your Immediate Management?
Obtain the perinatal history
Physical examination
Renal function tests (UEC)

M. O'Brien (✉)
The Royal Children's Hospital, Melbourne, VIC, Australia
e-mail: Mike.Obrien@rch.org.au

P. Godbole et al. (eds.), *Practical Pediatric Urology*,
https://doi.org/10.1007/978-3-030-54020-3_9

Ultrasound urinary tract to confirm the findings
MCUG: given his male gender and the presence of bilateral hydronephrosis to exclude Posterior Urethral Valves (PUV) or Vesico-ureteric Reflux (VUR).

His physical examination and renal function (Cr 28 μmol/l) were normal. An US urinary tract was performed on day 2 of life and showed persistent bilateral renal pelvis dilatation, with apparent improvement in the degree of dilatation. The MCUG showed normal urethral contour and no evidence of VUR (Fig. 9.1).

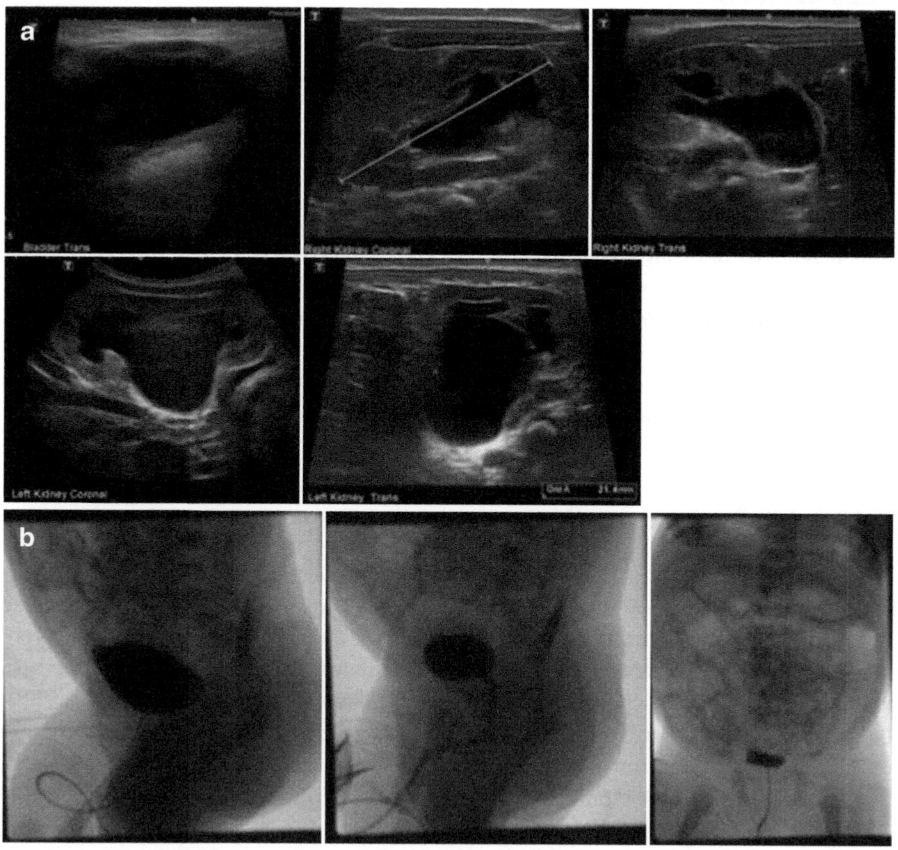

Fig. 9.1 (**a**) US Urinary Tract day 2 of life shows severe left hydronephrosis with APD 21 mm, and moderate hydronephrosis on the right with APD 12 mm. No evidence of ureteric dilatation and a sonographically normally appearing bladder. (**b**) MCUG: early bladder filling images demonstrated normal bladder wall appearance. No evidence of vesicoureteric reflux on either side. No evidence of posterior urethral valves, with prompt passage of contrast via the urethra and normal contour demonstrated

Questions 2. What Is the Differential Diagnosis?

1. *PUV*
2. *VUR*
3. *PUJO*
4. *Transient hydronephrosis*

Question 3. What Is the Long-Term Management and Follow-Up?
Conservative management and surveillance with repeated renal tract ultrasounds. No indication for antibiotic prophylaxis.

His renal pelvis dilatation improved on subsequent scans; however, at 6 months of age, he developed progression of the renal pelvicalyceal dilatation bilaterally with suspicion of left Pelvi-Ureteric Junction Obstruction (PUJO). He remained completely asymptomatic (Fig. 9.2).

Question 4. What Would You Do Next? What Follow Up Is Recommended?
A MAG-3 renogram to assess renal function.
Repeat US urinary tract to assess progression of dilatation
Follow-up with US only at 1 year and then at 2, 5, and 10 years of age
Repeat NM scan only of there is again progression of renal pelvis dilatation

The patient remained asymptomatic and the renal pelvis dilatation improved on subsequent imaging. The MAG 3 renogram showed almost equal split function and slow but adequate drainage after administration of Lasix.

9.1.1 Discussion

Antenatal hydronephrosis (AHN) has become one of the most commonly detected ultrasound (US) findings, associated with 1–5% of pregnancies [1, 2]. The underlying aetiology is varied, ranging from transient hydronephrosis to congenital anomalies of the kidney and urinary tract. The benefits of early detection and intervention in cases of urinary tract dilation include a reduction in renal damage due to obstruction and infection. However, the majority of antenatal hydronephrosis are secondary to non-obstructive causes. Many of these antenatally detected cases spontaneously resolve [3]. A list of the underlying conditions that can cause antenatal hydronephrosis is summarised below in Table 9.1.

The challenge remains to determine which of these prenatally detected infants will require surgery, prior to the development of symptoms or potentially irreversible renal damage, thus permitting a more tailored screening [3].

The presence of bilateral renal tract dilation, especially in males, raises concerns of bladder outlet obstruction, such as posterior urethral valves and, very rarely, urethral atresia. In females it is far less common, but other underlying conditions should be suspected, such as a persistent urogenital sinus, cloacal anomaly or a

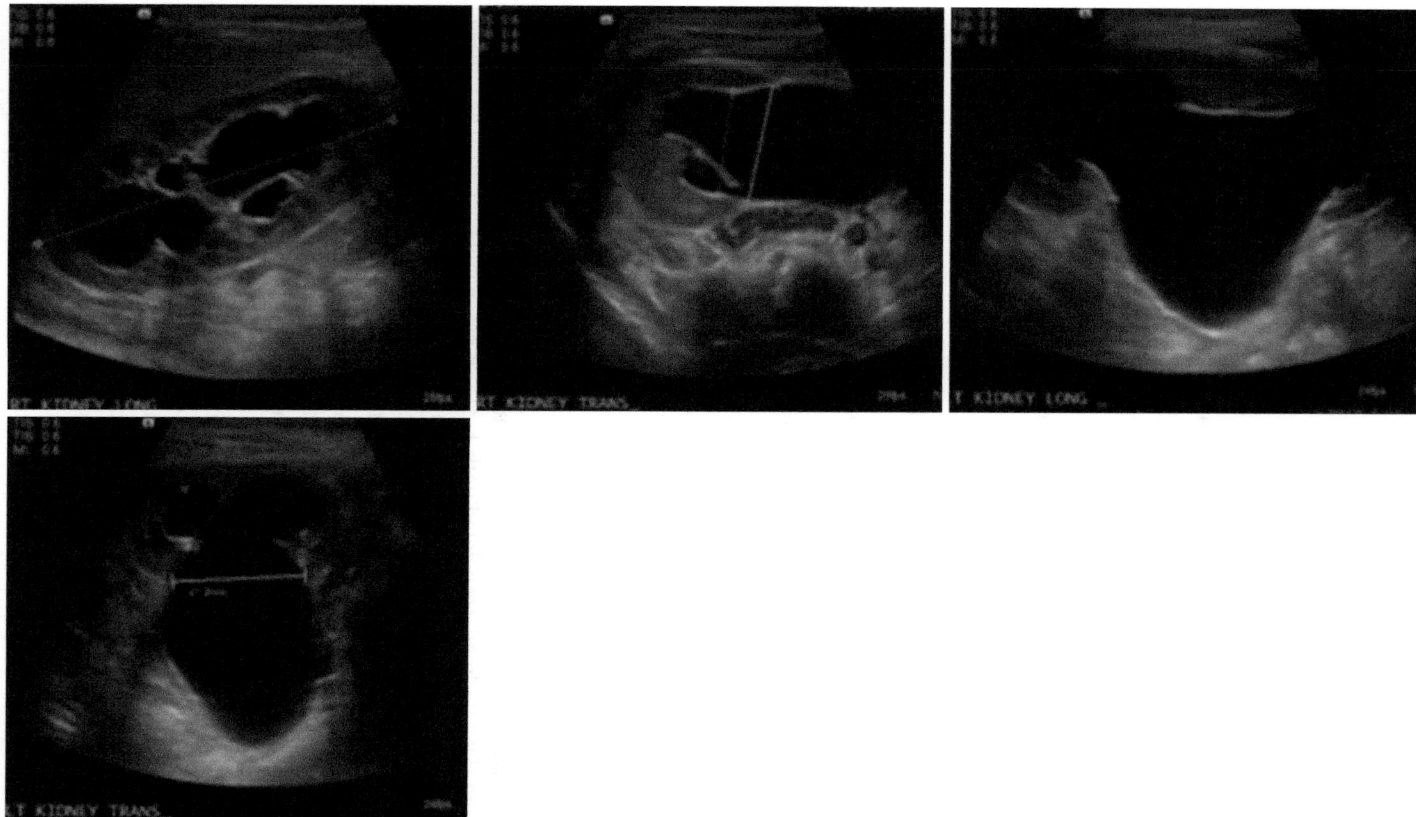

Fig. 9.2 US Urinary tract at 5 months of age shows increasing bilateral renal pelvis dilatation, 33 mm left (previously 21 mm) and 20 mm right (previously 12 mm), with cortical thinning and no ureteric dilatation. Bladder over distended with 97 ml

Table 9.1 Aetiology of urinary tract dilation detected on antenatal ultrasound [2, 4]

Condition	Frequency	Incidence in ANH (%)	Gender ratio
Transient/physiologic hydronephrosis	2–4/100	41–88	M:F = 1:1
Pelviureteric junction obstruction (PUJO)	1/1500	10–30	M:F = 2:1
Vesicoureteric reflux (VUR)	1/100	10–20	M:F = 1:5
Vesicoureteric junction obstruction (VUJO)	1/10000	5–23	M:F = 3–4:1
Duplex system	1–2/100	7	M:F = 1:4
Ureterocoele/ectopic ureter	1/10000	5–7	M:F = 1:6
Multicystic dysplastic kidney	1/3000	4–6	M:F = 1:1
Posterior urethral valves	1/8000	1–2	Male

spinal anomaly. After birth, these children should be commenced on prophylactic antibiotics and ultrasonography of the urinary tract should be performed within 24–48 h of life [5, 6]. In males, a urethral catheter should be inserted to ensure bladder drainage and renal function should be assessed. Following this, micturating cystourethrography is recommended to look for evidence of urethral obstruction and/or VUR to determine if urgent intervention is required. In all other cases, a postnatal US urinary tract should be performed within 3–7 of life to avoid underestimating the degree of urinary tract dilatation. A repeat US is recommended at 4–6 weeks of age.

In most cases of isolated antenatal unilateral hydronephrosis, the child is commenced on prophylactic antibiotics at birth, usually trimethoprim at the dose of 2 mg/kg weight each night, and further investigations are organised. An ultrasound of the urinary tract is repeated in the first week, ensuring that the baby is adequately hydrated and repeated after 2 and 6 weeks in most cases, and again at 3 months if abnormal. Functional imaging should be deferred ideally until 3 months of age to allow for renal maturation. A dynamic renal scan such as 99Tc-mercaptoacetyltriglycine (MAG3) is preferred for children with possible obstruction and it provides differential renal function as well.

In this case, the patient was managed accordingly, but no structural abnormality was identified. Once this was ruled out, the prophylactic Abs were stopped, and he was only monitored with regular US urinary tract [5–7].

The follow-up of patients with non-obstructive hydronephrosis still remains controversial. Children with renal pelvis APD > 12 mm are usually commenced on prophylactic antibiotics pending further investigations. In the absence of calyceal involvement only US is recommended for follow-up at the ages of 3 months, 1 year and then at 2, 5, and 10 years of age. In infants who develop significant increase in the degree of dilatation a NM isotope scan is also indicated. Patients with renal APD of 13–19 mm should have a similar follow-up by US, but imaging should also include isotope study at 2–3 months of age, to assess renal function. Children with severe hydronephrosis (>20 mm) should have their first functional imaging earlier, at 6–8 weeks of age, so that those with decreased function (<40%) can proceed to surgery [3].

Patients with transverse renal pelvis APD between 20 and 50 mm and good function continue to pose a problem, as they can either remain stable, resolve spontaneously, or eventually warrant surgery. Those with a severe degree of dilatation (>20 mm), calyceal involvement and with >40% function require close follow-up with US at 1, 3, and 6 months, 1 year and annually thereafter. A repeat NM scan is indicated in cases of progressive dilatation, potentially representing an obstructed system, which would finally benefit from surgery if the function were to decrease <40% or if they developed symptoms related to their urinary tract [3].

9.2 Case 2

A 2-week old male infant with an antenatal diagnosis of right hydronephrosis (6.5 mm) first identified at 24 weeks gestation and then increasing up to 14 mm at 34 weeks of GA. He was born at 36 weeks and treated for suspected neonatal sepsis. He was discharged on Prophylactic Abs and referred for further investigations. The US of the urinary tract done on day 5 of life showed persistent right renal pelvis dilatation of 25 mm. Normal physical examination and renal function (Cr 28 µmol/l) (Fig. 9.3).

Question 1. What Is the Main Diagnosis That Needs to Be Excluded and What Investigations Would You Perform to Confirm It?
The main diagnosis to exclude is a right PUJO

A NM scan should be requested to confirm the diagnosis and decide further management.

On MAG-3 there was evidence of reduction of the function of the right kidney with impaired drainage (Fig. 9.4).

The appearances of moderate right hydronephrosis, no evidence of ureteric dilatation and a reduction in differential renal function (33%) are consistent with a diagnosis of Partial Right PUJ Obstruction.

Question 2. What Is the Definitive Management for This Patient?
The patient should undergo an Anderson Hynes open dismembered pyeloplasty with insertion of JJ stent or a nephron-stent depending on the surgeon's preference. A perinephric drain may also be indicated.

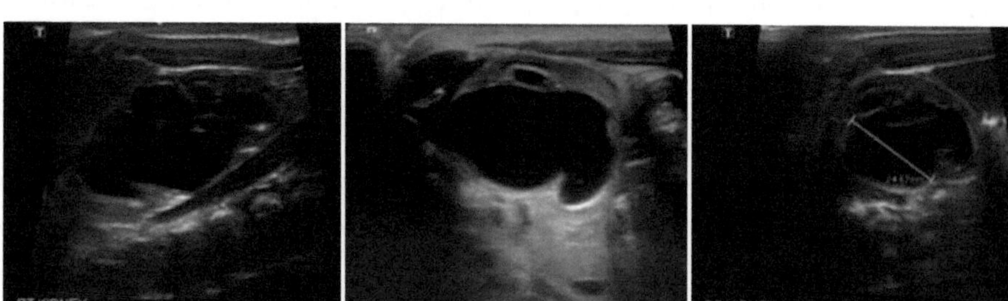

Fig. 9.3 Ultrasound urinary tract at 5 days and 4 weeks of life show right pelvicalyceal dilatation, with APD renal pelvis of 25 mm. Normal contralateral kidney and bladder

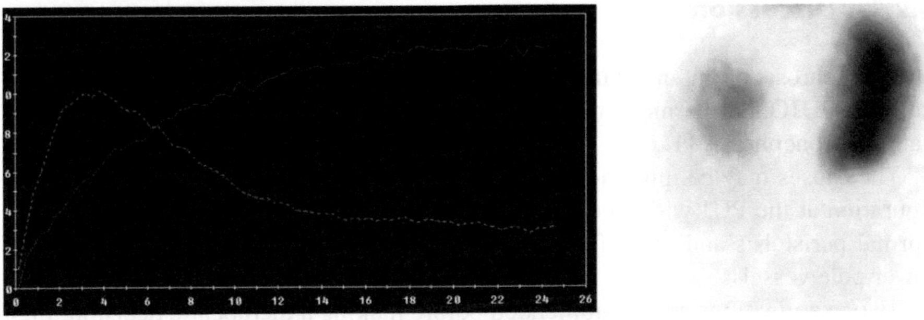

Fig. 9.4 MAG-3 done at 4 weeks of age. Clearance of activity into the dilated right pelvicalyceal system was slower than normal and although the intensity of tracer within the collecting system increased over time, there was no evident drainage into the ureter despite lasix administration and upright positioning. The renogram curve is shown below and the relative function of the right kidney is 33%

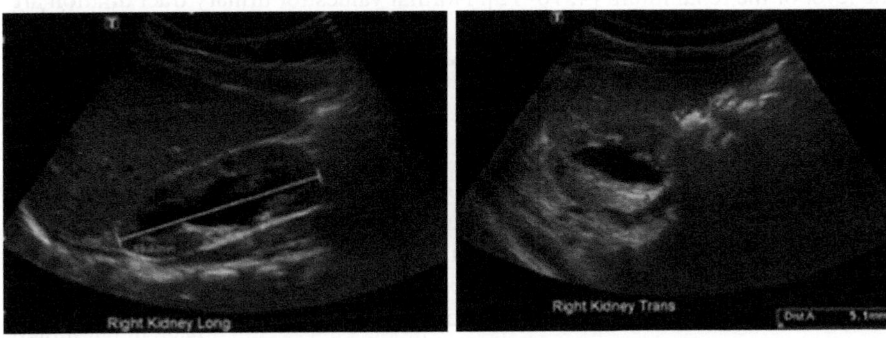

Fig. 9.5 US urinary tract 3 months after procedure: significant interval improvement of right renal pelvis dilatation with APD now 5 mm (previously 25 mm). There is persistent right global parenchymal thinning, but with maintained corticomedullary differentiation. Normal left kidney, slightly bigger than right

Postoperative recovery was uneventful. The histopathology report confirmed the diagnosis and the JJ stent was removed 6 weeks after surgery.

Question 3. What Follow Up Would You Recommend?

Follow up should include an US urinary tract 6 weeks after the removal of JJ stent, and at 6 and 12 months after the surgery. A repeat MAG-3 is indicated around 6 months after the procedure if the renal function was already compromised.

On review 3 months after the procedure he remained well and asymptomatic and a follow-up US urinary tract showed significant reduction of the right renal pelvis dilatation, with no other abnormalities identified (Fig. 9.5).

9.2.1 Discussion

Hydronephrosis on antenatal ultrasound is today the most common mode of presentation of PUJO. Furthermore, obstruction is the second most common cause of antenatal hydronephrosis [1, 6].

The causes may be intrinsic, due to an abnormal fibromuscular and neural configuration at the PUJ with a congenital adynamic segment [8, 9] which affects the normal peristalsis and urine flow, or extrinsic, due to compression from crossing lower pole vessels.

Two examinations are recommended before making a therapeutic decision. First a postnatal US of the urinary tract, to assess the APD diameter of the renal pelvis, the degree of calyceal dilatation, the appearance of the renal parenchyma (cortical thickness, corticomedullary differentiation, echogenicity, presence of cysts, etc.), the presence of ureteric dilatation and the bladder appearances [4]. The main US parameter is the transverse antero-posterior diameter (APD) of the renal pelvis at the level of the renal hilum [4, 10–12]. Normal values for urinary tract dilation are:

- Antenatal from 16–27 weeks of GA <4 mm
- Antenatal ≥28 weeks GA <7 mm
- Postnatal (>48 h) <10 mm

Secondly, a nuclear medicine scan should be requested in all patients with renal pelvis APD >15 mm or when there is evidence of parenchymal thinning and/or increased echogenicity, to assess the relative function of the affected kidney, and to look for features that would support or exclude obstruction. This should ideally be performed around 6–8 weeks of age to ensure further renal maturation and avoid overestimation of function due to increased background activity [13, 14]. In the vast majority of cases, the split renal parenchymal function given by the MAG3 renogram is reliable; therefore, an additional DMSA scan with the only purpose of assessing split renal function is not required. Nevertheless, a DMSA may be necessary in cases of a grossly enlarged kidney or conditions with poor parenchymal extraction of the radiopharmaceutical, with high background activity, such as very immature kidneys or severe chronic kidney disease.

The degree of hydronephrosis in the postnatal period is important. Spontaneous resolution takes place in approximately 50% of the cases with mild hydronephrosis, where as it is much less likely in cases with more pronounced dilatation, APD > 15 mm. No intervention is required in most cases, but it is more likely that the child will need surgery if the renal pelvis diameter is >30 mm [15–17]. According to the experience from Great Ormond Street hospital, published by Dhillon et al. in 1998 [3], patients can easily be divided into 3 groups based on the degree of renal pelvic dilatation on US. Patients with renal pelvis dilatation of <12 mm require simple follow-up with US (dilatation <12 mm); on the other hand, those with a gross dilatation (>50 mm) benefit from early surgical intervention. For the intermediate groups, with renal pelvis dilatation between 20 and 50 mm, surgery will be recommended for those with reduced function, symptoms, increasing dilatation and severe hydronephroses in solitary and bilateral systems.

Decreased split function at initial assessment is often used as an absolute indication for surgery, but when the dilatation of the pelvicalyceal system is not significant this may be due to a dysplastic kidney instead of a PUJO; therefore, each case should be considered separately. Another indication for surgery would be progressive increase of renal pelvis APD on follow-up US, as it could indicate a degree of impedance to urinary drainage and risk of renal function deterioration. If there is evidence of associated reduction of relative renal function, surgery is indicated.

The liklihood of pyeloplasty is also increased if the antenatal dilatation was severe, >15 mm, before the 20 weeks of gestation or if there is a large increase in the degree of dilatation between the first and third trimesters, even if the hydronephrosis appears to stabilize in the first few months of life [3].

Obstruction of the PUJ represents the most common malformation of the upper urinary tract causing hydronephrosis. US scans of the urinary tract and renal scintigraphy concur in most cases in providing a definitive diagnosis. Management can be debatable while investigations are done. In this case, the neonate was started on antibiotic prophylaxis and was referred for further assessment [5–7]. An US of the urinary tract and MAG-3 were performed when the patient was 6 weeks old and both confirmed the diagnosis of a PUJO. The operation of choice with time tested results and a success rate of >95–98% is the dismembered Anderson-Hynes pyeloplasty [18, 19]. The stenotic segment is excised and a wide water- tight, dependant anastomosis made after spatulating the ureteric end. Our institution's preference is to leave a trans-anastomotic stent in the form of a JJ stent, to avoid the potential complications of having an externalised nephrostomy tube. Evidence suggests that the presence of trans-anastomotic drainage tube favours less complications such as urinary leak, stenosis and need for redo-surgery [19].

In this case, an open pyeloplasty was performed at 2 months of age with excellent result and proven decrease in renal pelvis dilatation on follow up US.

9.3 Case 3

A 9-month-old girl referred for persistent postnatal bilateral hydronephrosis for further investigations and management. The patient had been diagnosed with mild bilateral hydronephrosis antenatally on the 20-week scan and US on day 4 of life had shown resolution of left hydronephrosis with only mild right renal pelvis prominence of 5 mm. Despite being started of prophylactic Abs after birth she developed a febrile *E. Coli* UTI at 2 weeks of age, which was treated with oral Abs with good clinical response (Fig. 9.6).

Question 1. What Investigations Would You Request After This Episode and Why?

US urinary tract to assess any possible progression of the dilatation and if new finding of ureteric dilatation was present.

NM scan to assess the renal function and potentially the presence of vesicoureteric reflux as well.

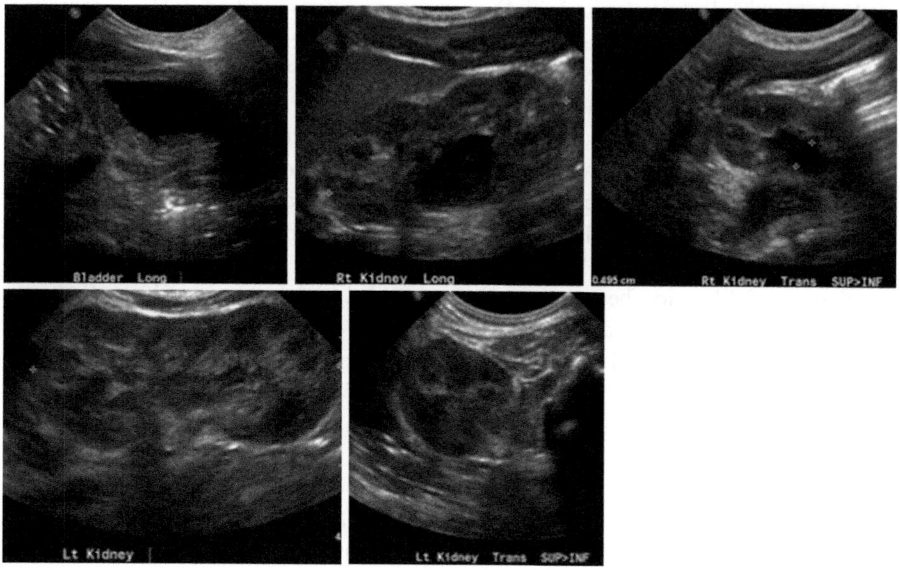

Fig. 9.6 US Urinary tract on day 4 of life. Resolution of left hydronephrosis and only mild right renal pelvis dilatation of 5 mm. Normal bladder and no distal ureteric dilatation

MCUG—debatable. The management would not change even with the diagnosis of VUR.

The US urinary tract showed again bilateral renal pelvis dilatation larger on the right (renal pelvis APD right 18 mm and left 5 mm). The dynamic NM scan demonstrated preserved differential function and there was no evidence of VUR (Fig. 9.7).

Question 2. How Would You Manage the Patient?
Commence patient on prophylactic Abs, due to the febrile UTI during the neonatal period and the underlying possibility of VUR as the cause for her symptoms.

Conservative management with US surveillance at 12 and 18 months of age.

On follow-up imaging, the patient developed progressive increase of the renal pelvis APD up to 25 mm at 1 year of age and 30 mm pre-void (19 mm post-void measurement) at 18 months of age. Unfortunately, a subsequent US urinary tract at 18 months of age showed again significant increase in the right renal pelvis dilatation up to 30 mm (Fig. 9.8).

Question 3. What Would You Do Next?
Repeat the dynamic NM scan to ensure there is no deterioration of renal function.

As she remained asymptomatic it was decided to continue conservative management and monitor with a repeat US 3 and 6 months after, in which the right renal pelvis dilatation was stable. With these findings, need for surgical intervention was ruled out and decision was made to stop the Ab prophylaxis. Subsequent follow-up US urinary tract showed stable persistent right renal pelvis dilatation, without other abnormal findings. A repeat NM scan at 4 years of age also confirmed preserved right renal function. When she was last reviewed at 6 years of age she remained well and asymptomatic with similar findings on US.

9.3.1 Discussion

The management of antenatally diagnosed hydronephrosis (HN) depends on its severity and the timing of diagnosis. It is generally accepted that renal pelvis dilatation in the third trimester is defined as APD > 7 mm. Postnatal data on MRI, not US, suggests that the normal APD in children is 3 mm at 1 year of age, 6 mm at 18 years, with the 99th percentile for children <5 years of age being <10 mm [2, 4] (Table 9.2).

A dilated urinary tract does not automatically infer obstruction of the urinary tract. Whereas hydronephrosis equates a dilated renal collecting system, obstruction cannot be proven on the basis of any single imaging study, hence the need for a period of observation to demonstrate deterioration over time.

Second trimester hydronephrosis is often followed-up so that progression of severity can be detected, and appropriate postnatal follow-up is planned. Postnatal resolution has been noted in up to 50% of antenatally diagnosed cases [9, 15, 16].

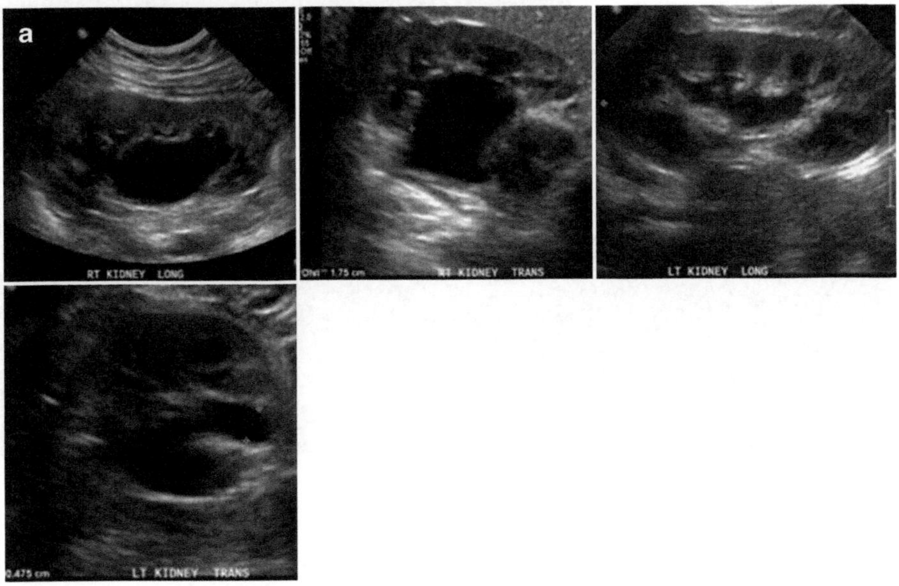

Fig. 9.7 (**a**) US at 4 months of age showing increase in right renal pelvis dilatation to 18 mm and prominent left renal pelvis. (**b**) DTPA at 5 months of age. Preserved differential function of 51% on the left and 49% on the right. No evidence of significant obstruction on the right. No evidence of VUR

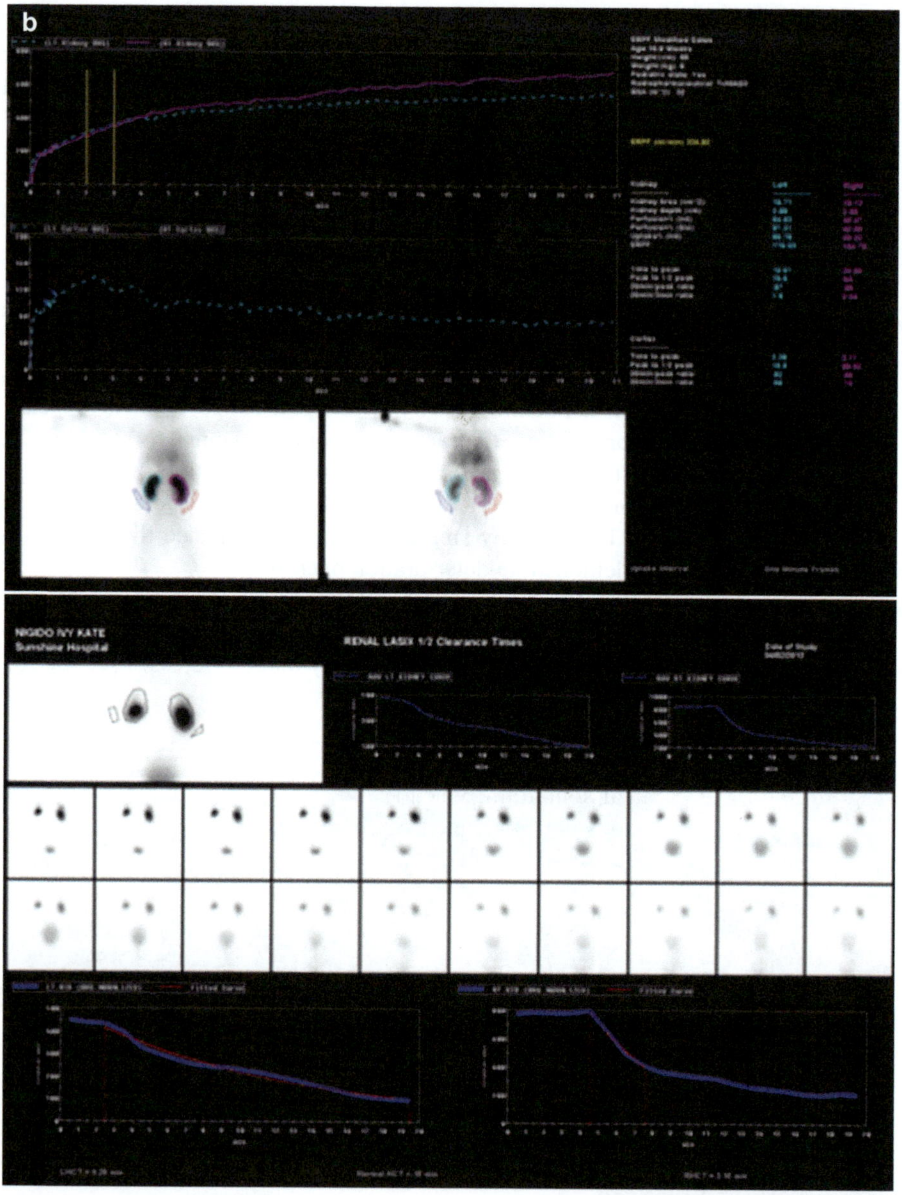

Fig. 9.7 (continued)

Of those that persist after birth, the majority will be low-grade [15, 16] (Table 9.3). However, if the antenatal renal pelvis APD is >15 mm in the third trimester there is an 88% chance of postnatal pathology [4]. Dias et al. [17], have shown that if prenatal APD is >18 mm in the third trimester and >16 mm postnatally, the sensitivity

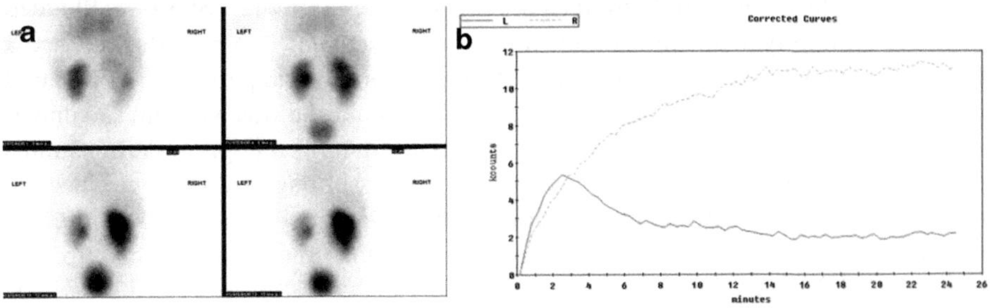

Fig. 9.8 (**a** and **b**) MAG-3 at 20 months of age. Preserved differential function of 52% on the right. The right kidney is enlarged with a medial photon deficient region. Activity is initially pooled in the right proximal collecting system, which appeared significantly dilated; following administration of diuretic the drainage on the right is slightly slower, with retained activity at the end of the study despite voiding

Table 9.2 Severity of antenatal hydronephrosis by APD [4, 8–10]

Degree of ANH	Second trimester (mm)	Third trimester (mm)	Postnatally (mm)
Mild	4 to <7	7 to <9	<15
Moderate	7 to ≤10	9 to ≤15	15–25
Severe	>10	>15	>25

Table 9.3 Distribution of antenatal hydronephrosis severity and likelihood of postnatal urinary tract pathology [4, 12, 15]

Degree of antenatal hydronephrosis	% of antenatal HN	% postnatal pathology
Mild	57–88	12
Moderate	10–30	45
Severe	1.5–13	88

and specificity of cut-off values to identify infants who would eventually require pyeloplasty for PUJO is 100 and 86%, respectively.

Postnatally, most cases resolve spontaneously without need for any intervention. About a third of infants with unilateral hydronephrosis (APD > 15 mm) and a differential function of >40%, remain stable on follow-up; almost 50% will progress to complete resolution or improvement to mild dilatation. Indications for surgery included worsening renal function, an increase in hydronephrosis (especially calyceal dilation) and a differential function of <40% on a MAG-3 scan [12, 15–17].

If the renal pelvis APD after birth is <15 mm, there is rarely a deterioration of renal function with time or need for intervention and many patients could be discharge after the initial scans. However, if the dilatation is >30 mm the likelihood of surgical intervention is high. The intermediate group of 15–30 mm pose the biggest challenge, as they need regular follow up [12, 16, 17].

In this case, the patient was diagnosed antenatally with mild bilateral hydronephrosis and the postnatal US urinary tract on day 4 of life had shown resolution of left hydronephrosis with only mild right renal pelvis prominence of 5 mm. She was monitored initially with ultrasound; however, subsequent imaging showed again bilateral renal pelvis dilatation larger on the right, with a renal pelvis APD of 18 mm right and 5 mm on the left. Due to the fact that the dilatation was >15 mm she underwent a MAG-3 scan to rule out obstruction. The MAG-3 renogram demonstrated good renal function without significant obstruction. Although subsequent US scans demonstrated some further progression of the dilatation on the right side, she remained asymptomatic and her differential renal function remained stable on the repeat MAG-3 scans.

The patient was managed conservatively and followed up with serial US urinary tract and NM scans, as there was not enough evidence on imaging to confirm obstruction and justify surgical intervention. To date, she remains asymptomatic with preserved renal function.

9.4 Case 4

A 5-years old male with antenatal diagnosis of mild left hydronephrosis identified at 20 weeks of gestational age. He was initially monitored with serial US of the urinary tract which showed stable mild left renal pelvis dilatation but was referred for further investigations at the age of 3 years for worsening left hydronephrosis.

Question 1. What Investigation(s) Would You Request?
MAG-3 or dynamic NM scan, to assess the renal function and determine if there is evidence of obstruction.

Repeat US urinary tract to assess the evolution of the renal pelvis dilatation

In this case, the MAG—3 scan showed preserved differential function and drainage. The patient remained asymptomatic and was followed up with US urinary tract after 6 and 12 months, both showing stable left renal pelvis dilatation and no other abnormalities.

A plan was made to continue conservative management and monitor him with yearly US. Unfortunately, he presented a few months after to the emergency department with severe left flank pain and vomiting. An urgent US urinary tract was performed, showing significant increase in the left renal pelvis and calyceal dilatation, with APD 32 mm (images not in system) (Figs. 9.9 and 9.10).

Question 2. What Is Your Main Differential Diagnosis and Which Investigations Would You Request to Confirm/Exclude That Diagnosis?
The most likely diagnosis is PUJO.

A MAG-3 scan was also performed, which again confirmed preserved renal function of the left kidney of 50%.

Cystoscopy and retrograde pyelogram study to assess the anatomy of the collecting system and drainage from the upper urinary tract in search of evidence of obstruction.

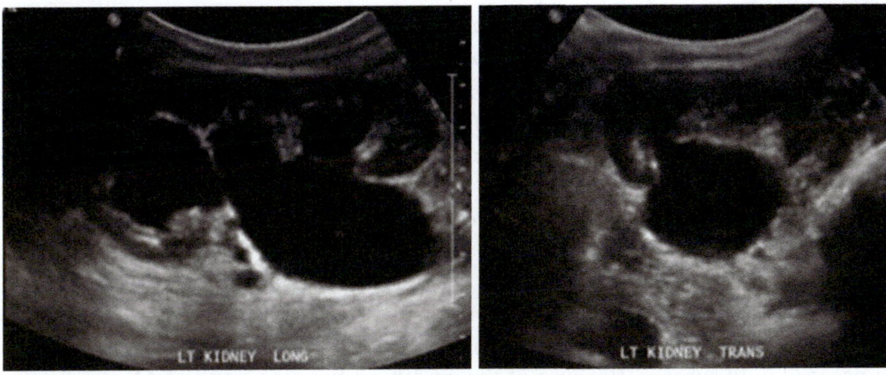

Fig. 9.9 US urinary tract at 5 years of age performed during the episode of abdominal pain, showing increased left renal pelvis and calyceal dilatation, with an APD of 32 mm

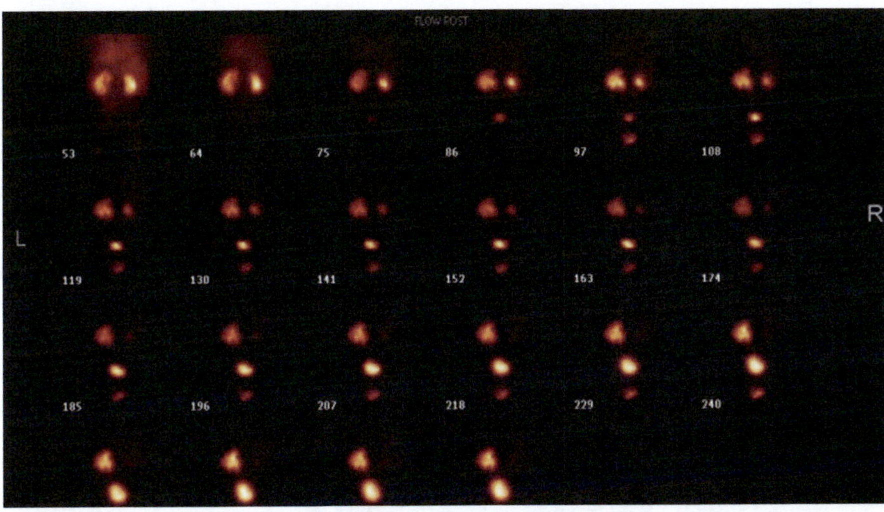

Fig. 9.10 Repeat MAG-3 scan showing preserved left renal function. There is delayed clearance from the left renal pelvis suggestive of a PUJ obstruction. The differential function measures 50% on the left and 50% on the right

Question 3

a. ***What is/are the best management option(s)?***
b. ***What would be your follow up plan?***

a. *This patient needs surgical management to avoid renal function deterioration. The main indication for surgery in his case are the symptoms and the progression of the dilatation on the US at the time of the symptoms, which are consistent with a PUJO. The technique and approach of choice are dependent on the surgeon's preferences and expertise, with different possibilities, ie: open vs minimally invasive pyeloplasty.*

In some centres, when the function is preserved, a cystoscopy with retrograde pyelogram is performed prior to proceeding with the definitive surgical intervention under the same GA. This allows assessment of the anatomy of the collecting system and the drainage from the upper urinary tract.

b. *The patient will require follow up around 3 and 6 months after the procedure with an US urinary tract. A repeat NM scan is indicated 6–9 months after in cases where the function of the kidney was already compromised before the surgery.*

In this case, due to the development of symptoms with increasing dilatation on the US during the episode of pain and high suspicion of a PUJO, decision was made to proceed with surgery. Because of the preserved function on the NM scan, a cystoscopy and retrograde pyelogram study was also performed to assess the anatomy and drainage of the left kidney, in order to confirm the upper urinary tract obstruction (Fig. 9.11).

We subsequently proceeded to a laparoscopic Anderson Hynes pyeloplasty without complications. Intraoperatively there was no evidence of lower pole crossing vessels and histopathology confirmed an intrinsic stenosis of the PUJ with increased peri-pelvic fibrosis.

Since the surgery, he has remained well, with no further episodes of pain and there has been significant decrease of his left renal pelvis dilatation of follow up US (Fig. 9.12).

9.4.1 Discussion

In this case, the patient was diagnosed antenatally with unilateral mild hydronephrosis and was monitored postnatally with serial US of the urinary tract, which

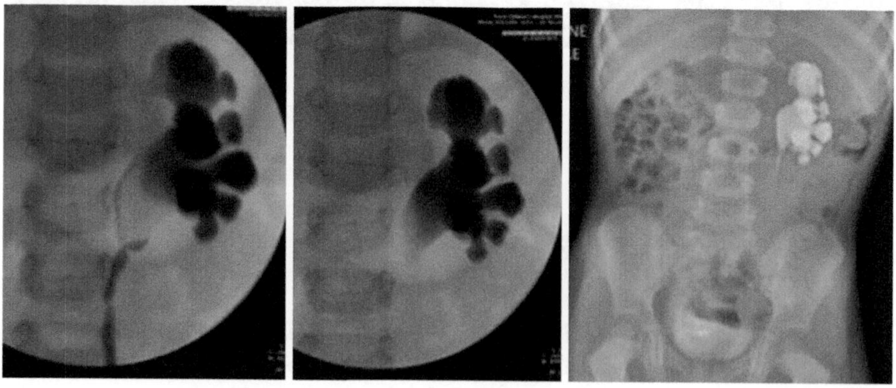

Fig. 9.11 Intraoperative findings on left retrograde pyelogram study and delayed abdominal X ray 1 h after procedure. Contrast was injected under direct vision, with evidence of an S-shape left PUJ and dilated renal pelvis. On the delayed abdominal X-ray, a large amount of contrast persists within the left pelvicalyceal system extending into the proximal left ureter, which appears narrowed; however, there was contrast within the urinary bladder

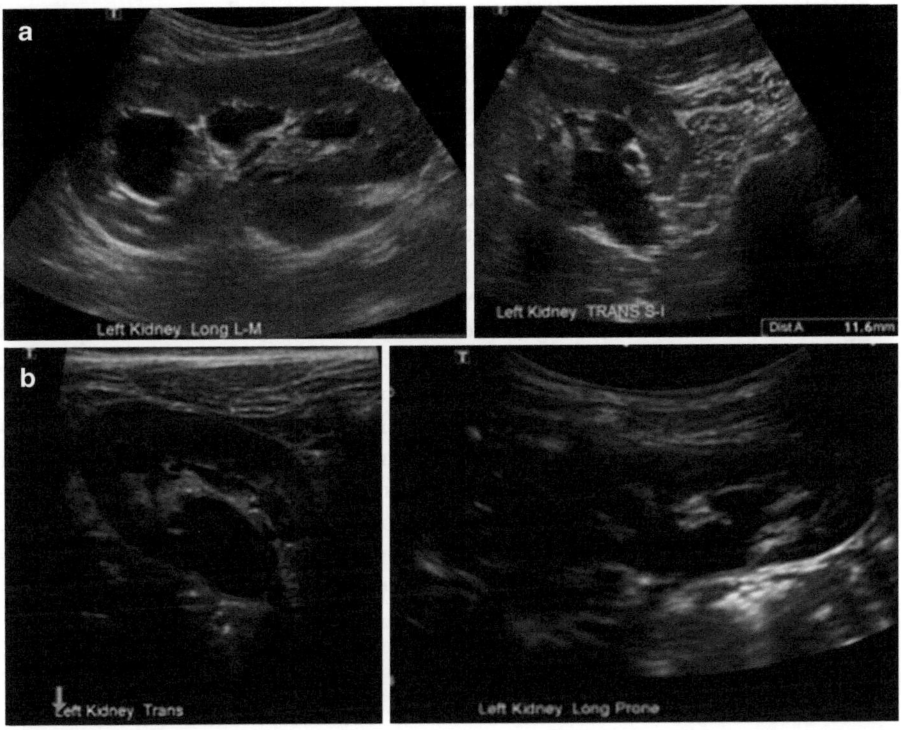

Fig. 9.12 (**a**) US urinary tract 4 months postop. Significant decrease in left pelvicalyceal dilatation, with renal pelvis APD 12 mm. (**b**) US urinary tract 9 months after surgery. Stable left renal pelvis dilatation, APD 10 mm

demonstrated stable mild left renal pelvis dilatation (APD 8–9 mm) until he was 3 years old and there was evidence of worsening left hydronephrosis with increase in the pelvicalyceal dilatation, APD 21 mm. Due to the severity of the dilatation, a MAG-3 was performed to rule out obstruction, but the left renal function was preserved. The patient was asymptomatic at that stage and subsequent US urinary tract demonstrated some improvement of the left renal pelvis dilatation. However, he became symptomatic and there was worsening left pelvicalyceal dilatation, with preserved renal function. Due to his symptoms and high suspicion of a PUJO, he could no longer be managed conservatively, and decision was made to proceed with surgical intervention. At our institution, in some cases we also perform a retrograde pyelogram study to assess the drainage and functional anatomy of the collecting system, the degree of pelvicalyceal dilatation, confirm the level of obstruction and determine if there is evidence of reduced and/or delayed elimination of contrast. Since the marked improvements in the quality of ultrasound examinations, the indications to perform retrograde pyelogram studies are more restricted, but there is still a role for this modality in some patients before deciding surgical intervention. Nowadays, this radiographic study is rarely necessary to diagnose UPJ obstruction, mainly because in most cases it does not change the surgical approach or planned procedure. However, RPG is still commonly performed before open pyeloplasty [8].

Because of his age, he underwent a laparoscopic pyeloplasty and histopathology confirmed an intrinsic stenosis of the PUJ with increased peri-pelvic fibrosis. He did not complain of further episodes of abdominal pain after the surgery and the renal pelvis dilatation decreased significantly on subsequent US urinary tract.

Indications for surgery in children with unilateral hydronephrosis are the presence of symptoms, failure of the dilatation to improve over time, and poor relative renal function or a reduction in function during follow up. The presence of pelvicalyceal system dilatation associated with renal colic in childhood should always suggest a PUJO and indicate surgical treatment. As mentioned before, the operation of choice is the dismembered Anderson-Hynes pyeloplasty due to its high success rate [18, 19]. The approach depends on surgeon's preference, although minimally invasive surgery is not commonly performed under 2 years of age. Open and laparoscopic dismembered pyeloplasty are comparable and effective methods for repair of PUJO. Operative time is the only variable that appears to be significantly different between both groups, with a shorter time for the open pyeloplasty [20]. Nevertheless, the type of repair should also consider family's preference for incision aesthetics and surgeon's comfort with either approach.

9.5 Case 5

An 8-years old male with no significant previous medical history and normal antenatal scans presented with central abdominal pain and haematuria. He subsequently developed further episodes of abdominal pain and an US of the abdomen and urinary tract was performed. He was referred for further investigations and management (Fig. 9.13).

Question 1

a. ***What does the US show?***
b. ***What other investigation might you consider and why?***

a. *The ultrasound shows severe left pelvicalyceal dilatation, with an APD of 39 mm.*
b. *A NM dynamic scan to assess the function of the kidney and decide further management.*

   An MRI/MRU could also be considered to identify the stenotic segment at the level of the PUJ or the abnormal vascular anatomy with lower pole crossing vessels. In some centres, MRU can also provide renal function. The downsides are the costs and the likelihood of needing a GA to perform the study.

The MAG-3 scan showed significant deterioration of left renal function with impaired drainage on the renogram (Fig. 9.14).

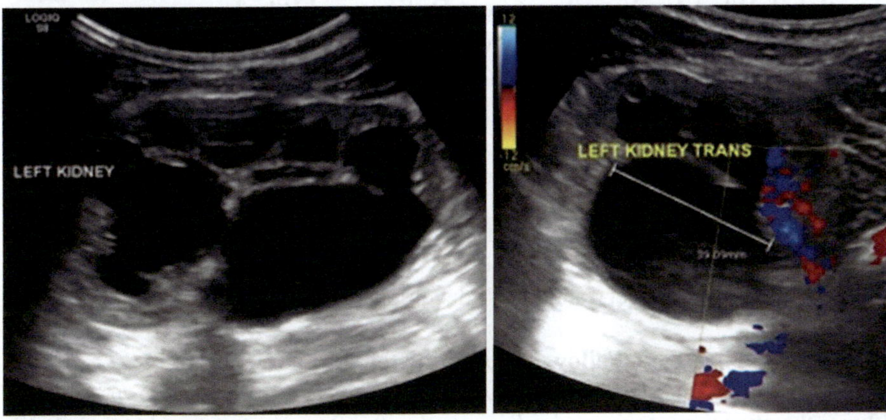

Fig. 9.13 US urinary tract performed during episode of abdominal pain

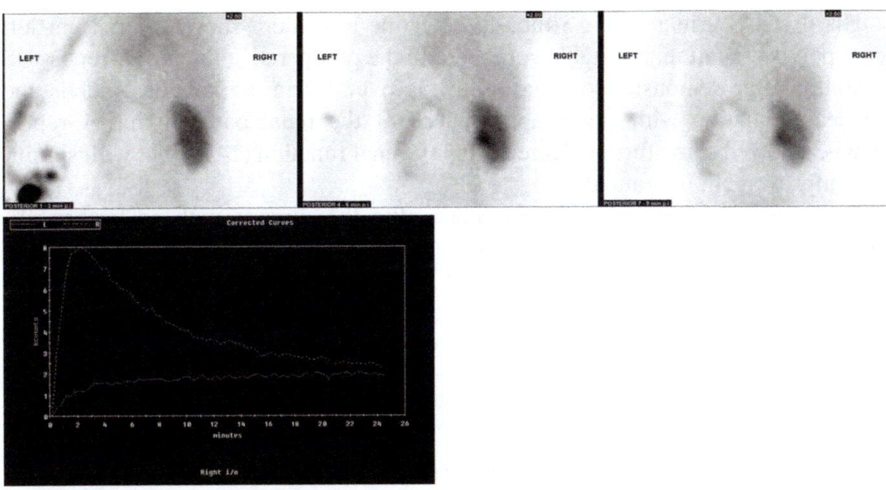

Fig. 9.14 MAG-3 scan after presentation. Markedly dilated left pelvicalyceal system and substantially reduced differential renal function (around 20%)

Question 2. What Is the Differential Diagnosis?

With the evidence of severe left pelvicalyceal dilatation and reduced function the most likely diagnosis is a PUJ obstruction. Because of the patient's age, the obstruction could be extrinsic due to Lower Pole Crossing Vessels.

Urinary tract lithiasis is also a possibility in patients that present with loin/abdominal pain and haematuria, however there is no evidence of stones in the collecting system on US.

Question 3. What Are Your Treatment Options and Why?
This boy should undergo surgical intervention to release the obstruction and preserve renal function. Considering his age, the approach should ideally be minimally invasive. If there is evidence of Lower Pole crossing vessels, he could benefit from a Vascular Hitch technique with transposition of the lower pole vessels (pyelopexy).

With these findings decision was made to proceed with surgical intervention. Intraoperatively there was evidence of lower pole crossing vessels causing obstruction for which a Laparoscopic Pyelopexy (Vascular Hitch) was performed. He recovered well from surgery and didn't develop further episodes of abdominal pain.

Question 4. What Type Follow Up Is Indicated and How Often?
The patient should undergo surveillance with serial US urinary tract at 3, 6, and 12 months after the surgery and subsequently after 2 years. A repeat MAG-3 should also be performed to reassess the renal function and the drainage through the PUJ, to determine if there are any improvements once the obstruction is relieved.

His first US urinary tract 3 months after the procedure showed persistent left renal pelvis dilatation, but stable compared to the preoperative images. A repeat US 6 months after demonstrated some mild improvement in the left renal pelvis and calyceal dilatation with stable appearances of the renal parenchyma. A repeat MAG-3 showed some further decrease in left renal function (14%), but with significant improvement in drainage.

He remained completely asymptomatic after the surgery, with no further episodes of abdominal pain, and serial follow up ultrasounds showed stable left pelvicalyceal dilatation with stable growth of the left kidney. His renal function also remained within normal limits.

9.5.1 Discussion

This patient presented with a symptomatic severe unilateral pelvicalyceal dilatation. The two most frequent aetiologies to explain flank pain with haematuria in older children are obstructive uropathy, in particular pelviureteric junction obstruction (PUJO), and urinary tract calculi. Older children may present with intermittent loin pain and a diagnosis is made on US scanning [9, 21].

The suspected condition in this case is a PUJO, because no lithiasis is visible and the ureter is not distended. In this age group the usual cause is lower pole crossing vessels, although an intrinsic defect may occur as well. A MAG—3 is mandatory to estimate the relative renal function of each kidney (in this case left kidney 20%). We can see non-homogeneous left renal perfusion and uptake, with poor washout of radiotracer after the lasix injection. A dynamic MRU or an angiography could delineate a more specific preoperative diagnosis, by depicting the anomalous vessels; however, the aetiological diagnosis should not change the therapeutic planning nor delay it, especially when there is evidence of reduced renal function [22, 23].

Surgical indications in older children with unilateral renal pelvis dilatation are symptoms, severe pelvicalyceal dilatation or worsening hydronephrosis on follow-up, poor renal function, and/or deterioration of renal function over time [9, 21]. Surgery is needed in this case because the left renal function is severely compromised, and the patient is symptomatic. At his age a minimally invasive approach should be offered. Intraoperatively there was evidence of lower pole crossing vessels causing obstruction for which a Laparoscopic Transposition of lower Pole Vessels (Chapman's Vascular Hitch) or Pyelopexy was performed. The Vascular Hitch is technically less demanding than a laparoscopic pyeloplasty and has lower complication rates. It is a safe, feasible, and attractive alternative to treat obstructed hydronephrosis due to crossing vessels [21, 22]. Careful patient selection is recommended, mainly based on the age of presentation and the intraoperative confirmation of this vascular anatomical variant. In some centres a preoperative MRU is performed to confirm the diagnosis. In this case, follow-up should include not only urinary tract US but also a dynamic scintigraphy to re-assess the renal function. The MAG-3 provides evidence of some further decrease in the left renal function despite significant improvement in the drainage, and the ultrasound shows some residual pelvicalyceal dilatation. His symptoms resolved completely. A delay in the diagnosis and treatment of a PUJO due to an anomalous vessel probably caused the renal damage. The presence of pelvicalyceal system dilatation associated with renal colic in childhood should always suggest an anomalous vessel and indicate the surgical treatment.

9.6 A. VUJO

9.6.1 Case 6

A 3-month old male with normal antenatal scans and no significant previous medical history is referred after developing a febrile *E. Coli* UTI at 3 weeks of age, for which he was treated with IV and oral Abs and was subsequently started on prophylactic Abs. He underwent an US urinary tract during the admission, which demonstrated moderate right hydroureteronephrosis (with distal ureter diameter of 14 mm and APD renal pelvis 17 mm) with significant calyceal dilatation. A nuclear medicine scan was also performed, with evidence of some compromise of right renal function down to 40% (Fig. 9.15).

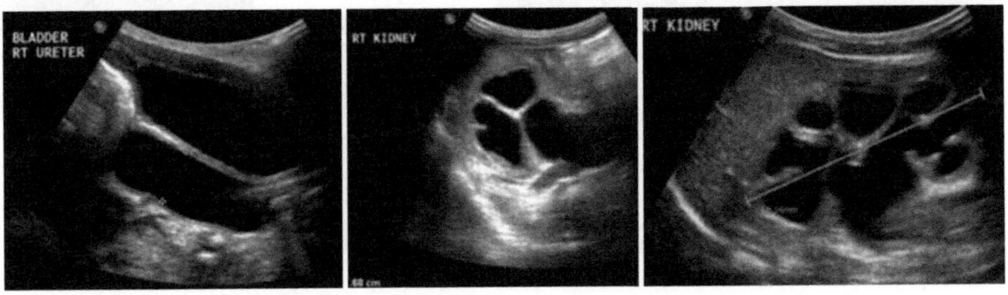

Fig. 9.15 (**a**) US urinary tract at 3 weeks of age. Right ureteric dilation 14 mm, moderate right pelvicalyceal dilatation with APD 17 mm. (**b**) DTPA at 4 weeks of age. The perfusion of the right kidney is reduced and the centrally photopenic area slowly accumulates radiotracer over the course of the study. The right ureter is very prominent. The right kidney contributes 40% of the overall renal function. The left kidney has good perfusion, cortical uptake parenchymal transit and drainage

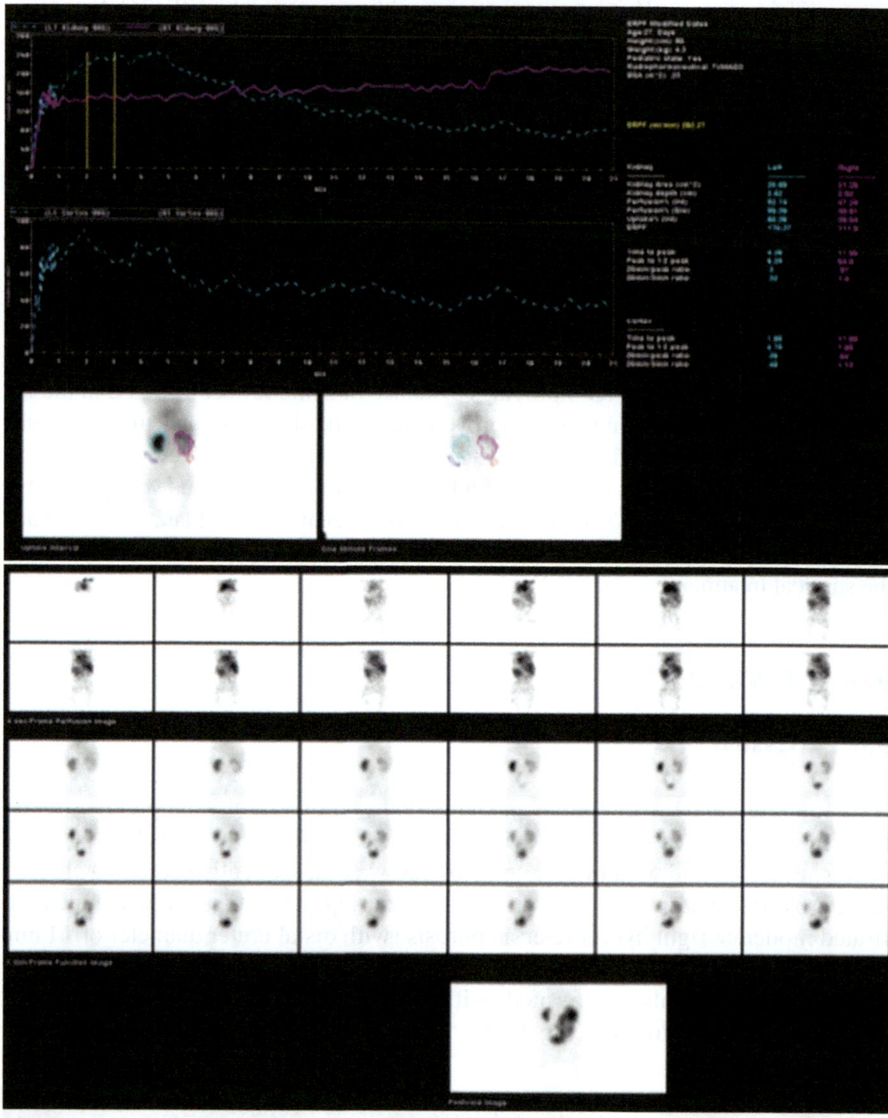

Fig. 9.15 (continued)

Question 1. What Is the Most Likely Diagnosis?

The most likely diagnosis is an obstructive megaureter due to the degree of upper urinary tract dilatation and the evidence of compromise of the right renal function; although VUR should also be considered.

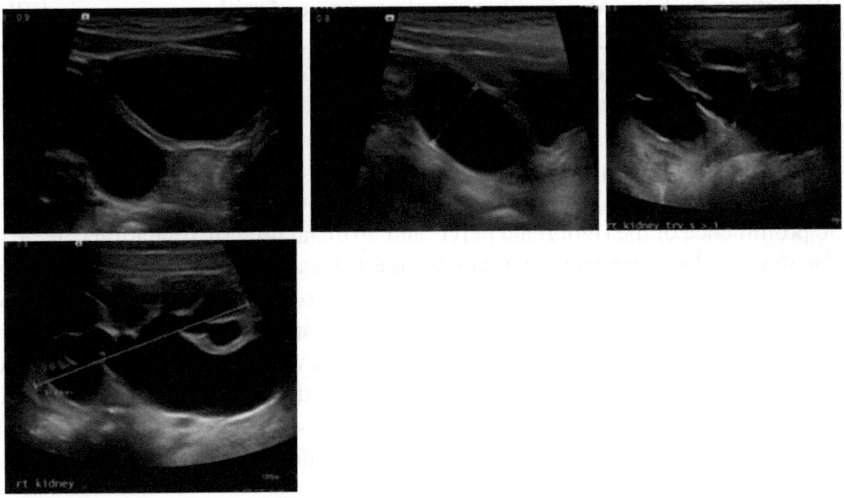

Fig. 9.16 Repeat US urinary tract at 3 months of age. Markedly dilated and tortuous right distal ureter up to 18 mm. Persistent severe right pelvicalyceal dilatation and worsening thinning of the cortex, with increased echogenicity. Right renal pelvis APD 14 mm

Question 2. What Is Your Initial Management and Why?

The patient should be started of prophylactic Abs to prevent any further UTIs and potential renal damage. A circumcision should be offered as well to reduce that risk and avoid long-term use of Abs. He should be followed-up with serial US at 3, 6, and 12 months of age and subsequently at 2, 5, and 10 years of age or until resolution or significant improvement of hydronephrosis.

Since prophylaxis was started, he remained asymptomatic; however, a repeat US of the urinary tract performed at 3 months of age showed some mild increase in the right distal ureteric dilatation to 17 mm and worsening calyceal dilatation with parenchymal thinning. On physical examination he was also found to have a right UDT (Fig. 9.16).

Question 3. What Would You Do Next and Why?

In this case, the worsening dilatation is an indication for surgical management which at his young age should be performed with a minimally invasive approach. The main options would be a cystoscopy and insertion of a JJ stent, or a cystoscopic endoureterotomy of the obstructed VUJ with insertion of a JJ stent. He should remain on Ab prophylaxis until the stent is removed.

He should undergo a circumcision under the same GA, to reduce his risk of UTIs and avoid the need for prophylactic Abs. His follow up should include an US urinary tract 6–12 weeks after the removal of the JJ stent and after 6 months, and a repeat NM dynamic scan to ensure the renal function is stable.

With these findings, decision was made to proceed with a cystoscopic balloon dilatation of the right VUJ and insertion of a JJ stent, right orchidopexy and circumcision to reduce his risk of further UTIs and further renal function deterioration. He remained on prophylactic Abs and the JJ stent was removed 3 months after (Fig. 9.17).

An US urinary tract performed at 10 months of age, 2 months after the JJ stent removal, demonstrated significant improvement of the right PC dilatation with only mild prominence of the right renal pelvis and no distal ureteric dilatation (Fig. 9.18).

He remained asymptomatic with no further UTIs and on Ab prophylaxis. He was reviewed 4 months after the procedure with an US urinary tract, which again showed right-sided hydroureteronephrosis, but reduced compared to the images performed before the VUJ dilatation. Subsequently a NM scan was also performed which confirmed stable right renal function, slightly reduced compared to the initial scan (35%). He was managed conservatively with follow up US urinary tract and the antibiotic prophylaxis was stopped after the first follow-up.

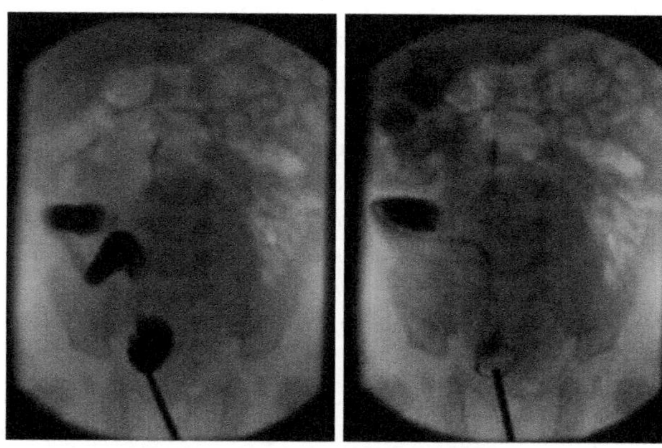

Fig. 9.17 Intraoperative findings on image intensifier for right VUJ Balloon dilatation and insertion of JJ stent. Significant right distal ureteric dilatation, with dilated tortuous ureter proximally and dilated collecting system

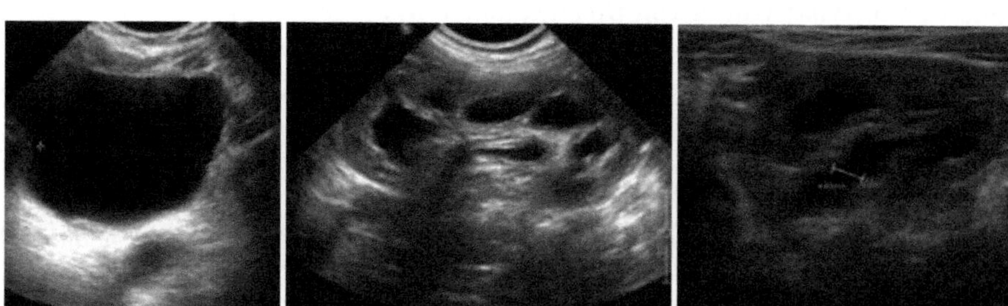

Fig. 9.18 US urinary tract after JJ stent removal. Mild right renal pelvis prominence, APD 4 mm, and no distal ureteric dilatation

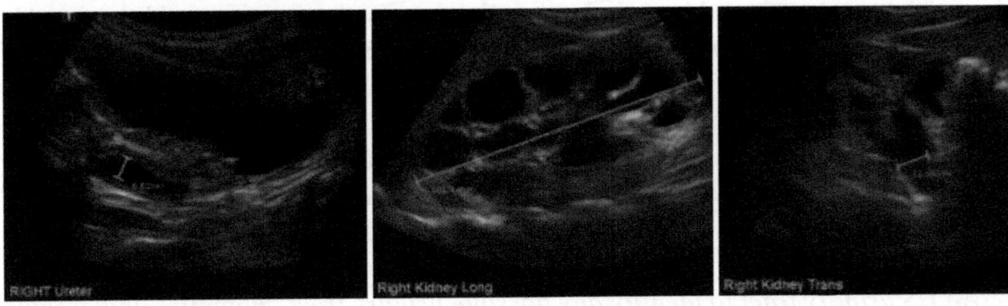

Fig. 9.19 US urinary tract 6 weeks after removal of the JJ stent. Right pelvicalyceal dilatation and global cortical thinning with significant improvement compared to the previous scan. The renal pelvis APD measures 11 mm pre-void and 14 mm post-void. There is also significant decrease in the ureteric dilatation, which measures 16 mm proximally and 6 mm distally, and increases to 20 mm post-void

The patient remained asymptomatic and UTI-free and the surveillance US at 3 and 4 years of age demonstrated stable right PC and ureteric dilatation.

He was reviewed again at 4½ and 5 years of age with repeat imaging. He was thriving, remained asymptomatic and was fully toilet trained. He had not developed any further UTIs. The NM scan showed stable right renal function; however, a repeat US urinary tract showed progression of the severe right pelvicalyceal dilatation with global parenchymal thinning and ureteric dilatation.

Question 5. What Would Be Your Management Now and Why?

Due to the progression of the upper urinary tract dilatation, in the context of reduced renal function, and the patient's age, the best way to proceed is with surgical correction of the VUJ obstruction to prevent any further progression of his condition and secondary deterioration of the renal function even further.

The options for surgical intervention include a minimally invasive approach, with the possibility of a repeat VUJ endoureterotomy, and ureteric reimplantation, which could be performed with open surgery or again with a minimally invasive approach with Laparoscopy or Robotic surgery.

Because of these findings, decision was made to proceed with a right ureteric reimplantation, and a Psoas-Bladder Hitch technique was used, leaving a JJ stent across the VUJ. He recovered well from surgery, without any complications and underwent cystoscopy for removal of the JJ stent 4 weeks after. He was followed up 3 months after the surgery with an US urinary which showed significant improvement of the right upper tract dilatation, with decreased PC and ureteric dilatation (Fig. 9.19).

9.7 Case 7

A 7-month old male, with no significant past medical history and normal antenatal scans, presented with 2 weeks history of decreased appetite, followed by vomiting and lethargy. Urine MC + S confirmed Citrobacter koseri infection; blood tests showed hyponatremia and hyperkalemia, slightly raised creatinine and leucocytosis with neoutrophilia. He was diagnosed with urosepsis requiring ICU management and IV antibiotics.

Question 1. What Investigations Would You Do Next and Why?
Because of the early presentation with urosepsis, male gender and the atypical bacteria causing the infection further investigations are required.

- *An US urinary tract to identify any possible urinary tract anomalies and exclude pyelonephritis or a complicated UTI*
- *A NM scan, depending on the US findings. DMSA to assess the renal function and possible scarring, ideally 6 months after the episode, or a MAG-3/DTPA to assess the renal function as well and determine possible obstruction of the upper urinary tract.*
- *MCUG, to assess for possible VUR, although the indication is controversial and may not influence management.*

As part of his diagnostic investigations an US urinary tract was performed which revealed severe left upper urinary tract dilatation, with renal pelvis APD of 24 mm and ureteric dilatation up to 30 mm distally, with layering debris in the lower pole calyx and ureter. He was treated with IV and oral ABS with good response, and was then discharged home on Px Abs. Once the infection was cleared a follow up US urinary tract and NM scan were performed to decide further management. The US urinary tract 2 weeks after showed persistent left pelvicalyceal and ureteric dilatation with improvement in renal pelvis dilatation down to 12 mm, but severe distal ureteric dilatation up to 25 mm. The NM scan showed preserved function of his left kidney of 45% and no evidence of vesicoureteral reflux (Fig. 9.20).

Question 2. What Would Be Your Initial Management with the Results of These Investigations?
The findings are suggestive of a left VUJO, with severe upper urinary tract dilatation but with preserved renal function, and the patient is symptomatic. Because of this the patient should be started on prophylactic antibiotics and should undergo surgical intervention to release the obstruction at the level of the VUJ and a

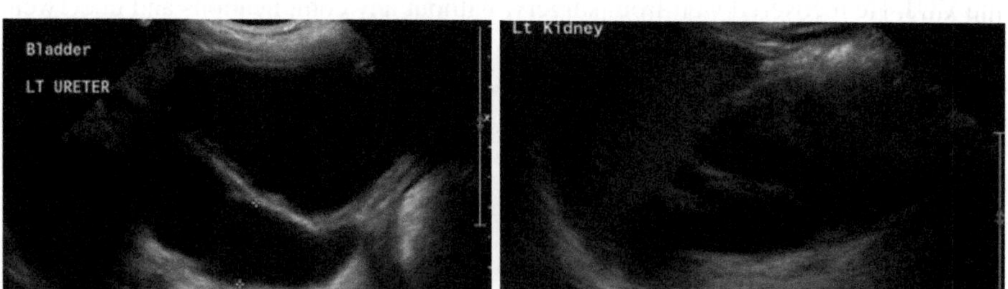

Fig. 9.20 US urinary tract showing severe left hydroureteronephrosis

circumcision; all of this to prevent further UTIs and prevent renal damage. At his age, there is indication for a minimally invasive approach and an attempt should be made to proceed with a cystoscopy and insertion of JJ stent to allow passive dilatation of the VUJ and circumcision to reduce his risk of further UTIs. The JJ stent can be left in situ for 3–6 months, but the patient should continue prophylactic Abs during this period. An alternative would be to proceed with endoscopic balloon dilatation of the VUJ, but this technique is not performed in all centres.

The patient underwent a cystoscopic insertion of JJ stent and circumcision at around 9 months of age. The JJ stent was left in situ for 6 months, with Ab prophylaxis cover. Follow up US and MAG—3 at that stage showed significant reduction in left renal pelvis dilatation, APD 9 mm, and reduced ureteric dilatation to 10 mm with JJ stent in situ, with consistently preserved left renal function and improved drainage compared to the previous study. His creatine remained normal (Fig. 9.21).

The patient underwent cystoscopy and JJ stent removal at 15 months of age without complications and antibiotic prophylaxis was stopped after the procedure. The patient remained asymptomatic and a repeat US urinary tract showed stable appearances of the left hydroureteronephrosis with some mild improvement in renal pelvis APD, now 5 mm, and distal ureteric dilatation 6 mm on last follow up (Fig. 9.22).

9.7.1 Discussion for Cases 6 and 7

Both patients had normal antenatal scans and presented with a febrile UTI and urosepsis, for which they underwent further investigations (US of the urinary tract and subsequently a dynamic NM renogram), which lead to the diagnosis of a Megaureter.

UTIs are the most common cause of fever due to bacterial infection in infants. In young children with febrile UTIs, especially males with atypical bacteria, an US of the urinary tract is usually performed within 48 h of diagnosis to confirm or exclude the presence of acute pyelonephritis and/or anatomical abnormalities [24]. Most patients will have a normal urinary tract, although in about 10–15% of the cases there is an underlying urinary tract abnormality responsible for the infection [25, 26], one of which is a VUJ obstruction. In such cases, further investigations are indicated, such as a DMSA or a MAG-3 depending on the US findings. The MAG-3 also has the ability to identify VUR in cases where voiding is achieved during the study. Nevertheless, reflux can be missed in 21–50% cases on indirect cystography [27, 28]. MCUG has a much higher sensitivity for the detection of VUR, up to 93%, however, we do not perform micturating cystourethrogram routinely at our institution, only when there is a suspicion of lower urinary tract obstruction or a urethral anomaly.

Nowadays, the clinical value of routine ultrasonography for young children with a first UTI is questionable because of the limited impact of those findings on clinical management, mainly because the proportion of children with clinically significant findings that would modify management is only 1–4% [24, 26]. Nevertheless, the diagnosis may lead to the use of antibiotic prophylaxis or even to an operative intervention. An example of this situation are patients with primary non-refluxing

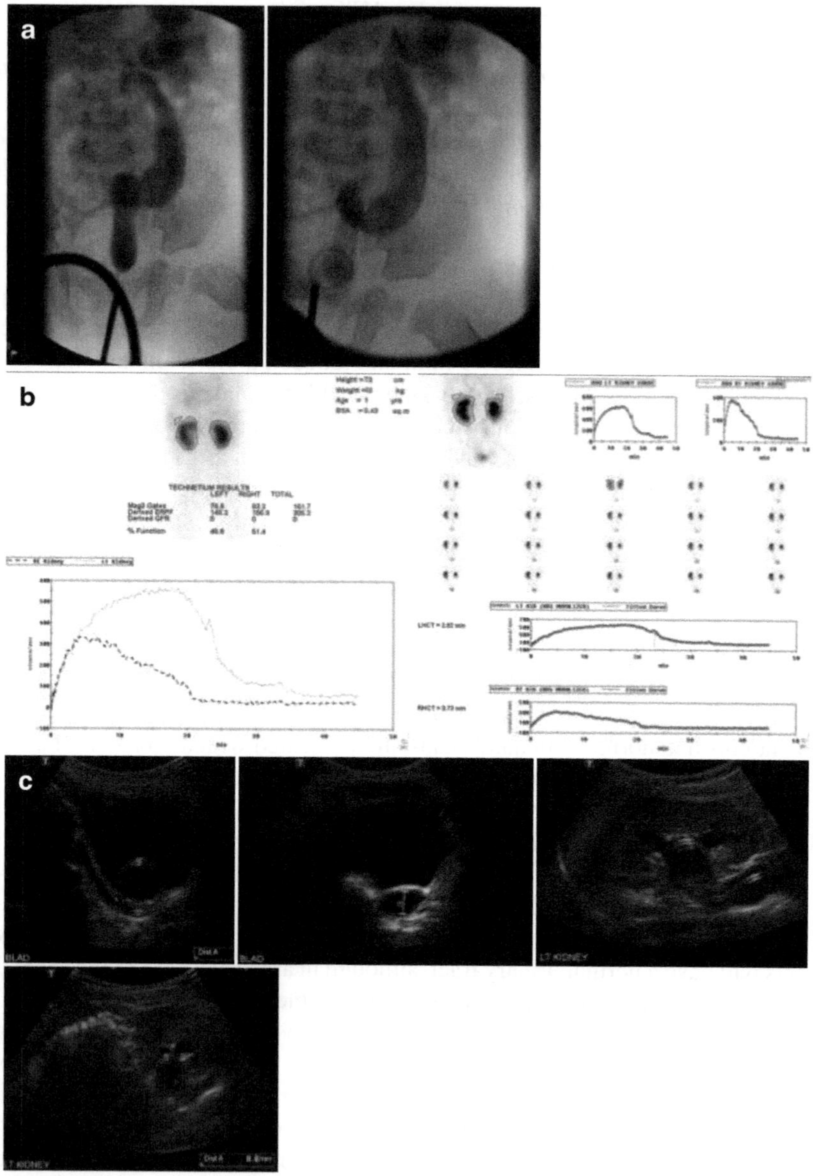

Fig. 9.21 (**a**) Intraoperative findings: Retrograde pyelogram with evidence of dilated left ureter and PC dilatation, and significant narrowing at the VUJ level JJ stent in situ. (**b**) US urinary tract and MAG-3 with JJ stent in situ: significant reduction in left renal pelvis dilatation, APD 9 mm, and reduced ureteric dilatation to 10 mm with JJ stent seen both in the renal pelvis and the bladder. (**c**) MAG-3 with JJ stent in situ. There is prompt and equal perfusion of the kidneys. The left kidney has less prominent medial photopenia than previously. There is normal cortical uptake and cortical transit. The left ureter is less tortuous than seen previously. Following intravenous administration of lasix there is prompt and near-complete drainage from the left collecting system and ureter. There is no evidence of vesicoureteric reflux during micturition. Differential renal function is preserved, of 49% on the left

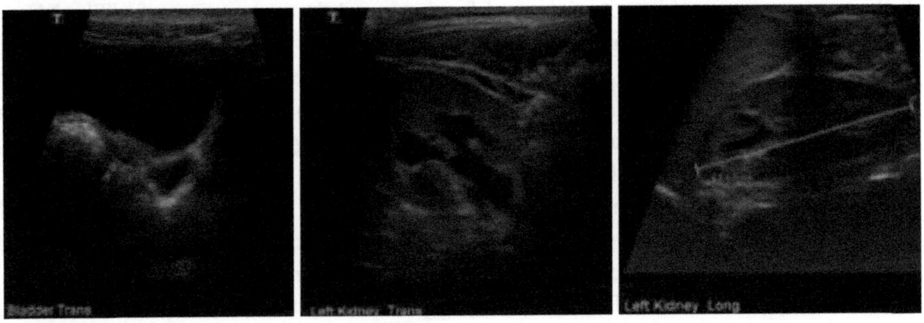

Fig. 9.22 US urinary tract after removal of JJ stent: stable appearances of the left renal pelvis (APD now 5 mm), and distal ureteric dilatation (6 mm) on last follow up

Table 9.4 The international Classification of Megaureter (Smith), modified by King [29]

Type	Primary	Secondary
Obstructed	Intrinsic ureteric obstruction	Intravesical obstruction or extrinsic lesions
Refluxing	Reflux is the only abnormality	Associated with BOO or neurogenic bladder
Non-refluxing/ non-obstructive	Idiopathic ureteric dilatation	Polyuria (Diabetes Insipidus)
Refluxing/ obstructive	Primary VUR with intrinsic obstruction	Associated with BOO or neurogenic bladder with a thickened bladder wall

megaureters in whom the hydronephrosis is likely to resolve spontaneously, but who also have a higher risk of infections and are therefore placed on prophylactic antibiotics and monitored [29].

A megaureter is characterized by a visibly dilated ureter of >10 mm to the level of the bladder. This may be associated with renal pelvis and calyceal dilatation based on the severity. Many of these will resolve spontaneously. According to the International classification by Smith, there are 3 types of megaureters: refluxing, obstructive, and non refluxing—non obstructive, all of which can be primary or secondary (Table 9.4) [29]. Megaureter is usually reserved for conditions in which the bladder and bladder outlet are normal (primary) but the ureter is dilated to some extent. Therefore, a more practical classification by King defines them as refluxing, obstructive, not refluxing-not obstructive, and both refluxing and obstructive.

Primary megaureter (PM) is a common cause of obstructive uropathy among neonates and young children, affecting up to 23% of newborns with antenatally diagnosed hydronephrosis [30]. PM is three to four times more common in boys than in girls and is bilateral in 25% of patients. The left ureter is involved more often than the right. Dynamic renography with Tc-99 m-MAG3 is indicated to assess the cortical renal function and confirm the level of urinary hold up with a full and an empty bladder. The diagnosis and treatment of an obstructive megaureter is still debatable. The indication to treatment is the presence of clinical symptoms, decrease of renal function, and dilatation. The aims of diagnosis, treatment, and long-term follow-up are the preservation of renal function and the prevention of UTIs. Many asymptomatic primary megaureters in infancy improve spontaneously and do not require surgical treatment. Because of this, many patients are currently managed conservatively [30]; these patients are followed up regularly and monitored with ultrasonography and nuclear renography until stable improvement or complete resolution of hydroureteronephrosis is noted.

Children with asymptomatic megaureters associated with preserved differential renal function can be managed conservatively. In these cases, circumcision [30, 31] and/or low-dose prophylactic antibiotics within the first year of life are recommended for prevention of UTIs while waiting for the dilatation to improve or resolve spontaneously. Close follow-up every 3 months with ultrasound is warranted, especially in cases with significant dilatation (>1 cm ureteral diameter). Improvement of many cases of upper urinary tract dilatation is more common when the degree of dilatation is less. Megaureters with associated mild renal pelvis dilatation are likely to resolve between 12 and 36 months of age; the ones with more severe pelvicalyceal dilatation may take longer to resolve, up to 72 months [29]. When the upper urinary tract is more severely dilated, patients may need antibiotic prophylaxis and/or a circumcision, because the larger dilatation of the upper urinary tract increases the risk of UTIs.

In some clinical scenarios, surgical management is necessary after failure of medical or conservative treatment: increasing hydroureteronephrosis, deteriorating renal function with permanent obstruction on scintigraphy, recurrent UTIs despite antibiotics, or presence of pain, pyonephrosis, or stones. Only 10–20% of megaureters require surgical treatment [29, 30]. In cases where surgical correction is required, the characteristic adynamic segment of the distal ureter just before its insertion into the bladder [8] can either be stretched/incised endoscopically using balloons or excised with or without tapering and reimplanted into the bladder wall. Traditionally, the surgical management of an obstructing megaureter has been via ureteric reimplantation with or without ureteral remodelling. Ureteral reimplantation has good results, with a success rate of 90–97% [30, 32, 33] and it's a safe procedure. The technique involves resection of the stenosis, remodelling-tapering if required and intravesical ureteric reimplantation. A minimally invasive alternative to this technique is the endoscopic balloon dilatation of the VUJ, with or without cutting atherotomes, with a reported success rate between 71 and 90% [33]. Other interventions may consist of simple drainage such as an ipsilateral ureterostomy, JJ stenting to passively dilate the VUJ [34]. However, most of these temporizing procedures have a modest success rate or work only until the child is old enough to have definitive surgery. In general, follow-up investigations using US and radionuclide imaging are performed between 6 and 9 months after surgery. After the first follow-up, prophylactic antibiotics are usually stopped if the child is toilet-trained.

In the first case, the patient was initially managed with prophylactic Abs, as he had only developed 1 UTI and his renal function was borderline (40%). However, there was increasing pelvicalyceal and ureteric dilatation on follow-up imaging. To prevent further deterioration of the renal function he underwent endoscopic balloon dilatation with JJ stenting to allow further passive dilatation of the VUJ and a circumcision to reduce his risk of UTIs. After the JJ stent was removed, the dilatation improved for a few months and he did not develop any further UTIs, although his renal function had slightly deteriorated further on imaging (35%). Despite the fact that he remained asymptomatic, UTI-free and with stable right renal function, subsequent US demonstrated further progression in the right upper urinary tract dilatation with severe pelvicalyceal dilatation and parenchymal thinning at the age of 5 years old. At this point it was decided, along with his parents, that conservative management was not a good option anymore and he underwent a right ureteric reimplantation without tapering, but excising the adynamic stenotic segment of the VUJ, which so far has proven to be successful. A 'Psoas Bladder—Hitch Procedure' was used in this case at the time of reimplantation, as it is a common ureteroneocystostomy technique used for the treatment of distal ureteric obstruction [35]. The technique of choice is debatable, although a Politano-Leadbetter Reimplantation augmented with a Psoas Bladder Hitch was preferred due to the large diameter of the ureter and its tortuosity, to stabilize a relatively long submucosal tunnel and allow excision of the stenotic segment of the distal ureter. The procedure involves bladder mobilisation by freeing the peritoneal attachments to develop the space of Retzius. With traction the bladder should reach superior to the iliac vessels. The ureter is identified and is transected proximal to the narrowed segment. An anterior cystostomy is then used to manually displace the bladder toward the ipsilateral ureter. The ureter is then delivered into the superolateral aspect of the dome of the bladder and the anastomosis performed, in a non-refluxing manner by placing it through a submucosal tunnel. The ipsilateral bladder dome is then anchored to the psoas major muscle with several absorbable sutures, taking care to prevent injury to the genitofemoral nerve. This technique includes three major advantages: mobilisation of the bladder with fixation above the iliac vessels to guarantee a tension-free ureteric anastomosis; formation of an adequate submucosal tunnel to prevent VUR, and implantation of the ureter into an immobilised part of the bladder to prevent kinking during bladder filling and emptying [35].

For the second case a similar approach was adopted, although his initial management was successful. Because of his age and the severity of his presentation, he was managed surgically with stenting of the VUJ and circumcision to reduce his risk of further UTIs. The JJ stent was kept in situ for 6 months and he remained on Ab prophylaxis until the stent was removed when he was 15 months old. The US performed after the JJ stent removal showed significant improvement of the left distal ureteric dilatation and almost complete resolution of the pelvicalyceal dilatation. Ureteric stents should be used as a temporising measure for children <1 year of age, until the child is old enough for a reimplant, if required during follow up [30, 34]. The complication rates from JJ stenting ranges from 12.7 to 40%, from UTIs to stent migration and damage to the VUJ. Cutaneous ureterostomies (loop or end stomas) are an alternative when an endoscopic modality has failed or cannot be performed, being a safe and effective temporizing procedure while awaiting definitive ureteral reimplantation [36].

9.8 Case 8

A 12-years old female presented with 3 months history of intermittent right-sided colicky abdominal pain, radiated to right hip and introitus, and haematuria.

Question 1

a. ***What are the differential diagnoses?***
b. ***What investigations would you request to confirm the diagnosis?***

a. *The main possible diagnoses are:*
   - *Primary obstructive megaureter that becomes symptomatic later in life. Can also present with abdominal pain and haematuria.*
   - *Distal ureteric stone causing upper urinary tract obstruction. This would explain the presentation with pain and haematuria.*
b. *A plain abdominal X ray, to look for a possible calcification in the pelvis which could be consistent with a stone at the level of the VUJ.*

   An US of the abdomen and pelvis and the urinary tract to identify the cause of the pain.

   Depending on the US findings, a NM dynamic scan to assess the renal function and determine if there is evidence of obstruction or a non-contrast CT KUB if stone still felt a clinical possibility.

A renal US showed right hydroureteronephrosis, with renal pelvis APD of 22 mm and distal ureter 25 mm. A Mag-3 scan was also performed, which showed preserved differential renal function (45% right) and prominence of the right ureter but no evidence of VUR.

Question 2. What Is Your Management for This Girl?
The patient has severe upper urinary trac dilatation likely due to a VUJ obstruction, with minimal reduction of the renal function, and is symptomatic. Her symptoms warrant some form of intervention. Considering that the renal function is preserved an option is to proceed with a minimally invasive approach and perform an endoscopic cutting balloon dilatation of the VUJ. An alternative is to proceed with a ureteric reimplantation, which can be done open or with laparoscopic/robotic surgery.

Because of her abdominal pain and ultrasound findings with severe ureteric dilatation, decision was made to proceed with treatment of her VUJO with cutting balloon endoureterotomy.

The procedure was performed endoscopically under II guidance with a Small Peripheral Cutting balloon and a JJ stent was left in situ for 4 weeks. During this period the patient remained on prophylactic antibiotics. At JJ stent removal a check cystoscopy was performed and UO was calibrated by distal ureteroscopy, allowing passage of a 9.5 Fr cystoscope easily (Fig. 9.23).

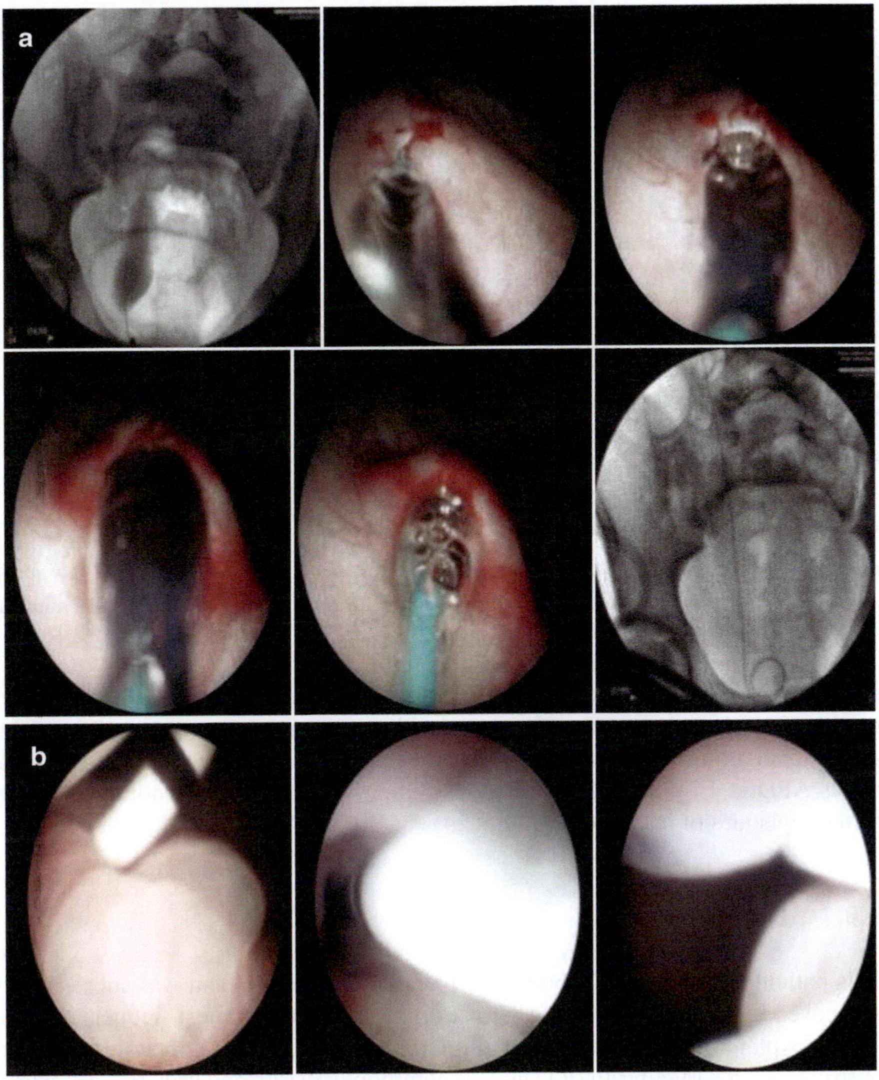

Fig. 9.23 (**a**) Intraoperative findings on fluoroscopy with contrast in the dilated distal ureter and evidence of tapering at the level of the VUJ. Cutting balloon endoureterotomy performed under direct vision and II guidance. (**b**) Intraoperative findings at repeat cystoscopy for removal of JJ stent. Right VUJ calibrated easily allowing passage of 9.5 Fr cystoscope along side of the JJ stent

Question 3. What Would Be Your Follow Up?

This patient should be reviewed 2–3 months after the stent removal with a repeat US. The ultrasound should be repeated at 6 and 12 months, because there is a risk of scarring at the level of the VUJ and recurrence of the obstruction. There is no indication for a repeat NM scan because the renal function was preserved, unless there is again increased ureteric dilatation or recurrence of the symptoms.

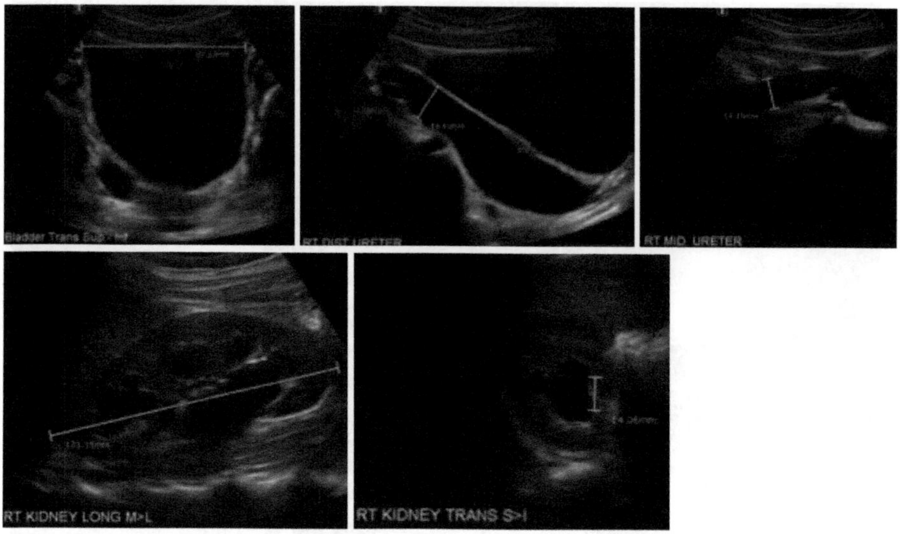

Fig. 9.24 US urinary tract 3 months after removal of JJ stent. Moderate right pelvicalyceal dilatation with APD 16 mm. Persistently dilated right ureter 19 mm distally and 16 mm in its mid portion. There is no significant cortical thinning

The patient was reviewed 6 weeks and 3 months after the JJ stent removal with a repeat US of the urinary tract, which showed significant improvement of the right-sided upper urinary tract dilatation, with ureteric dilatation at 19 mm and renal pelvis APD at 14 mm. Her pain had also improved, and she did not develop any further episodes of haematuria (Fig. 9.24).

9.8.1 Discussion

This patient presented with abdominal pain and haematuria and was subsequently diagnosed with right upper urinary tract dilatation. The two most frequent aetiologies to explain flank pain with haematuria in older children are upper urinary tract obstruction, in particular PUJO and less commonly VUJO, and urinary tract calculi [21]. In this case, the most likely underlying condition is a VUJO, because there is severe ureteric dilatation and there is no evidence of a visible calculus in the distal ureter. If the pain is under control and there is no evidence of on infected obstructed system, the patient does not need urgent surgical management and further investigations should be requested. A repeat US urinary tract demonstrated persistent severe right upper urinary tract dilatation and the MAG—3 showed slightly reduced right renal function (42%), with prominence of the right ureter and no evidence of VUR.

Surgical indications of VUJO/POM are the presence of symptoms, recurrent UTIs despite Ab prophylaxis, persistent severe upper urinary tract dilatation or worsening on follow-up, reduced renal function at presentation, and/or deterioration of renal function over time [29, 30]. A relative indication could be the presence of an obstructive drainage pattern on functional assessment, but probably associated to one of the indications mentioned above.

Surgery is indicated in this case because the patient is symptomatic, the severe upper urinary tract dilatation and mild compromise of the right renal function. We opted for an endoscopic approach for the management because of her age. At the time of JJ stent removal, the UO was calibrated by distal ureteroscopy, allowing passage of a 9.5 Fr cystoscope easily. This reassessment of the VUJ has been described as a direct measurement of success of the procedure [33]. The success rates of endoscopic management for primary obstructive megaureter range from 26 to 82% in the literature [34]. However, there is no data to determine which endoscopic modality is superior in management.

9.9 Case 9

A male patient born at term, is transferred on day 2 of life for further investigations and management of severe hydroureteronephrosis in a single left kidney. The patient had been diagnosed antenatally with right renal agenesis at 19 weeks and progressive left hydroureteronephrosis at 27 and 34 weeks of GA.

Question 1. What Would Be Your Initial Management and Investigations? Why?

Due to the presence of severe left hydroureteronephrosis and right renal agenesis, ie. Bilateral urinary tract pathology, it is necessary to exclude Posterior Urethral Valves and less likely urethral atresia. Because of this, an US urinary tract should be performed within the first 48 h of life to confirm the antenatal findings and assess the degree of upper urinary tract dilatation and the bladder appearances (wall thickness). The initial management should include insertion of a urethral catheter, assessment of renal function (UEC), commencement of prophylactic Abs, fluid resuscitation if necessary and correction of any possible electrolyte imbalance.

An US was done on day 1 of life, which showed a single left kidney with severe pelvicalyceal dilatation (renal pelvis APD 2.6 cm) and a dilated ureter up to 8 mm, and Cr on day 2 of life was raised up to 126 μ/l. A urethral catheter was inserted without difficulty with immediate urinary drainage and the patient was started on prophylactic antibiotics. He initially developed post obstructive diuresis with AKI and hypernatremia, requiring increased fluids. Even after the urethral catheter insertion, his creatinine remained persistently high for his age (Cr 107 μmol/l on day 5 of life) and there was persistent upper urinary tract dilatation on the repeat ultrasound (Fig. 9.25).

Question 2. What Would Be Your Management with These Findings?

Due to the severity of the upper urinary tract dilatation in his single kidney and the development of AKI, despite his bladder being on free drainage, the patient should undergo a cystoscopy for direct visualization of the posterior urethra and the bladder appearances, but also to assess the anatomy of the right VUJ to exclude

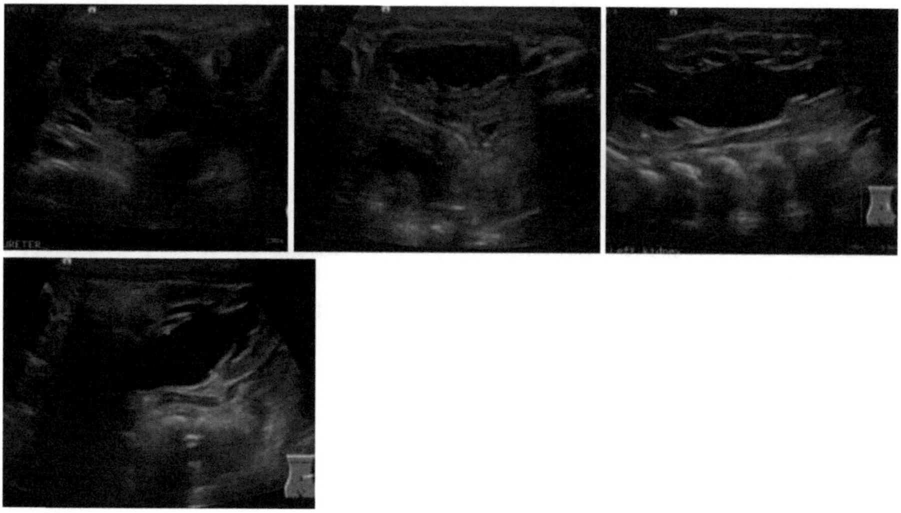

Fig. 9.25 US Urinary tract after insertion of urethral catheter showing a single left kidney with significant renal pelvis dilatation (APD 17 mm) and generalised thinning of the outlining cortical parenchyma. The left ureter was tortuous and dilated along its length up to 11 mm with a limited degree of bladder filling

obstruction. If there is evidence of PUV, the valves should be resected at the time of cystoscopy; if the urethra is normal and there is evidence of VUJO, a JJ stent could be inserted to allow passive dilatation of the VUJ. An alternative would be to perform a nephrostomy to allow free drainage from the single kidney and recovery of the renal function, to then perform an antegrade nephrostogram which would allow you to assess the VUJ. The disadvantage of the nephrostomy tube is the higher risk of infection and dislodgement due to it being an externalised catheter.

If the patient's condition is stable, there is time to perform an MCUG to assess the posterior urethra and the presence of right high grade VUR. If the MCUG is normal, a spinal US should be performed to exclude any associated spinal anomalies.

Due to the US findings with significant hydroureteronephrosis and the evidence of renal failure, decision was made to proceed to a cystoscopy. On cystoscopy, the bladder appeared trabeculated and the left UO appeared stenotic, however there was no evidence of bladder outlet obstruction. A retrograde pyelogram (RPG) and insertion of a JJ stent for treatment of a possible VUJ obstruction in a single kidney. A retrograde pyelogram study was performed to assess the anatomy of the collecting system and the drainage of contrast through the VUJ; the study confirmed the presence of an obstructed left VUJ for which a 3 Fr/8 cm JJ stent was inserted (Fig. 9.26).

Subsequently, his renal function improved with progressive decrease in his Cr down to 68 μ/l. A MCUG was performed, along with a spinal US, in view of the trabeculated appearance of the bladder, to rule out other anomalies. His spine appeared normal on US and the MCUG showed a normal bladder contour with no evidence of PUV and high grade left VUR likely due to the presence of the JJ stent.

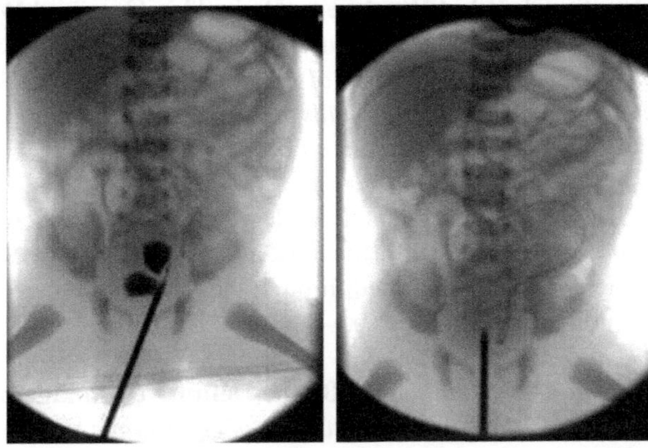

Fig. 9.26 RPG at the time of JJ stent insertion. Dilated distal ureter with change in calibre at the level of the VUJ

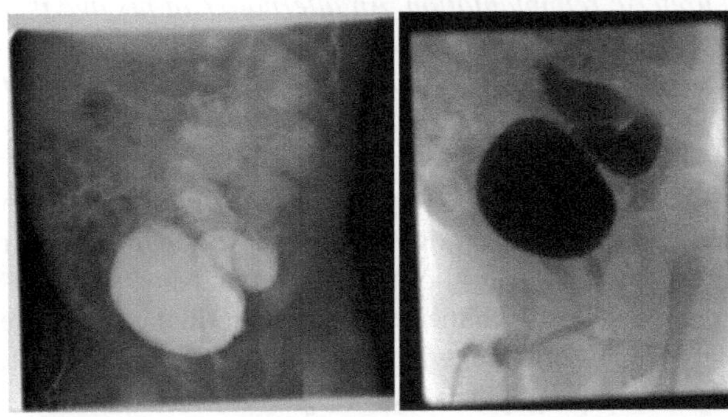

Fig. 9.27 Micturating cystourethrogram: normal bladder contour, high grade left VUR with JJ stent in situ. No evidence of PUV or urethral stricture

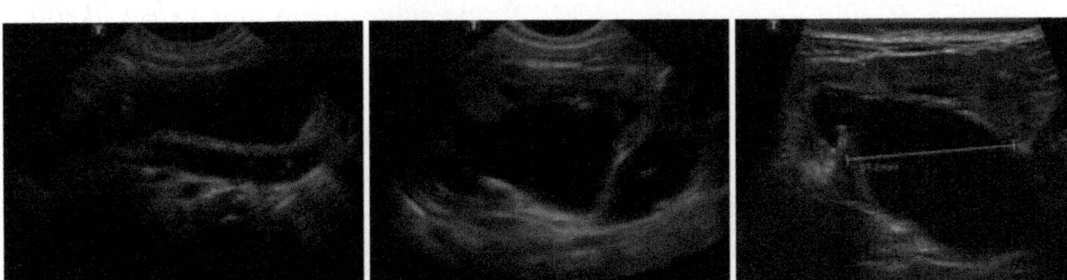

Fig. 9.28 US Urinary tract at 2 months of age. Severe hydroureteronephrosis with the distal end of the stent coiled in the distal left ureter. Worsening of left renal pelvis dilatation with thinning of the cortex

After this, the IDC was removed, and the patient successfully passed a trial of void. His Cr remained stable and he was discharged home on prophylactic Abs while the JJ stent was still in place (Fig. 9.27).

A follow up US Urinary tract was performed 2 months after, which showed increasing upper tract dilatation, with APD of 28 mm (previously 18 mm), with thinning of the cortex, and that the JJ stent had migrated up the distal ureter with the distal end not visible in the bladder anymore (Fig. 9.28).

Question 3. What Would You Do in This Case and Why?
Stent migration is a recognised complication after JJ stent insertion for management of a VUJO. Because of his young age a second attempt should be made to manage him with a minimally invasive approach and a second JJ stent should be inserted. He should remain on prophylactic Abs.

The patient subsequently underwent repeat cystoscopy and insertion of a new JJ a few weeks after. Unfortunately, a repeat X ray and USS confirmed that the second JJ stent had also migrated through the VUJO and there was persistent severe upper tract dilatation (Fig. 9.29).

Question 4. What Would Be the Definitive Management for This Patient?
Because of the 2 previous failures of endoscopic treatment and that this patient has a VUJ obstruction in a single kidney, he should undergo definitive management with a ureteric reimplantation. An alternative at his age is an endoscopic endoureterotomy, or the formation of an end ureterostomy, but this is also a temporising measure and he would finally require a ureteric reimplantation for the reconstruction of his urinary tract.

Decision was made to proceed with definitive treatment for his VUJ obstruction and he underwent an open left cross-trigonal ureteric reimplantation and left ureteroscopy for retrieval of the JJ stents. Postoperative US urinary tract showed progressive decrease in the left upper tract dilatation. He remained asymptomatic with stable renal function, with last Cr of 40 μ/l 3 months after the surgery, with no UTIs and off the prophylactic Abs (Fig. 9.30).

9.9.1 Discussion

This patient had an antenatal diagnosis of a single kidney with hydroureteronephrosis, and there was high suspicion of PUV due to the fact the underlying condition seemed to have affected both kidneys. He had been managed accordingly with insertion of an IDC, prophylactic Abs, assessment of renal function and transfer to a tertiary center for management. His initial US confirmed the presence of a single left kidney with severe pelvicalyceal and ureteric dilatation and his renal function at birth was abnormal, although the higher Creatinine levels were likely reflecting maternal renal function. Despite his bladder being on free drainage there was still severe upper urinary tract dilatation and his Cr remained high after 5 days, with the possibility of a VUJO as the cause of his acute renal injury. Because of this and his small age, decision was made to treat the obstruction with JJ stent to allow free drainage from the left kidney and assess if an improvement of the renal function would be possible. During the cystoscopy the urethra was also assessed to rule out PUV. Despite this, a MCUG was performed regardless in view of the trabeculated appearance of the bladder, to assess the anatomy and the posterior urethra and rule out VUR. A spinal US was also requested to ensure the cause was not a neurogenic

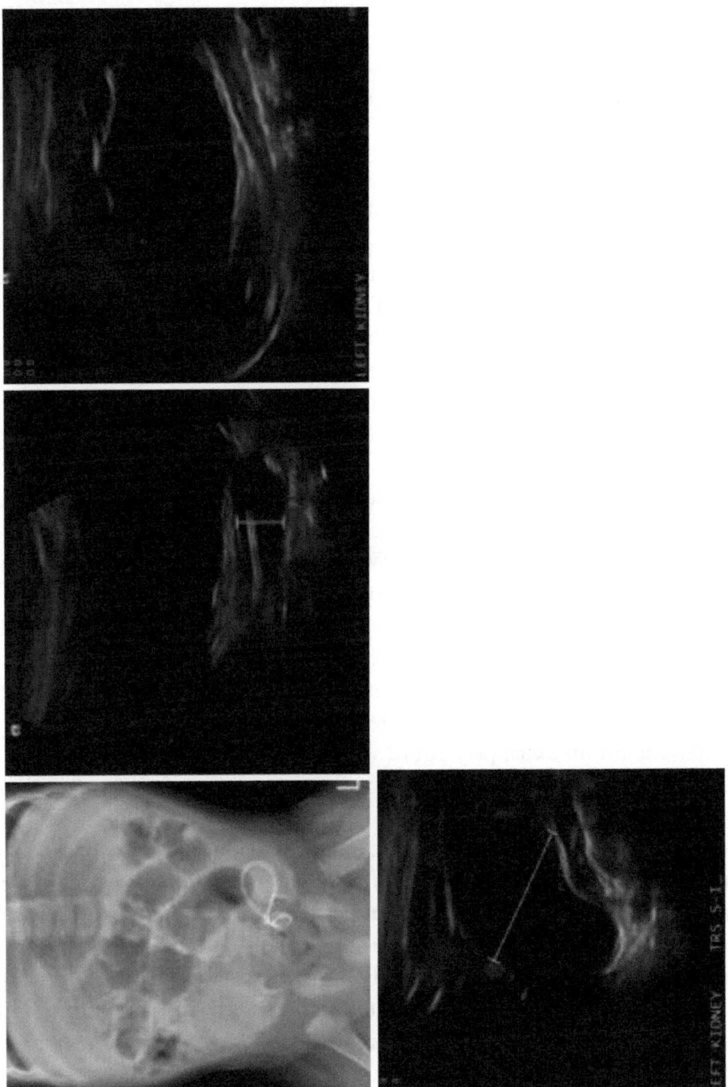

Fig. 9.29 Abdominal X ray and US Urinary tract: evidence of a second JJ stent also migrated and sitting in the distal ureter. Persistent left HUN, with distal ureteric dilatation of 9 mm and renal pelvis APD of 28 mm

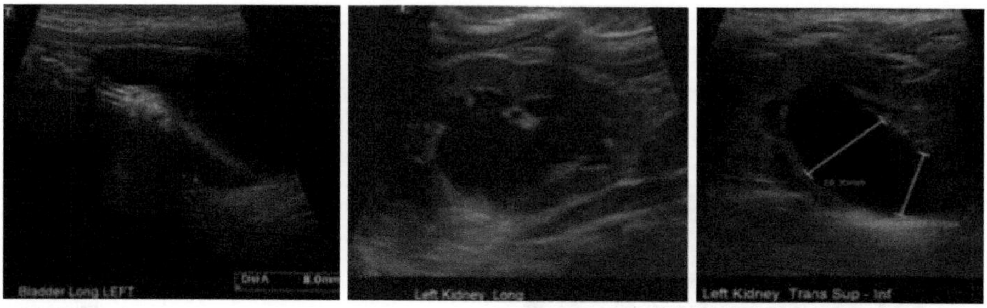

Fig. 9.30 US urinary tract 6 months postoperatively. Improved left renal pelvis dilatation with APD measuring 18 mm (previously 28 mm) and ureteric dilatation of 14 mm proximally (previously 18 mm) and 8 mm distally (previously 13 mm)

bladder, although his spine appeared normal on examination. His renal function improved with progressive decrease in his Cr down to 68 μ/l after the catheter was removed and he successfully passed a trial of void.

Unfortunately, this patient developed a rare but reported complication after JJ stenting [34] with 2 stents migrating up into the distal ureter and there was evidence of increasing upper urinary tract dilatation and thinning of the parenchyma, putting his single kidney at risk of further renal function compromise. After two failed attempts to manage his obstructive megaureter in less invasive manner, decision was made to proceed with open surgery, and he underwent a ureteric reimplantation when he was 6 months of age. We opted for a Cohen Technique as it is reported to be a safe technique with high success rates, despite his young age [30, 32]. In this case, the ureteric diameter was only 9 mm, and we ensured it could be safely reimplanted into the bladder with the appropriate length of the submucosal tunnel. An alternative of management would have been to perform a temporary cutaneous ureterostomy [36] and subsequently reconstruct the urinary tract, but this would have meant an extra procedure with no proven benefit. Cutaneous ureterostomies are indicated when endoscopic treatment has failed or cannot be performed.

This case illustrates how difficult it can be to confirm the diagnosis of an obstructive megaureter and why the management is so debatable. The indication to treat in this particular patient was mainly the deterioration of the renal function and the severe upper urinary tract dilatation with the subsequent findings on diagnostic cystoscopy and the RPG study. Because of his young age, the best and first option should be to attempt JJ stent and passive dilatation of the VUJ. As mentioned before, ureteric stents should be used as a temporising measure for children under 1 year of age, until the child is old enough for ureteric reimplantation, if required during follow up [34]. However, this modality was unsuccessful, and the patient developed complications in both occasions, making it safer to proceed with definitive treatment and open surgery.

9.10 Case 10

Four years old male with previous history of a left MCDK and right kidney with compensatory hypertrophy and hydroureteronephrosis, with normal posterior urethra and no evidence of VUR on MCUG, and 92% of right renal function on NM scan after birth. He subsequently developed mild HT and left ventricular hypertrophy, but with preserved renal function (Cr 0.4 mg/dl). He was referred after a follow up US urinary tract for further management (Fig. 9.31).

Question 1. What Does the US Urinary Tract Show?
The right kidney appears dysplastic and echogenic. There is moderate to severe right renal pelvis dilatation, APD 27 mm, and distal ureteric dilatation up to 16 mm. The left kidney was not visualised.

Question 2. What Is the MOST Likely Diagnosis?
The most likely diagnosis in this case is an obstruction of the vesicoureteric junction, which would explain the increasing right upper urinary tract dilatation.

The differential diagnosis is a VUJ stone, although there is no evidence of this on the US.

Question 3. What Is Your Immediate Management?
Even though the patient is asymptomatic, there is evidence of worsening dilatation in his functioning kidney with the possibility of a VUJ obstruction. This patient should not be managed conservatively and should undergo intervention to release

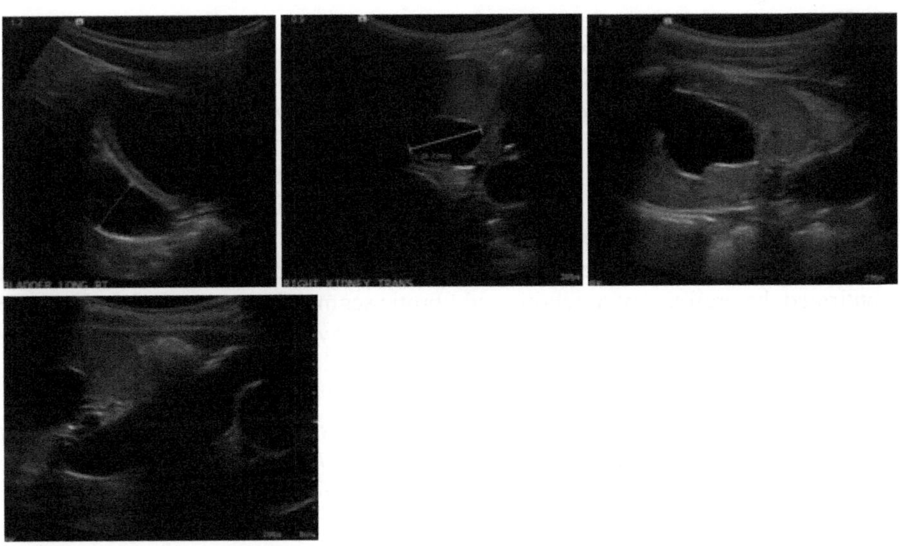

Fig. 9.31 US urinary tract

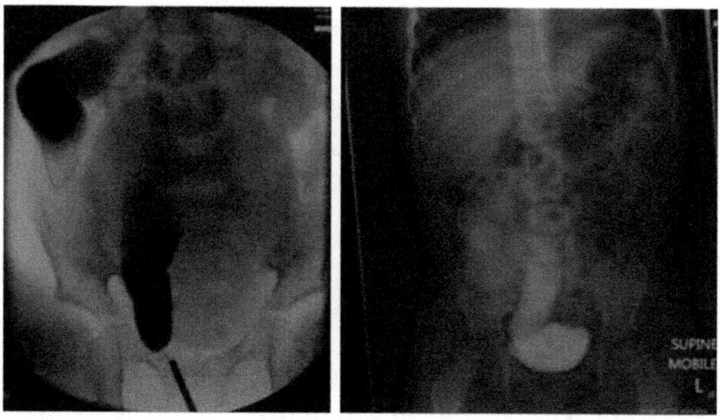

Fig. 9.32 Intraoperative findings and delayed X ray 75 min after injection of contrast showing significantly delayed drainage of the right kidney and ureter

the obstruction and prevent further damage of this single functioning kidney. The options of management are an endoscopic approach, with cystoscopic balloon dilatation of the VUJ, or a ureteric reimplantation.

In this case decision was made to proceed with a diagnostic cystoscopy, with a retrograde pyelogram and attempt at endoureterotomy with JJ stent insertion. On cystoscopy the right VUJ appeared narrow and initial catheterisation was possible, but the surgeon was unable to pass a 4.7 Fr JJ through the VUJ (Fig. 9.32).

What Does the Retrograde Pyelography and Delayed X Ray Show?

On retrograde pyelogram, the right ureter was grossly dilated and tortuous and there was minimal drainage of contrast into the bladder.

A delayed X ray was taken 1 hr after the procedure, showing a large amount of residual contrast in a dilated tortuous right ureter and some also in the bladder.

Question 4. What Would You Do Next?

Given that the option of endoscopic treatment was not possible and that this is an older patient, he should undergo a ureteric reimplantation.

Given the fact that he had a proven VUJO and we were unable to insert a JJ stent for dilatation of the VUJ, in the setting of a single functioning kidney, the patient underwent a right ureteric reimplantation with Politano-Leadbetter technique without complications. He recovered well postoperatively, and the histopathology report confirmed the presence of a stenotic and fibrotic segment at the level of the VUJ. He was discharged home on prophylactic Abs and antihypertensive treatment.

Question 5. What Would Be Your Follow Up for This Boy?

US urinary tract and repeat blood renal function tests at 3, 6, and 12 months and 2 years after the surgery. After this period, if the US appearances are stable, he could continue follow up with the nephrologist for his single kidney.

He remained asymptomatic and his renal function was stable (Cr 43 μmol/l). His first follow-up ultrasound 3 months after surgery showed stable left distal ureteric dilatation 17 mm, with significant improvement in renal pelvis dilatation down to 14 mm, and persistent diffuse parenchymal echogenicity. A repeat US 6 months after showed some mild improvement in the distal ureteric dilatation, down to 12 mm and stable renal pelvis dilatation, with a single simple cortical cyst. A NM scan was also performed, which confirmed normal right kidney perfusion and cortical function, with right hydroureteronephrosis but without evidence of significant functional obstruction. Subsequent USs of the urinary tract showed stable mild left hydroureteronephrosis with distal ureter measuring 8–10 mm and renal pelvis APD 10–14 mm. His hypertension remained well controlled and he didn't develop any further symptoms. He was last reviewed at the age of 9 years of age and his repeat US urinary tract showed stable mild prominence of the right renal pelvis (APD 7 mm) and distal ureteric dilatation, 16 mm (Fig. 9.33).

9.10.1 Discussion

This patient had a previous history of a left MCDK and a right dysplastic looking kidney with compensatory hypertrophy and pelvicalyceal and ureteric dilatation, with no function on the left side on a NM scan. He developed worsening right renal pelvis and ureteric dilatation on follow up with a suspected VUJ obstruction. Repeat functional imaging was not performed with the knowledge that the contralateral kidney was non-functioning.

Despite his age, in the setting of a single functioning kidney, an attempt was made to manage him endoscopically with cutting balloon dilatation and subsequent insertion of a JJ stent, but we were unable to cannulate the VUJ. This is a recognised, but infrequent, intraoperative complication [33]. A retrograde pyelogram study performed at the time of cystoscopy, confirmed the narrowing at the level of the VUJ with a grossly dilated and tortuous ureter, and minimal drainage into the bladder. He was old enough to undergo open surgery and a right ureteric reimplantation was performed. In his case, because of the degree of dilatation and to allow a straight channel for possible subsequent ureteral manipulation we opted for a modified Politano-Leadbetter technique. The surgery was successful, with subsequent improvement of the upper urinary tract dilatation and no significant functional obstruction on a MAG-3.

In this case, the management was also guided by the fact that the patient had a single functioning kidney with worsening dilatation. In cases where endoscopic treatment fails or is not possible, open surgery is indicated and the best option was a ureteric reimplantation. This type of reimplantation technique is a combined extra- and intra-vesical procedure [37, 38], which involves identification and mobilisation of the ureter outside the bladder and then opening the bladder to further dissect the ureter and detach it from its mucosal insertion. The ureter is re-tunneled in the bladder wall passing through a more cranial and medial part and creating a submucosal tunnel in the direction of the bladder neck, but through a different hiatus. The new ureteric opening is located superior and medial to the original one and the tunnel should be of at least 3 times the diameter of the ureter. The benefit of this is that you maintain the normal anatomic position with a straight channel for possible subsequent ureteral manipulation and that it allows for a longer submucosal

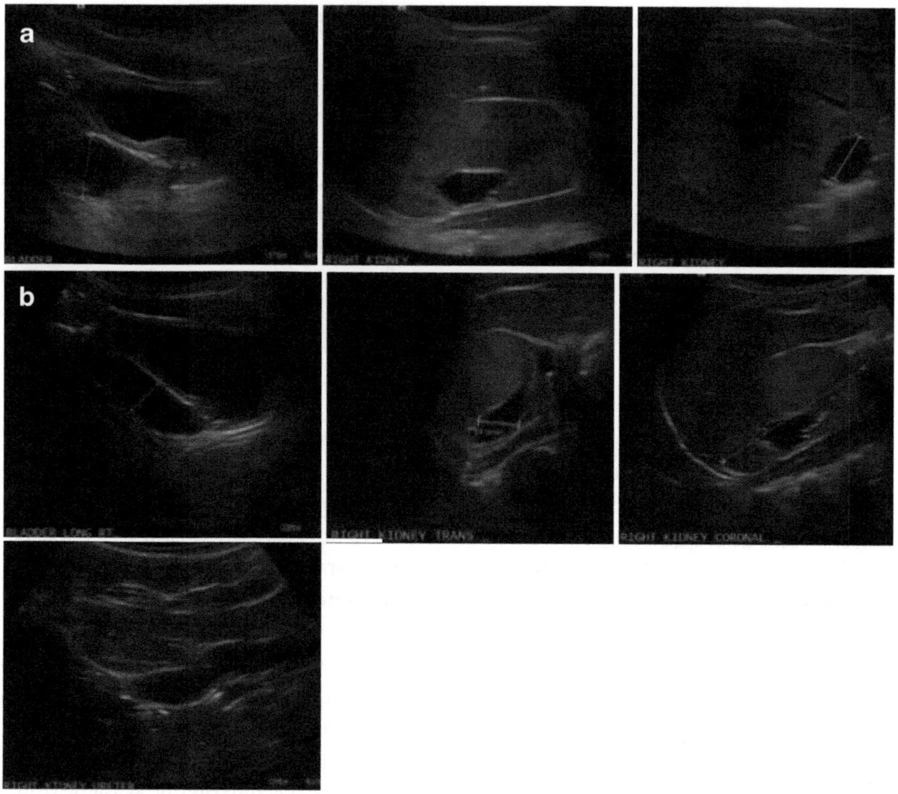

Fig. 9.33 (**a**) US urinary tract 3 months postop. Localised bladder wall thickening in the region of the right VUJ, at the site of recent implantation. Solitary dysplastic right kidney with persisting, non-progressive ureteric and renal pelvis dilatation. (**b**) US urinary tract at 5 years of age. Normal bladder appearances. Right renal parenchyma remains echogenic with loss of corticomedullary differentiation and evidence of cortical scarring. Stable mild right renal pelvis dilatation, APD 14 mm, and right distal ureteric dilatation up to 12 mm. (**c**) MAG-3 at 5 years of age. There is prompt perfusion of the right kidney and normal concentration of radiopharmaceutical in the cortex, with normal cortical transit and clearance into a dilated collecting system and drainage to the dilated ureter on this side. Following administration of lasix there is prompt drainage of activity from the right renal collecting system to the dilated ureter and bladder. The left kidney shows no function. (**d**) US 2 years post-surgery: Dysplastic echogenic right kidney with stable renal pelvis and ureteric dilatation, and good bladder emptying. The pre-void renal pelvic measurement is 14 mm, reduces to 10 mm on the postvoid imaging. There is a 12 mm lower pole cyst, is unchanged. A mild ureteric dilatation is noted measuring up to 8 mm. (**e**) US urinary tract at 9 years of age. Diffusely echogenic right kidney, with persistent mild prominence of the renal pelvis (APD 7 mm) and distal ureteric dilatation 16 mm

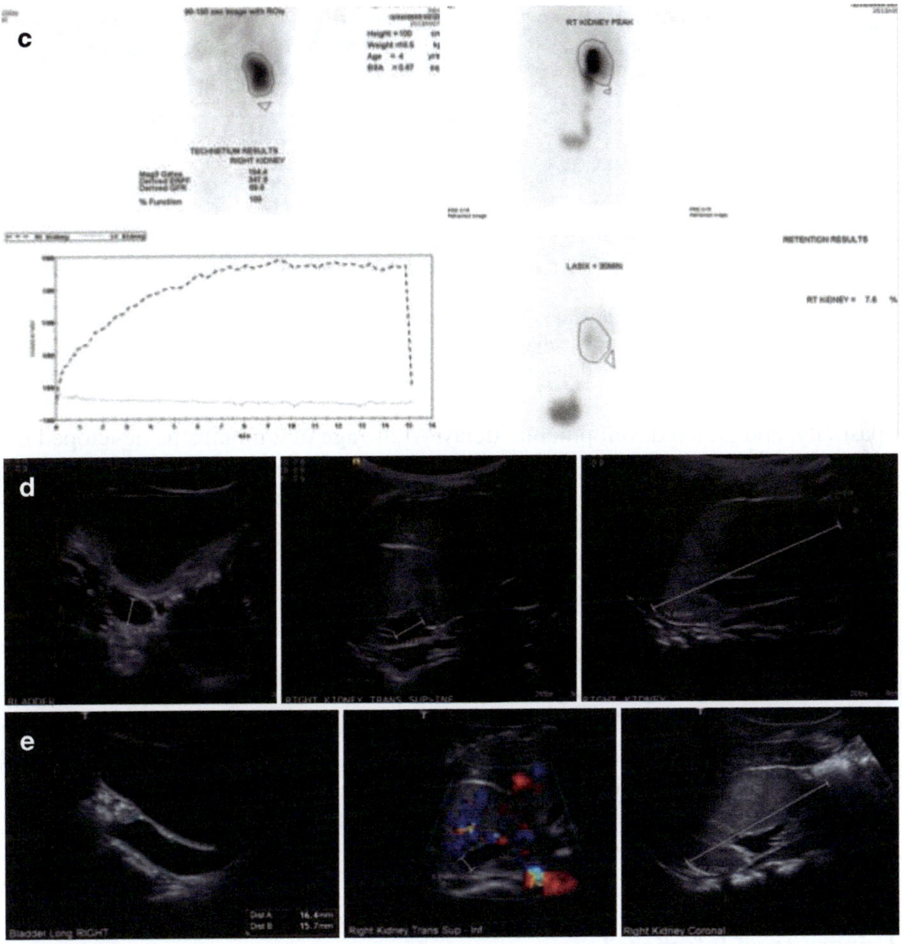

Fig. 9.33 (continued)

tunnel; however, there is a potential risk of kinking at the proximal entry into the bladder muscle, especially when the bladder is full and if the ureter is placed in the more mobile lateral portion of the bladder [35]. This procedure is still widely used during bladder augmentation for Mitrofanoff formation and for ureteric reimplantation of transplanted kidneys [38].

9.11 B. Duplex Kidney

9.11.1 Case 11

A 7-years old male is referred by the general paediatrician for recurrent UTIs. He was born premature at 30 weeks, due to maternal APH, but his antenatal morphology scan was normal. He also has cerebral palsy and left hemiplegia with leg

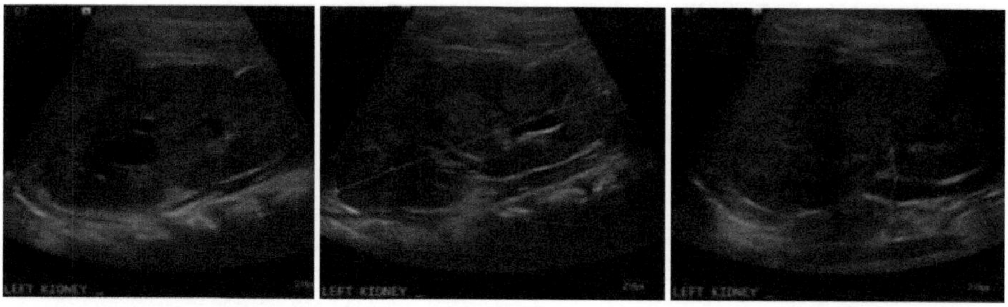

Fig. 9.34 US urinary tract at the time of presentation with a febrile UTI. Left duplex kidney with mild upper and lower moiety pelvicalyceal dilatation. The proximal upper moiety ureter is also mildly dilated. No distal ureteric dilatation

spasticity, and global developmental delay. At the age of 2 months he developed his first febrile UTI (Klebsiella Oxytoca and *Enterococcus faecalis*), and subsequently developed another episode at the age of 9 months (*E. Coli*), after which he underwent further investigations and was started on prophylactic Abs (Fig. 9.34).

Question 1

a. ***What does the US urinary tract show?***
b. ***What is the differential diagnosis?***

a. *The US urinary tract demonstrated a left duplex kidney with mild prominence of both pelvicalyceal systems, but without evidence of distal ureteric dilatation.*
b. *The main differential diagnosis is lower moiety vesicoureteric reflux because of the presence mild upper urinary tract dilatation.*

Question 2. How Would You Have Managed the Patient After the First 2 Urinary Tract Infections?
UTIs in duplex kidneys could be related to lower moiety VUR, especially if there is evidence of mild upper urinary tract dilatation. To prevent further UTIs the patient should be started on Abs prophylaxis, which should continue until he is 12 months old; a circumcision should be considered as well and offered to the family to avoid long term use of Abs.

He was managed conservatively with antimicrobial prophylaxis and monitored by the general paediatrician, remaining asymptomatic, with no further UTIs. His chemoprophylaxis was stopped at the age of 3 years old and he was fully toilet-trained by the age of 4½ years. At age of 5 years, the patient developed lower urinary tract infections again and underwent a repeat US urinary tract, which demonstrated a duplex left kidney with persistent minor fullness of the upper and lower moiety renal pelvis, but without ureteric dilatation. None of the episodes of infections presented with fevers (Fig. 9.35).

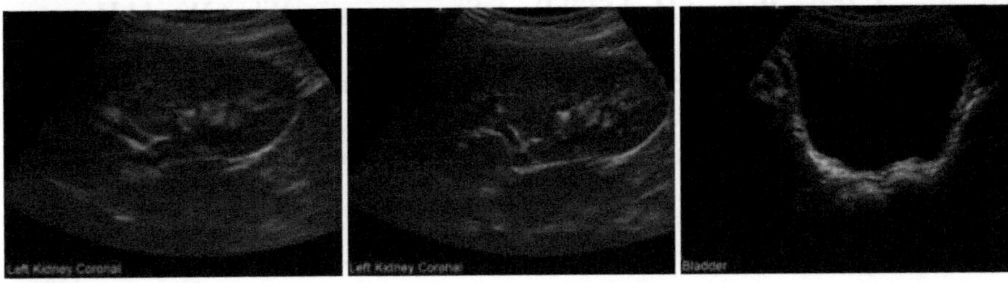

Fig. 9.35 US urinary tract at 5 years of age. Duplex/bifid morphology of the left kidney with persistent minor fullness of the upper and lower moiety calyceal systems, without distal ureteric dilatation and with complete bladder emptying

Question 3

a. ***What else would you like to know from his clinical history and physical examination?***
b. ***What other investigations could you request to confirm or exclude one of the differential diagnosis?***

a. *There is no information about his voiding, stooling, and drinking habits; bladder and bowel dysfunction are well known associated risk factors for UTIs at his age.*

   It was reported by the parents that he was fully toilet-trained before the age of 5yo; however, there is no indication of his voiding frequency, especially during the school time; the appearances of his urinary stream; the characteristics of his stools (for example with a Bristol Chart to assess for constipation), and his fluid intake or the type of fluid he usually drinks. On physical examination, it is important to examine his genitalia, in particular his foreskin and meatus.
b. *Due to the recurrence of the infective episodes and the persistent mild lower moiety renal pelvis dilatation, VUR should be excluded. This patient is now too old to easily undergo a MCUG, therefore the alternatives are a NM dynamic scan with indirect cystography, which would help determine the renal function and may confirm the presence of VUR or a DMSA to assess the presence of renal scarring (as an indirect sign of VUR).*

   A uroflow could also be performed during the clinic consultation to assess his flow patterns for signs of bladder overactivity or obstruction.

Because of the subsequent infections, a NM scan with indirect cystography was requested, which confirmed the presence of a left duplex system with equal function of both moieties and the presence of left lower moiety VUR. The differential renal function was preserved.

Interestingly, after that last episode at 6 years of age he did not develop any further UTIs and by the time he was reviewed by our team he had been asymptomatic for over 12 months. Therefore, decision was made to continue to conservative management with regular follow up with US surveillance.

Question 4. If the Patient Had Still Been Symptomatic, What Would Have Been Your Management Then?

There are 2 options of management in this case, and these should be discussed and agreed with the family. An attempt could be made to manage him conservatively again, but if this fails, he should undergo more definitive treatment.

(a) *Conservative management:*
   - *The first thing to address is any possible bladder or bowel dysfunction. The parents need to ensure he is voiding frequently, at least 6–7 times/day, and that he is drinking plenty of fluids, ideally only water. They should also determine how often he is opening his bowels and assess the type of stools to ensure he is not constipated. They should be given a bladder diary that includes a Bristol Chart to better document this.*
   - *Advice should be given regarding timed and regular voiding, adequate fluid intake and avoiding bladder irritants such as caffeinated and carbonated drinks*
   - *Control of constipation with laxatives may be necessary*
   - *There is some limited evidence for the benefit of Cranberries (because of Anthrocyanadin), Probiotics and D-mannose (interferes in vitro with bacterial adhesion).*
   - *Antibiotic prophylaxis can be considered for a short period if the UTIs are occurring too often, to break the cycle and allow time for the rest of the management to be effective*

(b) *Surgical management:*
   - *Endoscopic treatment of the VUR with a bulking agent—first line choice. May be a challenging procedure due to the anatomy of both UOs and their location, but it has a reported success rate of up to 80–85%.*
   - *Ureteric reimplantation as a more definitive procedure with a success rate of up to 97%*

9.11.2 Discussion

This patient had normal kidneys on antenatal scans but presented with febrile UTIs in infancy and was diagnosed with a duplex kidney. He was initially managed conservatively with prophylactic Abs and regular monitoring. Due to a favourable progression the prophylaxis was stopped at the age of 3 years old, but he developed further UTIs a couple of years after. This triggered further investigations to assess for possible associated VUR or bladder dysfunction as the cause for the UTIs. A NM scan with indirect cystography confirmed a left duplex system with lower moiety VUR and preserved differential function. After this, he remained UTI free again, and decision was made to just monitor him.

VUR is the most common associated anomaly found in duplex kidneys and it is present in almost 70% of these patients who present with a UTI [39–41]. In duplex systems, VUR almost always occurs into the lower-pole moiety due to its abnormal placement within the bladder [39].

There are certain factors that contribute to reflux resolution in single-system ureters, including patient age, grade of reflux, postnatal presentation, and the presence or absence of associated voiding dysfunction [41]. However, the natural history of VUR in association with duplex systems is not completely clear. Some studies conclude that the resolution rates for low grades (I–III) is comparable to the ones seen in single systems, although other studies state that the resolution is at least three times less in duplex systems and that it may take longer [40]. Despite this, most patients with duplex kidneys and low grade VUR can initially be managed conservatively with antibiotics and careful observation. Parents should be counselled that it may take longer for the reflux to resolve and for young females with high-grade VUR there may be an increased risk for infections. An alternative in boys is the possibility to perform a circumcision which can reduce the risk of infections and prevents the use of long-term antimicrobial prophylaxis [31, 42]. Nevertheless, the absolute indication for definitive surgery in individuals with low-grade VUR is not different from those with single systems and similar VUR, and surgical correction is successful in the majority of cases [32].

9.12 Case 12

A 7-months old boy with antenatal diagnosis of hydronephrosis identified at 20 weeks of gestation is referred for further management after he underwent a repeat US of his urinary tract. He was born term, was thriving and had remained asymptomatic since birth (Fig. 9.36).

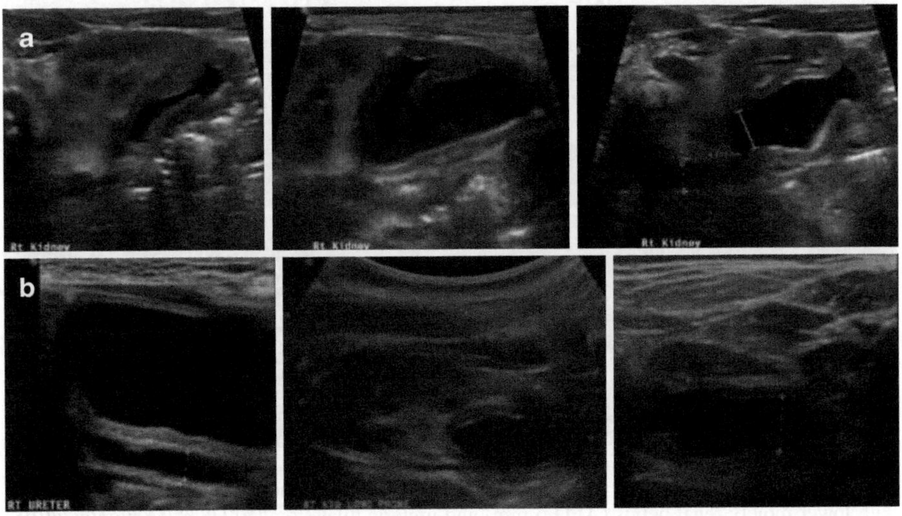

Fig. 9.36 (**a**) US urinary tract on day 4 of life. (**b**) Repeat US urinary tract at 4 months of age

Question 1. What Do the US Images Show?

The first US shows a right duplex kidney with lower moiety dilatation, APD 7 mm, and thinned cortex. The lower moiety ureter is dilated and tortuous proximally, but there is no evidence of distal ureteric dilatation.

The second one shows persistent right lower moiety dilatation, APD 10 mm, with thinning of the cortex and proximal ureteric dilatation. Now there is evidence of distal ureteric dilatation up to 6 mm.

Question 2. How Would You Manage Him with These US Findings?

The patient should be managed conservatively, although a circumcision could be offered to the family because of the presence of upper urinary tract dilatation, to reduce his risk of infections. Since he has remained asymptomatic there is no indication for antibiotic prophylaxis.

He should undergo regular follow up and surveillance with US to assess the degree of dilatation and its progression. A NM scan could have also been done when he was referred to assess the function of the lower moiety and potentially also determine the presence of VUR.

Due to the fact that he had remained asymptomatic decision was made to continue to monitor him with serial US urinary tract. A repeat US performed at 9 months of age showed stable appearances of the right duplex kidney with lower moiety renal pelvis and proximal ureteric dilatation.

Unfortunately, 2 months after his last appointment the patient developed 2 febrile UTIs requiring admission for treatment with IV Abs. After the last episode a repeat US demonstrated no progression in the degree of upper urinary tract dilatation (Fig. 9.37).

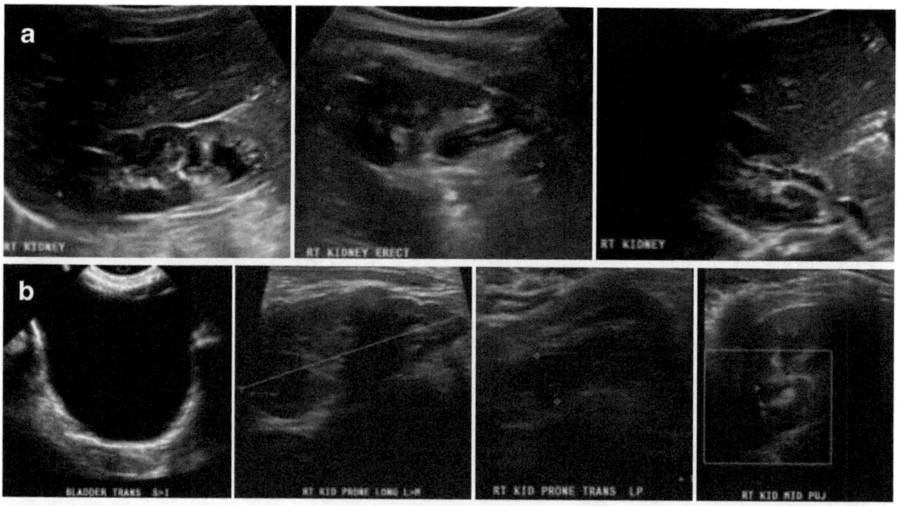

Fig. 9.37 (**a**) US urinary tract at 9 months of age. Stable appearances of the right duplex kidney with lower moiety renal pelvis (APD 6 mm) and ureteric dilatation. (**b**) US at 14 months of age after the second febrile UTI. Stable appearances of the right duplex kidney with lower moiety renal pelvis (APD 9 mm) and ureteric dilatation. Persistent cortical thinning of the lower moiety. No evidence of distal ureteric dilatation

Question 3. How Would This Change Your Management?

The patient should be started on prophylactic Abs to prevent any further UTI and renal damage.

Although he is over 12 months of age a circumcision should be offer to the family with the potential benefit of reducing the risk of further infections.

A NM scan, ideally with indirect cystography, should be performed as well to assess the renal function, mainly of the lower moiety, and to determine if there is VUR or not. An alternative, but more invasive, is to perform a MCUG which should only be done in cases of failure of treatment, when no VUR was detected with indirect cystography, to decide if surgical management is required.

In his case a NM scan with indirect cystography was performed to assess the differential function of the duplex kidney, and to determine the presence of VUR (Fig. 9.38).

Question 4. What Does the NM Scan Show?

Appearances are consistent with a right duplex kidney. There is normal perfusion, cortical function and drainage from the right upper moiety. The right lower moiety

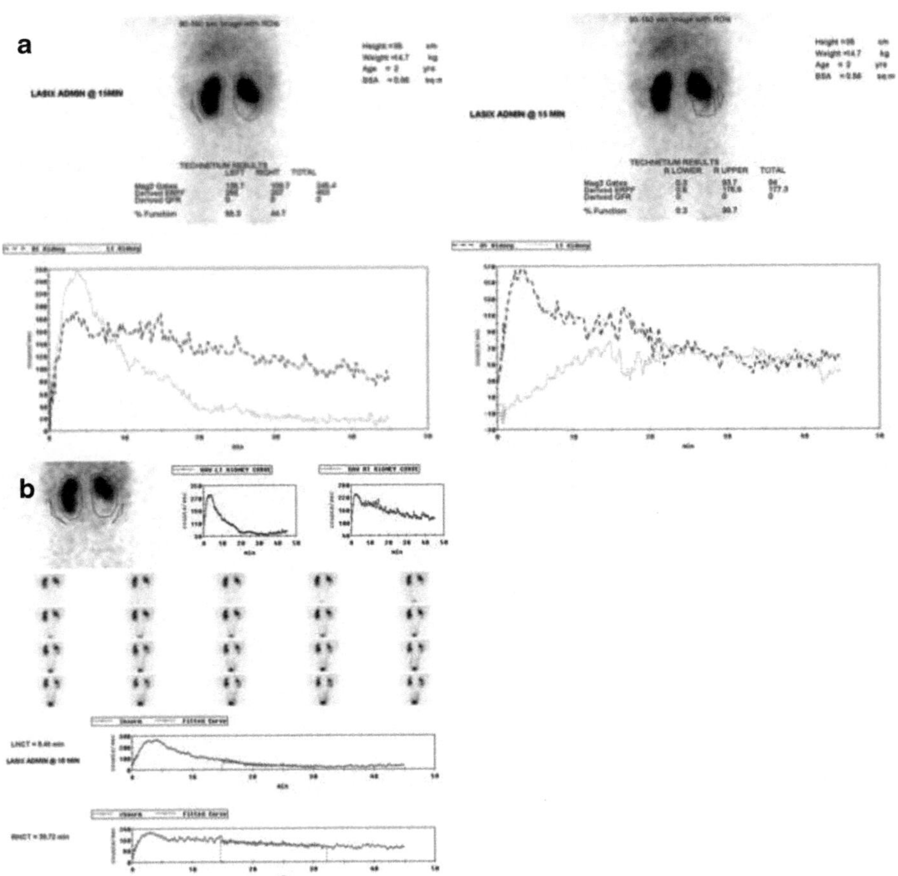

Fig. 9.38 MAG-3 with IRC after 2 febrile UTIs. (**a**, **b**) Right duplex kidney with very poorly functioning right lower moiety

is very poorly functioning with most likely severe vesicoureteric reflux. Differential function of the right kidney is 45%, with < 1% function in the lower moiety.

Question 5. Would These Findings Change Your Management?

Not if the patient remains asymptomatic with the conservative treatment, because the lower moiety has no function to preserve. The prophylaxis should be continued for at least 6–12 months or until he is toilette trained to prevent any further UTIs.

If the medical treatment fails, surgical management should be offered with the possibility to start with an endoscopic approach to treat the reflux (which has a change of failure of 20–30%) or more definitively with minimally invasive surgery to perform a partial nephroureterectomy of the non-functioning lower moiety.

His Ab prophylaxis was continued until the age of 2½ years old when he became toilette trained. During this period, he did not develop any further UTIs and didn't require any further interventions. Subsequent US urinary tract demonstrated stable appearances of right duplex kidney, with no evidence of lower moiety or ureteric dilatation (Fig. 9.39).

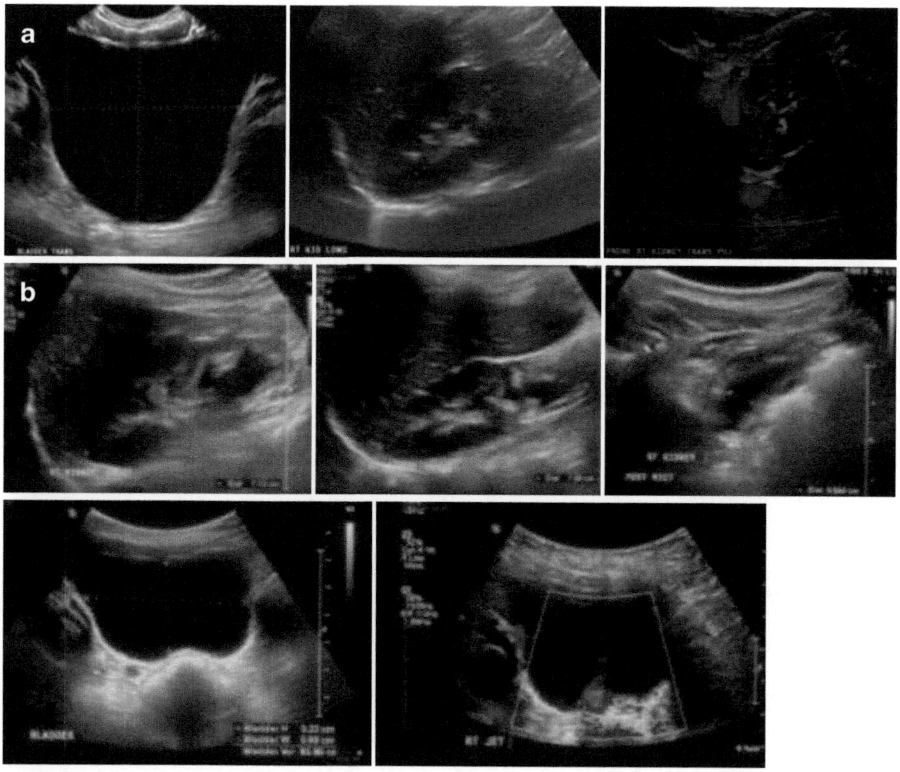

Fig. 9.39 (**a**) US urinary tract at 2 years of age. Mild cortical thinning of lower moiety of the duplex right kidney, but without PC dilatation nor ureteric dilatation. Normal bladder appearances and complete emptying. (**b**) US urinary tract at 3 years of age. Right duplex kidney with mild dilatation of the lower moiety calyces and renal pelvis, APD 6 mm. No right ureteric dilatation. Normal bladder appearances and complete emptying

9.12.1 Discussion

This patient had an antenatal diagnosis of a duplex kidney with lower moiety dilatation, which was suspected to be due to VUR. His postnatal ultrasounds confirmed a right duplex kidney with dilatation of the lower moiety and proximal ureter, but there was no evidence of distal ureteric dilatation. He was managed conservatively and remained asymptomatic until he was almost 1 year old when he developed 2 febrile UTIs. After this he was commenced on Ab prophylaxis and a NM scan with indirect cystography demonstrated a duplex kidney with preserved differential renal function, but with a non-functioning lower moiety and severe vesicoureteric reflux. His Ab prophylaxis was continued until he became toilette trained and he remained UTI-free after this. His follow-up US demonstrated complete resolution of the right lower moiety dilatation.

As previously mentioned, VUR is the most common associated anomaly in duplex kidneys, being present in up to 70% of the patients who present with a UTI, and it almost always occurs into the lower-pole moiety [39–41]. A shift in the management of primary VUR towards less aggressive options has also been applied when managing VUR in duplex systems, knowing that duplication per se is not an indication for surgical management [40, 41, 43]. Previously, patients with certain associated congenital anomalies had been subject to more aggressive treatments based on the assumption that their clinical outcome was poorer [41]. Many studies have reported high rate resolutions for VUR in duplex systems (up to 85% for low grades), although it may take longer to resolve, and low rate of complications of around 10% (mainly UTIs, renal scarring) [39–41]. Low grade VUR in a duplex system has an outcome similar to that in a single system and it should be managed conservatively. However, resolution tends to occur markedly later in patients with duplex kidneys. Most studies have noted a much lower resolution rate for high grade VUR in duplex systems, which is almost zero in grade IV–V reflux [39]. Nevertheless, most groups conclude that the likelihood of undergoing surgery in general, or due to absolute indications (such as breakthrough infections or new renal scars) was significantly higher for VUR in duplex systems [40, 41, 43].

In this patient, one of the arguments could have been to perform a circumcision to reduce the patient's risk of UTIs and eventually avoid the need for prophylactic Abs [31, 42]. This is common practice in many centres in male patients with upper urinary tract dilatation. The biggest influence can be made in patients <1 year of age. The patient should have also been started on prophylactic antibiotics at birth knowing that his risk of UTIs was higher due to the presence of lower moiety dilatation due to VUR. However, he managed to remain asymptomatic for several months and only developed a UTI when he was almost 1 year old. Despite this, after the infections he was managed conservatively only with Ab prophylaxis and his upper urinary tract dilatation resolved, probably correlated with a resolution of his VUR as well.

9.13 Case 13

A 9-months old girl with normal antenatal scans and no significant past medical history presents with recurrent febrile UTIs at the age of 5 months, requiring various admissions for IV Abs. The results of the initial investigations are presented below (Fig. 9.40).

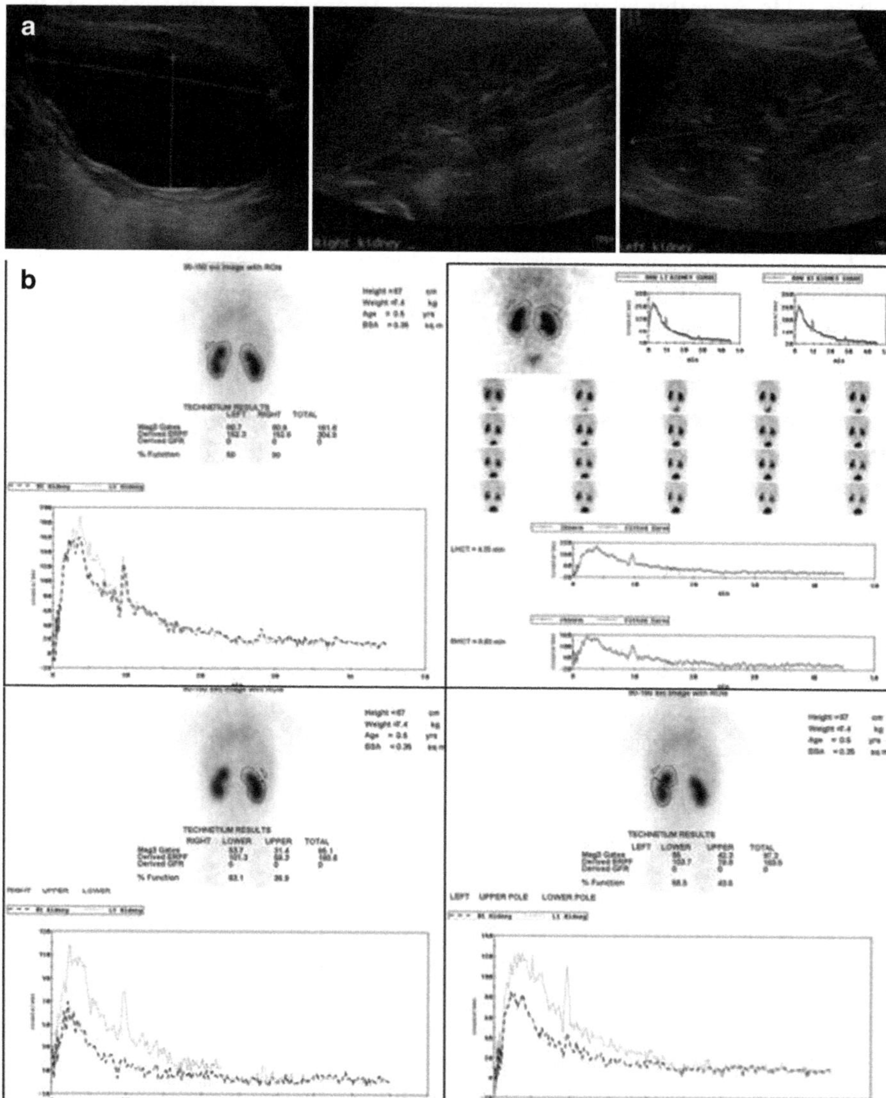

Fig. 9.40 (**a**) US urinary tract at the time of presentation, 5 months of age. (**b**) MAG-3 at 5 months of age. (**c**) MCUG at 5 months of age

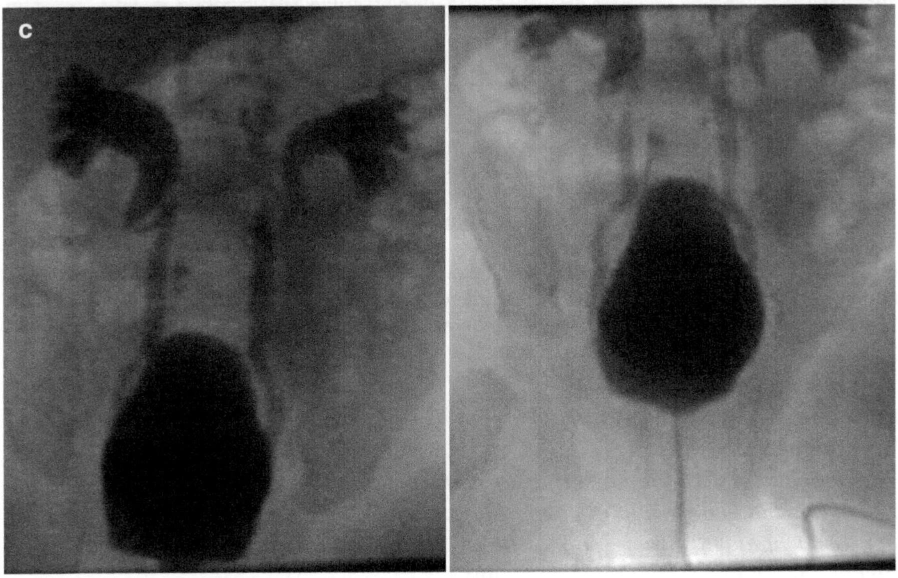

Fig. 9.40 (continued)

Question 1. What Do these Investigations Show?

a. *US urinary tract: normal appearances of both kidneys without upper urinary tract dilatation. Normal bladder.*
b. *NM dynamic scan: both kidneys have a duplex configuration with preserved differential renal function and normal drainage. There is evidence of bilateral lower moiety vesicoureteric reflux on indirect cystography. The differential function for each moiety is: left upper 44%, left lower 56%, right upper 37% and lower 63%.*
c. *MCUG: Normal bladder contour. Upon voiding there is bilateral reflux of contrast into the renal pelvis, which appear slightly drooping bilaterally (classical appearance of drooping lilies).*

The results of these investigations demonstrated bilateral duplex kidneys with VUR into both lower moieties.

Question 2. How Would You Manage the Patient?

The patient should be commenced on prophylactic antibiotics because of the findings, her age and the history of recurrent UTIs.

Other alternatives should be discussed with the parents, such as endoscopic treatment, to avoid long-term Abs and especially if the conservative management fails.

She was started on Ab prophylaxis but developed subsequent breakthrough febrile UTIs, even after changing different types of prophylactic Abs.

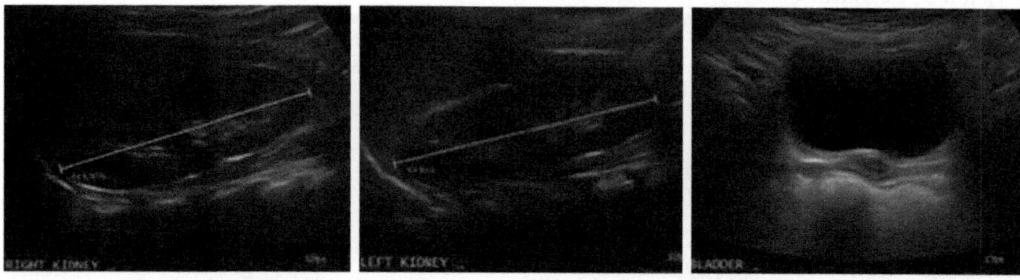

Fig. 9.41 US urinary tract 2 months after the procedure (11 months of age). Both kidneys have normal corticomedullary differentiation and there is no evidence of pelvicalyceal dilatation. The bladder is partly distended, with a small region of increased echogenicity at the VUJs consistent with Deflux material

Question 3. What Would Be Your Next Management Option When Medical Treatment Fails?

The patient should undergo surgical treatment and the probable best next option at her age is the endoscopic injection of a bulking agent. Because she is <1-year of age open bladder surgery should be avoided. Once definitive treatment is completed, the Ab prophylaxis can be stopped.

These options should be discussed and agreed with the family.

Due to failure of medical treatment, the patient underwent cystoscopy and bilateral deflux injections with STING technique at the age of 9 months. Shortly after this the prophylaxis was stopped and she was reviewed 2 months after the procedure with a repeat US urinary tract, which showed no abnormalities of the urinary tract (Fig. 9.41).

She remained well for about 6 months when she started having febrile UTIs again. The Ab prophylaxis was restarted, but despite this she continued to have recurrent episodes and required further admissions for IV Ab. Furthermore, a repeat ultrasound 6 months after demonstrated evidence of cortical thinning of both lower moieties, but without PC dilatation (Fig. 9.42).

Question 4. Would Your Management Change at This Point? If Yes, Why and What Would You Do Next?

The child has been managed both medically and endoscopically, with a minimally invasive approach, and both options have failed. Because of this, a more definitive and successful treatment should be chosen. In her case, now that he is almost 2 years of age, open bladder surgery is a very good and safe alternative, therefore a ureteric reimplantation should be the next step in management. She should remain on antimicrobial prophylaxis at least until the procedure, but ideally it should be stopped after the first postoperative follow-up.

Due to her failed management and the US findings decision was made to proceed with further surgical intervention. At the age of 22 months she underwent a bilateral common sheath trans-trigonal ureteric reimplantation with the Cohen technique, with insertion of JJ stent through all reimplanted ureters. She remained as an inpatient in IV abs and underwent cystoscopy with removal of all 4 JJ stents 5 days after.

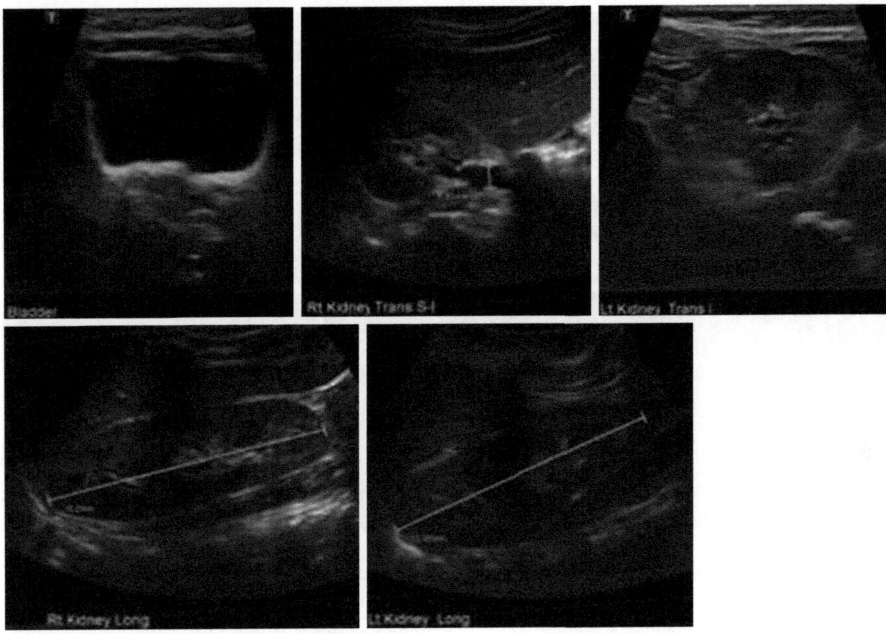

Fig. 9.42 US urinary tract 6 months after procedure (14 months old). Minimal thinning of the parenchymal thickness at the lower moieties. No pelvicalyceal dilation. The bladder is underfilled. No distal ureteric dilatation

She recovered well after both procedure and didn't develop any complications. She was discharged home on prophylactic Abs and reviewed with a repeat US 2 months after the procedure, at which time the prophylaxis was stopped. The US demonstrated good interval growth of both duplex kidneys, with no further progression of the lower moieties cortical thinning and no PC dilatation. Subsequent US showed similar findings. She has remained well and asymptomatic since the surgery and has not developed any further UTIs. She has not required further chemoprophylaxis either (Fig. 9.43).

9.13.1 Discussion

This patient had normal antenatal scans but presented with febrile UTIs in infancy and was diagnosed with bilateral duplex kidneys, with lower moiety VUR bilaterally. She was initially managed conservatively, but developed breakthrough UTI despite the Ab prophylaxis. With this there was an indication for surgery and because of her age decision was made to proceed with endoscopic treatment, with bilateral Deflux® injections. Unfortunately, the procedure was again unsuccessful, and she developed further febrile UTIs despite having restarted the prophylaxis, and there was evidence of cortical thinning of both lower moieties on US. After this, the best option left was to proceed with open surgery to reimplant both ureters of both

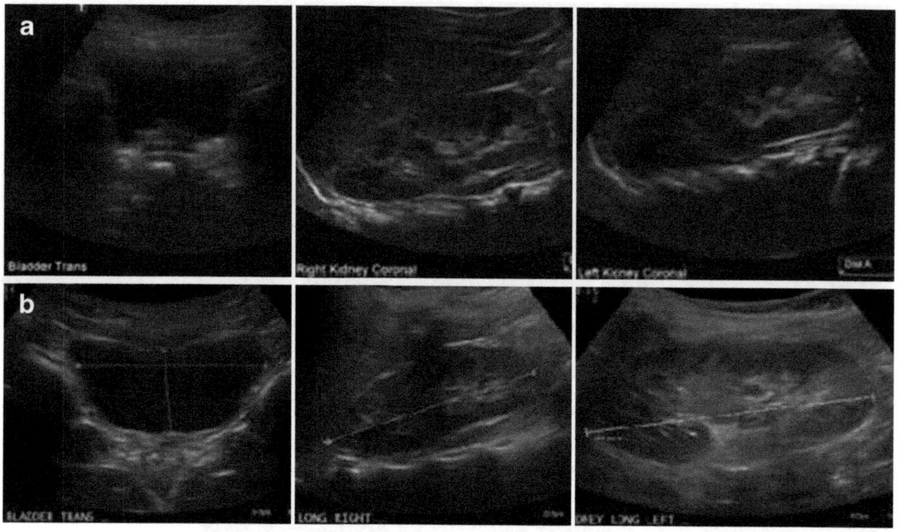

Fig. 9.43 (**a**) US urinary tract 2 months after ureteric reimplantation (2yo). Interval growth of both duplex kidneys, without pelvicalyceal dilatation. Under-filled bladder, no ureteric dilatation seen. (**b**) US urinary tract at 3½ years of age. No evidence of upper urinary tract dilatation of either duplex kidney. Minimally distended bladder, complete emptying

kidneys in the bladder. Fortunately, she was old enough to undergo this procedure safely and the surgery was successful.

In this case, the US was normal, but the MAG-3 with IRC had demonstrated bilateral lower moiety VUR. Although it is not common practice at our centre, a MCUG was also performed which again confirmed the presence of bilateral high grade VUR into both lower moieties. It was important to know whether the lower moieties were functional or not, as the answer would determine the choice of treatment. If the lower moieties are functional, a "preserving" treatment should be proposed: medical, endoscopic, or surgical [41]. In her case, an initial attempt was made to manage her conservatively, but this failed and there was enough indication to treat her surgically. We opted for endoscopic surgery first because of his age and knowing that this can have up to 80–85% success rates [44, 45]. Many studies have reported that the STING or HIT procedure is a safe and effective alternative for patients with refluxing duplex systems, although many patients require more than one injection [43, 44]. Unfortunately, in her case the UTIs recur despite restarting the Abs and we opted for open surgery, knowing that her high grade VUR would have almost no chances to resolve spontaneously and that a second injection still had a high chance of failure due to the same. She underwent a common sheath bilateral trans-trigonal ureteric reimplantation with no complications. This procedure can have up to a 98% success rate [41]. Many studies have concluded that the presence of a duplication anomaly does not adversely affect surgical outcome [41, 46]. Adequate tunnel width and long intravesical tunnels were noted to be the most important technical aspects [41]. An alternative to this, when both moieties have preserved function, is a uretero-ureterostomy or uretero-pyelostomy from the lower to the upper moiety systems, but this may carry higher complication rates [47].

9.14 Case 14

A 6-months old girl with normal antenatal scans presented at 2 months of age with a febrile UTI and was subsequently diagnosed with a right duplex kidney identified on US urinary tract. She developed further UTIs at 4 and 6 months of age.

Question 1

a. ***What is your initial management?***
b. ***Would you request other investigations? If yes, which ones?***
a. *The patient should be started on prophylactic Abs with trimethoprim 2 mg/kg, cephalexin 5–7.5 mg/kg or Nitrofurantoin 1–2 mg/kg, per dose at night.*
b. *The patient should undergo a NM dynamic scan to assess the renal function. If voiding is achieved, an indirect cystography could also be performed at the same time to determine if there is VUR or not. An alternative is to perform a MCUG to exclude VUR, but it is an invasive procedure that requires bladder catheterization which can be very traumatic at this age. This is not routinely performed at our institution.*

She was started on prophylactic Abs after the second infection and a NM scan was requested, which at 5 months of age confirmed the US findings of a right duplex kidney with preserved differential function, but reduced function of the right upper moiety, with no evidence of obstruction or VUR.

The differential function 46% on the left and 54% on the right. The differential function of the upper moiety of the duplex right kidney was 33% and of the lower moiety 67%; this represents 18% and 36% of total renal function respectively. The relatively small upper pole moiety showed no evidence of pelvicalyceal dilatation or obstruction and there is no evidence of significant reflux on the right.

Question 2. How Would You Manage the Patient with These Results?
The medical treatment in this case has failed, as she developed further UTIs despite the Ab prophylaxis, and there is evidence of right renal damage with reduced renal function of the upper moiety. The cause of the UTIs has not clearly been identified, so there are 2 options of management from here:

1. *An MCUG, to exclude VUR*
2. *A cystoscopy to assess the anatomy of the urinary tract and determine the location of both right UOs if possible. The advantage in this case is that if the UOs are visible it could also be a therapeutic procedure (i.e. if the lower moiety UO is visible and has a golf hole appearance, bulking agent could be injected for treatment of VUR)*

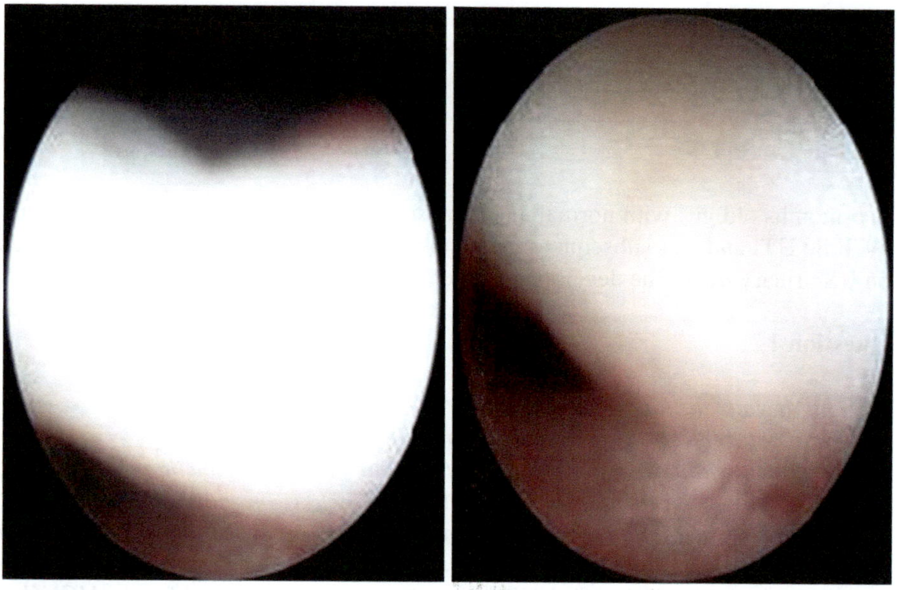

Fig. 9.44 Cystoscopy at 7 months of age. Right upper moiety UO located at the level of the bladder neck

Because of the recurrent UTIs in the context of a duplex right kidney with reduced function of the upper moiety, decision was made to proceed to a diagnostic cystoscopy to assess the anatomy of the urinary tract. Intraoperatively, the bladder appeared normal; however, the right lower moiety UO was placed very medially and the upper moiety one was located at the bladder neck. She underwent endoscopic incision of the right upper moiety UO through the bladder neck to facilitate drainage of that moiety into the bladder (Fig. 9.44).

She recovered well from surgery and remained on prophylactic Abs. She developed further breakthrough febrile UTIs until she was 13 months old, which subsequently stopped. She underwent repeat USS at the age of 11 and 18 months of age, which showed similar appearances of the right duplex kidney without upper tract dilatation and with normal bladder appearances (Fig. 9.45).

Her Ab prophylaxis was stopped by the time she became toilette trained at around 20 months of age. But unfortunately, only a few weeks after the Abs were ceased, she developed another febrile UTI with a multi-resistant *E. coli* and required admission for IV Abs treatment. The repeat US during the admission did not identify any abnormalities nor any complications such as pyelonephritis (Fig. 9.46).

She continued to develop further UTIs, some febrile, despite prophylaxis and rotating courses of Abs. Despite being toilet-trained she had ongoing issues with day and night-time urinary incontinence, which became more evident when she was around 3 years old.

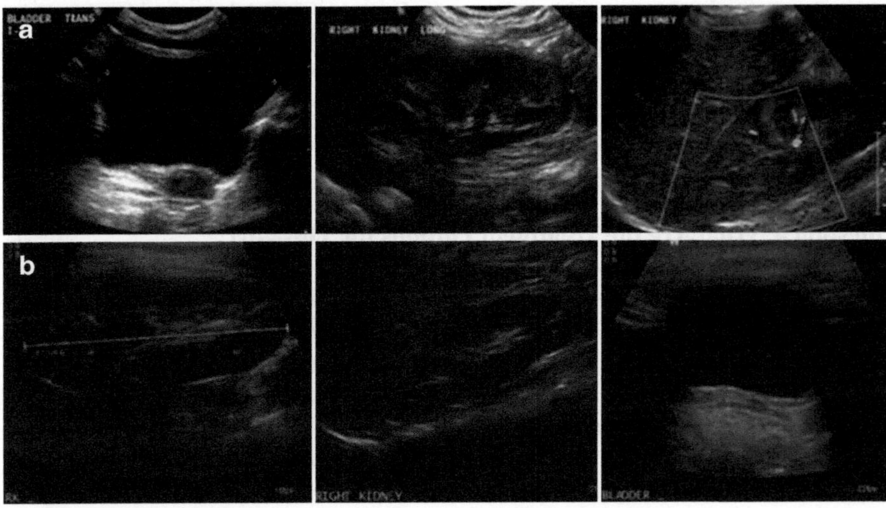

Fig. 9.45 (**a**) US urinary tract at 11 months of age. Normal bladder appearances, no distal ureteric dilatation. Right duplex kidney, no PC dilatation. (**b**) Repeat renal tract ultrasound at 18 months of age. Right duplex kidney, no pelvicalyceal dilatation. Normal left kidney and bladder appearances

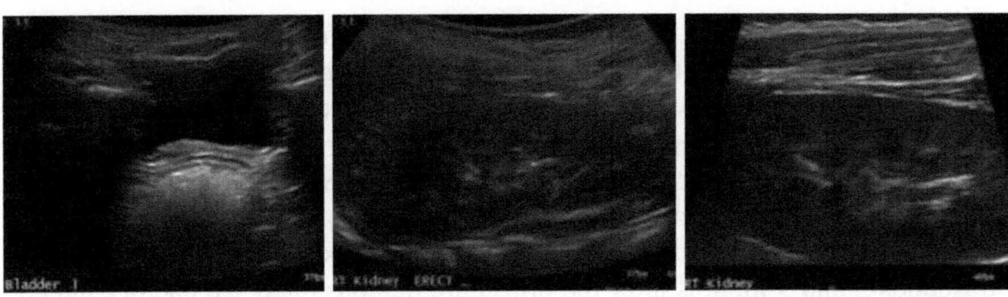

Fig. 9.46 Repeat US urinary tract at 20 months of age during the episode of UTI. Right duplex kidney, no pelvicalyceal dilatation

Question 3. What Would Your Next Step in Management Be at This Point?

The patient needs further investigations to decide definitive treatment as she is having recurrent UTIs despite medical management. Any evident signs of voiding dysfunction and constipation should be addressed as well.

The patient requires a repeat MAG-3, ideally with IRC, to reassess the renal function (particularly of the right upper moiety) and determine if there is evidence of obstruction on the drainage curve or VUR on indirect cystography. An MRI urogram could also be of help in particular if we are suspecting a duplex kidney with an ectopic ureter, which would explain the presence of incontinence as well. Unfortunately, at her age, this procedure requires a GA. An alternative is to repeat a cystoscopy to re-assess the anatomy of the urinary tract and the position of both right UOs. This, as well, involves a GA.

Further investigations were done between the age of 2 and 3 years old, with serial US demonstrating similar appearances of the duplex kidney and a NM scan with no evidence of significant renal scarring, loss of function or obstruction.

She had a repeat cystoscopy due to recurrence of UTIs and persistent day-time urinary incontinence at 4 years of age. Findings similar to previous with a right upper moiety UO opening into the BN.

Question 4. What Are the Treatment Options for This Girl?

This patient should undergo definitive surgery to prevent further renal damage due to the recurrent UTIs and the partial obstruction of the upper moiety. The initial procedure with incision of the upper moiety UO into the bladder neck had failed to improve the drainage of that system and the long-term urinary stasis with intermittent blockage were the reasons for the recurrent UTIs and the incontinence, as there was still function in the right upper moiety.

Considering that there is still function in the upper moiety the surgery should aim to preserve the remaining function of that moiety and reconstruct the abnormal urinary tract, either via a right distal side-to-end uretero-ureterostomy from the obstructive ureter to the normal ureter, or via a right conjoint trans-trigonal ureteric reimplantation, although this latter one has a risk of damaging the blood supply of the normal ureter during the dissection and re-tunnelling in the bladder.

With these findings and considering the preserved function of the right upper moiety, decision was made to proceed to a right distal uretero-ureterostomy, which was performed when she was 4 years old. In order to ensure safety of the lower moiety ureter, the normal ureter was catheterised via cystoscopy prior to the open procedure to facilitate its identification intraoperatively. She recovered well and was discharged a few days after. Her day-time incontinence resolved, and she did not develop any further UTIs, for which the chemoprophylaxis was stopped. Follow-up ultrasounds 3 and 9 months after the procedure demonstrated satisfactory interval growth of both kidneys, with stable mild cortical thinning of the right upper moiety and no upper urinary tract dilatation (Fig. 9.47).

9.15 Case 15

A 3-months old girl with antenatal diagnosis of a right duplex kidney identified at 32 weeks of GA is referred for further investigations and management. She was started on Px Abs at birth and underwent a repeat US scan at 6 weeks of age, which again demonstrated a duplex right kidney with dilatation of the upper moiety renal pelvis and ureter without a ureterocoele. A NM dynamic scan was also performed at 2 months of age, which confirmed a right duplex kidney with preserved differential function (53% on the right) and 38% function of the upper moiety (Fig. 9.48).

Question 1. How Would You Manage This Patient? Why?

The patient should be managed conservatively, because she remains asymptomatic and UTI-free with the antimicrobial prophylaxis which was commenced after birth.

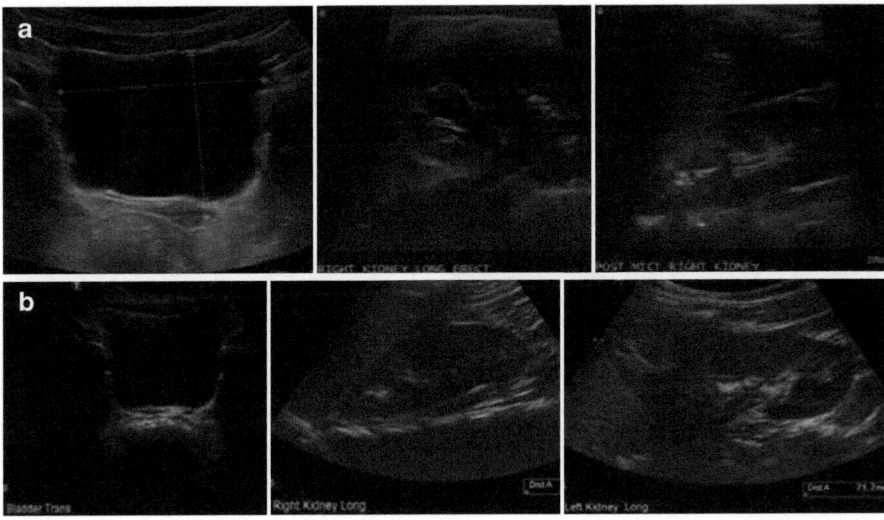

Fig. 9.47 (**a**) US urinary tract 3 months after the procedure. Satisfactory interval growth of both kidneys. Right duplex with mild prominence of the upper moiety in pre-void state and showing complete decompression in post-void state. Mild cortical thinning of the upper moiety. Normal left kidney and bladder. (**b**) Repeat US urinary tract 9 months after the procedure. The right duplex kidney has normal corticomedullary differentiation and no upper tract dilatation, and there is stable mild upper moiety cortical thinning. Normal left kidney and bladder appearances

The prophylaxis should continue until she is at least 12 months of age. The patient should be followed up with regular US at 3, 6, and 12 months of age; subsequently every 2 years until the age of 5 years. A repeat NM scan is not required unless the patient becomes symptomatic or there is progressive dilatation of the upper urinary tract on ultrasound.

She remained well and asymptomatic and was reviewed again 6 weeks after with a repeat US urinary tract, which demonstrated stable appearances of the right upper moiety renal pelvis and ureteric dilatation (Fig. 9.49).

Shortly after the US, and despite chemoprophylaxis, the patient suffered 2 febrile UTIs, requiring admission for IV Abs for the second episode. During the admission, a repeat US was performed with evidence of some slight increase in the upper moiety renal pelvis and ureteric dilatation and layering debris in the distal ureter. The patient responded well to a course of Abs and the prophylaxis was changed (Fig. 9.50).

Question 2

a. ***How would these findings change your management?***
b. ***What would you do next?***

a. *The patient has become symptomatic and there is increasing upper urinary tract dilatation on the ultrasounds, which means that the medical treatment has failed, and she will need more definitive treatment to prevent further UTIs and to avoid*

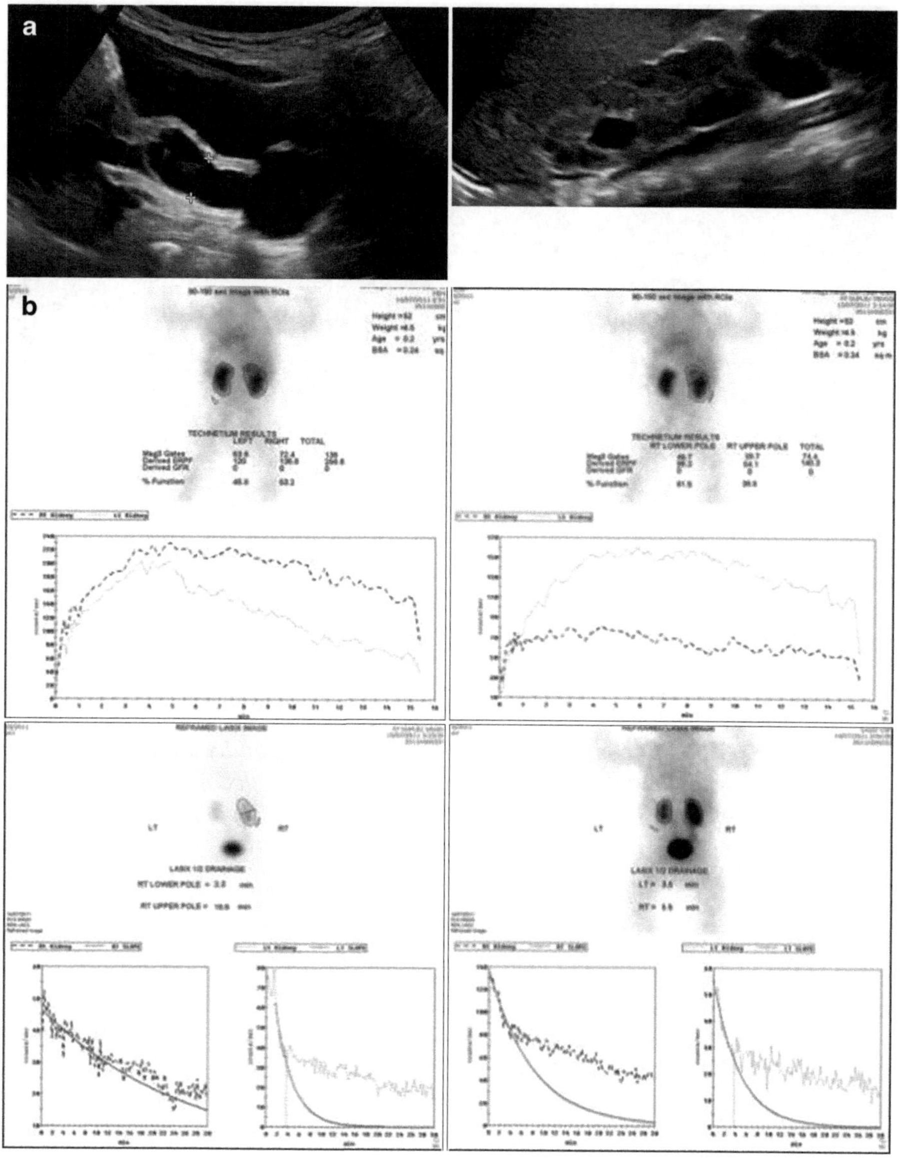

Fig. 9.48 (**a**) US urinary tract at 6 weeks of age. Right duplex kidney with upper moiety pelvi-calyceal dilatation, renal pelvis APD Distal ureteric dilatation up to 10 mm. (**b**) MAG-3 scan at 2 months of age. The right kidney has a configuration suggestive of a duplex system with features consistent with obstruction of the upper pole moiety ureter. The differential function measures 47% on the left and 53% on the right. The differential function of the right upper pole moiety is about 38% and the lower moiety about 62%

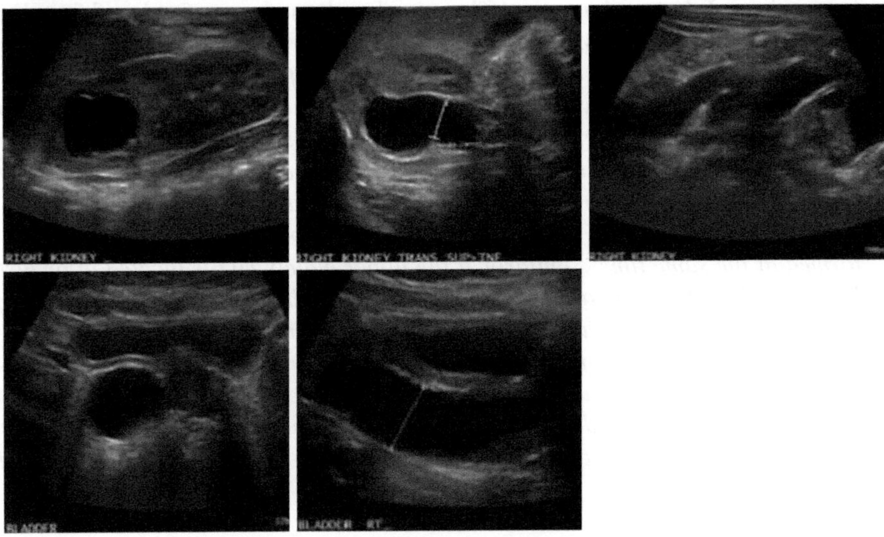

Fig. 9.49 US urinary tract at 4 months of age. The right kidney is a duplex kidney, with significant dilatation of a dysplastic appearing upper moiety and a dilated and tortuous proximal ureter. TheAPD is 10 mm and the surrounding parenchyma is thinned and echogenic with loss of cortico-medullary differentiation, and a dilated upper moiety ureter was noted behind the bladder measuring up to 14 mm

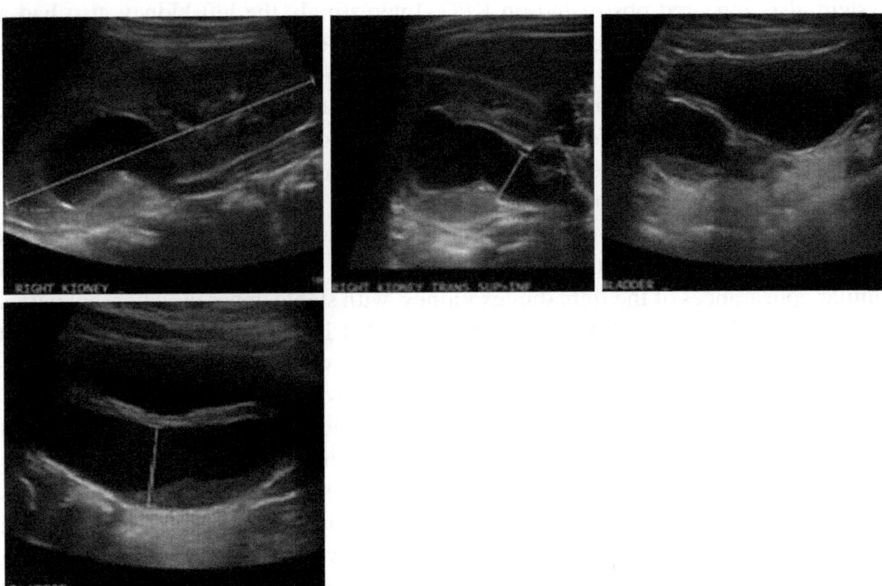

Fig. 9.50 US urinary tract during episode of febrile UTI. The dilated right upper moiety is again demonstrated, with a renal APD of 9.5 mm. There is now however increased in echogenicity of the parenchyma with thickening of the urothelium with echogenic particles demonstrated within the dilated system. The entire ureter is again demonstrated to be markedly dilated up to 15.4 mm with presence of debris within

further loss of the renal function. There is already evidence of reduced function and obstruction on the MAG-3, likely due to an ectopic upper moiety ureter. However, at this age, this a diagnosis difficult to confirm.

b. *The best way to proceed would be to perform a diagnostic cystoscopy which also has the potential to be therapeutic. This allows assessment of the anatomy of the urinary tract and the position of both right UOs to decide further treatment. If the configuration of the lower moiety UO is suspicious of VUR, this could potentially be the cause of the UTIs, and injection of a bulking agent could be performed at the same time. Similarly, if the upper moiety UO is located in or just below the bladder neck, an "cut-back" incision of the opening into the bladder can be made. Similar techniques of endoscopic internal urinary diversions have been described as temporary de-obstructive measurements, such as the transvesical or transurethral ureteric incisions with laser or puncture with a 5 Fr needle, and subsequent dilatation with a cutting balloon. These allow at least temporary drainage of the obstructive moiety to prevent further UTIs and renal damage.*

Due to these breakthrough UTIs decision was made to proceed with further operative management. Four weeks after the infection and once she had fully recovered, she underwent a diagnostic cystoscopy with a retrograde pyelogram study to assess the anatomy of the urinary tract. Intraoperative findings on cystoscopy demonstrated that the right upper moiety UO was located right at bladder neck and appeared obstructed at this position despite being widely open. The upper moiety collecting system also appeared obstructed on RPG. Interestingly the left kidney also had a duplex configuration. Because of these findings we decided to perform a cut back of the right upper moiety UO into the bladder neck to allow drainage of the moiety. She recovered well from the procedure and did not develop any further UTIs. A repeat US urinary tract performed 6 weeks after demonstrated stable appearances of the dilated right upper moiety with minimal overlying parenchymal scarring and a significantly dilated right ureter (Fig. 9.51).

Even though the patient initially continued to have recurrent UTIs until she was 12 months old, the follow up ultrasounds at 9 and 13 months of age demonstrated similar appearances of the right duplex kidney, with stable upper moiety renal pelvis and ureteric dilatation. A DMSA scan performed at 11 months of age showed again preserved differential function of 49% on the right, with moderately reduced activity in the upper moiety, which contributes 32% of overall function (Fig. 9.52).

The patient remained asymptomatic for the following 2 years and subsequent follow up ultrasounds demonstrated some improvement in the right upper moiety renal pelvis and ureteric dilatation. The Ab prophylaxis were stopped when she was around 3 years old, after she had started toilette training. According to her parents, she seemed to be constantly dribbling urine and developed urgency and frequency when she was around 4 years old. There was no history of voiding dysfunction and she had managed to spend a few periods of a few months dry in between voids. She was treated for suspected bladder overactivity, with only mild improvement of her symptoms (mainly the urgency and the frequency) for a short period of time. At the

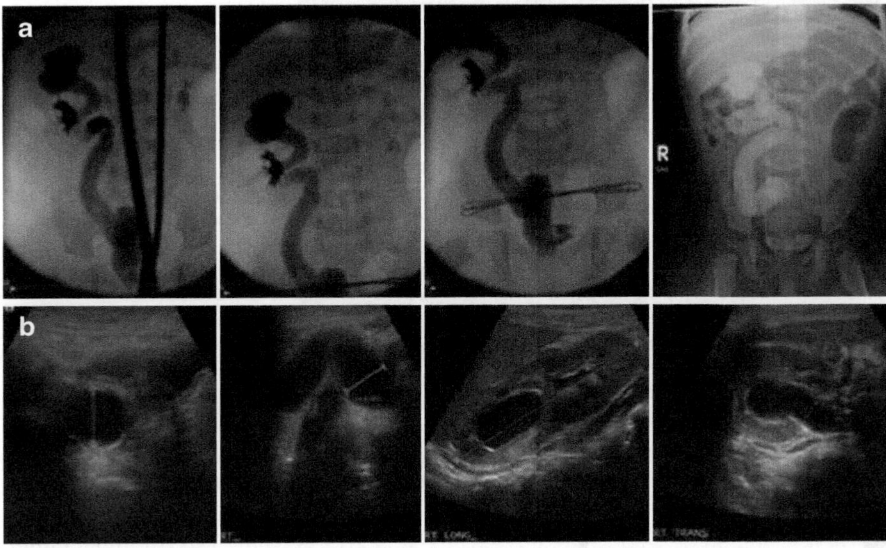

Fig. 9.51 (**a**) Cystoscopy and right RPG after febrile UTI. On RPG, the right lower moiety appeared normal; however, the upper moiety renal pelvis was grossly dilated with a tortuous dilated ureter, which did not drain. Limited views of the left kidney suggest a normal calibre duplex or possibly a bifid collecting system with a single normal calibre distal left ureter seen. With these findings, she underwent a cut back of the right upper moiety UO into the bladder neck with the resectoscope. A delayed X-ray of the abdomen, 2.5 h after, showed significant retention of contrast in a markedly dilated pelvicalyceal system and tortuous dilated ureter of the right upper moiety collecting system. (**b**) Repeat US urinary tract 6 weeks after initial diagnostic cystoscopy. Duplex right pelvicalyceal system with dilated upper moiety and minimal thinning of the cortex, unchanged in appearance since previously. The right upper moiety ureter is dilated throughout its length up to 16 mm.

age of 5 years her constant dribbling of urine had worsened, and decision was made to repeat the cystoscopy and RPG study to assess the right upper moiety and ureter and the location of both right UOs, in order to decide management. On cystoscopy, the upper pole UO was identified at bladder neck; the lower pole UO was located intravesical but also close to BN. The left UO appeared orthotopic. The RPG again demonstrated a dilated right upper moiety renal pelvis and ureter (Fig. 9.53).

Question 3. What Is Your Definitive Management for This Patient? Why?
This patient needs definitive surgery for the treatment of his partially obstructed right upper moiety ureter which is the likely cause for her incontinence and previous UTIs. In her case, because of her older age, the best way to proceed is with a trans-trigonal common sheath ureteric reimplantation.

With these findings and considering the likelihood of the incontinence to be related to the ectopic ureteric orifice with a functioning upper moiety, decision was made to proceed with a right trans-trigonal common sheath ureteric reimplantation, which was performed when she was almost 6½ years old. A 3.5 Fr feeding tube was

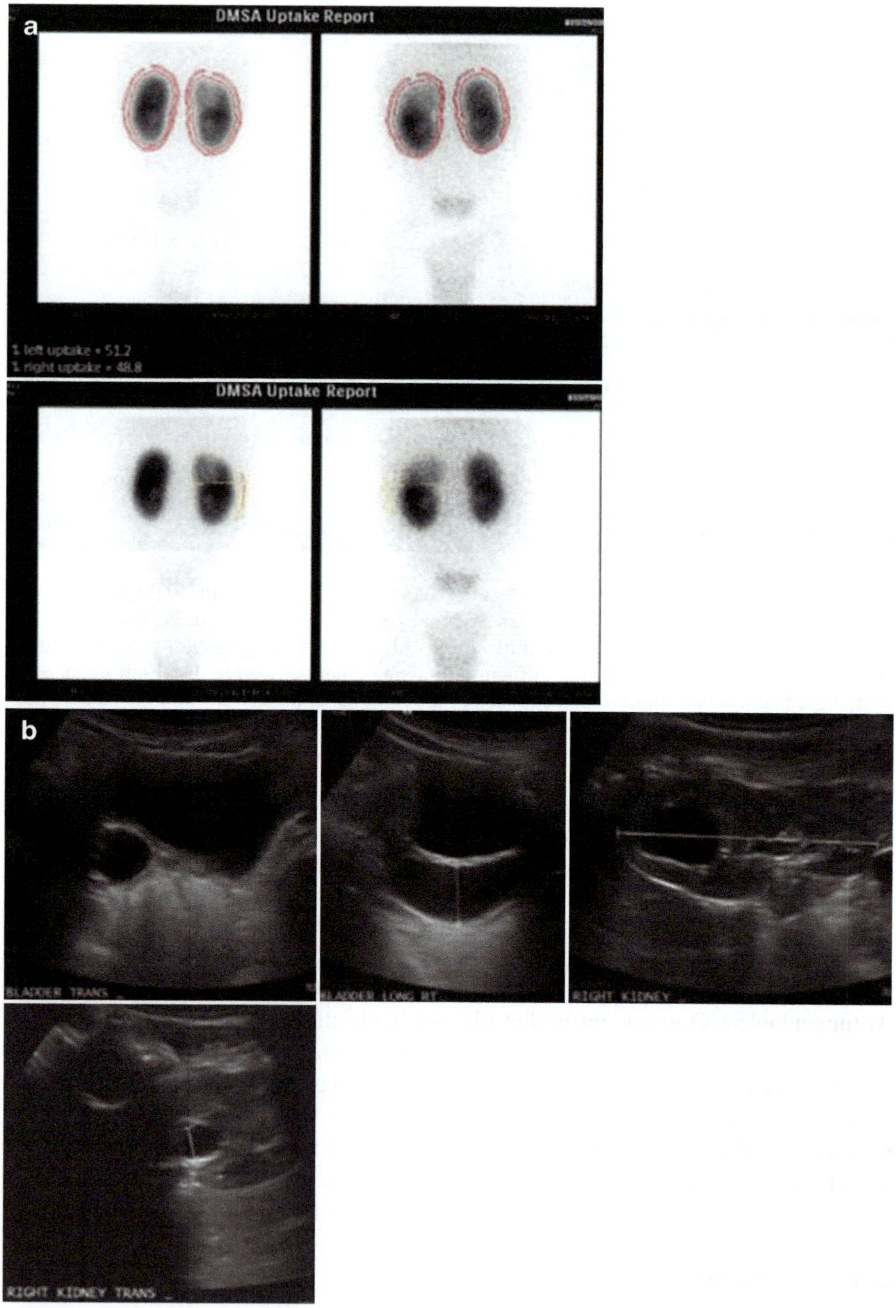

Fig. 9.52 (**a**) DMSA done at 11 months of age. The differential function is 51% on the left and 49% on the right. The right kidney has a duplex morphology. There is moderately reduced activity in the upper moiety, which contributes 32% of overall function with the lower pole 68%. (**b**) US Urinary tract at 13 months of age. Duplex right kidney with moderate upper moiety pelvicalyceal dilatation (APD 8 mm) with thinned overlying cortex. Right renal pelvis APD 8 mm. The right upper moiety ureter remains distended throughout its course, measuring 15 mm distally

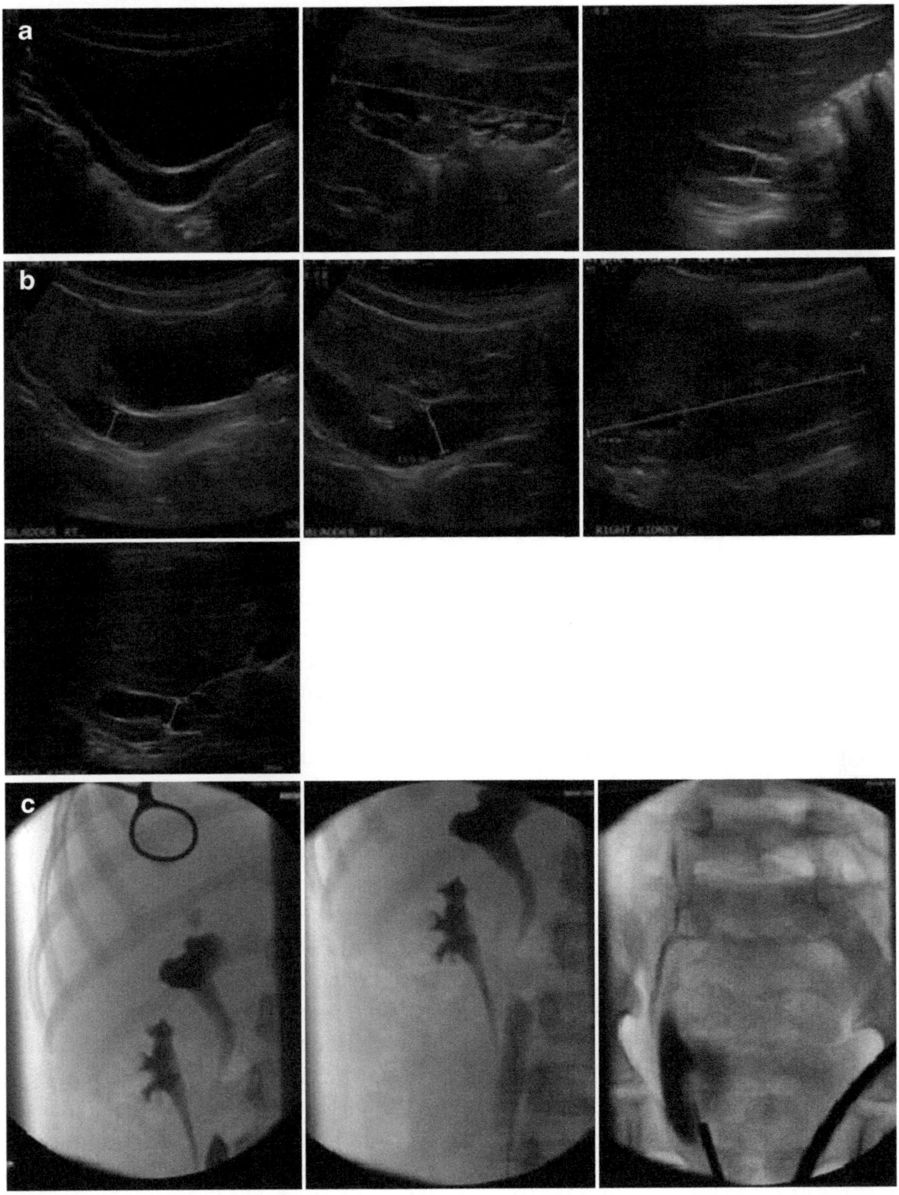

Fig. 9.53 (**a**) US urinary tract at 2 ½ years of age. Duplex kidney with stable mild dilatation of the upper moiety renal pelvis and parenchymal thinning. Persistent distal right ureteric dilatation is stable, up to 9.6 mm. (**b**) US urinary tract at 4 years of age. Duplex right collecting system, with dilated upper moiety renal pelvis, measuring 10 mm. The right upper moiety calyces are dilated on pre and post-void imaging. Dilated distal right ureter up to 12 mm. (**c**) Cystoscopy with RPG at 5½ years of age. The RPG demonstrated a right duplex kidney with a dilated upper moiety renal pelvis and ureter draining into the bladder neck

left in situ draining the small lower pole ureter and a 12 Fr Malecot catheter was used as a suprapubic catheter. Both were left on free drainage and removed 5 days after the procedure. The patient voided without difficulties and was discharged home on a course of oral Abs due to a possible urine infection detected on day 2 postoperatively when she developed fevers.

The patient was reviewed 3, 6, and 12 months after the surgery with US urinary tract which initially demonstrated mild dilatation of the upper moiety renal pelvis, APD 7 mm, and ureter; but subsequently showed complete resolution of the upper moiety collecting system dilatation. She had ongoing urinary incontinence immediately after micturition likely due to bladder dysfunction and postponed voiding. On physical examination, she was also discovered to have labial adhesions which were suspected to be contributing to the dribbling post-void and were managed with topical vaseline. With time, her symptoms improved and the frequency and quantity of her accidents decreased (Fig. 9.54).

9.15.1 Discussion for Cases 14 and 15

Both patients had a duplex kidney, the second one diagnosed antenatally, and presented with febrile UTIs, after which they were commenced on prophylactic Abs to prevent further infections. In both cases the initial NM demonstrated mild decrease in the upper moiety function, but no evidence of obstruction or VUR. Interestingly, only one of them had significant upper urinary tract dilatation on the US which progressed during surveillance at the same time that the patient developed further UTIs. In an attempt to assess the anatomy of the urinary tract and determine the location of the ureteric openings, a diagnostic cystoscopy was performed. In both cases it demonstrated an ectopic insertion of the upper moiety ureter draining the bladder neck, and both patients underwent endoscopic incision of the right upper moiety UO into the bladder neck to facilitate drainage. In both cases the endoscopic treatment was unsuccessful, as both developed further breakthrough UTIs, but also urinary incontinence. Due to the failure of both the medical and initial surgical managements, decision was made to proceed with open surgery to prevent further UTIs and renal damage, but also because the incontinence was thought to be related to the ectopic insertion of the ureter in the distal urinary tract. The differences in operative management were more related to the surgeons preference than an absolute indication for one or the other procedure. Both girls had complete resolution of their symptoms on follow up, with improvement of the upper urinary tract dilatation for the second patient, and the antimicrobial prophylaxis could be ceased shortly after the surgery. The evaluation and management of young female patients who present with recurrent UTIs and urinary incontinence after toilet training can often be difficult [48]. Many conditions can contribute to these symptoms, including dysfunctional voiding and detrusor instability, as well as an ectopic ureter. Ureteral ectopia has been used to describe any ureter that empties either at the bladder neck or caudally [49, 50]. If the ureteric bud arises in a more proximal position during development, the ureteral orifice can ultimately be incorporated into one of the

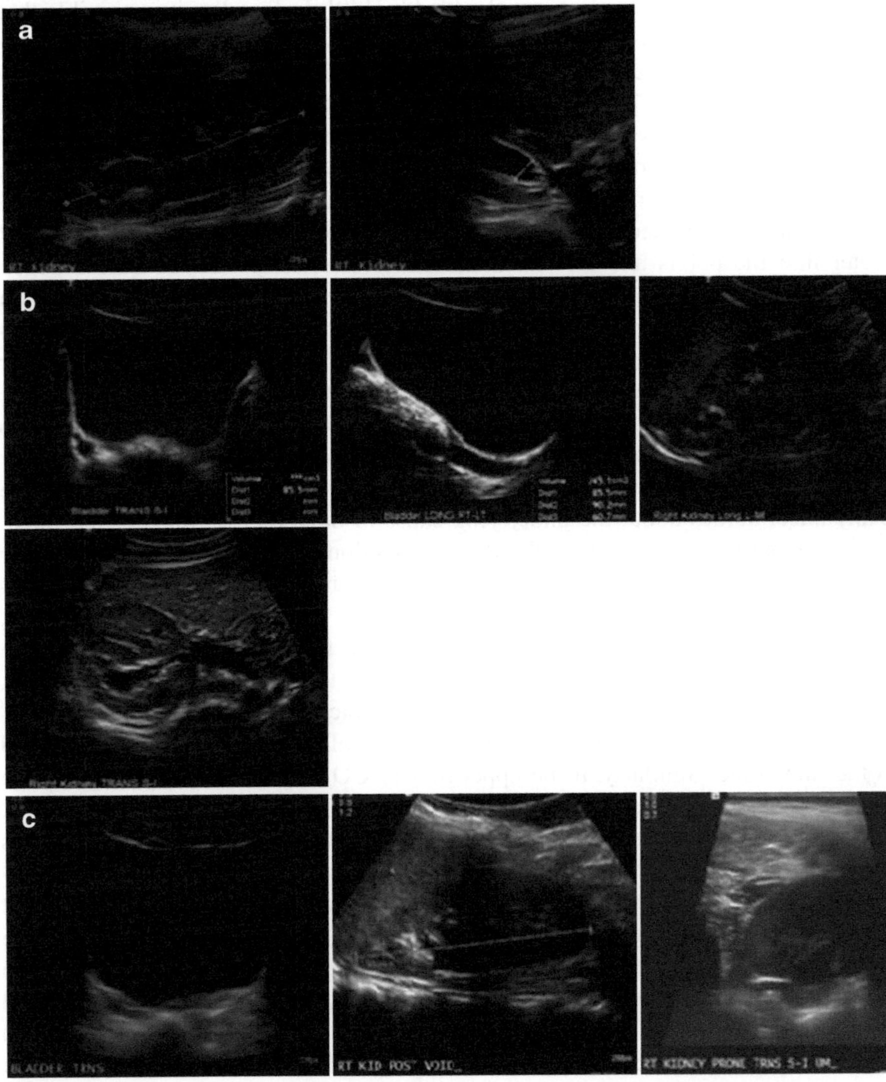

Fig. 9.54 (**a**) US urinary tract 3 months after surgery. Duplex right kidney with mild dilatation of the upper pole moiety, APD 7 mm. Bladder was under-filled and no distal ureteric dilatation could be seen. (**b**) US urinary tract 6 months after ureteric reimplantation. Right duplex kidney with improved mild central calyceal dilatation of right upper moiety of collection system (renal pelvis APD 6 mm) with mildly dilated distal right ureter up to 7 mm. Mild renal cortical thinning and increased cortical echogenicity of the upper pole moiety similar to previous. (**c**) US urinary tract 12 months after ureteric reimplantation. There is mild dilatation of the collecting system in the upper moiety of the right kidney with associated cortical thinning. No ureteric dilatation on either side. Two ureteric jets were identified

Müllerian structures instead of into the bladder [49]. In females, it is possible that the orifice may be distal to the urethral sphincter allowing continuous urinary incontinence. As ectopic ureters usually drain poorly functioning renal segments with low urine production, these patients may also present with intermittent incontinence as well [50]. In patients who are suspected to have ureteral ectopia, ultrasonography has been a first-line tool for evaluation. Dilatation of the upper moiety in duplex kidneys with a normal lower moiety is a common finding in cases of an ureterocoele and in some cases of ectopic ureters. Today, ultrasound may be able to trace a dilated ureter into the pelvis and into an abnormally low position beyond the bladder. Unfortunately, many cases of ureteric ectopia will often have no abnormality on initial imaging studies; such as the first case. Nevertheless, the absence of an ureterocoele in the bladder in these cases provides a high suspicion of an ectopic ureter [48]. Alternatively, many of these cases are associated with VUR into the ectopic ureter and upper moiety instead of obstruction [48]. Many patients will also undergo an MCUG to ensure there is no associated VUR to the lower moiety as the cause for the UTIs, as this may determine the surgical intervention of choice. Because of the many uncertainties about the underlying cause of their UTIs, a diagnostic cystoscopy was performed to confirm the ectopic position of the UO and decide further treatment. In both cases the upper moiety UO appeared to be draining into the bladder neck, which would explain the symptoms with intermittent drainage of urine, the lack of dilatation on US in one of them and normal drainage curve on the MAG-3. The cystoscopy also allows for immediate treatment in specific situations. If the configuration of the lower moiety UO is suspicious of VUR, this could potentially be the cause of the UTIs, and injection of a bulking agent could be performed at the same time. Similarly, if the upper moiety UO is located in or just below the bladder neck, an "cut-back" incision of the opening into the bladder can be made. Similar techniques of endoscopic internal urinary diversions have been described as temporary de-obstructive measurements [51], such as the transvesical or transurethral ureteric incisions with laser or puncture with a 5 Fr needle, and subsequent dilatation with a cutting balloon. These allow at least temporary drainage of the obstructive moiety to prevent further UTIs and renal damage. In the second case, the patient initially developed further UTIs after the procedure, however those resolved completely when she turned 1 year of age. This could be explained in 2 ways: (1) the upper moiety obstruction was treated with the bladder neck incision and the drainage and urinary stasis in the upper moiety improved, or (2) there was preoperative VUR to the lower moiety, which resolved with time.

Management of the upper segment of the ectopic ureter most often involves surgical treatment [47] to ensure drainage from the upper moiety and protect the renal function. Main indications for surgery in these cases are presence of symptoms, such as incontinence, and recurrent UTIs, failure of medical treatment, progressive upper urinary tract dilatation, with a functioning upper moiety. The procedure is dependent on the function of the upper moiety and the presence of associated lower moiety VUR or not. If the aim is to preserve functioning renal parenchyma, feasible options are a pyelo-ureterostomy, an uretero-ureterostomy or a common-sheath ureteric reimplantation [42]. In the first case, a uretero-ureterostomy was preferred over a common sheath reimplantation to avoid damaging an otherwise normal insertion of the lower moiety ureter in the bladder and because it is a less invasive procedure. In order to facilitate identification of the lower moiety ureter during the dissection of an upper moiety ureter which is not very dilated, catheterisation of the lower moiety UO via cystoscopy prior to the procedure is routinely performed at our institution.

According to the clinical situation, a uretero-ureterostomy may be used at the level of either the upper or lower ureter [47]. The general principle of uretero-ureterostomy is to anastomose the upper moiety ureter to the lower moiety ureter in an end-to-side fashion, excising and spatulating the dilated distal segment of the dilated upper moiety ureter and leaving the ureteric stump ligated as distally as possible to prevent complications. There may be a theoretical concern that uretero-ureterostomy might lead to a situation in which 'yo-yo' reflux promotes continued urinary stasis and urinary infection [47]. In addition, as the upper moiety ureter is often very dilated, anastomosis of this large, thick-walled ureter to a delicate lower moiety ureter might be considered difficult. Surgery to save a small upper pole can risk the larger and usually healthy lower pole if a ureteric stricture develops at the anastomosis. However, the risk of these complications is low [47]. Follow-up after surgery must include ultrasounds of the urinary tract and functional imaging should be considered at 6 months in cases where the function of the upper moiety was already compromised or there were multiple episodes of UTIs.

As mentioned before, confirming the underlying aetiology of urinary incontinence in toilette trained children with a duplex kidney and ectopic ureter is not always easy [48]. In the second case the patient had managed to achieve toilette training at a reasonable age and had spent periods of time without any accidents, so the history was not typical of an ectopic ureter. She also had some improvement initially with the anticholinergic medication, which also delayed the definitive treatment. In females, the ureteric orifice may be distal to the urethral sphincter allowing continuous urinary incontinence. But if the ectopic ureter drains a poorly functioning renal moiety with low urine production, these patients may also present with intermittent incontinence as well [48, 49]. In her case it was believed that the intermittent incontinence was probably due to the fact that the UO was located directly in the bladder neck.

9.16 Case 16

A 5-months old female with normal antenatal scans presented at 7 weeks of age with a short history of fevers and lethargy and was diagnosed with a *Klebsiella pneumoniae* UTI. She completed a course of IV and PO Abs. She underwent further investigations and was commenced on Px Abs after completing treatment (Fig. 9.55).

Question 1

a. ***What does the urinary tract US show?***
b. ***What other investigations would you request?***

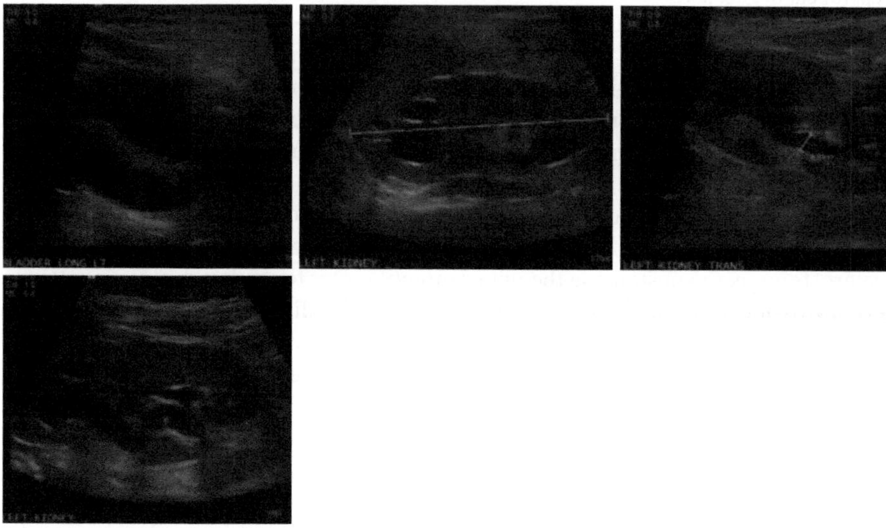

Fig. 9.55 US urinary tract at 3 months of age after the first UTIs

a. *There is a markedly dilated left ureter (12 mm). The left kidney has a duplex configuration and there is upper moiety dilatation with thinning of the cortex.*
b. *A NM scan with indirect cystography, if possible, to confirm the ultrasound finding of a* ***left*** *duplex kidney and determine the differential renal function, with the contribution of each moiety, and to assess for possible VUR. An alternative is to perform an MCUG, although in her case because of the possible ectopic insertion of the upper moiety ureter an obstructive cause is more likely to be the cause of her UTIs. Although VUR to the lower moiety can't be excluded.*

The ultrasound demonstrated a duplex left kidney with dilated upper moiety and a dilated left upper moiety ureter with an apparent ectopic insertion. A NM scan with indirect cystogram confirmed the diagnosis of a left duplex kidney with preserved differential function, with 40% function of the upper moiety.

Question 2. What Is Your Initial Management?
The patient should be commenced on prophylactic Abs and undergo regular surveillance with urinary tract US, with follow up appointments at 6, 9, and 12 months of age. She should remain on antimicrobial prophylaxis for at least 6 months or until she is 1 year of age.

She subsequently developed 1 further episode of a UTI, without fevers, but remained well and asymptomatic after. She underwent regular follow up with serial US at 6 and 9 months of age, which demonstrated interval growth of the left duplex kidney with stable upper moiety renal pelvis and ureteric dilatation. Due to her favourable progress her Abs were stopped when she was 9 months old. A few weeks

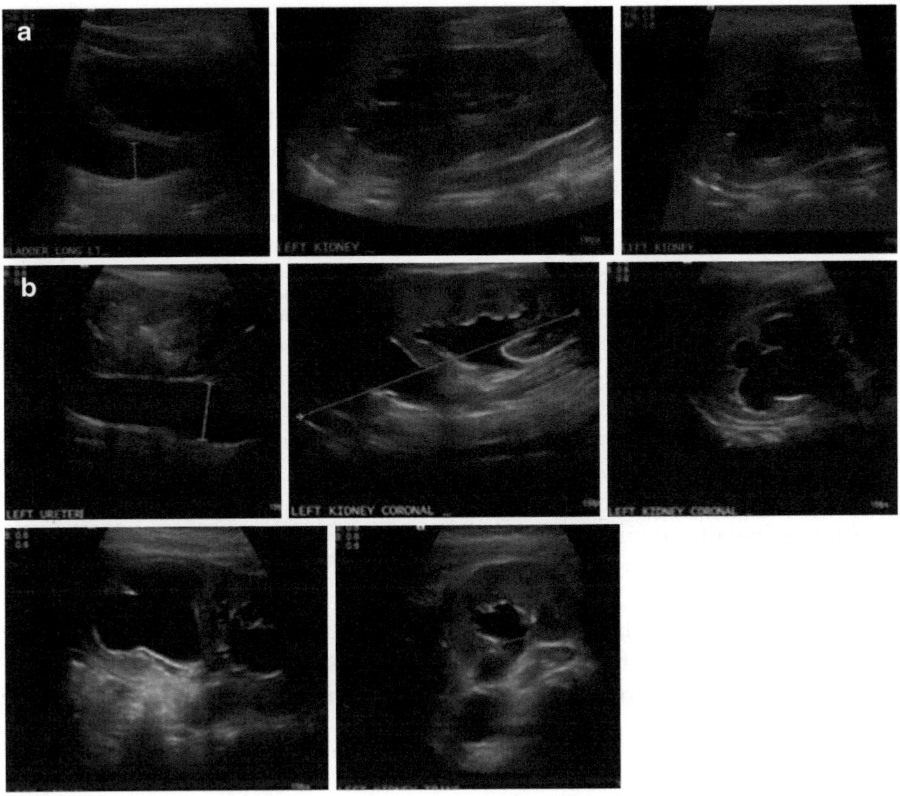

Fig. 9.56 (**a**) US urinary tract at 6 months of age. Duplex left kidney with persistent dilatation of the upper moiety collecting system. The distal insertion of the upper moiety ureter is ectopic below the level of the trigone and could not be clearly visualised, possibly inserting into the vagina. (**b**) US urinary tract at 1 year of age. Mild increase in the left renal cortical echogenicity and progressive dilatation of the upper moiety pelvicalyceal, renal pelvis APD 11 mm. There is new mild dilatation of the left lower moiety pelvicalyceal system, APD 7 mm. Persistent left upper moiety ureteric dilatation up to 20 mm

after the Abs were stopped, she presented to ED with another febrile UTI due to a multi-resistant *Pseudomonas aeruginosa*, requiring admission for IV antibiotic treatment. The repeat US Urinary tract at 12 months of age demonstrated increase in the left upper moiety renal pelvis and ureteric dilatation (Fig. 9.56).

Question 3. How Would You Manage Her Now?

Because of the recurrence of the UTIs as soon as the Abs were stopped and the atypical bacteria, but also the increasing upper moiety dilatation on US, the patient should not be managed conservatively anymore and should undergo definitive surgical treatment. In her case the urinary tract ultrasounds demonstrate a possible low insertion of the upper moiety ureter, raising the possibility of an ectopic ureter.

At her age, the options of surgical approach would be to perform an open uretero-ureterostomy or alternatively a common sheath ureteric reimplantation.

Due to the recurrence of the UTIs and the progressive dilatation on US, decision was made to proceed with surgical intervention; the prophylactic Abs were restarted until de procedure was performed. She underwent a left open uretero-ureterostomy at 13 months of age and although initially well, developed a UTI within 1 week from surgery.

Question 4. What Is Your Post-Operative Management and Follow Up?
The patient should stay on prophylactic Abs until the first review with a urinary tract US 6–8 weeks after the surgery. Subsequent follow ups should include ultrasounds 3 and 6 months after the surgery and then yearly until she is toilette trained. A repeat NM scan could be considered based on the previous history of reduced function of the upper moiety and recurrent UTIs.

She was initially continued on Px Abs after the procedure, but this were stopped 2 months after the surgery when she was reviewed with a repeat US urinary tract which demonstrated significant improvement of the left upper moiety renal pelvis and ureteric dilatation. She remained asymptomatic, with no further UTIs and was successfully toilet trained at the age of 3 years old. Subsequent US at 18 months, 2 and 3 years of age confirmed the previous findings with no evidence of left upper moiety collecting system dilatation (Fig. 9.57).

9.16.1 Discussion

This patient had no previous history but presented early in infancy with a febrile UTI, which triggered further investigations that lead to the diagnosis of a left duplex kidney. The US demonstrated a dilated left upper moiety and ureter with likely an ectopic insertion, with preserved function on the NM scan (40% upper moiety). As this was the first UTI she was started on prophylactic Abs and monitored with serial US, in which the dilatation of the left upper urinary tract remained stable. Due to her favourable progress the chemoprophylaxis was stopped when she was 9 months old, but only a few weeks after she developed a severe febrile UTI and there was increasing dilatation on her US. This was considered a failure of the medical treatment, as she developed further breakthrough UTIs and progressive dilatation on US. Because of her young age and the degree of dilatation of the left upper moiety ureter, decision was made to proceed with a left open uretero-ureterostomy instead of a ureteric reimplantation. The surgery proved to be successful, as she did not develop any further UTIs once the antibiotics were stopped and there was significant improvement of the left upper moiety renal pelvis and ureteric dilatation of her follow up imaging.

In this case the main reasons for surgical treatment were the breakthrough UTIs and the increasing left upper moiety urinary tract dilatation. The US had demonstrated severe distal ureteric dilatation and gave the impression of a very low ectopic ureteric insertion, which also favoured a more definitive management option. Many

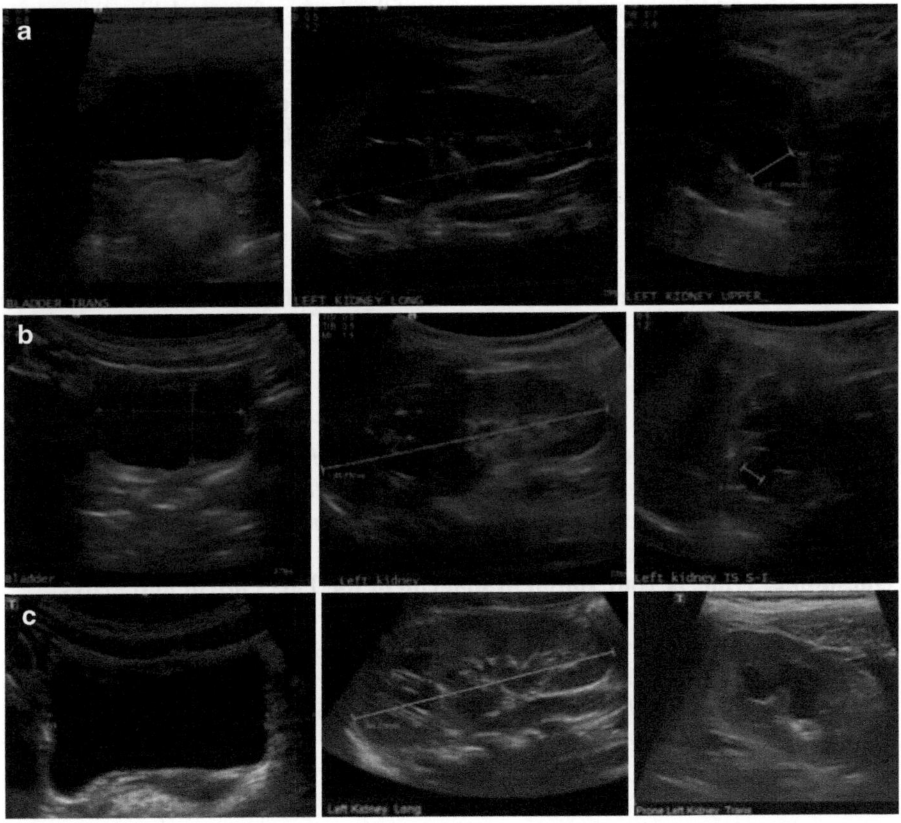

Fig. 9.57 (**a**) Urinary tract US 2 months after the procedure. Duplex left kidney with improved upper moiety pelvicalyceal dilatation, with a renal pelvis APD of 10 mm, and proximal ureteric dilatation and tortuosity. There is progressive generalised thinning of the upper moiety cortical parenchyma. No distal ureteric dilatation. (**b**) US urinary tract at 18 months of age. Interval growth of left duplex kidney with a lesser degree of upper moiety pelvicalyceal dilatation, with APD 6.5 mm, and improvement in the parenchymal thickness. No distal ureteric dilatation seen. (**c**) US urinary tract at 3 years of age. There is stable mild thinning of the upper moiety parenchyma with mildly decreased pelvicalyceal dilatation compared to previous. No evidence of distal ureteric dilatation

patients will also undergo an MCUG to ensure there is no associated VUR to the lower moiety as the cause for the UTIs. This was not performed in this case mainly due to the lack of dilatation of the lower moiety or its ureter. In this case, an uretero-ureterostomy was preferred over a common sheath reimplantation because of the young age of the patient and her small bladder, and the large ureteric dilatation.

Uretero-ureterostomy is an increasingly used alternative for children with pyeloureteral duplication in whom the obstructed moiety has significant functionality [52]. It is the technique of choice for children without VUR to the lower moiety, like this case, to avoid introducing reflux into a functional but anatomically abnormal upper pole moiety. However, a few centres have begun using uretero-ureterostomies for the management of duplex anomalies irrespective of the degree of ureteral dilatation, upper moiety functionality, or presence of ipsilateral VUR [52–54]. After surgery, infection of the residual ureteral stump is a concern and it can occur in up to 12% of cases [52]. The patient had a single UTI shortly after the surgery, but this was not suspected to be related to the ureteric stump. Regardless, no further episodes occurred after.

9.17 Case 17

A 4-weeks old girl with antenatal diagnosis of right duplex kidney identified on the 20-week morphology scan undergoes a urinary tract US at 2 weeks of age and is referred for further management (Fig. 9.58).

Question 1. What Does the Ultrasound Show?
The right kidney appears to have a duplex configuration with a dilated upper moiety. The right upper moiety ureter is tortuous and dilated throughout its length up to 12 mm and there is evidence of a moderate size right ureterocoele.

Question 2. What Is Your Initial Management for This Patient and Why?
The patient should be commenced on Px Ab and should undergo endoscopic incision of the ureterocoele with the aim to drain the right upper moiety. The ureterocoele has to be treated because there is a risk of bladder outlet obstruction due to the its size, but also to release the obstruction of the upper moiety of the right kidney, in order to preserve its function.

She was born term and was started on antibiotic Px after birth. A postnatal US at 2 weeks of age confirmed a right duplex kidney with upper moiety dilatation (renal

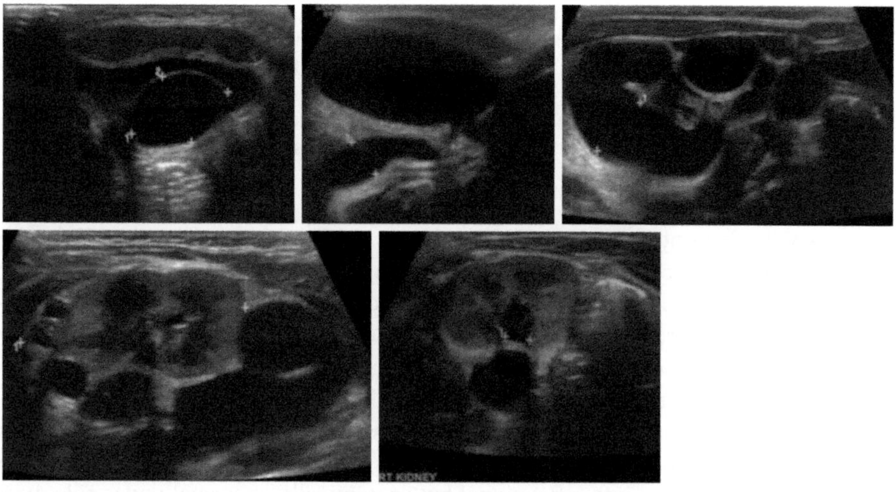

Fig. 9.58 Urinary tract US at 2 weeks of age. Images of the bladder, right kidney and right ureter

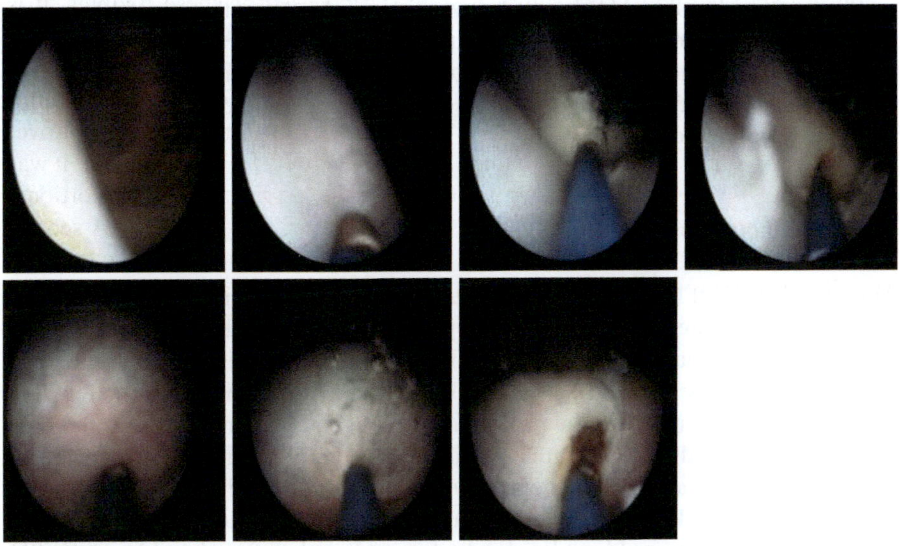

Fig. 9.59 Endoscopic ureterocoele incision. Intraoperatively there was evidence of a large right ureterocoele entering the bladder neck, which was incised with a 3.5 mm Bugby diathermy. Drainage of debris from the obstructive system was demonstrated after a second incision

pelvis APD 5 mm) and also demonstrated a moderate size ureterocoele (18 × 18 × 12 mm) and dilated tortuous right upper moiety ureter. Due to the size of the ureterocoele, with the risk of bladder outlet obstruction, and the obstruction of the upper moiety of the right kidney, decision was made to proceed with an endoscopic incision of the right ureterocoele, which was performed when she was 6 weeks old. She was discharged home on the same day and recovered well from the procedure (Fig. 9.59).

Question 3. What Is Your Postoperative Management Plan?

The patient should remain on antibiotic prophylaxis ideally for another 6 weeks until the first follow up. She should undergo a repeat ultrasound at 6 weeks and subsequently a NM scan to assess the function of the right upper moiety and potentially also exclude VUR. Subsequent surveillance should include a urinary tract US 3 and 6 months after the procedure, and at 2 and 3 years of age.

She remained on prophylactic Abs and did not develop any UTIs. She underwent a urinary tract US 3 months after the procedure, which showed improvement in the right upper moiety PC dilatation, with persistent proximal and distal ureteric dilatation and a moderate size right ureterocoele. A NM scan was also requested to assess the function of the upper moiety. Due to her favourable progress her antibiotics were stopped, and she was monitored with regular US urinary tract. A repeat US at 11 months of age demonstrated again a right duplex kidney with a dysplastic upper moiety and dilated ureter and ureterocoele, similar in size compared to the previous scan.

She remained well and UTI-free and was reviewed again at the age of 18 months, 2 and 3 years and by that time she was toilette trained as well. Serial US urinary tract demonstrated good interval growth of the right kidney remaining lower moiety with no upper moiety PC dilatation and some mild upper moiety ureteric dilatation and mostly collapsed ureterocoele.

9.17.1 Discussion

This female patient had an antenatal diagnosis of a duplex kidney and the postnatal US also demonstrated dilatation of the upper moiety associated with a large ureterocoele. She was managed with prophylactic Abs and endoscopic incision of the ureterocoele due to its size and its potential to cause bladder outlet obstruction. The ultrasounds preformed after the procedure demonstrated improvement in the right upper urinary tract dilatation, with a persistent moderate size right ureterocoele; she remained UTI-free and the chemoprophylaxis was stopped when she was almost a year old. The right kidney appeared smaller with slightly reduced function (42%) and the upper moiety could not be clearly demonstrated on functional imaging. She was toilette trained at around 3½ years of age and all her follow up US urinary tract demonstrated resolution of the right upper moiety pelvicalyceal dilatation, with only mild ureteric dilatation and a mostly collapsed ureterocoele.

Ureterocoeles are most commonly associated with the upper pole of a complete ureteral duplication; single system ureterocoeles are less common and they usually affect males [49, 55]. Asymptomatic neonates without severe hydroureteronephrosis can be treated conservatively and be started on antibiotic prophylaxis until they undergo further investigations by 3–6 months of age [52]. The risk of UTIs in patients receiving antibiotic prophylaxis is <10% before 6 months of age [56]. On the other hand, cases with severe upper urinary tract dilatation can be treated by an upper urinary tract approach or by endoscopic decompression depending on upper pole function and the presence of VUR to the lower moiety. The ureterocoele moiety function is generally negligible and scintigraphic assessment is enough, as it is a reliable means of assessment of the function of each moiety. Endoscopic decompression is the approach of choice for intravesical ureterocoeles and it allows for a definitive treatment in at >90% of patients [52, 55, 56] and, in the remaining ones, it can be combined with conservative management or endoscopic treatment of possibly associated VUR. Preoperative VUR tends to persist after ureterocoele decompression, but <50% of patients with reflux develop urinary tract infections [55, 56]. Nevertheless, those patients are more likely to require secondary procedures. Non-functioning or poorly functioning upper poles can be left *in situ* if the patient is asymptomatic, or in cases of lower urinary tract reconstruction and after endoscopic decompression. This patient was asymptomatic, but the main reason for treating her early in life was the size of the ureterocoele and the associated upper urinary tract dilatation, as there was no confirmation of the function of the upper moiety at that stage. The main worry with large ureterocoeles is that they can cause bladder outlet obstruction and subsequently contralateral upper urinary tract dilatation as well, with the risk of compromising the overall renal function [57]. In her case the obstruction of the upper moiety also represented a risk for UTIs, despite the Ab prophylaxis.

9.18 Case 18

A 7-months old girl with normal antenatal scans and no significant previous medical history presented with febrile UTIs, one due to Citrobacter Freundii infection. She initially responded to oral Abs but then required admission for intravenous AB treatment. An US urinary tract was performed during the admission, which demonstrated a left duplex kidney, with echogenic mildly dilated upper moiety and ureteric dilatation, and large left ureterocoele with significant debris in it (Fig. 9.60).

Question 1. What Is Your Initial Management for This Patient?
The patient should be started on antimicrobial prophylaxis as soon as the treatment is completed and should undergo an endoscopic incision of the ureterocoele ideally once the infection is cleared, to decompress it and allow drainage from the left upper moiety to prevent further UTIs and preserve renal function.

She completed a course of antibiotics and was started on chemoprophylaxis on discharge. Once she had recovered from the infection, she underwent endoscopic incision of the ureterocoele with adequate collapse of it (Fig. 9.61).

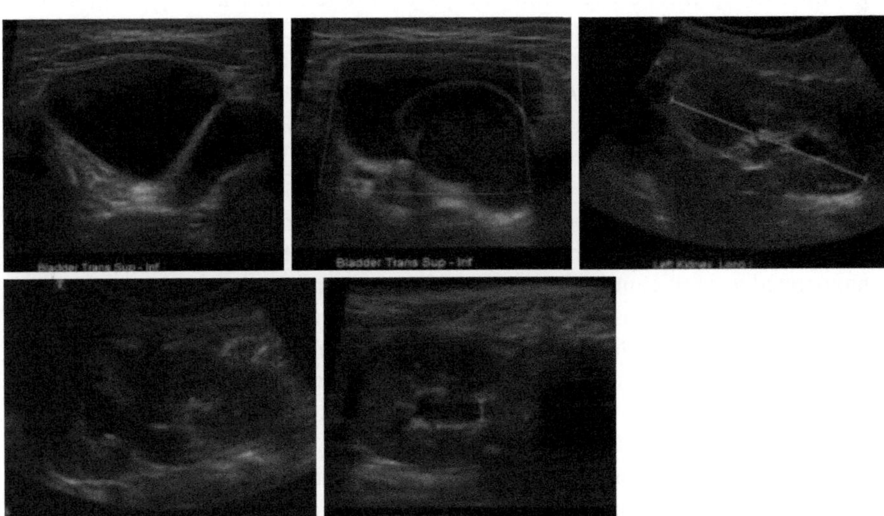

Fig. 9.60 US urinary tract at 7 months of age during episode of febrile UTI. Duplex left kidney with moderate upper moiety pelvicalyceal dilatation, renal pelvis APD 9 mm, and mild prominence of the lower moiety renal pelvis, APD 4 mm. Large left sided ureterocoele filled with mobile debris and dilated left distal ureter

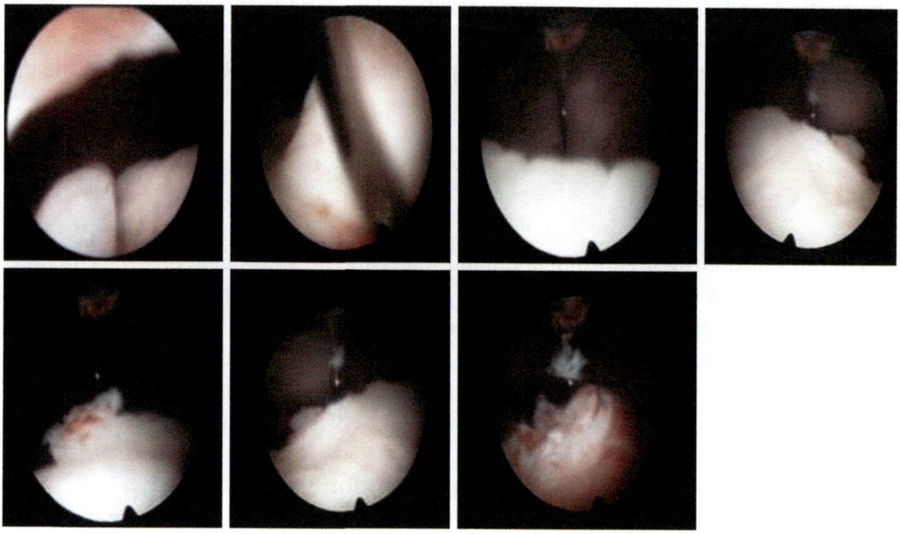

Fig. 9.61 Cystoscopic incision of ureterocoele. Intraoperatively a large left ectopic ureterocoele was identified, protruding through the bladder neck. The ureterocoele was incised multiple times until adequate collapse was achieved

Question 2. What Is Your Postoperative Management and Follow Up Plan?
The patient should remain on prophylactic Abs at least until the first follow up after the procedure, usually within six to 8 weeks. Imaging surveillance should include an US of the urinary tract 2 weeks after the procedure to ensure decompression of the ureterocoele, and subsequently, at three and 6 months, and then yearly until the patient is toilette trained to assess the progression of the upper urinary tract dilatation. A NM scan, ideally with indirect cystography, should also be performed to assess the function of each moiety and eventually also confirm or exclude the presence of VUR.

She was continued on prophylactic antibiotics and remained well after the procedure, with no further UTIs. A repeat ultrasound 2 weeks after the endoscopic incision demonstrated a significant improvement in the left upper moiety and ureteric dilatation and a partially collapsed ureterocoele. A NM scan was also performed and confirmed the presence of a left duplex kidney with a poorly functioning upper moiety (20%) and high-grade lower moiety VUR. She was reviewed again at 11 months of age with a repeat urinary tract US, which demonstrated again a left duplex kidney with minimal dilatation of upper and lower moieties, with some upper moiety cortical thinning, with intermittent left upper moiety ureteric dilatation, distally up to 8 mm, and a collapsed ureterocoele. She remained asymptomatic with no further UTIs during this period and remained on the antimicrobial prophylaxis.

Unfortunately, at 1 year of age she developed another febrile UTI, again due to Citrobacter Freundii. She was treated with oral Abs with good response and continued on Ab prophylaxis after. A repeat ultrasound was requested after the infection

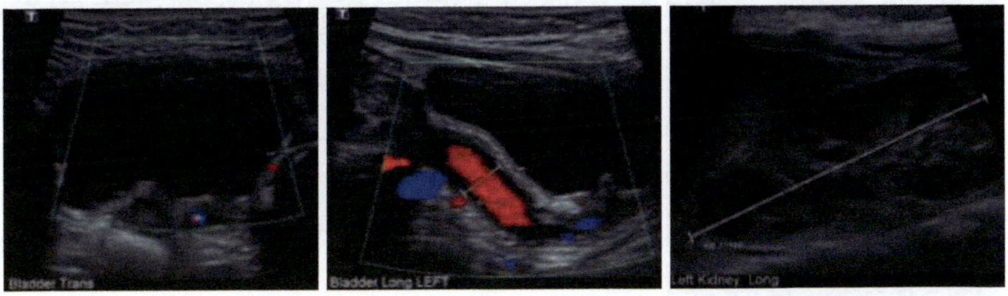

Fig. 9.62 US urinary tract 3 month after UTI. The left duplex kidney is larger with interval growth noted. No significant dilatation of either moiety. Left distal ureteric dilatation stable, 8 mm. Left ureterocele is smaller, appears collapsed

to assess any possible progression of the dilatation. After this, she subsequently developed 3 more UTIs (*K. pneumoniae*, *E. cloacae*, and *E. coli*) despite AB prophylaxis and changes to the type of Abs (Fig. 9.62).

Question 3. What Is Your Management Now and Why?
In this case the medical treatment has failed, and the patient requires surgical management to prevent further UTI and loss of kidney function. Because there is still evidence of left upper urinary tract dilatation on the ultrasound, the UTIs could be explained by the high-grade lower moiety VUR or the possibility that there is still some degree of obstruction of the upper moiety, although the ureterocoele appears collapsed on the most recent imaging. In her case, because of the presence of VUR, she should undergo a common-sheath ureteric reimplantation with excision of the remnant of the ureterocoele and repair of the bladder wall.

Due to failure of medical treatment, the evidence of lower moiety VUR and the presence of residual function of the upper moiety decision was made to proceed with surgical management. At the age of 15 months she underwent a conjoined left ureteric reimplantation with excision of the remnant of the ureterocoele and repair of the bladder wall. A left lower moiety ureteric and a urethral catheter were left in place to ensure safe bladder drainage, which were removed 3 days after the surgery.

She recovered well from the procedure and was discharge home a few days after on Px Abs. She was reviewed again 2, 6, and 9 months after the surgery with a urinary tract US which initially demonstrated some mild increase in the left upper urinary tract dilatation, but subsequently only minor prominence of the upper moiety renal pelvis, with stable distal ureteric dilatation.

Her prophylactic Abs were stopped after the first follow up appointment and she remained well and asymptomatic with no further UTIs (Fig. 9.63).

9.18.1 Discussion

This female infant had normal antenatal scans but was diagnosed with a left duplex kidney and a large ureterocoele while being investigated for an atypical febrile UTI

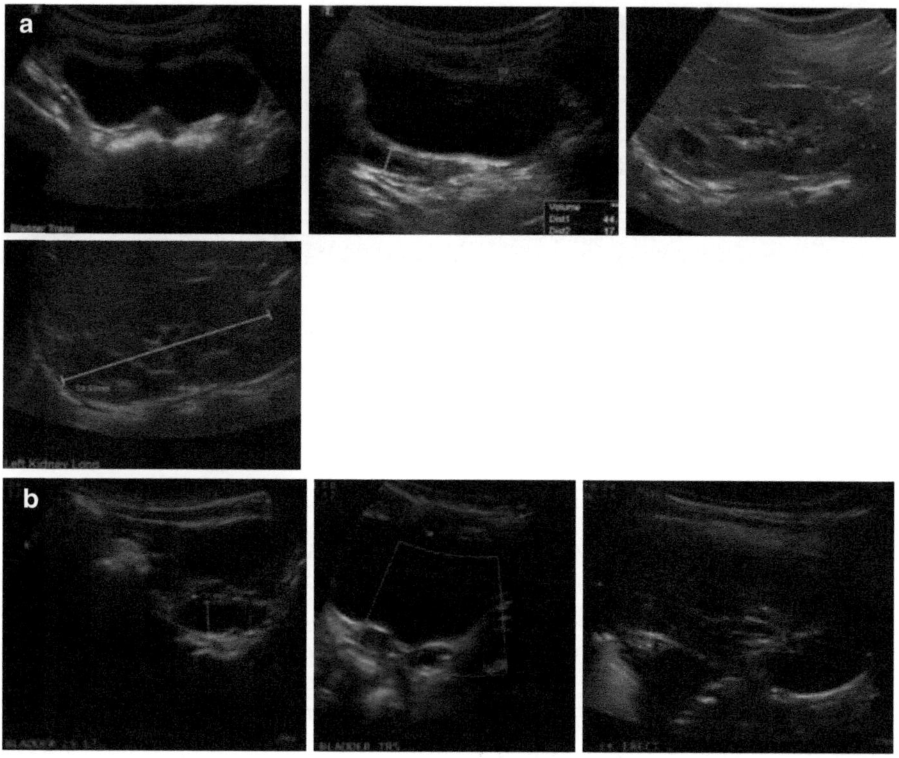

Fig. 9.63 (**a**) US urinary tract 2 months after surgery. Left duplex kidney with mild increase in upper moiety renal pelvis dilatation up to 6 mm and persistent distal ureteric dilatation up to 10 mm. Ureterocoele not identified. (**b**) Repeat US urinary tract 9 months after the surgery. Left duplex kidney with irregular cortical thinning within the upper moiety and minor prominence of the upper moiety renal pelvis (3 mm). Persistent but stable left distal ureteric dilatation 10 mm. Bladder wall focal irregularity related to previous ureterocoele repair

at 7 months of age. She was started on antibiotic prophylaxis and underwent endoscopic decompression of the ureterocoele, but developed further UTIs despite medical and minimally invasive treatment, with subsequent significant improvement in the left upper moiety and ureteric dilatation and a collapsed ureterocoele on follow up imaging, The functional imaging demonstrated a poorly functioning left upper moiety, but also high grade VUR to the lower moiety, which was likely the cause of her recurrent UTIs. Because of this, even though she was only 14 months old, she underwent reconstructive surgery to allow drainage of the upper moiety and correct the VUR at once, to prevent further renal function deterioration and avoid UTIs.

As mentioned before, patients with duplex system ureterocoeles and severe upper urinary tract dilatation can be treated by an upper urinary tract approach or by endoscopic decompression depending on the upper pole function and the presence of VUR to the lower moiety. Preoperative VUR tends to persist after ureterocoele decompression, but <50% of patients with reflux develop urinary tract infections

[55, 56, 58]. In her case, the lower moiety VUR was diagnosed after the endoscopic decompression and she developed breakthrough UTIs, making her a candidate for a secondary procedure. In this patient it is highly likely that the recurrent UTIs were due to the lower moiety VUR or a combination of both the upper urinary tract stasis of urine from the upper moiety and the VUR. Interestingly, the UTIs only started when she was over 6 months old, which is less frequent, and with time, her infections became more difficult to eradicate and to prevent even with different antibiotics. Because of her age and the fact that there was functional parenchyma to preserve from the upper moiety, in the context of a duplex kidney with an upper moiety ureterocoele and lower moiety VUR, we opted for a lower urinary tract approach and reconstructive surgery was performed when she was over 12 months old. An alternative in this case would have been to treat the VUR with a minimally invasive approach as well. There is evidence to suggest that endoscopic puncture may be used irrespective of the presence of reflux, and that minimally invasive techniques may be used to treat children with VUR either inherent to a duplex system or resulting from previous endoscopic puncture [52, 59–61]. Some studies have shown spontaneous resolution of the preoperative VUR in up to 71% of cases during follow-up, and good results with endoscopic injection of a bulking agent in symptomatic patients with persistent VUR after the initial procedure [59]. It has also been reported, that a small number of patients develops "de-novo" VUR after decompression. The VUR in these patients may also resolve spontaneously, but about 50% of cases may need further surgical correction, which can be attempted with endoscopic injection first [52, 59]. Regardless of the type of VUR, these patients should be managed conservatively with prophylactic antibiotics, except for patients with persistent VUR and breakthrough UTI. And this was the case with our patient.

9.19 Case 19

A 3-months old female with antenatal diagnosis of a non-complicated left duplex kidney presented with a febrile UTI and required admission for treatment with IV Abs. A urinary tract US was performed after birth and she was referred for further management (Fig. 9.64).

Question 1. What Does the Ultrasound Show?
The left kidney has a duplex configuration, with dilatation of the upper moiety collecting system with the renal pelvis APD 16 mm. There is marked dilatation and tortuosity of the upper moiety ureter extending into the pelvis, with an associated ureterocoele. There is marked thinning of the upper moiety parenchyma.

Question 2. What Is Your Initial Management?
The patient should be started on Px Abs and undergo further investigations: a repeat urinary tract US to reassess the degree of dilatation of the left upper moiety and a NM scan to determine the differential renal function of each moiety.

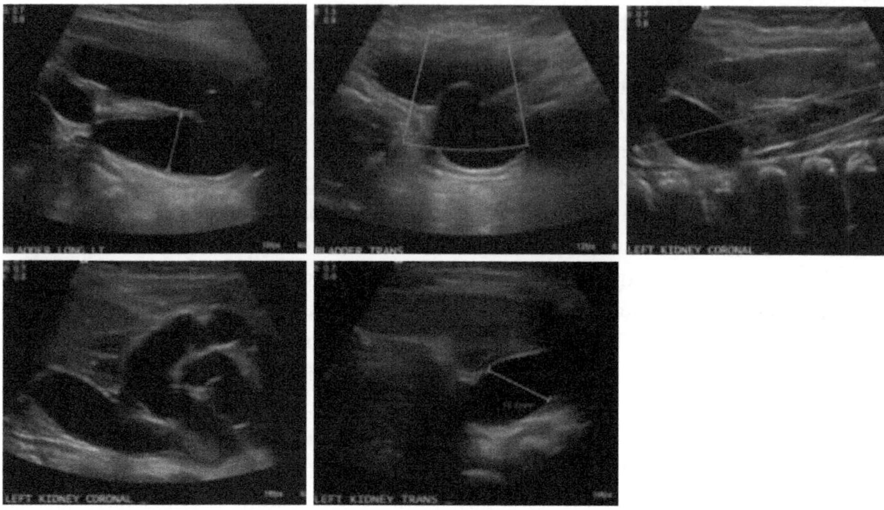

Fig. 9.64 Urinary tract US 2 weeks after birth

The ultrasound demonstrated a left duplex kidney with dilatation of the upper moiety collecting system, with a tortuous and dilated ectopically inserted ureter (up to 14 mm) and an associated ureterocoele. With the US findings she was started on Px Abs in the neonatal period and a NM scan was also requested, which confirmed the presence of a left duplex kidney with a poorly functioning and obstructed upper moiety (2%). A repeat US at 3 months of age, at the time of the UTI, showed stable appearances of the dilated left upper moiety PC system and ureter, with some debris in the upper urinary tract and bladder (Fig. 9.65).

Question 3. Would You Perform any Other Investigations and Why?
Because of the US findings with significant upper moiety renal pelvis and ureteric dilatation, but the apparent ectopic insertion of the ureter and associated ureterocoele, a diagnostic cystoscopy could be of help to assess the anatomy of the urinary tract, confirm the presence of a ureterocoele and determine the position of each UO.

She recovered well from the infection after a course of antibiotics and underwent a diagnostic cystoscopy 1 week after, to assess the urinary tract and determine if a ureterocoele or other cause for the upper moiety obstruction could be identified and treated. On cystoscopy, a right upper moiety ureterocoele could not be identified, nor a normal UO. The lower moiety UO was positioned low in the trigone but remained above the bladder neck and there was a single orthotopic right UO.

She continued the Ab prophylaxis remaining UTI-free and asymptomatic and was reviewed 2 months after the procedure with an US urinary tract, which again demonstrated stable appearances of the left duplex kidney with dilated upper moiety renal pelvis and ureter (Fig. 9.66).

Despite AB prophylaxis and changes in the type of Abs, she subsequently developed further febrile UTIs, one of them due to a multi-resistant *K. pneumoniae*. A repeat US urinary tract performed when she was 11 months old, showed some mild progression of the upper moiety collecting system dilatation, with increase in the distal ureteric dilatation up to 22 mm (Fig. 9.67).

Question 4. What Is Your Definitive Management for This Girl and Why?

This patient requires surgical management, because of the breakthrough UTIs and increasing dilatation on ultrasound. The medical treatment has failed and there is no option for endoscopic treatment, as there is no ureterocoele and the upper moiety

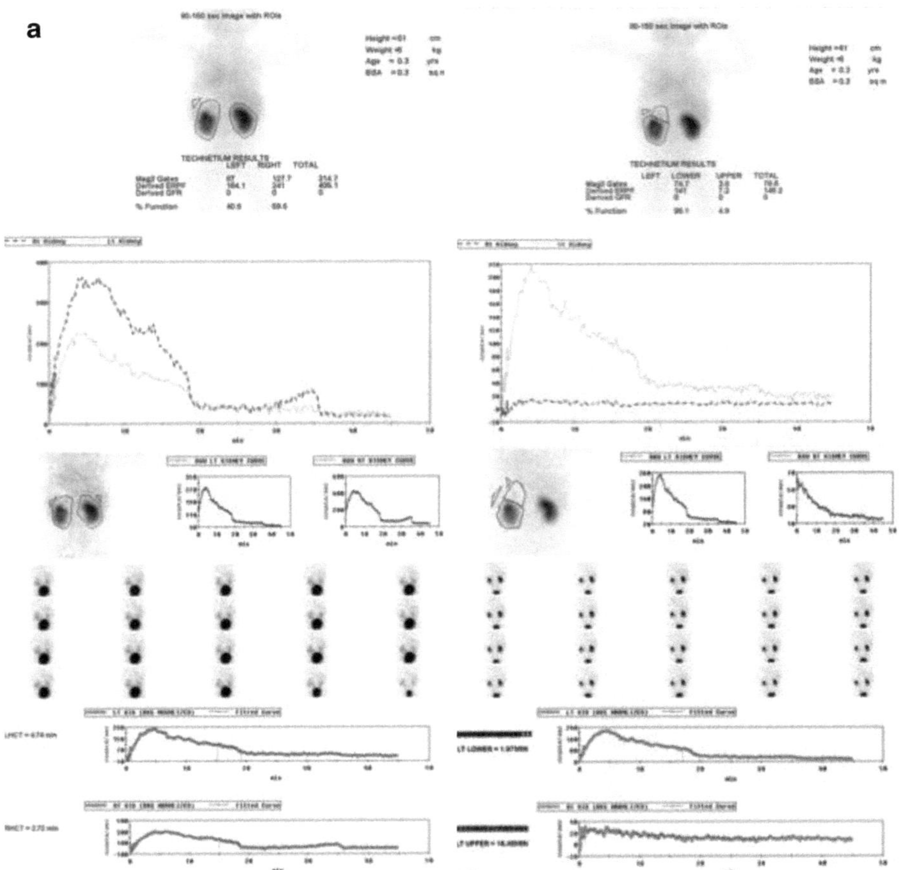

Fig. 9.65 (**a**) MAG-3 at 3 months of age. The left kidney shows features of a duplex kidney with a poorly functioning and obstructed upper moiety. The differential function measures 41% on the left and 59% on the right. The differential function of the upper moiety measures 2% and lower moiety about 39% of overall renal function. (**b**) Repeat US at 3 months of age during admission for UTI. Echogenic debris is now noted within the collecting system and ureter of the left upper moiety. The upper moiety ureter remains tortuous and dilated up to 15 mm, as well as the PC system, with a renal pelvis APD of 14 mm, and the parenchyma remains thin and echogenic with loss of corticomedullary differentiation. The lower moiety appears normal

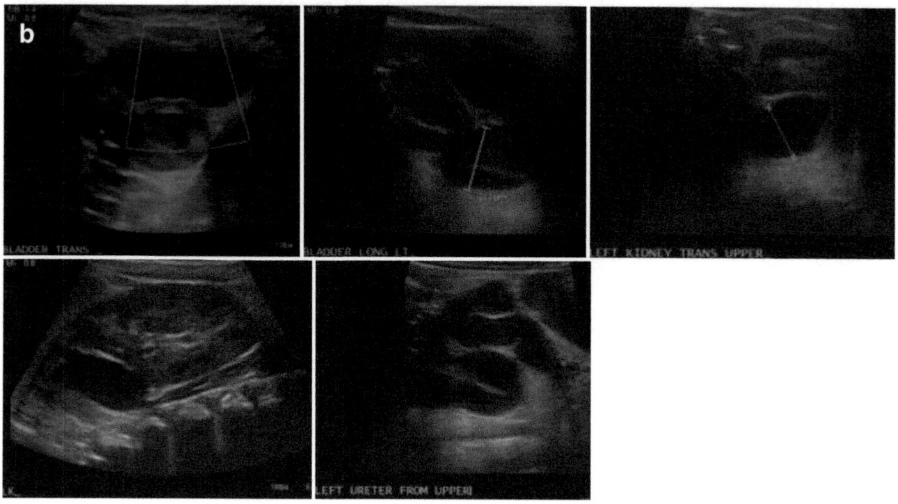

Fig. 9.65 (continued)

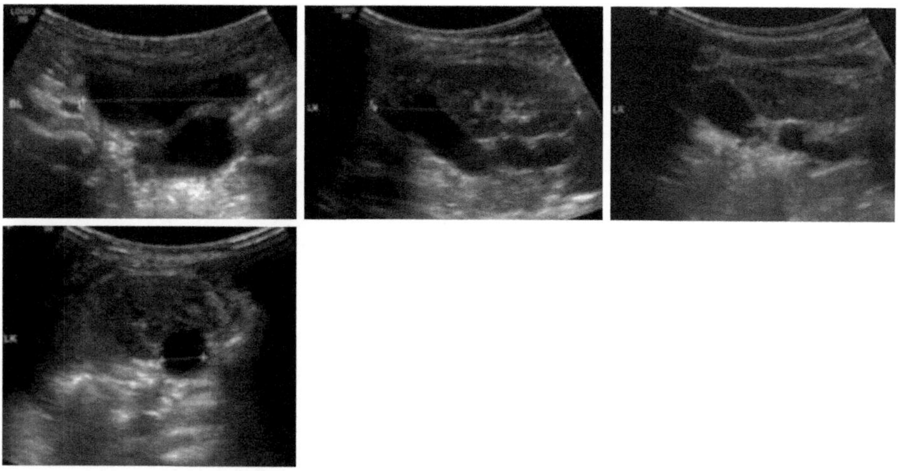

Fig. 9.66 US urinary tract 6 weeks after diagnostic cystoscopy. Persistent but stable left upper moiety renal pelvis dilatation, APD 12 mm, with parenchyma thinning and mild increase in the distal ureteric dilatation up to 20 mm

UO could not be identified on cystoscopy. Considering the lack of function of the upper moiety the best option would be to perform an upper pole heminephrectomy. The patient is almost 1 year of age and could undergo a minimally invasive technique, with a retro or transperitoneal approach, although in many centres this surgery is still performed open at her age.

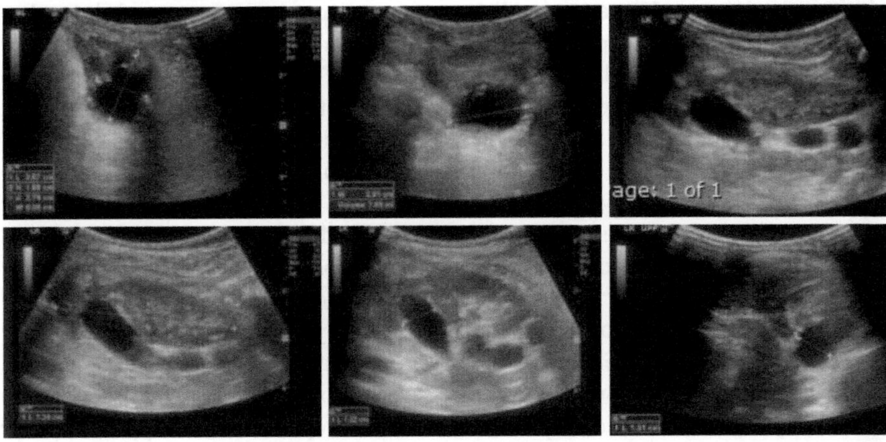

Fig. 9.67 US urinary tract at 11 months of age. Left duplex kidney with persistent upper moiety renal pelvis dilatation, APD 12 mm, and mild increase in the distal ureteric dilatation up to 22 mm

Because of the recurrent UTIs and persistent upper moiety collecting system dilatation in the context of a non-functioning and obstructive upper moiety, she underwent a laparoscopic retroperitoneal upper pole heminephrectomy when she was 1 year old. She recovered very well from surgery and was discharged 24 h after. She remained well and asymptomatic, with no further UTIs, and was reviewed 3 and 6 months after the procedure with an US urinary tract. On US, there was interval growth of both kidneys, with normal appearances on the right. The remaining left lower moiety had no upper urinary tract dilatation and there was no collection at the upper pole on the bed of the partial nephrectomy. Six months after she was toilette trained and remained asymptomatic. A repeat urinary tract US at 2 and 3 years of age demonstrated good interval growth of both kidneys, without upper urinary tract dilatation and normal bladder appearances, with complete emptying. A NM scan was also performed to assess the function of the remaining left kidney.

9.19.1 Discussion

In this case the patient had an antenatal diagnosis of a left duplex kidney and presented with a febrile UTI, despite being on prophylactic Abs since birth. The postnatal ultrasounds demonstrated dilatation of the left upper moiety collecting system, with a possibly ectopic ureteric insertion and a ureterocoele, and the function of the upper moiety was negligible on the MAG-3 (2%). She underwent a diagnostic cystoscopy to confirm the ultrasound findings and with the plan of decompressing the ureterocoele endoscopically. Interestingly, an ureterocoele could not be identified and she continued conservative management with AB prophylaxis. Unfortunately, she developed further breakthrough febrile UTIs, and decision was made to proceed with surgery. We opted for a minimally invasive upper tract approach and she underwent a laparoscopic retroperitoneal upper pole heminephrectomy, which is our institutions preference at this age. She remained UTI free after the procedure and the remaining left lower moiety appeared normal on the follow-up ultrasounds.

Upper tract approaches to duplex system anomalies are usually indicated when the affected moiety has no function, when the patient suffers from recurrent UTIs, when there is high grade VUR to the lower moiety, and/or when a primary lower urinary tract approach has already been attempted and failed [52]. These approaches traditionally included pyelopyelostomy, ureteropyelostomy, and open or minimally invasive heminephrectomy [52]. The technique of choice depends on the age of the patient and the function of the affected moiety. Pyelo/uretero-pyelostomies are rarely used because of their higher risk of complications and no real advantages over a heminephrectomy, which can offer very good outcomes when performed with minimally invasive techniques [62–65]. Heminephrectomy is appropriate for children with ectopic ureters and duplex system ureterocoeles without VUR and its success rate is around 85% [52, 62, 64, 66, 67], and it may also be considered for non-functioning refluxing lower moieties. There are several advantages of minimally invasive approaches compared with open surgery. First, the affected moiety is not directly manipulated as it is with open surgery, which requires mobilization of the kidney from the surrounding structures for exposure, risking torsion of the renal pedicle and consequent injury or thrombosis of the vessels of either moiety [52, 62]. In contrast, a laparoscopic approach is performed with the kidney in situ with minimal traction on the pedicle [63, 64]. Secondly, minimally invasive approaches offer a shorter hospital stay and improved cosmesis with comparable operative duration [66]. Transperitoneal and retroperitoneal laparoscopic heminephrectomy are comparable with respect to operative duration, hospital stay, and analgesic requirements and both are superior to open surgery in these respects [62, 63]. Conversion to open surgery is still required in up to 10% of cases due to bleeding/vascular injury, damage to surrounding structures and peritoneal breach [62, 64, 66]. Possible immediate complications after minimally invasive upper moiety heminephrectomy are urine leak/urinoma, haematoma and UTIs. Long-term complications include cyst formation at the surgical bed; functional loss of the ipsilateral remaining moiety; UTIs caused by persistent VUR; de-novo VUR; infections of the ureteric stump; hypertension, and need for additional surgery (completion nephrectomy, excision of the ureteric stump) [52, 62, 64, 66, 67]. Our patient has not developed any of these complications so far.

9.20 E. VUR

9.20.1 Case 20

A 5-years old female with a previous history of febrile UTIs from the age of 1 year is referred for further investigations after a urinary tract US demonstrated scarring and thinning of the cortex of the upper and mid poles of the left kidney, and mild left

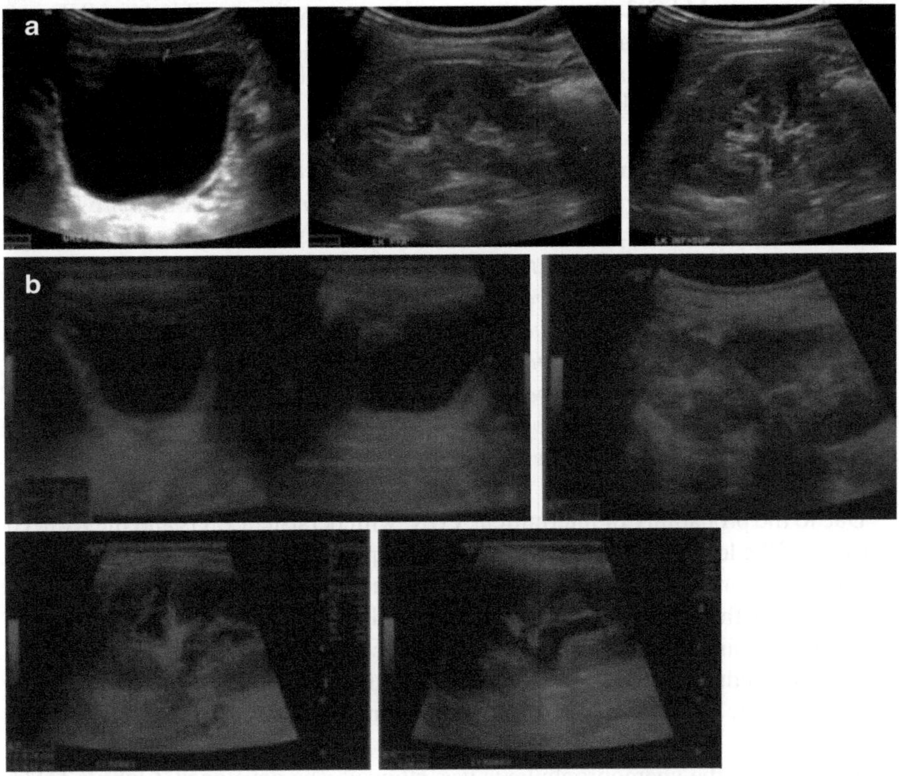

Fig. 9.68 US urinary tract at 5 years of age. (**a**) Focal cortical thinning is seen at the upper and mid poles of the left kidney, suggestive of focal scar. Mild left renal pelvis prominence, APD 8 mm. (**b**) Repeat US urinary tract at 5½ years of age. Stable appearances of both kidneys with mild left renal pelvis prominence. No evidence of distal ureteric dilatation seen

renal pelvis dilatation. She was toilette trained since she was 2½ years old, voiding around 6 times/day and remained dry day and night. She did not have any issues with constipation (Fig. 9.68).

Question 1. What Would You Do Next and Why?

The history of recurrent UTIs, without voiding dysfunction, and evidence of scarring of the left kidney on the ultrasound raises the possibility of VUR as the underlying cause for the infections. The patient should be commenced on prophylactic antibiotics and should also undergo further investigations. A NM scan should be performed; either a DMSA, to confirm the presence of scarring as an indirect indicator of VUR, or a MAG-3 with indirect cystography to assess the renal function and determine if VUR is present or not, although it can be missed in 21–50% cases. At her age, an indirect cystogram is a less invasive and better tolerated option compared to an MCUG.

In this case a MAG-3 scan was requested to assess for possible left VUR and unfortunately, she continued to have febrile UTIs after the assessment. This showed Slightly reduced left renal function, 42%. An indirect cystogram was performed with no demonstrable reflux.

Question 2. What Is Your Management for This Girl?

As mentioned before there is possibility that this patient has VUR and she has not responded to the initial preventive treatment and has had further breakthrough UTIs. The failure of medical treatment and evidence of scarring with reduction of the left renal function justifies performing another procedure to prevent further UTIs and reduction of the renal function. The best option in her case is to proceed with a diagnostic cystoscopy, with the possibility to perform an injection of a bulking agent into the UO if the appearances are consistent with VUR. Otherwise, if there is no evidence of a golf hole UO, a urethral catheter could be inserted to perform an MCUG later the same day.

Due to the probability of intermittent VUR, with persistent UTIs and the reduced function of the left kidney, decision was made to proceed with endoscopic treatment and also to start her on Px Abs. She underwent a cystoscopy and injection of Deflux© to both UOs at the age of 5½ years old and recovered without complications. She remained well and asymptomatic and continued on Px Abs until 3 months after the procedure, when she was reviewed with a repeat US urinary tract which didn't show any evidence of upper tract dilatation or further scarring of the left kidney (Fig. 9.69).

Shortly after the chemoprophylaxis was stopped, she developed 3 febrile UTIs, and her Abs were restarted. After this, she managed to remain asymptomatic again for about 3 months, but she had recurrent febrile UTIs as soon as the prophylaxis was stopped. A repeat US urinary tract 6 months after demonstrated interval growth of both kidneys and no upper tract dilatation, but persistent focal scarring of the upper and lower poles of the left kidney (Fig. 9.70).

Due to the recurrent febrile UTIs while off Abs and the persistent renal scarring with lack of indirect signs of VUR on the MAG-IRC, she underwent a micturating cystourethrogram to assess for VUR and decide further management with those findings (Fig. 9.71).

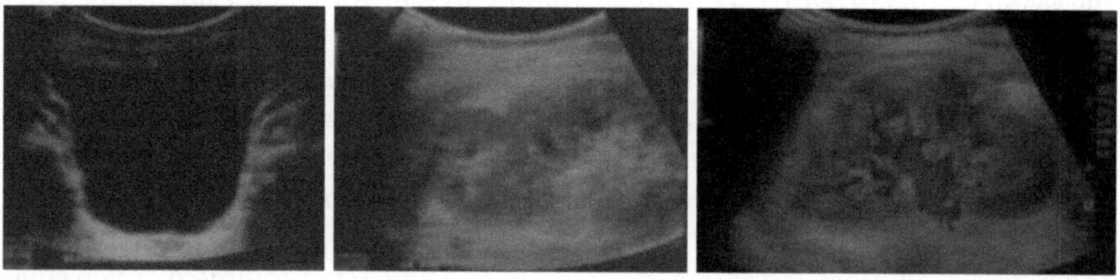

Fig. 9.69 US urinary tract 3 months after the procedure. Stable kidney appearances with no upper urinary tract dilatation

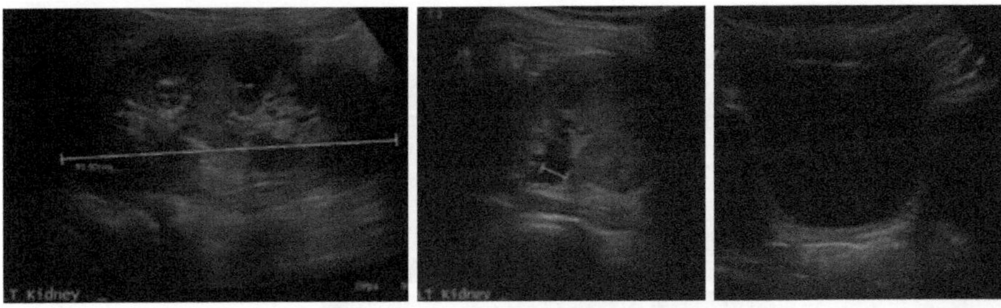

Fig. 9.70 US urinary tract at 6 years of age. Both kidneys measure 8.9 cm. Right kidney has normal appearances. Left kidney with minor focal cortical thinning in the upper and lower poles in keeping with focal scarring. No pelvicalyceal or ureteric dilatation on either side, only mild prominence of the left renal pelvis (APD 6 mm). Complete bladder emptying

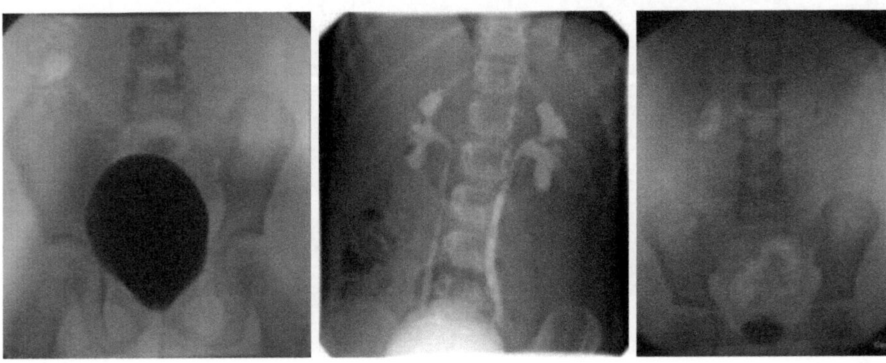

Fig. 9.71 MCUG at 6½ years of age

Question 3. What Does the Micturating Cystourethrogram Show?

There is evidence of bilateral VUR with mild dilation of the ureter and pelvicalyceal system, slightly worse on the left, in keeping with grade III VUR. Both systems emptied almost completely on micturition with no obstruction. Smooth bladder outline without filling defects.

The MCUG demonstrated bilateral Grade III VUR, with good bladder emptying and no other abnormality.

Question 4. What Is the Best Option for Definitive Management for This Girl?

This patient is a candidate for definitive surgery, because both the medical and endoscopic treatment have failed. In some cases, a repeated Deflux injection can be offered; however, at her age the preference is to proceed with reconstructive surgery to correct the VUR. In her case, the best approach would be an open ureteric reimplantation with the Cohen technique with a success rate of around 96%. These treatment alternatives should be discussed with the parents before a decision is made.

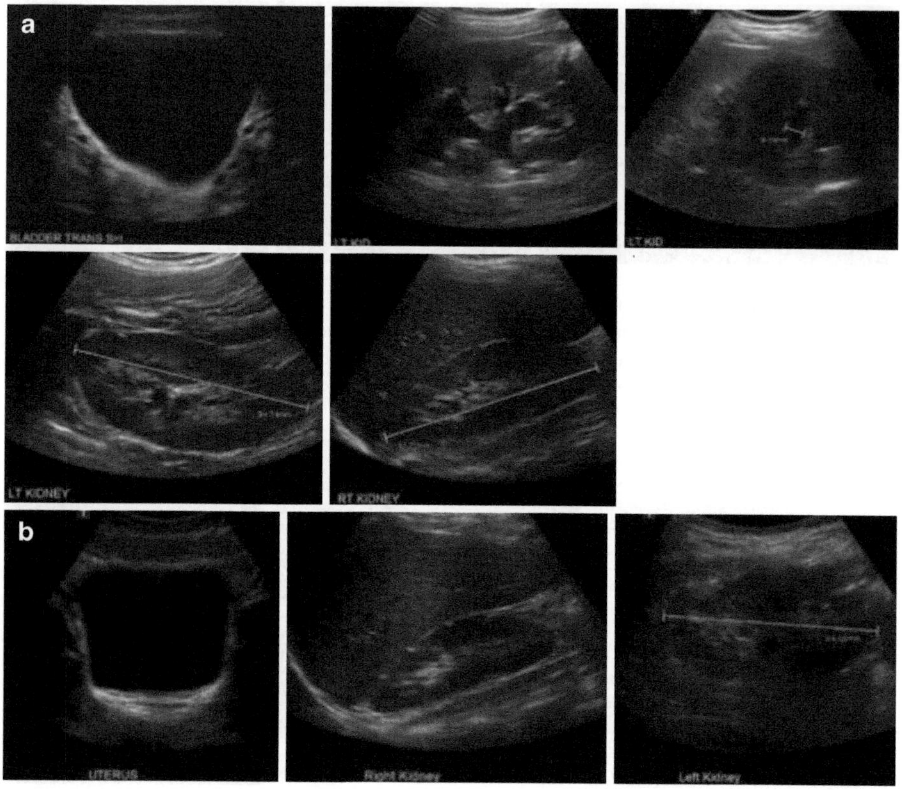

Fig. 9.72 (**a**) US urinary tract 3 months after surgery. Normal appearances of the right kidney, no upper urinary tract dilatation. Minor focal cortical scarring noted at the upper and lower poles of the left kidney. Mild prominence of the left renal pelvis pre-void, APD 8 mm, which resolves post-micturition. (**b**) US urinary tract 1 year after surgery. Normal bladder and complete emptying. Normal right kidney appearances. The left kidney demonstrates focal areas of cortical loss or scarring with an irregular contour. No upper urinary tract dilatation on either side

Options of repeat injection of Deflux© or ureteric reimplantation were discussed largely with parents and it was agreed to proceed with open surgery. She underwent a bilateral cross-trigonal Cohen ureteric reimplantation when she was almost 7 years old and was reviewed 6 weeks after the procedure with an US urinary tract, with evidence of persistent mild prominence of the left renal pelvis, which resolved after micturition, and stable cortical scarring in the upper and lower poles. She remained well and asymptomatic, with no further UTIs after the surgery. A repeat US urinary tract 12 months after the procedure again demonstrated stable cortical scarring in the upper and lower poles of the left kidney, with complete resolution of the left renal pelvis dilatation (Fig. 9.72).

9.20.2 Discussion

This 5-years old girl presented with recurrent febrile UTIs, scarring of the upper and mid poles and slightly reduced left renal function (42%) on NM scan, and mild left renal pelvis dilatation, raising the possibility of left VUR. She had no evidence of voiding dysfunction and was fully toilette trained when she was referred to our institution. The initial investigations aimed to exclude vesicoureteric reflux, but because of her age, a NM scan with indirect cystography had to be performed, as it is a less invasive and better tolerated option compared to an MCUG, although VUR can be missed in up to 21–50% cases [27, 28]. Because of the persistent UTIs with evidence of renal scarring and the fact that VUR could not be ruled out completely, she was started on prophylactic Abs and underwent endoscopic treatment with injection of a bulking agent to both UOs, because the right side also appeared abnormal. As it is our usual practice, the prophylactic Abs were stopped shortly after the procedure, but her UTIs recurred whenever an attempt was made to stop the chemoprophylaxis. In order to confirm the presence of VUR and decide further management she underwent a MCUG, which is the gold standard for the diagnosis. Interestingly, the MCUG demonstrated bilateral grade III VUR, with good bladder emptying and no other abnormalities. The surgical options were discussed with the parents, and it was decided to proceed with open surgery.

Bacterial urinary tract infections (UTIs) are one of the most common causes for children to be admitted to hospital, such that between 3 and 7% of girls and 1–3% of boys will require treatment [68]. Urinary tract infections are more common in females in all age groups except in the elderly. Females are also at higher risk for recurrent UTIs, likely due to the shorter length of the urethra, and its close proximity to the anus [68]. *Escherichia coli* is the most common cause of UTIs in both children and adults. The most significant risk factor for a child to develop pyelonephritis is the presence of vesicoureteric reflux (VUR), although the presence of bladder and bowel dysfunction is an important risk factor as well. Boys typically present with a higher grade of VUR and more severe renal damage when compared to girls. There are certain factors that contribute to reflux resolution, including patient age, grade of reflux, postnatal presentation, and the presence or absence of associated voiding dysfunction [69]. Lower resolution rates occur in patients with higher grade of VUR, older age at diagnosis, postnatal presentation and voiding dysfunction.

It is now accepted that in the absence of infection VUR rarely results in renal damage. This has shifted management from a primarily surgical approach to more conservative medical treatment consistent of antibiotic prophylaxis and management of voiding dysfunction if present [68–70]. The biggest consequence of recurrent febrile UTIs is the development of renal scars with the risk of long-term loss of kidney function and hypertension. The immune response of the child, along with a quick introduction of antimicrobial treatment, are fundamental for the clearance of the infection and to prevent renal scarring. This is the reason why only a part of the children with recurrent UTIs will develop renal scars and this will occur even if these children receive antibiotic prophylaxis, as demonstrated by the RIVUR trial

(Randomized Intervention for Children with Vesico-Ureteric Reflux) [70]. In this study, the incidence of UTI was significantly reduced in patients on antibiotic prophylaxis, but the rate of renal scarring was similar between the treatment and the placebo groups. This study also showed that early initiation of treatment with antibiotics was effective at preventing pyelonephritis, but there was no difference in the rate of renal scarring in children. Treatment of bladder and bowel dysfunction decreases the number of UTIs, but it is not clear if it reduces renal scarring.

In regards to the surgical management, this can be done endoscopically with injection of bulking agents into the UO, or via reconstructive surgery to correct the VUR with ureteric reimplantation. Absolute indications for surgical correction are breakthrough febrile UTIs and new renal scars or deterioration of renal function [69, 71, 72]. Relative indications include non-compliance with or contraindication to medical treatment; persistent VUR with no improvement; complex anatomy; parental preference (to avoid continuous antibiotic therapy and imaging); VUR grade, and bilateralism [69, 71, 72]. Interestingly, surgical correction of VUR has not proven to diminish the rate of renal scar formation [71, 72]. In this case, the surgical options were discussed with the parents, who were offered repeat endoscopic treatment and reconstructive surgery. There is evidence that repeated injections increase the success rate of the procedure, up to 90% depending on the technique used (HIT > STING) and the initial severity (grade) of the reflux, with better results for grades I–III [69, 71, 72]. Reconstructive surgery consists of a ureteric reimplantation with an anti-reflux mechanism, which can be performed open or with minimally invasive approaches and has a success rate of up to 92–98% depending on the technique used [73]. The most common surgical treatment is the intravesical repair described by Cohen, where the ureters are placed in a trans-trigonal submucosal tunnel, whose length should be 5 times the diameter of the ureter. It was agreed with the parents to proceed with open surgery to ensure a more definitive procedure.

9.21 Case 21

A 2-days old male with antenatal diagnosis of bilateral hydronephrosis who was born at term and commenced on Ab prophylaxis after birth, is referred to you for further management. His perinatal history is otherwise unremarkable, and his physical examination is normal.

Question 1. What Is Your Initial Management for This Patient and Why?
This male patient has an antenatal history of bilateral hydronephrosis and the main diagnosis that needs to be ruled out is posterior urethral valves, although there is no mention of the bladder and ureteric appearances or the amniotic fluid volume and lung development on the antenatal scans.

Because of this, the patient should undergo a repeat urinary tract US within the first 48 h of life and if there is evidence of persistent bilateral renal pelvis and ureteric dilatation a urethral catheter should be inserted. Blood tests should also be performed to assess the renal function (UEC). Depending on the ultrasound findings, if there is evidence of bilateral hydroureteronephrosis the patient should undergo a MCUG to exclude bladder outlet obstruction, due to PUV and less likely urethral atresia, and eventually transfer the patient for further management to a urology unit if the diagnosis is confirmed.

He underwent an US urinary tract on day 2 of life which again demonstrated bilateral renal pelvis dilatation, but with distal ureteric dilatation as well. Due to these findings, with bilateral renal pelvis and ureteric dilatation, he also underwent a MCUG. He remained UTI free and his renal function was normal, with a creatinine of 37 μmol/l. A repeat US urinary tract at 2 weeks of age again demonstrated bilateral renal pelvis dilatation, with distal ureteric dilatation (Fig. 9.73).

Question 2. What Does the MCUG Show?
The MCUG demonstrates bilateral grade V vesicoureteric reflux. Normal urethra, with no evidence of PUV, and normal bladder appearances. Both ureters are dilated and tortuous and there is pelvicalyceal distension on both sides, worse on the left. Both ureters drained, the right more quickly than the left.

Question 3. Would You Request any Further Investigations?
Yes, a NM dynamic scan to assess the differential renal function, mainly because of the thinning of the cortex and dysplastic appearances of the left kidney on US, in the context of high grade bilateral VUR.

An US of the spine may also be considered to rule out spinal anomalies, although the physical examination was normal, and the bladder outline was also normal on both the US and the MCUG.

Due to the appearances of a dysplastic left kidney on US and the high grade VUR he also underwent a NM scan at 2 months of age, which demonstrated bilateral hydronephrosis and tortuous, dilated ureters secondary to VUR, with no evidence of ureteric or bladder outlet obstruction, and confirmed a small poorly functioning left kidney (17%) with retrograde filling of the collecting system consistent with high grade VUR. An US of the spine was not performed due to absence of abnormal findings on physical examination of the spine and the normal bladder outline on both the ultrasound and the MCUG.

Question 4. With These Results, What Is Your Management for this Patient?
In the absence of UTIs the VUR can be managed conservatively with prophylactic Abs until he is old enough to undergo a circumcision under GA, to reduce his risk of UTIs and prevent further renal damage. A diagnostic cystoscopy could be performed at the same time to confirm the radiological findings. The Ab prophylaxis could be stopped after the procedure, although in some centres the preference is to continue with it until the patient is 1 year old because of the natural history of VUR.

The patient should undergo regular surveillance with urinary tract US at 3, 6, and 9 months of age to assess the upper urinary tract dilatation and the growth of the dysplastic kidney. He should also be referred to the nephrology team for regular monitoring of his renal function.

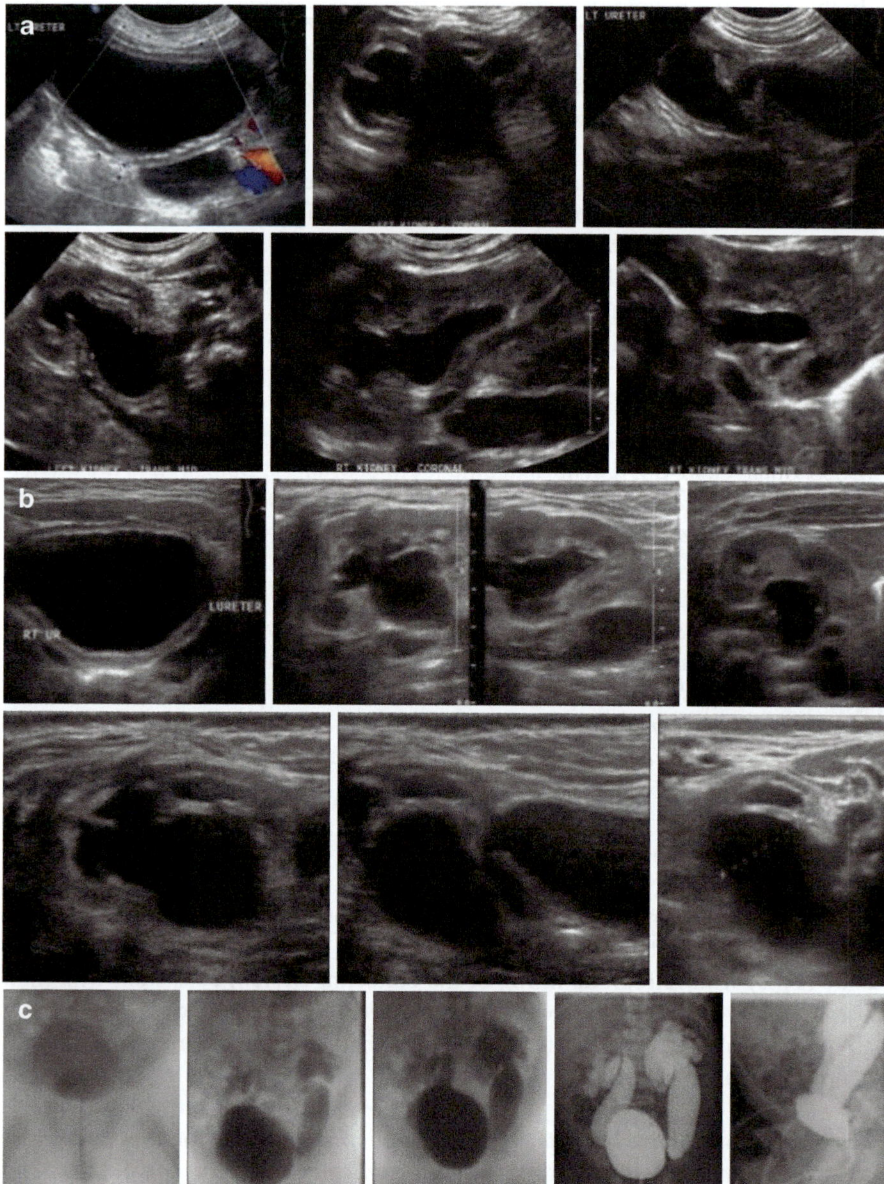

Fig. 9.73 (**a**) US urinary tract day 2 of life. Small left kidney with thinned parenchyma and severe renal pelvis dilatation, with a dilated and tortuous ureter. Mild right renal pelvis dilatation, APD 5 mm, with normal parenchyma. (**b**) US urinary tract at 2 weeks of age. Mild right renal pelvis dilatation, APD 10 mm, with normal surrounding parenchyma and only minimal distal ureteric dilatation. The left kidney only has a rim of very thin cortex, appears dysplastic and has persistent renal pelvis dilatation, APD 15 mm; the left ureter is tortuous and dilated down to the bladder. Normal bladder outline. (**c**) MCUG at day 5 life

He remained asymptomatic with stable renal function (Cr 26 μmol/l) and UTI free on the prophylactic Abs and underwent a repeat US at 5 months of age, with stable appearances of the smaller dysplastic left kidney and mild renal pelvis dilatation of the hypertrophic right kidney, and subsequently a cystoscopy and circumcision at 6 months of age, to reduce the risk of urinary tract infections. On cystoscopy, the posterior urethra was not dilated but there was evidence of non-obstructive type III PUV. The bladder mucosa appeared normal, without trabeculations, polyps or diverticula. Both UOs had golf hole configuration, with the left larger than the right. US urinary tract 3 and 6 months after the procedure demonstrated further reduction in size of the dysplastic left kidney and compensatory hypertrophy on the right, with only mild right renal pelvis dilatation. He remained well with no UTIs and stable renal function (Cr 28 μmol/l) and his Abs were stopped when he was 12 months old (Fig. 9.74).

He remained well and without UTIs, with stable renal function and was fully toilette trained at around 3 years of age. He was then reviewed yearly and subsequently every 2 years with regular US urinary tracts and BP checks, remaining asymptomatic (Fig. 9.75).

9.22 Case 22

A 6-weeks old male with antenatal diagnosis of a possible left duplex kidney and hydronephrosis is referred after a urinary tract ultrasound performed on day 7 demonstrated a single system left kidney with renal pelvis dilatation, with an APD of 13 mm. He was started on Px Abs at birth, remained well with no UTIs and was thriving. A repeat US at 6 weeks of age demonstrated a mildly dilated left renal pelvis, APD 4 mm, with less pronounced calyceal dilatation, and globally slightly reduced left renal parenchyma. There was new evidence of a dilated left distal ureter, up to 5 mm, and the right kidney appeared normal (Fig. 9.76).

Question 1. What Is Your Initial Management for This Patient?

The patient should remain on prophylactic Abs and further investigations should be requested, because of the reduced left renal size and evidence of left renal pelvis dilatation with distal ureteric dilatation as well. The possible underlying cause for these findings is left VUR and in this scenario it is important to ascertain the function of the left kidney to decide further management.

In this case, because of the evidence of upper urinary tract dilatation, the parents should also be offered a circumcision to reduce his risk of urinary tract infections.

With these findings, decision was made to proceed with a NM scan with indirect cystography to assess the renal function and for possible VUR and to repeat the US urinary tract at 3 months of age. On the MAG-3 there was evidence of reduced function of the left kidney and left VUR. During the study, the activity within the collecting system increased during an episode of voiding confirming the presence of left-sided vesicoureteric reflux. The differential function measures 24% on the left and 76% on the right.

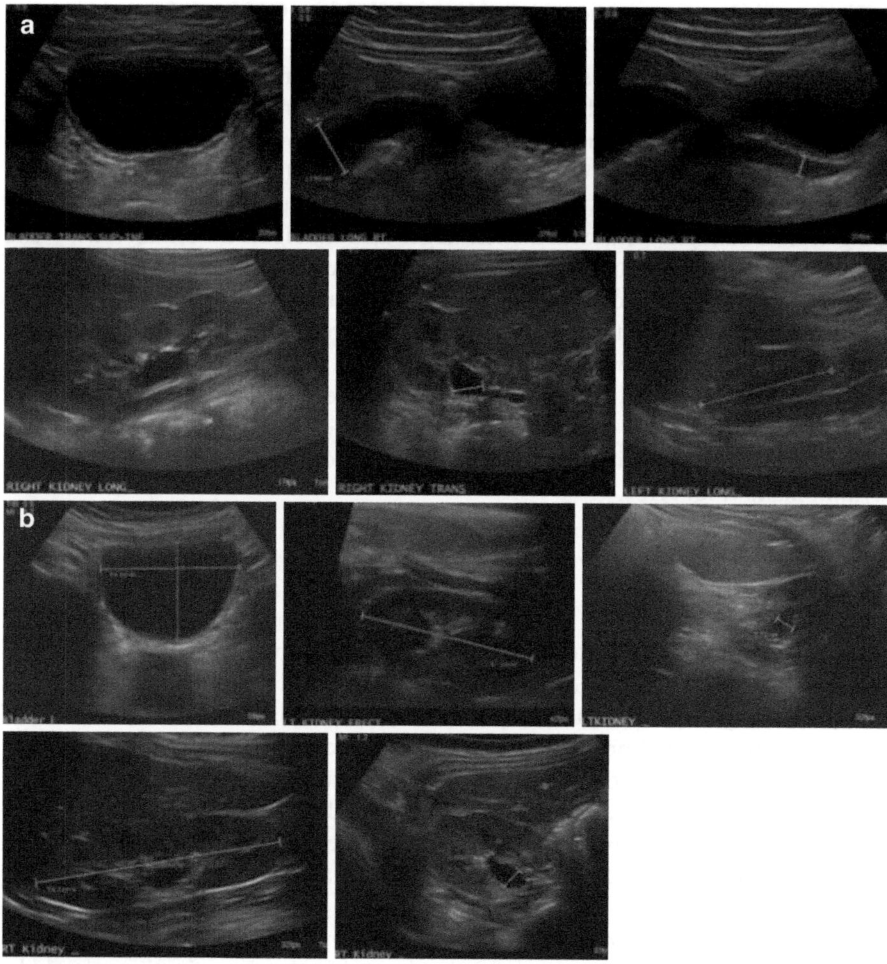

Fig. 9.74 (**a**) US urinary tract at 5 months of age. Normal bladder appearances. The right kidney is mildly echogenic, with compensatory hypertrophy, preserved corticomedullary differentiation and mild renal pelvis dilatation, APD 8 mm. There is proximal and mid ureteric dilatation up to 13 mm. The left kidney is dysplastic and smaller, with loss of corticomedullary differentiation. (**b**) US urinary tract at 15 months of age. Stable size and appearance of the dysplastic left kidney with loss of corticomedullary differentiation. The right kidney is normal in appearance with mild renal pelvis dilatation, APD 7 mm. The moderately distended bladder demonstrates a smooth contour

US urinary tract at 3 months of age showed Interval growth of both kidneys. The left kidney shows reduction of the corticomedullary differentiation and the renal cortex is diffusely thinned, with persistent renal pelvis (APD 14 mm) and ureteric dilatation up to 7 mm.

Because of the presence of upper urinary tract dilatation on the ultrasound and the compromised function of the left kidney likely secondary to the VUR, he underwent a circumcision at 4 months of age to reduce the risk of UTIs. He recovered well after the procedure and his Abs were stopped.

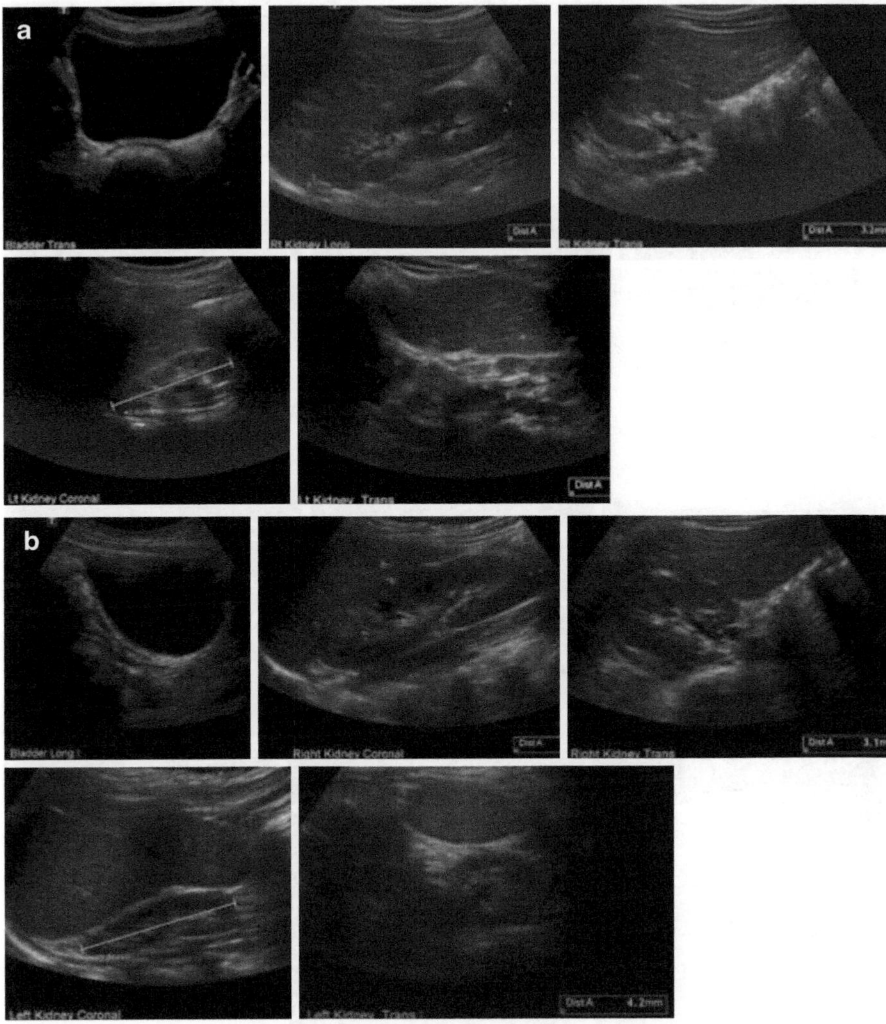

Fig. 9.75 (**a**) US urinary tract at 3 years old. Good interval growth of the right kidney, with no pelvicalyceal dilatation. Small dysplastic left kidney with echogenic parenchyma with loss of corticomedullary differentiation, showing minimal interval growth. Mild prominent looking left extrarenal pelvis. No distal ureteric dilatation, normal bladder appearances. (**b**) US urinary tract at 5 years of age. The right kidney demonstrates interval growth and there is only mild prominence of the right renal pelvis, APD 3 mm. The left kidney demonstrates echogenic parenchyma with loss of corticomedullary differentiation and persistent mild prominence of the left renal pelvis, APD 5 mm. The bladder is smooth walled

Question 2. What Is Your Follow Up Plan for This Patient?

The patient should undergo regular surveillance with urinary tract US at three, six and 12 months of age, then yearly until he is toilette trained and at the age of 5 years. No further investigations are required unless the patient becomes symptomatic or there is evidence of increasing upper urinary tract dilatation on ultrasound.

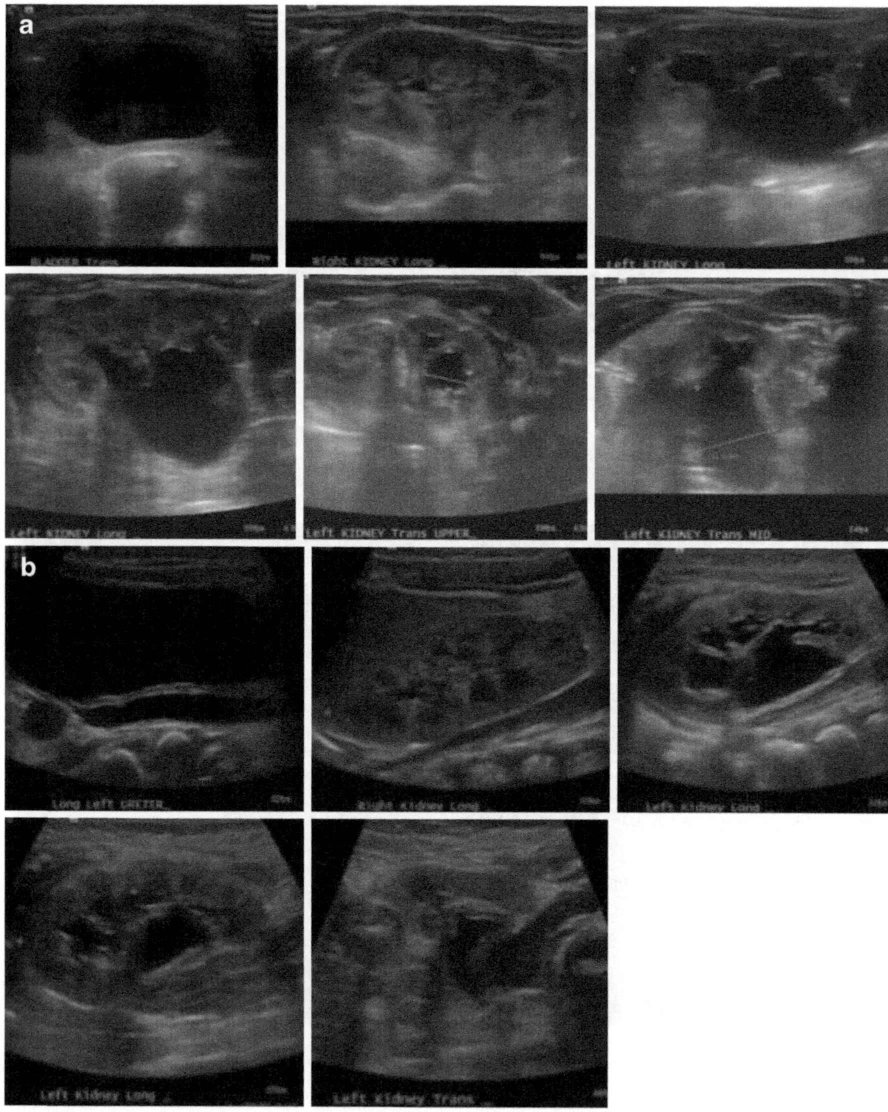

Fig. 9.76 (**a**) US urinary tract on day seven of life. The right kidney measure 4.3 cm and the left 3.9 cm. Normal right kidney appearances, without upper urinary tract dilatation. Single system left kidney with pelvicalyceal dilatation, renal pelvis APD 8 mm, and extrarenal pelvis 13 mm. No distal ureteric seen and normal bladder outline. (**b**) Repeat US at 6 weeks of age. The right kidney measures 5.3 cm and the left 4.4 cm. Mildly dilated left renal pelvis, APD 4 mm, with less pronounced calyceal dilatation, and globally slightly reduced left renal parenchyma. Intermittently dilated left distal ureter, up to 5 mm. Normal appearances of the right kidney

He remained UTI-free and asymptomatic and subsequent follow up ultrasounds demonstrated reduction in the left renal pelvis and ureteric dilatation with interval growth of both kidneys. He was toilette trained during the daytime on last follow up at 2½ years of age (Fig. 9.77).

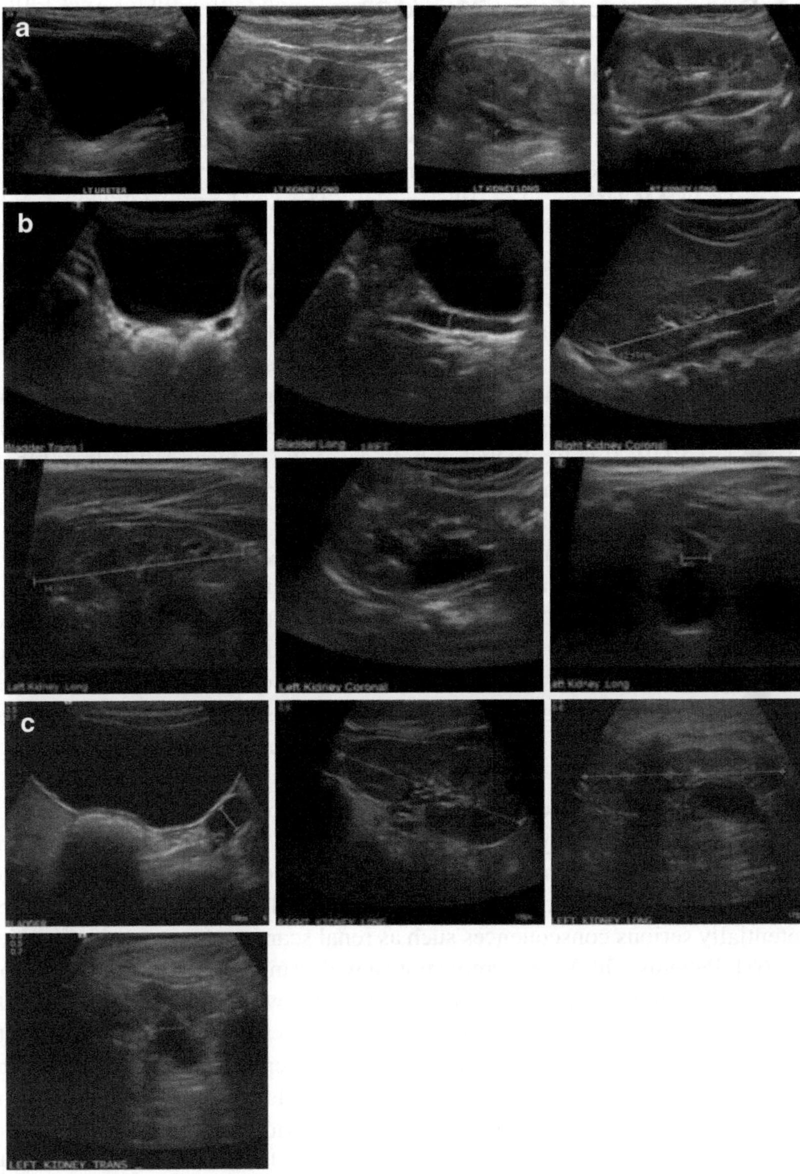

Fig. 9.77 (**a**) US urinary tract 3 months after circumcision. Interval growth of both kidneys, with the left persistently smaller than the right with slightly echogenic and thinned cortex. There is no significant renal pelvis dilatation on either side. Normal bladder appearances. (**b**) US urinary tract at 12 months of age. Normal appearances of the right kidney. There is moderate thinning of the left renal parenchyma and mild left pelvicalyceal dilatation, renal pelvis APD 7 mm. The left distal ureter is mildly dilated up to 7 mm. (**c**) US urinary tract at 2 years of age. There is mild left pelvicalyceal dilatation, APD 5 mm, with urothelial thickening and a baggy extra renal pelvis. Mild global renal cortical thinning and the corticomedullary differentiation is mildly reduced. The pre-void renal pelvis APD is 5 mm. Persistent mild left distal ureteric dilatation, 7 mm. Normal right kidney

9.22.1 Discussion for Cases 21 and 22

In the first case, because of the antenatal diagnosis of bilateral hydronephrosis with further evidence of distal ureteric dilatation and a dysplastic left kidney on the post-natal ultrasound, the main diagnosis to exclude is bladder outlet obstruction due to PUV. In order to achieve this, the child underwent an US urinary tract at birth and subsequently an MCUG to assess the urethra. The voiding cystogram showed a normal posterior urethra and confirmed the presence of bilateral high grade VUR. To complete the diagnostic assessment, functional imaging also needed to be performed to determine if there was any compromise of the renal function. The left kidney in fact, appeared smaller and poorly functioning (17%) with high grade VUR on the MAG-3 scan. In the second case, the ultrasound findings of left ureteric and renal pelvis dilatation and a smaller left kidney triggered further investigations, which then demonstrated significant reduction in the function of the left kidney (26%) and left VUR. It is likely that in both cases the reduced left kidney function was secondary to an abnormal induction of the ureteric bud during embryological development producing an abnormal vesicoureteric junction responsible for the VUR, but also to reflux nephropathy. Both boys were commenced on antimicrobial prophylaxis at birth and subsequently underwent a circumcision when they were old enough to have a safe procedure. After this, they remained UTI-free and asymptomatic, and only required regular monitoring of his renal function and ultrasounds to assess their progress. In both cases, the follow up ultrasounds demonstrated decrease in the upper urinary tract dilatation, although there was further reduction in the size of the dysplastic left kidney and compensatory hypertrophy of the right one for the first boy.

Vesicoureteric reflux, or retrograde flow of urine from the bladder into the ureter, is the most frequent uropathy in the pediatric age [69, 70]. It can be either primary due to a congenital malformation or a delay of development of the vesicoureteral junction, or secondary due to anatomical or functional vesical or ureteral factors. It has potentially serious consequences such as renal scarring, hypertension, and renal failure [68]. Patients with VUR demonstrate a wide range of severity, and a majority of patients will not develop renal scars and probably will not need any intervention [71–74]. The main goal in the management of patients with VUR is the preservation of kidney function by minimizing the risk of pyelonephritis. By defining and analysing the risk factors for each patient (age, sex, reflux grade, lower urinary tract dysfunction [LUTD], anatomic abnormalities, and kidney status), it is possible to identify those patients with a potential risk of upper UTIS and renal scarring [69, 74]. VUR has been shown to resolve spontaneously in around 68% of cases, with higher resolution rates with grades I–III (up to 93%) and at a more rapid pace, but only about 30% in children with high-grade reflux (IV–V) [75]. The rate of resolution also depends on the gender of the child (boys > girl) and the presence of bladder and bowel dysfunction, and its management.

Controversy persists over the optimal management of VUR, particularly the choice of diagnostic procedures, the treatment (medical, endoscopic, or open surgical), and the timing of treatment [71, 72]. Preventing UTIs by using prophylactic antimicrobials is generally the first treatment step. However, there is also a proven benefit from performing a circumcision, to reduce the risk of urinary tract infections [31, 42, 69, 75, 76] and therefore avoid the use of Ab prophylaxis. As mentioned before, indications for surgical treatment are recurrent symptomatic breakthrough UTIs, poor compliance to medical treatment, and presence of new scars or deterioration of renal function with time. In these cases, the patients were initially commenced on prophylactic Abs and subsequently underwent a circumcision, remaining asymptomatic and UTI-free with stable renal function even after stopping the prophylaxis. Because of this, no further surgical intervention was required.

9.23 Case 23

A 3-months old male with antenatal diagnosis of left hydronephrosis, persistent after birth, developed urosepsis and secondary meningitis due to a Klebsiella UTI at 2 weeks of age. He was treated with IV and oral Abs for a course of 3 weeks. A urinary tract ultrasound was performed during the admission (Fig. 9.78).

Question 1. What Does the Ultrasound Show?

Both kidneys demonstrate increased echogenicity, with loss of corticomedullary differentiation, but no evidence of focal scarring. The left kidney demonstrates left pelvicalyceal dilatation and proximal ureteric dilatation with debris in the collecting system and urothelial thickening. There is mild prominence of the right renal pelvis.

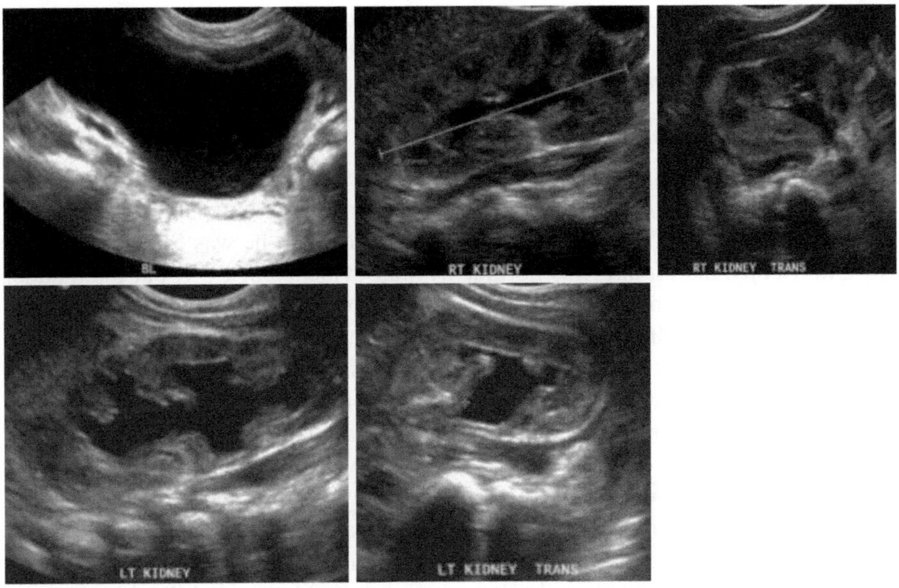

Fig. 9.78 US at 2 weeks of age during episode of UTI

Question 2. What Is Your Initial Management for This Patient?

The patient should be commenced on prophylactic Abs and should undergo further investigations to decide further management. A urinary tract ultrasound should be repeated at 6 weeks and 3 months of age to assess the progression of the upper urinary tract dilatation. Because of the previous UTI and the ultrasound findings the patient should undergo a NM dynamic scan, ideally with indirect cystography, in order to assess the renal function and exclude or confirm the presence of VUR as the underlying cause of the UTI.

The urinary tract US performed during the admission demonstrated left pelvicalyceal dilatation, with APD 13 mm, and distal ureteric dilatation with urothelial thickening, as well as mild prominence of the right renal pelvis with mobile debris in both collecting systems. The patient was commenced on antimicrobial prophylaxis after completing treatment and remained well after the episode, with no further UTIs. A repeat ultrasound 2 weeks after the infection showed persistent left pelvicalyceal dilatation, with a renal pelvis APD of 10 mm, and moderate left distal ureteric dilatation. A subsequent urinary tract ultrasound at 3 months of age demonstrated some mild progression of the left pelvicalyceal and distal ureteric dilatation. The NM scan demonstrated reduced function of left kidney (25%) with high-grade reflux.

Question 3. What Is Your Definitive Management for This Patient?

The patient should undergo a circumcision to reduce his risk of further UTIs and a diagnostic cystoscopy can be performed at the same time to assess the anatomy of the urethra and bladder, and the appearances of both UOs. The Ab prophylaxis can be stopped at that point and he should undergo regular surveillance with a repeat ultrasound 6–8 weeks after the procedure and at nine and 12 months of age; then yearly at least until he is toilette trained and subsequently at 5 years of age. No repeat NM scan is required in this case, unless there is progressive upper urinary tract dilatation, or the patient becomes symptomatic with recurrent UTIs.

With these findings decision was made to proceed with a diagnostic cystoscopy to assess the anatomy of the urethra and bladder, and a circumcision to reduce his risk of further UTIs. The procedure was performed when he was 5 months of age. On Cystoscopy, his urethra was normal without evidence of PUV, but his bladder appeared large and cone shaped, with multiple trabeculations. The left UO was laterally placed and "golf hole"; the right orthotopic and slit like. He underwent further investigations, with a spinal US due to the bladder appearances on cystoscopy and a repeat US urinary tract. His spine appeared normal on US; however, the left pelvicalyceal dilatation had increased from 6 to 15 mm and there was evidence of mild right renal pelvis dilatation of 6 mm. A follow up at 9 months of age US demonstrated again improvement in the left renal pelvis and ureteric dilatation, with stable appearances on the right. He remained well and asymptomatic, with no UTIs after stopping the Px Abs. Unfortunately, the urinary tract US at 1 year of age showed significant increase in the left renal pelvis dilatation, APD 13 mm, and extrarenal pelvis 28 mm, but with a full bladder, with global cortical thinning and reduced corticomedullary differentiation (Fig. 9.79).

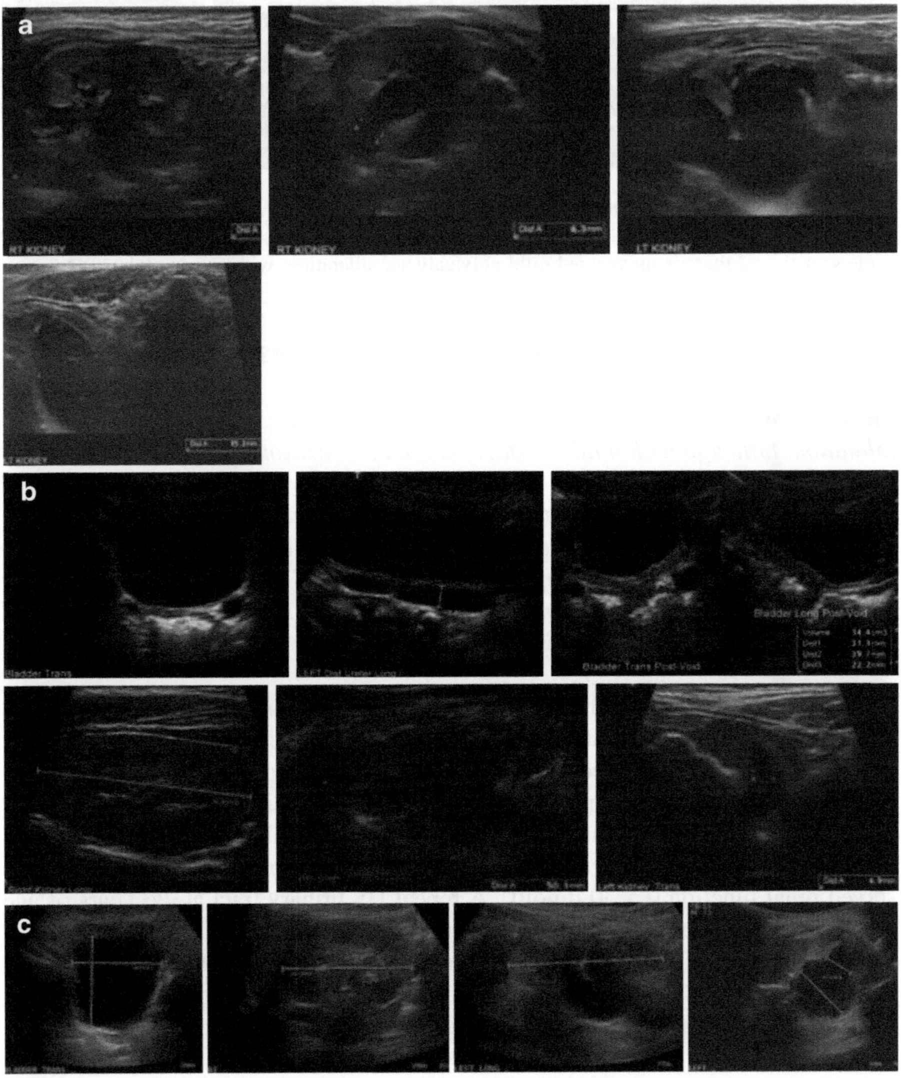

Fig. 9.79 (**a**) Ultrasound 6 weeks after the procedure. Right kidney demonstrates mild renal pelvis dilatation, APD 6 mm, with normal corticomedullary differentiation. Worsening left pelvicalyceal dilatation with parenchymal thinning, renal pelvis APD 15 mm. No distal ureteric dilatation. (**b**) US urinary tract at 9 months of age. Both kidneys demonstrate interval growth. Normal right kidney appearances, with only mild prominence of the renal pelvis (APD 4 mm). Left kidney demonstrates cortical scarring in the lower pole and mild prominence of the renal pelvis, APD 5 mm. Both distal ureters are dilated with the right measuring 7 mm and the left 8 mm. (**c**) US urinary tract at 12 months of age. Normal right kidney with no upper urinary tract dilatation. The left kidney is abnormal with marked global cortical thinning and reduced corticomedullary differentiation. Renal cortical scarring is noted involving the lower pole and there is marked left pelvicalyceal dilatation. The pre-void intrarenal renal pelvis APD is 13 mm, but there is also a large extrarenal pelvis of 28 mm

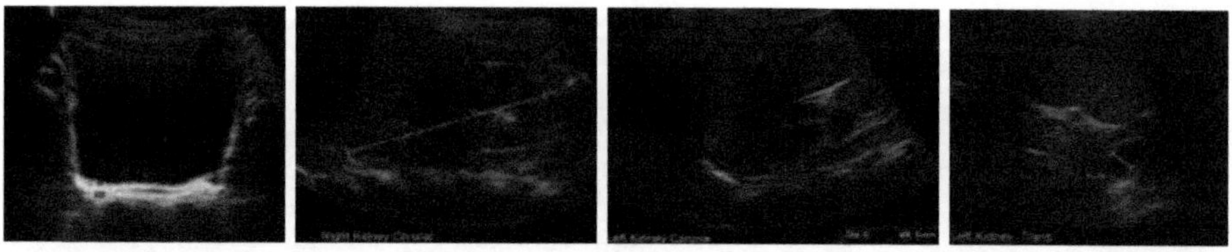

Fig. 9.80 US urinary tract at 2½ years of age. Interval renal growth of both kidneys. Normal right kidney appearances, without upper urinary tract dilatation. The small scarred left kidney has shown some growth and there is unchanged mild pelvicalyceal dilatation, with renal pelvis APD 6 mm. No distal ureteric dilatation seen

Question 4. How Does This Change Your Management? What Would You Do Next?

There is now evidence of increased left renal pelvis dilatation and distal ureteric dilatation, although with a full bladder on the last ultrasound. These findings have been intermittent during follow up, although with an APD of the renal pelvis of 28 mm, upper urinary tract obstruction should be excluded. In order to do this, a NM scan should be repeated to assess the renal function and the drainage curves. Ideally, a urinary tract ultrasound should be repeated 3 months after to ensure the upper urinary tract dilatation remains stable and the APD of the renal pelvis should be measured after the patient has voided.

Because of the increase in the renal pelvis dilatation a repeat NM scan was performed to rule out obstruction. This showed some further decrease of the left kidney function to 17% and associated left VUR, but no evidence of obstruction. A repeat ultrasound demonstrated again improvement in left renal pelvis dilatation, APD now 8 mm, but with persistent global thinning and reduced corticomedullary differentiation.

The patient remained asymptomatic and UTI free for over 12 months, with preserved renal function (Cr 30 μmol/l). A repeat US urinary tract at 2½ years of age demonstrated stable appearances of the smaller and scarred left kidney with stable mild prominence of renal pelvis (7 mm) and no distal ureteric dilatation. Due to his favourable progression he was referred to the nephrologist to continue monitoring with serial US and assessment of his BP and renal function (Fig. 9.80).

9.23.1 Discussion

This male infant had antenatal diagnosis of left hydronephrosis, but also developed severe uropesis and secondary meningitis at only 2 weeks of age. His US demonstrated significant left upper urinary tract dilatation an there was reduced function of left kidney (25%) with high-grade reflux on the MAG-3 with IRC. Because of these findings he was commenced on prophylactic Abs once the infection was treated and underwent a circumcision to reduce his risk of further UTIs [31, 42]. A diagnostic cystoscopy was performed under the same GA, which demonstrated a normal urethra and a left "golf hole" UO consistent with VUR. We opted not to treat the left VUR at that point and to manage him conservatively, knowing that the main risk of

UTIs is in uncircumcised males with VUR and that the resolution rates are higher in males, as mentioned before [69, 75]. He remained asymptomatic after stopping the prophylactic Abs, but his follow-up imaging demonstrated intermittent increase in the left upper urinary tract dilatation, with global cortical thinning, and some further decrease of the left kidney function to 17% with persistent left VUR; there was no evidence of obstruction. Because he was still UTI-free and asymptomatic we opted to manage him conservatively and monitor him with frequent US.

The incidence of VUR is much higher among children with urinary tract infections (30–50%, depending on age). Furthermore, among all children with UTIs, boys are more likely than girls to have VUR (29% compared with 14%) [74, 77, 78]. Boys also tend to have higher grades of VUR diagnosed at younger ages, although their VUR is more likely to resolve. Dilating VUR increases the risk of developing acute pyelonephritis and renal scarring. Approximately 10–40% of children with symptomatic VUR have evidence of renal scarring resulting from congenital dysplasia, acquired post-infectious damage, or both [74]. Furthermore, patients with higher grades of VUR present with higher rates of renal scarring.

Guidelines for the management of UTIs in male infants indicate that these patients should undergo further investigations, which include an US urinary tract, and an MCUG to confirm or rule out the presence of VUR and a DMSA scan to assess for renal scarring if they present with atypical or recurrent UTIs [73, 79–82]. In most paediatric urology textbooks, fluoroscopic MCUG is understandably recommended as the routine imaging study of choice in children with an episode of UTI, as VUR is detected in up to 30% of cases [24, 27, 28]. However, in recent days, a less invasive approach is being favour and most patients undergo a NM scan with indirect renal cystography (IRC) to assess for VUR, unless there is a suspicion of PUV as the underlying cause. In IRC, when the upper urinary tract is drained and most of the tracer is contained in the bladder, the patient is scanned before, during and after voiding. Any increase in radioactivity over the ureters or kidneys indicates VUR [13]. The main advantage of IRC over conventional MCUG is that it is performed under more physiological conditions, as unpleasant catheterization is prevented. It has a low radiation burden and it also provides functional, morphological and uro-mechanical information, by assessing the effect of a full and empty bladder on the drainage from dilated upper tracts. The functional assessment of the urinary tract includes renal parenchymal integrity, split renal function, drainage, timing, and completeness of bladder emptying. The major disadvantage of IRC is the estimated percentage of false-negative results in terms of VUR, which can be up to 22–51%, depending upon technical aspects, the timing of the study and the patient's age and cooperation [27, 28]. However, its specificity is extremely high, of up to 97%.

9.24 Case 24

A 9-years old female with previous medical history of recurrent UTIs since the age of 5 years is referred for further investigations and management, after failure of medical treatment by the general practitioner. She usually presented with urgency, frequency, dysuria and haematuria and the infections were usually due to *E. coli*, but she only had the first febrile UTI at the age of 9 years old. An US urinary tract performed when she was 8 years old could not identify any abnormalities nor a cause for the infections.

Question 1. What Other Information Would You Like to Know About Her Symptoms and Why?
Because she presented late in life, with lower urinary tract infections and only had an episode of pyelonephritis at the age of 9 years, and the urinary tract US appears normal, her UTIs could be related to other associated problems such as constipation and/or voiding dysfunction. Because of this, it is important to gather as much information possible related to her bladder and bowel function and drinking habits. She should ideally fill in a bladder diary and a Bristol Chart.

She was fully toilette trained and voided frequently, had regular bowel motions and had good fluid intake, but suffered from intermittent urinary urgency and incontinence which were initially thought to be related to bladder overactivity (OAB). She was initially treated with anticholinergics, with significant improvement of the overactivity symptoms, but her UTIs continued.

Question 2. Would You Request Other Investigations and Why?
Yes, a NM dynamic scan with indirect cystography to assess the renal function and exclude or confirm the presence of VUR. She is too old to undergo an MCUG, which is a much more invasive procedure and has the disadvantage of the radiation exposure.

A MAG-3 with IRC demonstrated left VUR with preserved differential renal function.

Question 3. With This Information and the Results of the Investigations, What Is Your Management for This Patient?
The patient has failed medical management and should undergo surgical treatment. As the initial approach, a minimally invasive technique should be offered. She should undergo injection of a bulking agent into the ureteric opening to treat the VUR. If this fails, she is old enough to perform reconstructive surgery to correct the VUR. Both options should be offered to the parents.

Because of this and the findings on the NM scan, decision was made to proceed with endoscopic treatment for the VUR when she was 9½ years old. She underwent a diagnostic cystoscopy which demonstrated that the bladder was slightly trabeculated and that both orthotopic UOs distended significantly to the flow and allowed passage of the cystoscope through the VUJs. An endoscopic injection of deflux® into both UOs with a combined HIT and STING technique was performed to treat the VUR (Fig. 9.81).

She recovered well from the procedure and did not develop any further UTIs. Since her OAB symptoms had also improved, her anticholinergic medication was also stopped. She was reviewed 4 weeks after the procedure with an US urinary tract, which demonstrated normal bladder and kidney appearances without upper

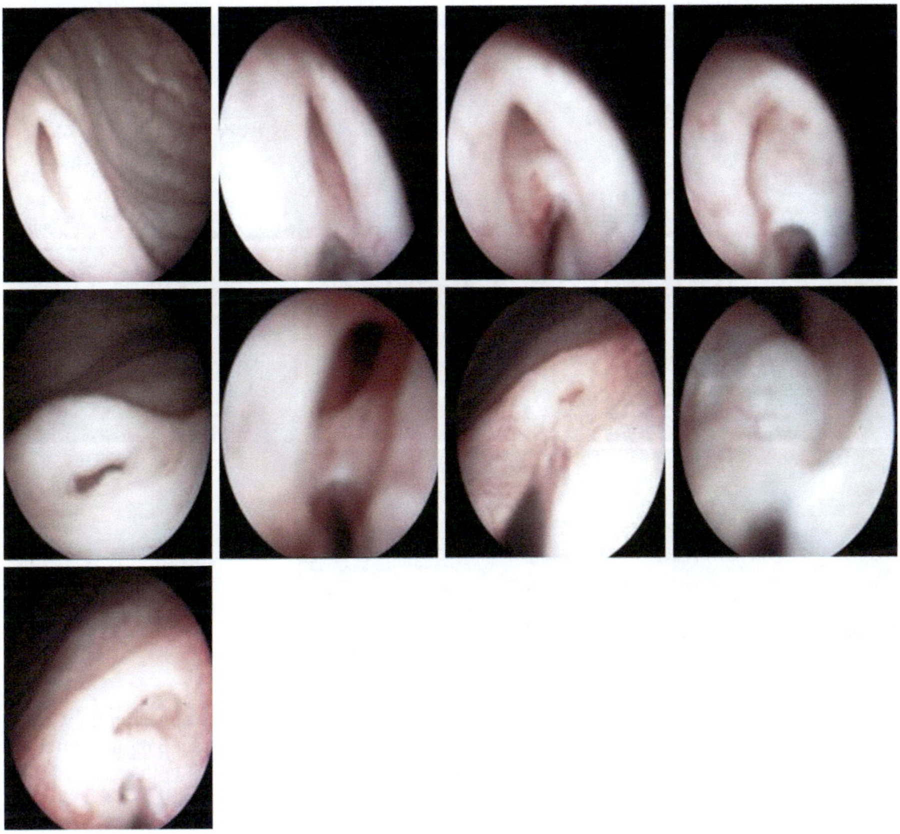

Fig. 9.81 Cystoscopy and injection of deflux® at 9½ years of age. The bladder was slightly trabeculated and that both orthotopic UOs distended significantly to the flow and allowed passage of the cystoscope through the VUJs. To treat the VUR, deflux injection into both UOs with a combined HIT and STING technique was performed

urinary tract dilatation. A repeat US urinary tract 6 months after again demonstrated normal appearances of the urinary tract and she did not develop any further issues (Fig. 9.82).

9.24.1 Discussion

This girl presented with a long-standing history of UTIs and symptoms of bladder overactivity (OAB).

She initially underwent an US, which was normal, and subsequently an NM scan with indirect cystography, which demonstrated left VUR with preserved differential renal function. Despite treatment with anticholinergics and prophylactic Abs her UTIs continued. Because of failure of medical treatment, surgical treatment was indicated; however, these children should also be advised to void frequently and drink abundant fluids as part of the management of a possible voiding dysfunction.

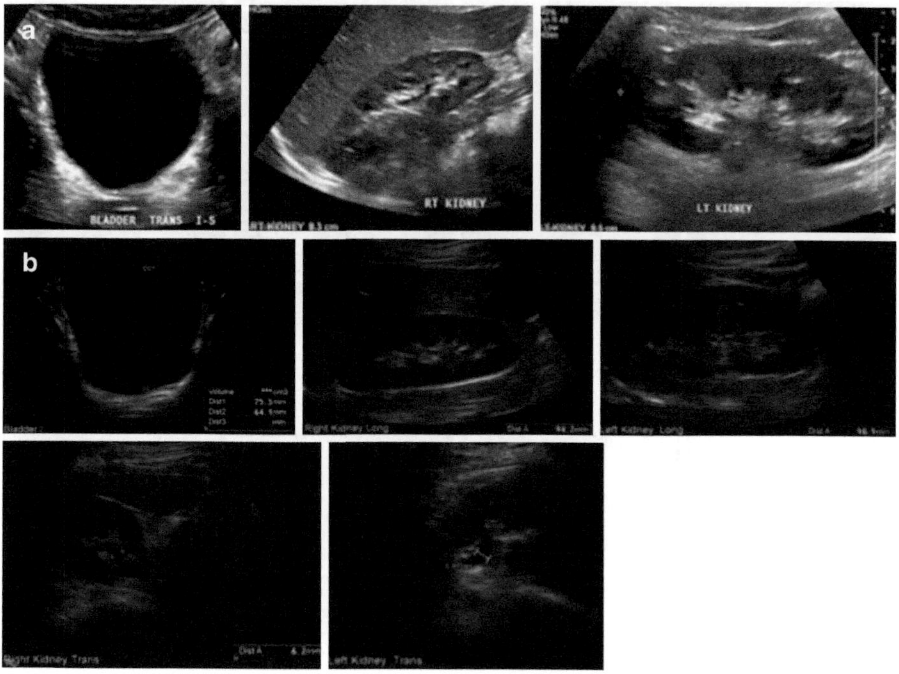

Fig. 9.82 (**a**) US urinary tract 4 weeks after the procedure. Normal kidney appearances without upper urinary tract dilatation. Complete bladder emptying. (**b**) US urinary tract 6 months after the procedure. Interval growth of both kidneys. There is borderline prominence of both renal pelvises, right APD 6 mm and left 7 mm, which doesn't change post-void

We opted for endoscopic treatment initially and she underwent injection of a bulking agent to both UOs, with a combined HIT and STING technique to ensure a better success rate. She did not develop any further UTIs and her OAB symptoms also improved.

In cases where there is poor compliance or failure of medical treatment, breakthrough UTIs, evidence of deterioration of renal function or progression of renal scarring, or when there is parental preference to avoid continuous antibiotics, surgery has an indication [68, 69, 71–74]. The main goal of surgery for VUR is to stop the recurrence of febrile UTIs, prevent renal scarring and avoid long-term complications of VUR [73, 80, 81]. Surgery can be approached with endoscopic injection of bulking agents, open ureteric reimplantation, and minimally invasive approaches such as laparoscopic/robotic ureteric reimplantation. The endoscopic injection of bulking agents gained popularity in the last 2 decades, including the use of different materials over the years, and has become an alternative to long-term antibiotic prophylaxis and surgical intervention in the treatment of VUR in children [71, 80, 81]. Currently, dextranomer/hyaluronic acid microspheres (Deflux®) is the most commonly used agent. The goal of the procedure is to inject the bulking agent in the submucosal intramural tunnel to downgrade or resolve the VUR. The injected bulking agent elevates the ureteral orifice and the distal ureter so that coaptation is increased. The lumen is thus narrowed, preventing reflux of urine into the ureter while still allowing the urine's antegrade flow. The endoscopic management has migrated from the STING technique (subureteric Teflon injection), which originally used polytetrafluoroethylene (PTFE/Teflon) injected below the ureteric orifice at the 6 o'clock position to generate a "crescent shaped" orifice, to the HIT technique (hydrodistention of the ureteric orifice), in which the injection of bulking agent is located in the mid to distal submucosal tunnel at the 6 o'clock position. More recently, the double HIT technique is the preferred one (modified HIT technique with proximal and distal intraluminal submucosal injections) [80, 81]. Several studies have demonstrated resolution rates of 70–90% with the endoscopic treatment, and the highest success is seen in lower grades [71, 75, 81]. Nevertheless, rates of correction appear to be lower than those reported with surgical reimplantation techniques particularly for high grade VUR (92–98% as mentioned before). Furthermore, when compared with long-term low-dose antibiotic prophylaxis alone, endoscopic correction with or without antibiotics may make little or no difference to the likelihood of either symptomatic, febrile UTI or progressive renal damage [68, 71, 72].

9.25 Case 25

A 6-months old male with 2 previous non-febrile UTIs at 4 and 5 months of age presented to the emergency department with 1-day history of high temperatures and irritability and was diagnosed with a febrile UTI. A urine culture confirmed a Klebsiella oxytoca infection, but he was well and was treated with a course of oral Abs with good response.

Question 1. What Is Your Initial Management for This Patient?
The patient should be commenced on prophylactic Abs once the infection is resolved. Because of the recurrent UTIs, the atypical bacteria, and his gender, the patient should undergo further investigations. A urinary tract US should be requested to assess for any possible urinary tract anomalies, such as a renal duplication or upper urinary tract dilatation. Functional imaging is also indicated, either a DMSA to exclude renal scarring or a MAG-3, ideally with indirect cystography, to determine the renal function and assess for VUR.

A urinary tract US was organised and demonstrated mild dilation of the right pelvicalyceal system, with a normal left kidney and bladder. With these findings and the previous history of UTIs, he was started on Px Abs and a NM scan with indirect cystography was performed to assess the renal function and rule out VUR. The MAG-3 scan demonstrated significant reduction in the right renal function (22%) and confirmed the presence of bilateral VUR, worse on the right.

Question 2. What Are the Treatment Options and Why?
Because of the recurrent UTIs, the evidence of bilateral VUR and the compromise of the right renal function this patient should not be managed conservatively and the VUR should be treated. In this case, endoscopic treatment with a bulking agent should be offered, and a circumcision could be performed at the same time. The

prophylactic Abs should continue at least until the procedure or can be ceased after 12 months of age.

Due to the recurrent UTIs and bilateral VUR with compromise of the renal function decision was made to proceed with endoscopic treatment for the VUR and a circumcision under the same GA when he was 8 months of age. On diagnostic cystoscopy the right UO was orthotopic, but appeared very patulous, and the left was laterally placed. Deflux® material was injected with a combined HIT/STING technique on the right and STING technique on left. He recovered well after the surgery and remained asymptomatic without further UTIs, under Ab Px.

Question 3. What Is Your Follow Up Plan for This Patient?
He should be reviewed 6–8 weeks after the procedure with a urinary tract US to assess the upper urinary tract dilatation and ensure there is no evidence of obstruction secondary to the procedure. Further follow up urinary tract US should be performed 6 months after and subsequently once a year until he is toilette trained, and then at 5 years of age. A repeat NM scan is not required unless he develops symptoms again or there is evidence of progression of the upper urinary tract dilatation on the ultrasounds.

He was reviewed with a urinary tract US 2 months after the procedure, which demonstrated some mild improvement of the pelvicalyceal dilatation of the smaller right kidney and compensatory hypertrophy on the left. The chemoprophylaxis was stopped when he was 15 months old and he continued to thrive and remained asymptomatic with normal BP and stable appearances on subsequent US urinary tract until the age of 5 years when he was fully toilette trained and discharged to continue follow up with the nephrology team (Fig. 9.83).

9.25.1 Discussion

This male infant had normal antenatal scans but presented with recurrent UTIs and an US of his urinary tract demonstrated mild dilation of the right pelvicalyceal system. The NM scan demonstrated reduced right renal function (22%) and confirmed the presence of bilateral VUR, worse on the right. He was started on prophylactic Abs, but also underwent a circumcision and bilateral endoscopic treatment for the VUR. In this case, because of the reduced kidney function with high grade VUR, and the recurrent UTIs, a combined management approach was used, and the patient received both medical and surgical management. He was initially started on antibiotic prophylaxis, but subsequently underwent endoscopic treatment because of the findings on the functional imaging. A circumcision was offered at the same time to reduce his risk of UTIs.

In this case, a MAG-3 with IRC was preferred to assess the renal function and confirm the presence of VUR. According to most guidelines, however, because of her age, the recurrence of the UTI and the atypical microorganisms, an MCUG could have been recommended [74, 77–80]. The objective of conservative therapy

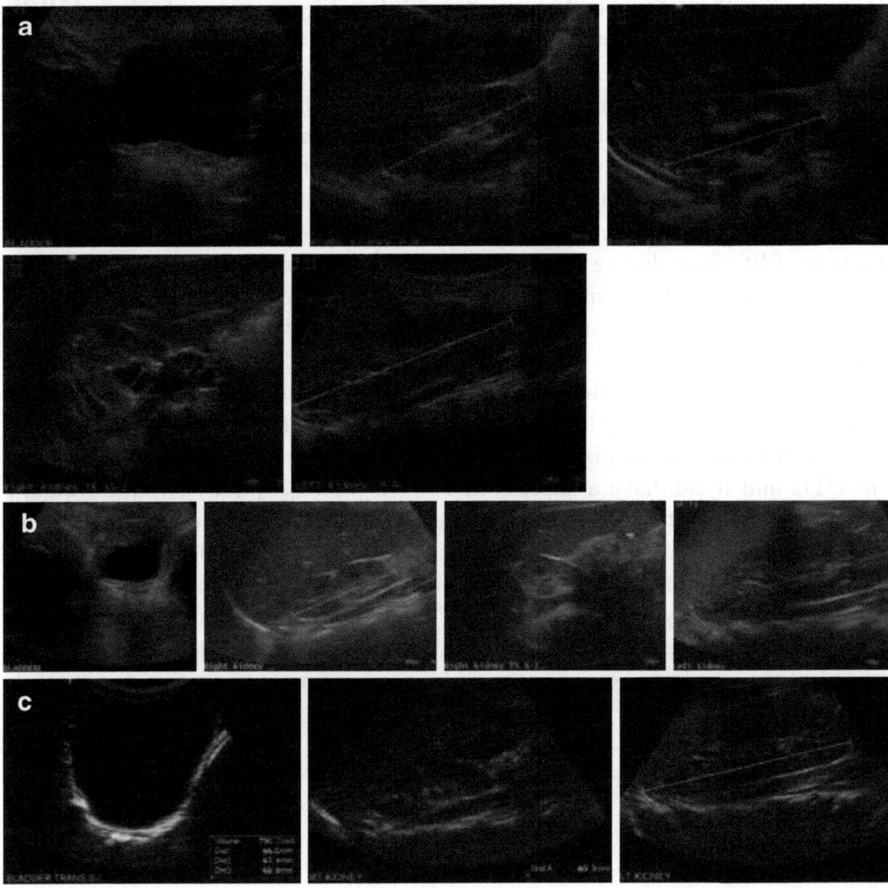

Fig. 9.83 (**a**) US urinary tract 2 months after the procedure. Right kidney with diffuse cortical thinning and loss of corticomedullary differentiation. Right renal pelvis is prominent measuring 8 mm. Compensatory hypertrophy of the left kidney with no upper urinary tract dilatation. (**b**) US urinary tract at 3 years of age. Persistently smaller right kidney with diffuse cortical thinning and scarring, with loss of corticomedullary differentiation. Minor urothelial thickening, but no pelvicalyceal dilatation. Compensatory hypertrophy of the left kidney with normal appearance. (**c**) US urinary tract at 5 years of age. Smaller right kidney with global cortical thinning and scarring, without pelvicalyceal dilatation. Normal appearing left kidney with compensatory hypertrophy. No distal ureteric dilatation and complete bladder emptying

is prevention of febrile UTI, which in this case was not deemed reasonable due to the evidence of reduced renal function and the previous recurrent UTIs the patient developed. Conservative therapy is based on the understanding that VUR can resolve spontaneously, mostly in young patients with low-grade reflux, and that VUR does not damage the kidney in the absence of UTI and the presence of normal lower urinary tract function. Circumcision during early infancy may be considered part of the conservative approach because the procedure has been shown to be effective in reducing the risk of infection even in normal children [44]. Circumcision should be considered in boys with higher risk of UTIs, as it decreases periurethral colonization with bacterial pathogenic flora [76]. In boys recurrent UTIs and VUR, circumcision with or without antibiotic prophylaxis prevents recurrent and febrile urinary tract infections [31, 44, 76]. Conservative management should be dismissed in all patients with breakthrough or recurrent febrile UTIs and compromised renal function, and intervention should be considered. Several studies have demonstrated that circumcision in boys with severe uropathy is efficacious, as it significantly decreases the bacterial colonization rate in boys with and without VUR compared to antibiotic prophylaxis. Circumcision is most effective when performed during the first year of life for reducing the incidence of UTI and antibiotic prophylaxis alone is not sufficient for decreasing bacterial colonization on the preputium, therefore circumcision is essential in such patients even when treated with antibiotic prophylaxis [31].

As mentioned before, surgery for VUR has one main objective, which is the prevention of renal scarring by stopping the recurrence of febrile UTIs. Endoscopic injection of bulking agents is an excellent alternative for young infants with recurrent UTIs and it can have a success rate of 70–90% [73, 80, 81]. However, the long-term success rates appear to be lower than with surgical reimplantation techniques and, when compared with low-dose antibiotic prophylaxis alone, endoscopic correction with or without antibiotics makes little or no difference to the likelihood of either symptomatic, febrile UTI or progressive renal damage [71, 72]. Nevertheless, endoscopic injection is a good alternative when long-term prophylaxis wants to be avoided or when the child is too young to undergo reconstructive surgery safely.

9.26 Case 26

A 1-week old term baby boy with antenatal history of bilateral hydronephrosis and distended bladder, developed four-days history of vomiting, feeding intolerance, progressive weight loss, poor urinary stream and fevers, with secondary acute kidney injury (AKI) with Cr 144 μmol/l and urea of 17 mmol/L. He was transferred from a peripheral hospital for further investigations and management. During the admission he was diagnosed with urosepsis secondary to *E. coli* infection, and meningitis. He underwent an US urinary tract which demonstrated a thick-walled bladder, with bilateral distal ureteric and pelvicalyceal dilatation, worse on the right, with echogenic kidneys (Fig. 9.84).

Question 1. What Is Your Main Differential Diagnosis?
The main diagnoses that need to be excluded in this case are:

- *Posterior urethral valves with secondary urosepsis and acute kidney injury*
- *Vesicoureteric reflux with secondary urosepsis and acute kidney injury*
- *Urethral atresia with secondary urosepsis and acute kidney injury (less likely)*
- *Prune Belly Sd. (even less likely)*
- *Spinal anomaly/dysraphism (spina bifida)*

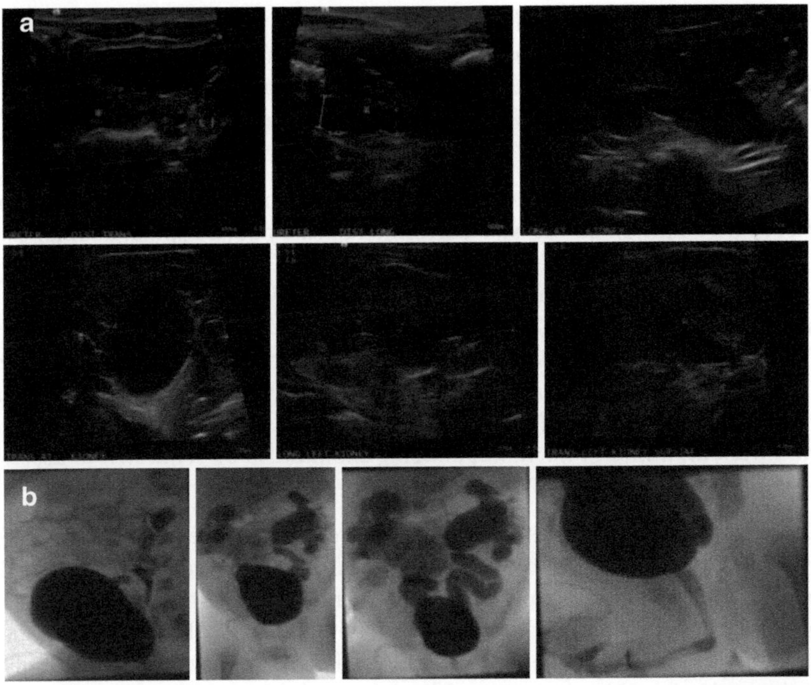

Fig. 9.84 (**a**) Urinary tract US on week one of life. Partially filled bladder. The left kidney demonstrates markedly reduced corticomedullary differentiation and multiple small cysts within the echogenic renal cortex. There is mild left pelvicalyceal dilatation with an APD 6 mm and proximal ureteric dilatation, and a minimally dilated left distal ureter, up to 2 mm. The right kidney has generalised parenchymal thinning and the cortex is echogenic with loss of corticomedullary differentiation. There is gross right pelvicalyceal dilatation, with a renal pelvis APD of 23 mm, and there is a moderate amount of mobile debris seen within the dilated pelvicalyceal system. The right ureter is noted to be dilated both proximally and distally up to 7 mm. (**b**) MCUG at 2 weeks of age

Question 2. What Is Your Initial Management for This Patient?

The first and main intervention in the case of suspected posterior urethral valves is the insertion of a urethral catheter to release the potential bladder obstruction, and also help with the clearance of the infection; this will improve his renal function. The patient needs long-term IV/PO antibiotics to treat both infections (21 days as per guidelines) and subsequently prophylactic Abs to prevent further UTIs. Once the more severe infection and AKI have been treated and he has remained well for at least 48 h, a MCUG should be performed to confirm or exclude the diagnoses mentioned above. A spinal US may also need to be requested depending on the MCUG findings if there is no evidence of PUV and the bladder appears abnormal and/or there is high grade bilateral VUR.

A urethral catheter was inserted without fdifficulties on admission and he was treated with IV/PO Abs for a period of 3 weeks. His AKI was also managed by the nephrology team with IV fluids and correction of his electrolytes. Because of his presentation with urosepsis and AKI, and the US findings with the possibility of posterior urethral valves (PUV) as the underlying cause, he underwent a MCUG after completing a few days of IV Abs.

Question 3. What Does the MCUG Show?

The bladder has normal contour and shape. Bilateral grade V vesicoureteric reflux, with tortuous/dilated ureters and severe dilatation of the pelvicalyceal systems. Normal appearance of the posterior urethra during void. No dilatation or filling defect identified to suggest posterior urethral valve.

The cystourethrogram ruled out PUV but demonstrated bilateral high grade VUR. An US of the spine was also performed to rule out any spinal anomalies.

Question 4. How Would You Manage This Patient with a Diagnosis of Bilateral High Grade VUR?

The patient should be commenced on antimicrobial prophylaxis and should undergo a circumcision to prevent further UTIs. A repeat US urinary tract should be performed at 6 weeks, and 3 and 6 months of age to assess the progression of the upper urinary tract dilatation. Functional imaging should also be requested to assess the differential renal function.

Once he completed treatment and had recovered from the sepsis and AKI, with Cr decreasing (Cr down to 50 μmol/l and subsequently 39 μmol/l) and improved feeding, he underwent a circumcision prior to his discharge from the hospital. He was commenced on Ab prophylaxis and remained well without any further UTIs. A repeat US urinary tract 2 months after the admission showed persistent severe right pelvicalyceal dilatation and only mild prominence of the right renal pelvis, with some mild improvement in the distal ureteric dilatation. He also underwent a NM scan to assess the function of both kidneys and a repeat US urinary tract 4 weeks after to reassess the upper urinary tract dilatation, to ensure there was no evidence of associated obstruction. The NM scan showed preserved differential renal function and persistent right VUR, and there was persistent bilateral renal pelvis dilatation, but improved on the right (right APD 16 mm) with mild bilateral prominence of the distal ureters on US (Fig. 9.85).

The patient remained asymptomatic and UTI-free on prophylactic Abs, with stable renal function (Cr 31 μmol/l), and was reviewed again with a repeat US

Fig. 9.85 (**a**) US urinary tract at 4 months of age. Bladder underfilled, with mild bilateral distal ureteric dilatation of 9 mm on the left and 4 mm on the right. Persistent right pelvicalyceal dilatation, with renal APD 29 mm, and generalised parenchymal thinning with loss of corticomedullary differentiation. There is mild left renal pelvis prominence, APD 5 mm and the left kidney demonstrates increased parenchymal echogenicity with reduced corticomedullary differentiation. (**b**) MAG-3 at 4 months of age. There is patchy concentration of radiopharmaceutical in the cortex of the right kidney with there is of photopenia in the upper and lower poles consistent with reflux nephropathy. Uptake in the left kidney is also patchy but better preserved than on the right. At the end of the initial imaging period there is pooling in both collecting systems and both ureters appear prominent. Following intravenous administration of Lasix there is good drainage from the left but significant retention on the right. There is reflux to the right ureter on the dynamic micturating images. Differential renal function is preserved with 46% on the right and 54% on the left. (**c**) Repeat US urinary tract at 5 months of age. Moderate right pelvicalyceal dilatation, with renal pelvis APD 16 mm, and increased cortical thinning. Mild left pelvicalyceal dilatation and increased cortical echogenicity. Left renal pelvis APD 5 mm. The distal ureters are intermittently prominent, and the bladder outline is normal

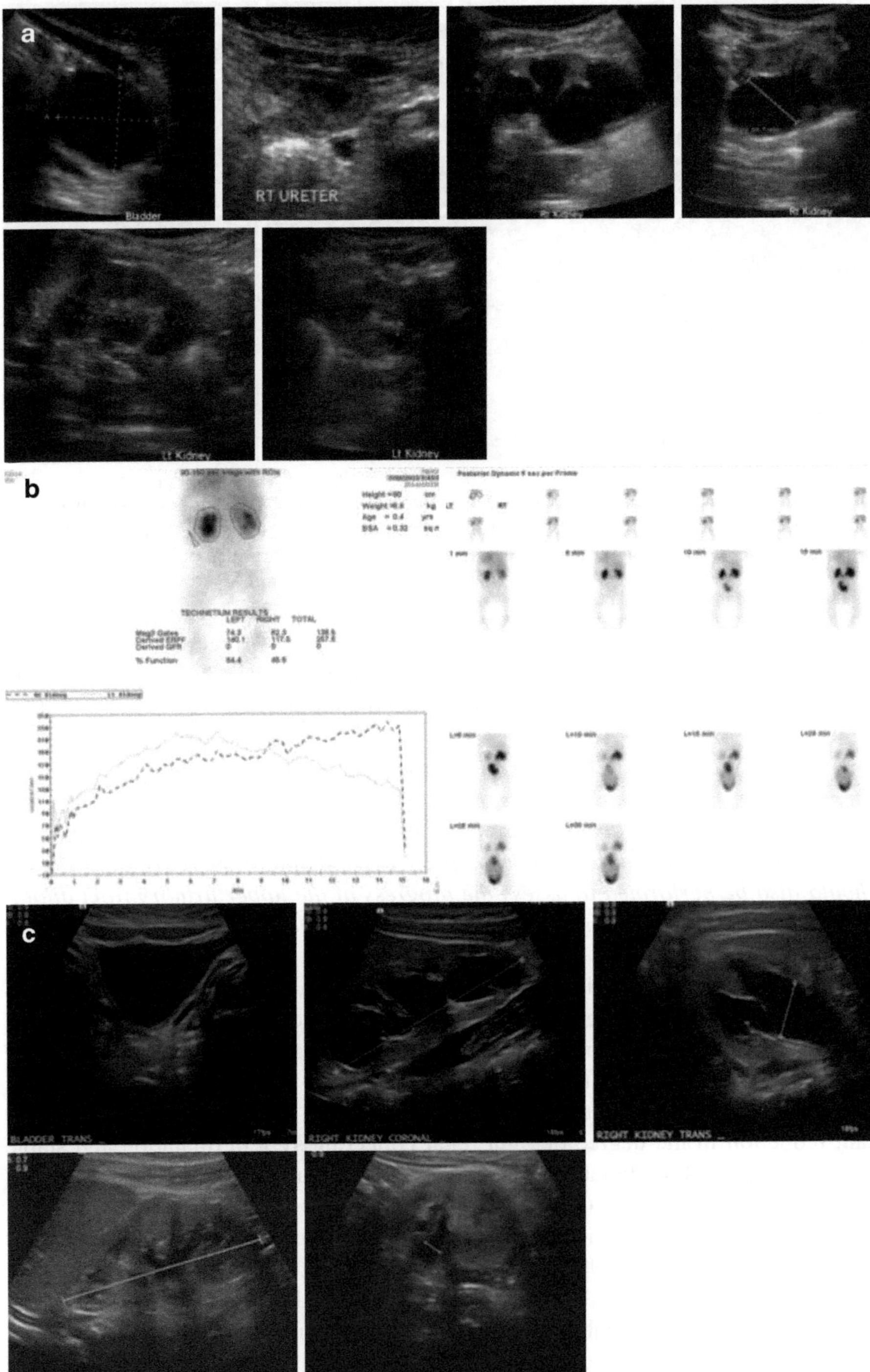
a
Bladder
RT URETER
Rt Kidney
Rt Kidney
Lt Kidney
Lt Kidney
b
TECHNETIUM RESULTS
c
BLADDER TRANS
RIGHT KIDNEY CORONAL
RIGHT KIDNEY TRANS

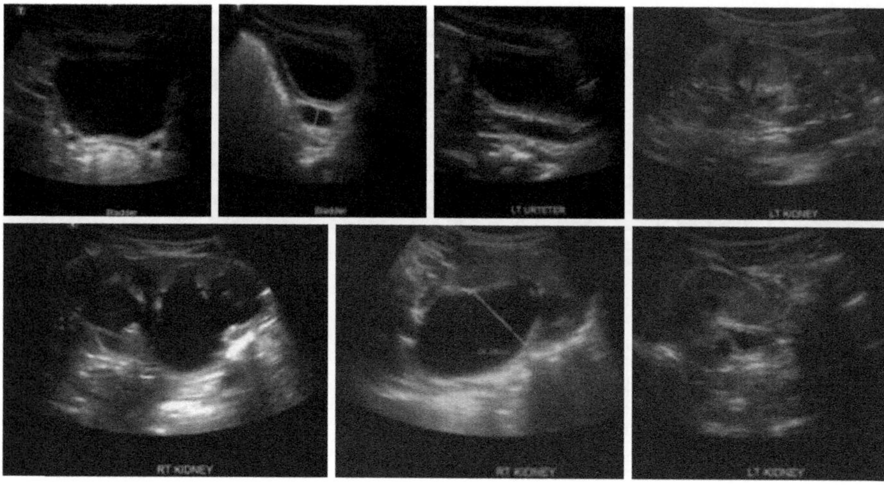

Fig. 9.86 US urinary tract at 7 months of age. Interval growth of both kidneys, with persistent increased parenchymal echogenicity. The right kidney demonstrates cortical thinning and severe right pelvicalyceal dilatation, with renal pelvis APD 29 mm. Mild left renal pelvis dilatation, APD 5 mm. Bilateral distal ureteric dilatation, worse on the left, up to 7 mm

urinary tract at 7 months of age, which demonstrated severe right pelvicalyceal dilatation (renal pelvis APD 29 mm) with persistent mild distal ureteric dilatation, and mild progression of the left upper urinary tract dilatation (Fig. 9.86).

Question 5. Would this Change Your Management for the Patient? Why?
Yes, the patient should undergo a repeat NM dynamic scan to reassess the function of the right kidney and ensure there is no evidence of obstruction, because of the evidence of further increase in the right pelvicalyceal dilatation. A urinary tract US should also be performed to assess the progress of the upper urinary tract dilatation. The patient should remain on prophylactic Abs at least until he is 1 year of age.

Because of the increase in the right renal pelvis dilatation, a repeat NM scan was performed to reassess the renal function. Although there had been a slight reduction in the right renal function to 42%, VUR was not demonstrated. No further investigations were undertaken at that point as he remained asymptomatic and he was reviewed again 6 months after with an US urinary tract, which again showed significant reduction in the degree of right renal collecting system dilatation and stable mile left renal pelvis dilatation, with ongoing bilateral renal scarring and altered parenchymal echogenicity (Fig. 9.87).

He remained well and did not develop any UTIs. His renal function and BP also remained stable. A repeat US urinary tract performed at 2 years of age demonstrated stable right pelvicalyceal dilatation, with renal pelvis APD 16 mm and parenchymal thinning, and mild left renal pelvis dilatation, APD 9 mm, with some major calyceal prominence, without distal ureteric dilatation. Due to his good progress and absence

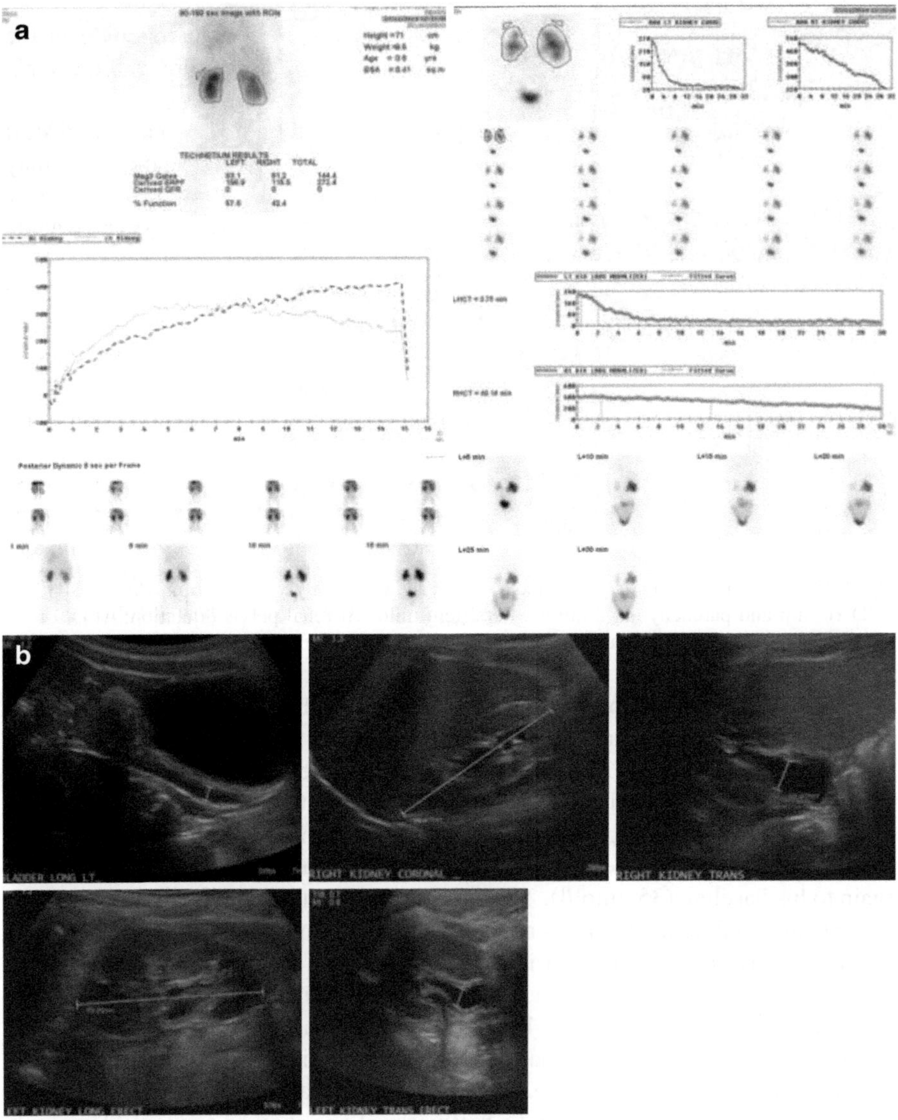

Fig. 9.87 (**a**) MAG-3 with IRC at 7 months of age. Patchy cortical uptake is again demonstrated bilaterally, worse on the right. Right renal function has decreased slightly. Differential function is 42% on the right and 58% on the left. Right-sided drainage is slow. No vesicoureteric reflux was demonstrated on today's study. (**b**) US urinary tract after 12 months of age. There is patchy heterogeneous cortical echogenicity bilaterally and the cortex appears irregular and thinned due to scarring at the upper and lower poles. There is marked reduction in the degree of right pelvicalyceal dilatation, renal pelvis APD now 10 mm. The left kidney demonstrates mild renal pelvis dilatation, APD 5 mm. Mildly dilated distal ureters, right 3 mm and left 4 mm

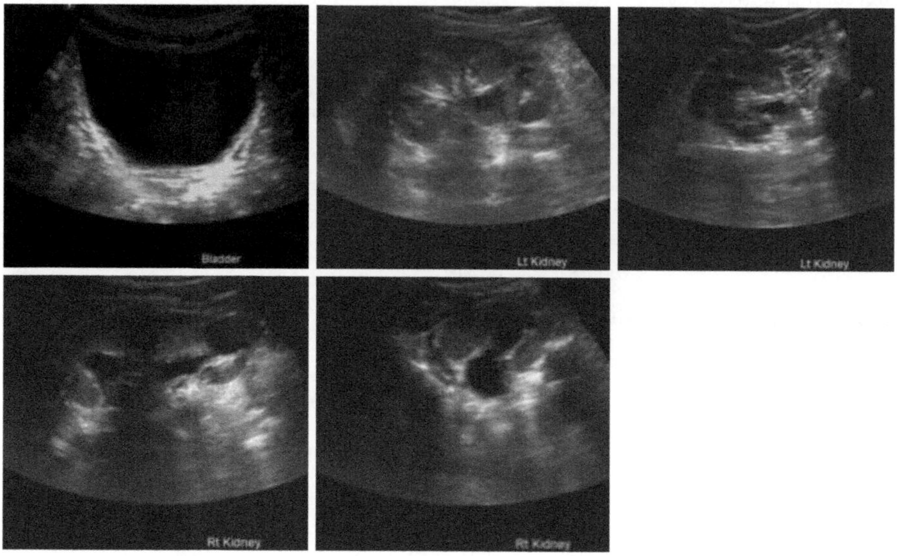

Fig. 9.88 US urinary tract at 2 years of age. Stable right pelvicalyceal dilatation, with renal pelvis APD 16 mm and parenchymal thinning. Persistent mild left renal pelvis dilatation, APD 9 mm, with some major calyceal prominence. No distal ureteric dilatation

of symptoms, the chemoprophylaxis was ceased, and he started toilette training when he was around 3 years old (Fig. 9.88).

During the following 12 months he developed issues with intermittent deterioration in his renal function with increased Cr up to 75–85 μmol/l and urea 6.1–8.9 mmol/l, and multiple admissions for febrile illnesses suspected to be UTIs, but without any proven infections. Once these were treated, his Cr would normalise again to his baseline (35 μmol/l). The patient also developed issues with postponed voiding and holding manoeuvres and his toilette training had to be postponed for a few months. Various repeat US urinary tract performed locally demonstrated stable appearances of both kidneys with stable mild upper urinary tract dilatation bilaterally. He was reviewed again at 4 years of age and had remained well during a period of about 6 months. He had started toilette training again but was having intermittent urinary incontinence. His Cr was stable at 35 μmol/l, as well as his BP. A renal US performed at 3 and a half years of age showed some mild progression of the bilateral distal ureteric and renal pelvis dilatation, with some increase in the right calyceal dilatation compared to the previous scans. A subsequent US urinary tract demonstrated some further increase in the upper urinary tract dilatation with incomplete bladder emptying and significant post-void residual volumes, and he suffered from 2 febrile UTIs requiring admission for IV Abs. His issues with urinary incontinence worsened and he also developed increased frequency and urgency (Fig. 9.89).

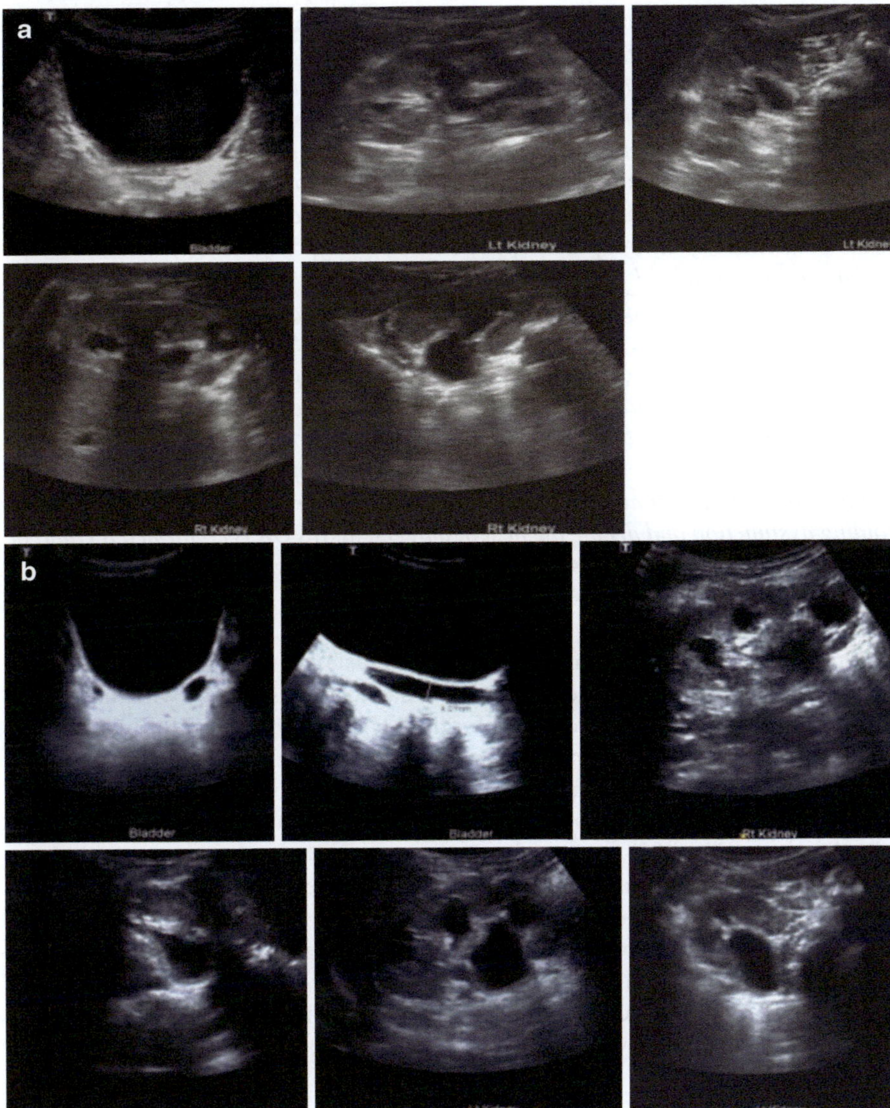

Fig. 9.89 (**a**) US urinary tract at 3½ years of age. Mild to moderate collecting system dilatation bilaterally, worse on the left with right renal pelvis APD of 17 mm and left APD 9 mm. No obvious ureteric dilatation. (**b**) US urinary tract at 4 years of age. There is global cortical thinning bilaterally, with mild increase in pelvicalyceal dilatation, with renal pelvis APD of 13 mm on the right and 17 mm on the left. Both distal ureters are dilated up to 9 mm on the left. Evidence of incomplete bladder emptying with post-void residual volume of 127 ml (pre-void volume 240 ml)

Question 6. What Is Your Definitive Management for This Patient and Why?
In this case, the medical treatment has failed as he developed further UTIs, progressive upper urinary tract dilatation and symptoms of voiding dysfunction, all likely related to his underlying high grade VUR. Because of this, he should undergo surgical treatment and the first option can be an endoscopic injection of a bulking agent into de UOs. Reconstructive surgery is also an alternative, although it is a much more invasive approach especially considering the lack of evidence for the real underlying cause of his symptoms (i.e. VUR vs voiding dysfunction).

An alternative would be to repeat the NM scan (or even an MCUG, although contraindicated at his age) to reassess the presence of VUR and the differential renal function. However, a diagnostic and potentially therapeutic cystoscopy is a much easier option considering the possibility of treating the VUR immediately. The disadvantage is the requirement of GA for the procedure.

A video-urodynamic study could also be performed to assess his bladder dynamics during filling and emptying, and if there is evidence of persistent VUR. This study could also help determine if the VUR is responsible for his urinary symptoms and voiding dysfunction and decide the best management. If VUR is confirmed it could be corrected either with endoscopic or reconstructive surgery, as mentioned above.

Because of his worsening symptoms and deterioration of his bladder function with recurrent UTIs, his chemoprophylaxis was restarted to try and prevent further UTIs and decision was made to proceed to a diagnostic cystoscopy with the view of also performing endoscopic treatment for his VUR and to assess if his bladder dysfunction also improved. The procedure was performed when he was 4½ years old and the cystoscopy demonstrated a non-trabeculated, cone shaped bladder, with orthotopic gapping UOs; he underwent injection of deflux® into both UOs without complications (Fig. 9.90).

He recovered well from the procedure and was discharged on prophylactic Abs for 3 months. He remained well and asymptomatic with no further UTIs and his urinary incontinence improved, with resolution of the urgency and frequency. A repeat US urinary tract demonstrated stable appearances of the bilateral upper urinary tract dilatation, which improved after voiding with almost complete bladder emptying, and his Ab Px was stopped again (Fig. 9.91).

9.26.1 Discussion

In this case, the main underlying condition to exclude in the presence of bilateral upper urinary tract dilatation and urosepsis in the neonatal period, is PUV. The child was managed accordingly with the insertion of a urethral catheter for bladder decompression and stabilization of his renal function, and subsequently underwent further investigations to confirm the diagnosis. A MCUG demonstrated high grade bilateral VUR and he was commenced on prophylactic Abs and underwent a circumcision to prevent further UTIs. His initial MAG-3 demonstrated preserved differential renal function and right VUR; however, repeat functional imaging indicated

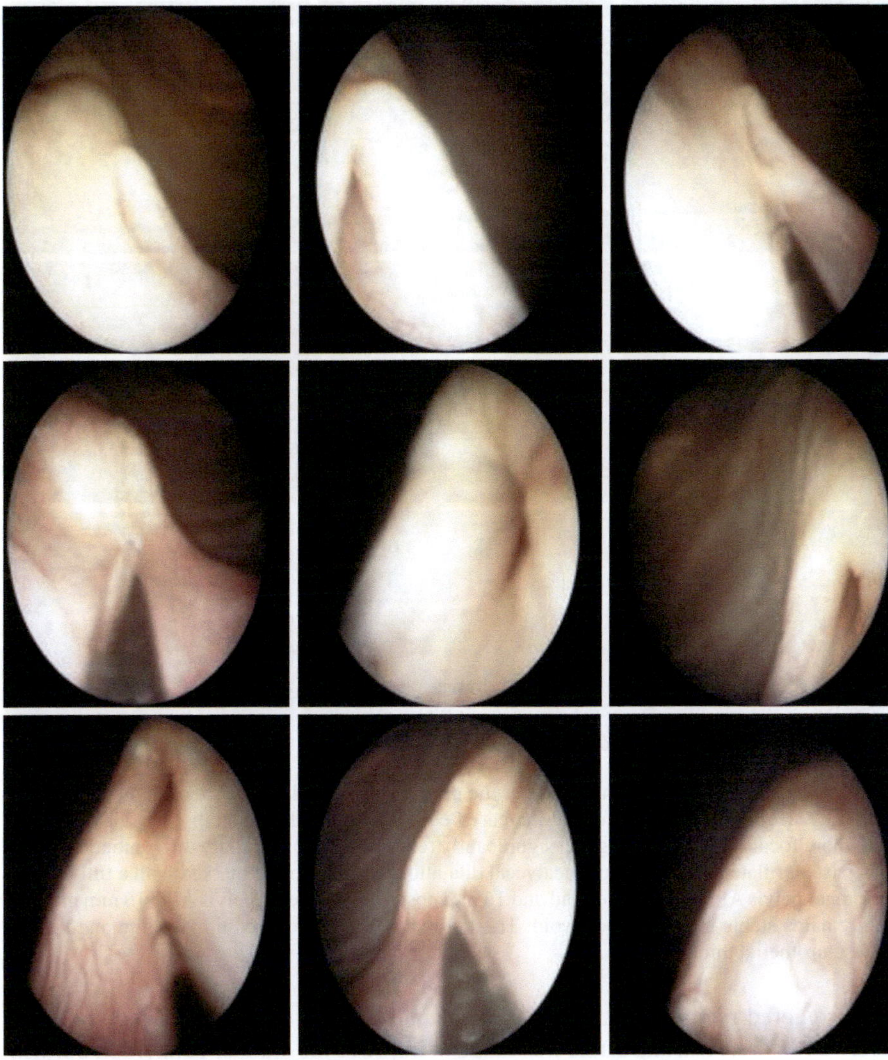

Fig. 9.90 Cystoscopy and injection of bulking material into the UOs at 4½ years of age. Evidence of a cone shaped bladder, non-trabeculated, with orthotopic gapping UOs

some deterioration in his right renal function with progression of the right pelvicalyceal dilatation. The patient remained asymptomatic the first 2 years of life and was therefore managed conservatively. Most of his issues appeared when he started toilette training and he developed holding manoeuvres with secondary urinary incontinence due to incomplete bladder emptying. Although it was not clear if the VUR was the reason for his voiding dysfunction, with the so called "Jo-Jo" mechanism and constant refilling of the bladder immediately after micturition, or if the bladder dysfunction was causing a worsening of his underlying primary VUR. This

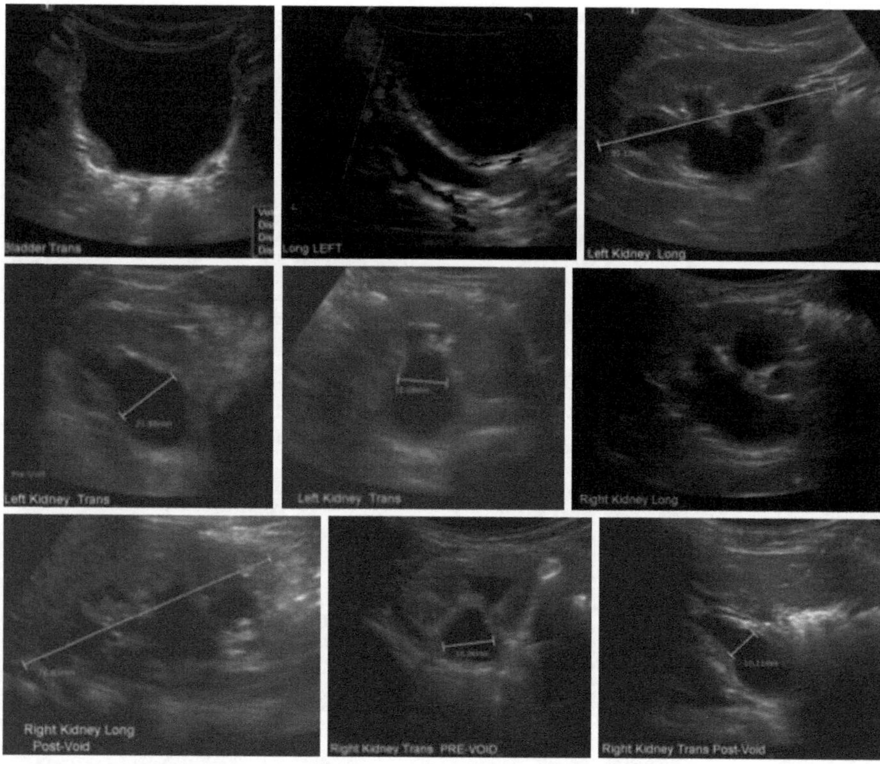

Fig. 9.91 US urinary tract 3 months after the procedure. There is evidence of deflux material at both VUJ. Both kidneys demonstrate increased echogenicity and a generalised cortical thinning with more focal areas of scarring and significantly reduced corticomedullary differentiation. There is persistent bilateral moderate pelvicalyceal dilatation, which is more marked with a full bladder. Left renal pelvis APD 22 mm pre-void and 16 mm post-void; left renal pelvis APD 16 mm pre-void and remains stable at 10 mm post-void. The left distal ureter is dilated up to 7 mm and there is diffuse urothelial thickening

also triggered recurrence UTIs, which meant he could not be managed conservatively anymore. A strong effort was made to improve his bladder behaviour, but with the risk of further deterioration of his renal function we opted to treat the VUR in this case. Because we were unsure of the underlying mechanism for the symptoms we decided to proceed with endoscopic injection of a bulking agent and perform a diagnostic cystoscopy prior. This would allow us to also determine if the correction of the VUR would have an impact in his bladder function as well. This seemed to be the case as his urinary incontinence improved with time. He also remained UTI-free after the procedure. An alternative in his case could have been to perform Urodynamic studies to assess the bladder behaviour prior to surgery, but with the recurrent UTIs and quick deterioration of his renal function with each episode, treatment needed to be more aggressive.

An important aspect of VUR management is the treatment of voiding dysfunction, as it is associated with an increased risk of recurrent UTIs and a reduced probability of VUR resolution [80, 82]. Most patients present with high bladder capacity and incomplete bladder emptying. Over 40% of patients with high grade VUR have associated bladder/bowel dysfunction and they usually have persistent VUR, renal damage and recurrent UTIs during follow-up [68, 82]. Most patients with Lower Urinary Tract Dysfunction (LUTD) have voiding phase symptoms and a minority presents isolated OAB, although many children have a combination of both types of symptoms [69, 82]. Voiding phase problems are associated with higher rates of VUR and persistent VUR in children with LUTD at follow-up. Patients with LUTD have a higher rate of renal damage, as also noted in young children with high grade VUR. LUTD is also a risk factor for recurrent UTIs, but the overall recurrence rate is higher in girls than in boys [82]. Treatment of bladder and bowel dysfunction should include behavioural therapy, biofeedback (particularly for school-age children), anticholinergic medications, alpha blockade, and constipation management. Only behavioural measurements were attempted in this case, but failed, and decision was made to proceed with endoscopic treatment worried about further renal damage.

9.27 F. Multicystic Dysplastic Kidney

9.27.1 Case 27

A 3-months old female with antenatal diagnosis of a left cystic kidney, identified on the 20 weeks GA scan, is referred for further investigations and management. She was monitored with antenatal scans every 4 weeks before birth and underwent 2 further US urinary tract at 12 days and 5 weeks of life (Fig. 9.92).

Question 1. Please Describe the Typical Sonographic Characteristics of a MCDK on These Ultrasounds

The classical findings on imaging are:

- *Reniform-shaped multicystic mass occupying renal fossa*
- *Lobulated outer contour due to cysts of variable size*
- *Wide range of sizes: up to 15 cm in length in newborn period, but may be only 1–2 cm after years of involution*
- *Cysts of varying sizes that are not connected*
- *Poorly defined intervening echogenic parenchyma without normal corticomedullary architecture*
- *The classic type has a random configuration of cysts, whereas the hydronephrotic type presents with a discernible, dilated renal pelvis surrounded by cysts.*

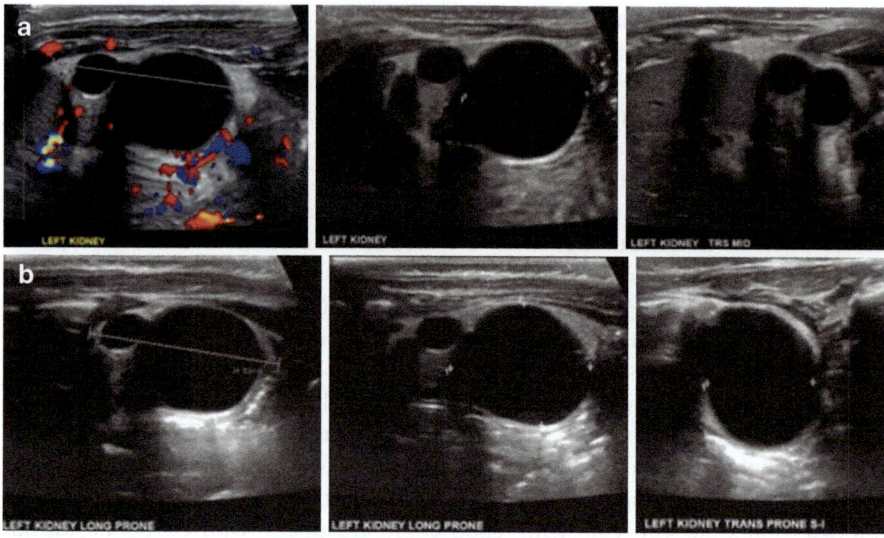

Fig. 9.92 (**a**) US day 12 of life. (**b**) US urinary tract at 5 weeks of age

In this case there is presence of cysts of various sizes connected by insubstantial fibrous tissue; no functional renal tissue can be identified. Both ultrasounds demonstrate appearances suggestive of a hydronephrotic MCDK. The first US shows a left MCDK with at least 3 large cysts of varying size and echogenic surrounding renal parenchyma. The second ultrasound demonstrated multiple cysts with minimal left renal parenchyma.

Question 2. What Is Your Management for This Girl and Why?

The patient should be managed conservatively, as long as she remains symptomatic, and does not require surgical intervention. The natural history is for the MCDK to progressively involute and not cause any complications.

The patient should be referred to the nephrology team and continue surveillance with US and monitoring of the BP. Further investigations are not required unless the patient becomes symptomatic or there is progressive increase in the size of the kidney or the cysts. Some centres advocate performing a NM scan (DMSA) for documentation of lack of renal function.

She remained well after birth and asymptomatic. She also had a finding of a nasal infantile haemangioma that was treated with propranolol and resolved completely. A repeat US was performed when she was 6 months of age, which again demonstrated a left multicystic dysplastic kidney and a normal right kidney. She was reviewed again at 2 years of age with a repeat US urinary tract. She had progressed well, was thriving and had not developed any UTIs nor other symptoms. Her BP remained within normal limits as well as her renal function, and her left MCDK seemed to be involuting on US images (Fig. 9.93).

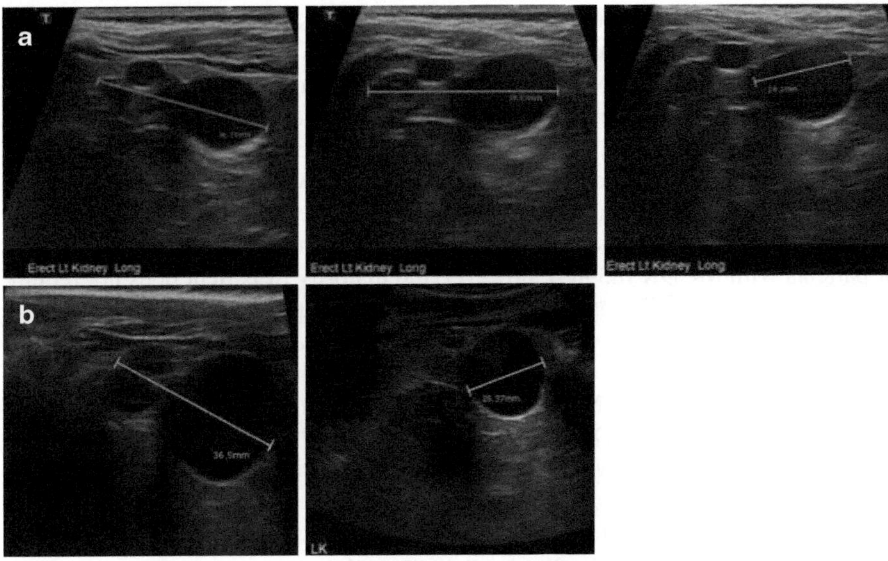

Fig. 9.93 (**a**) US urinary tract at 6 months of age. The left kidney measures 3.9 cm (<5th centile) and is composed of multiple cysts of varying sizes, largest measuring approximately 24 × 16 × 19 mm. The cysts are all simple in nature with no septations, loculations or debris. The intervening parenchyma is echogenic and dysplastic with no evidence of normal renal surrounding tissue. There is evidence of compensatory hypertrophy of the right kidney, which measures 6.2 cm (95th centile). (**b**) US urinary tract at 18 months of age. The left kidney is replaced by multiple anechoic variably sized cysts with no normal intervening parenchyma, the largest one measuring 26 × 23 mm. The left kidney measures 3.6 cm (previously 3.9 cm). Compensatory hypertrophy of the normal right kidney with interval growth to 7.6 cm (>95th centile); previously 6.2 cm

9.27.2 Discussion

This girl was diagnosed antenatally with a dysplastic kidney and the postnatal US confirmed a left MCDK, which seemed to be involuting on follow-up imaging. She remained asymptomatic and was therefore managed conservatively.

Multicystic dysplastic kidney (MCDK) is the most common form of renal cystic disease in children, reported to occur in 1/2400–1/4300 live births [83, 84], and most cases are diagnosed antenatally. Routine postnatal US is performed to confirm the diagnosis, with the classical US features of multiple, non-communicating cysts of varying size, separated by dysplastic parenchyma and the absence of a normal pelvicalyceal system. However, in few instances it will be difficult to differentiate between MCDK and hydronephrosis based on the US alone. The value of further investigations for confirming the diagnosis is debatable. In the presence of classical ultrasound appearances and a normal contralateral kidney, a nuclear medicine scan is not necessary [83–85]. An associated contralateral anomaly has been reported in up to 40% of patients, with VUR being most commonly encountered (15–25%), followed by PUJO (4–5%), VUJO and ureterocoele. Many patients used to be screened with MCUG, since there is a higher possibility of contralateral reflux even with normal US [85]. Although US is a poor tool for assessment of VUR, almost all cases that could be missed will be likely of low grade and with a high rate of spontaneous resolution [83]. A NM scan should be used to obtain additional prognostic information from the contralateral urinary tract in patients who had upper urinary tract dilatation on postnatal imaging. MCDK might persist without any change, increase in size, or undergo spontaneous involution, which occurs in most cases. Complications of MCKD include hypertension and infection, and the risk of malignancy in this lesion is considered remote. Hypertension has been reported in 0–3% of patients with MCDK [83–85], however, the majority of patient does not require surgical intervention. The association of MCDK with neoplastic transformation is rarely encountered and several studies reported no malignancy in large series of patients with MCDK. Only case reports of either a Wilms' tumor or renal cell carcinoma in association with MCDK have been documented [84, 85].

Most patients with MCDK will not require any sort of intervention, as most of the cases tend to involute over time with the fastest rates during early life, although the involution rates vary from 20 to 75% [83–85]. The main factor that determines involution is the in size on US, with the major prognostic indicator for spontaneous involution being an initial size of ≤5 cm on presentation.

A conservative approach to MCDK cases is still recommended and routine nephrectomy is not indicated, as the risk of complications is extremely low. The surgical treatment of MCDK should be considered in only few selected conditions, such as a very large kidney (>6 cm), when the retained mass appears to be growing, when there is a history of recurrent UTIs, and if hypertension or other symptoms develop [83, 85].

References

1. Elder JS. Management of antenatal hydronephrosis. In: Puri P, editor. Newborn surgery. 4th ed. Florida: CRC Press; 2018. p. 1029–47.
2. Capolicchio J-P, Braga LH, Szymanski KM. Canadian Urological Association/pediatric urologists of Canada guideline on the investigation and management of antenatally detected hydronephrosis. Can Urol Assoc J. 2018;12(4):85–92.
3. Dhillon HK. Prenatal diagnosed hydronephrosis: the great Ormond street experience. Br J Urol. 1998;81:39–44.
4. Nguyen HT, Herndon CD, Cooper C, et al. The Society for Fetal Urology consensus statement on the evaluation and management of antenatal hydronephrosis. J Pediatr Urol. 2010;6:212–31.
5. Silay MS, Undre S, Nambiar AK, Dogan HS, Kocvara R, Nijman RJM, Stein R, Tekgul S, Radmayr C. Role of antibiotic prophylaxis in antenatal hydronephrosis: a systematic review from the European Association of Urology/European Society for Paediatric Urology Guidelines Panel. J Pediatr Urol. 2017 Jun;13(3):306–15.
6. Islek A, Güven AG, Koyun M, Akman S, Alimoglu E. Probability of urinary tract infection in infants with ureteropelvic junction obstruction: is antibacterial prophylaxis really needed? Pediatr Nephrol. 2011;26:1837–41.
7. Roth CC, Hubanks JM, Bright BC, et al. Occurrence of urinary tract infection in children with significant upper urinary tract obstruction. Urology. 2009;73:74–8.
8. Babu R, Vittalraj P, Sundaram S, Shalini S. Pathological changes in ureterovesical and ureteropelvic junction obstruction explained by fetal ureter histology. J Pediatr Urol. 2019;15(3):240.e1–7.

9. Growth T, Mitchell M. Ureteropelvic junction obstruction. In: Coran C, editor. Pediatric surgery, vol. 1. 7th ed. Saunders: Elsevier; 2012. p. 1411–25.
10. Chow JS, Koning JL, Back SJ, Nguyen HT, Phelps A, Darge K. Classification of pediatric urinary tract dilation: the new language. Pediatr Radiol. 2017;47:1109–15.
11. Toiviainen-Salo S, Garel L, Grignon A, Dubois J, Rypens F, Boisvert J, Perreault G, Decarie JC, Filiatrault D, Lapierre C, Miron MC, Bechard N. Fetal hydronephrosis: is there hope for consensus? Pediatr Radiol. 2004;34:519–29.
12. Hodhod A, Capolicchio J-P, Jednak R, El-Sherif E, El-Doray AE-A, El-Sherbiny M. Evaluation of urinary tract dilation classification system for grading postnatal hydronephrosis. The J Urol. 2016;195:725–30.
13. Mendichovzky I, Solar BT, Smeulders N, Easty M, Biassoni L. Nuclear medicine in pediatric Nephro-urology: an overview. Semin Nucl Med. 2017 May;47(3):204–28.
14. Gordon I. Pathophysiology of renal function and its effect on isotope studies in the workup of hydronephrosis. World J Urol. 2004 Dec;22(6):411–4.
15. Lee RS, Cendron M, Kinnamon DD, et al. Antenatal hydronephrosis as a predictor of postnatal outcome: a meta-analysis. Pediatrics. 2006;118:586–93.
16. Ahmad G, Green P. Outcome of fetal pyelectasis diagnosed antenatally. J Obstet Gynaecol. 2005;25:119–22.
17. Dias CS, Silva JM, Pereira AK, et al. Diagnostic accuracy of renal pelvic dilatation for detecting surgically managed ureteropelvic junction obstruction. J Urol. 2013;190:661–6.
18. O'Reilly PH, Brooman PJ, Mak S, Jones M, Pickup C, Atkinson C, Pollard AJ. The long-term results of Anderson–Hynes pyeloplasty. BJU Int. 2001;87(4):287–9.
19. Smith KE, Holmes N, Lieb JI, Mandell J, Baskin LS, Kogan BA, Walker RD 3rd. Stented versus nonstented pediatric Pyeloplasty: a modern series and review of the literature. J Urol. 2002;168(3):1127–30.
20. Gatti JM, Amstutz SP, Bowlin PR, Stephany HA, Murphy JP. Laparoscopic vs open Pyeloplasty in children: results of a randomized, prospective. Controlled Trial J Urol. 2017;197(3 Pt 1):792–7.
21. Lopez PJ, Acuna C. Abdominal pain—urological aspects. In: Godbole P, Koyle M, Wilcox D, editors. Guide to pediatric urology and surgery in clinical practice. London: Springer; 2011. p. 157–64.
22. Polok M, Toczewski K, Borselle D, Apoznanski W, Jedrzejuk D, Patkowski D. Hydronephrosis in children caused by lower pole crossing vessels–how to choose the proper method of treatment? Front Pediatr. 2019;7:83.
23. Esposito C, Bleve C, Escolino M, Caione P, Gerocarni Nappo S, Farina A, Caprio MG, Cerulo M, La Manna A, Chiarenza SF. Laparoscopic transposition of lower pole crossing vessels (vascular hitch) in children with pelviureteric junction obstruction. Transl Pediatr. 2016;5(4):256–61.
24. Hoberman A, Charron M, Hickey RW, Baskin M, Kearney DH, Wald ER. Imaging studies after a first urinary tract infection in young children. N Engl J Med. 2003;348:195–202.
25. Giorgi LJ Jr, Bratslavsky G, Kogan BA. Febrile urinary tract infections in infants: renal ultrasound remains necessary. J Urol. 2005;173(2):568–70.
26. Samnakay N, Barker A. Urinary tract infections: Australasia. In: Godbole P, Koyle M, Wilcox D, editors. Guide to pediatric urology and surgery in clinical practice. London: Springer; 2011. p. 157–64.
27. Craig JC, Knight JF, Sureshkumar P, Lam A, Onikul E, Roy LP. Vesicoureteric reflux and timing of micturating cystourethrography after urinary tract infection. Arch Dis Child. 1997;76:275–7.
28. McDonald A, Scranton M, Gillespie R, Mahajan V, Edwards GA. Voiding cystourethrogram and urinary tract infections: how long to wait? Pediatrics. 2000;105:E50.
29. McLellan DL, Retik AB, Bauer SB, et al. Rate and predictors of spontaneous resolution of prenatally diagnosed primary nonrefluxing megaureter. J Urol. 2002;168:2177–80.
30. Shokeir AA, Nijman RJM. Primary megaureter: current trends in diagnosis and treatment. BJU Int. 2000;86:861–8.

31. Bader M, McCarthy L. What is the efficacy of circumcision in boys with complex urinary tract abnormalities? Pediatr Nephrol. 2013;28(12):2267–72.
32. Jude E, Deshpande A, Barker A, Khosa J, Samnakay N. Intravesical ureteric reimplantation for primary obstructed megaureter in infants under 1 year of age. J Pediatr Urol. 2017;13(1):47.e1–7.
33. Ortiz R, Parente A, Perez-Egido L, Burgos L, Angulo JM. Long-term outcomes in primary obstructive Megaureter treated by endoscopic balloon dilatation. Experience after 100 cases. Front Pediatr. 2018;6:275.
34. Doudt AD, Pusateri CR, Christman MS. Endoscopic Management of Primary obstructive megaureter: a systematic review. J Endourol. 2018;32(6):482–7.
35. Stein R, Rubenwolf P, Ziesel C, Kamal MM, Thüroff JW. Psoas hitch and Boari flap ureteroneocystostomy. BJU Int. 2013 Jul;112(1):137–55.
36. Kitchens DM, DeFoor W, Minevich E, Reddy P, Polsky E, McGregor A, Sheldon C. End cutaneous ureterostomy for the management of severe hydronephrosis. J Urol. 2007 Apr;177(4):1501–4.
37. Politano V, Leadbetter W. An operative technique for the correction of vesicoureteral reflux. J Urol. 2017;197(2):S94–S100. (Reprinted from J Urol, 79: 932–941, 1958)
38. Steffens J, Stark E, Haben B, Treiyer A. Politano-Leadbetter ureteric reimplantation. BJU Int. 2006 Sep;98(3):695–712.
39. Lee PH, Diamond DA, Duffy PG, Ransley PG. Duplex reflux: a study of 105 children. J Urol. 1991;146:657.
40. Afshar K, Papanikolaou F, Malek R, Bagli D, Pippi-Salle JL, Khoury A. Vesicoureteral reflux and complete ureteral duplication. Conservative or surgical management? J Urol. 2005;173(5):1725–7.
41. Thomas JC. Vesicoureteral reflux and duplex systems. Adv Urol. 2008;2008:651891.
42. Singh-Grewal D, Macdessi J, Craig J. Circumcision for the prevention of urinary tract infection in boys: a systematic review of randomised trials and observational studies. Arch Dis Child. 2005;90:853–8.
43. Hensle TW, Reiley EA, Ritch C, Murphy A. The clinical utility and safety of the endoscopic treatment of vesicoureteral reflux in patients with duplex ureters. J Pediatr Urol. 2010;6(1):15–22.
44. Rossini CJ, Moriarty KP, Courtney RA, Tashjian DB. Endoscopic treatment with Deflux for refluxing duplex systems. J Laparoendosc Adv Surg Tech A. 2009;19(5):679–82.
45. Aboutaleb H, Bolduc S, Khoury AE, Upadhyay J, Bägli DJ, Farhat W. Polydimethylsiloxane injection versus open surgery for the treatment of vesicoureteral reflux in complete duplex systems. J Urol. 2003;170(4, Pt2):1563–5.
46. Ellsworth PI, Lim DJ, Walker RD, Stevens PS, Barraza MA, Mesrobian HGJ. Common sheath reimplantation yields excellent results in the treatment of vesicoureteral reflux in duplicated collecting systems. J Urol. 1996;155(4):1407–9.
47. Choi H, OH SJ. The management of children with complete ureteric duplication: selective use of uretero-ureterostomy as a primary and salvage procedure. BJU Int. 2000;86:508–12.
48. Hanson GR, Gatti JM, Gittes GK, Murphy JP. Diagnosis of ectopic ureter as a cause of urinary incontinence. J Pediatr Urol. 2007;3(1):53–7.
49. Peters CA, Mendelsohn C. Ectopic ureter, ureterocele, and ureteral anomalies. In Campbell-walsh urology, 12th ed. Published January 1; 2016. Ch 134, p. 3075–3101.e3.
50. Handler TF, Shapiro E. Incontinence in a child with a duplex kidney: case report. Rev Urol. 2002;4(Winter, 1):44–8.
51. Ortiz R, Parente A, Burgos L, Angulo JM. Endoscopic urinary diversion as initial Management of Symptomatic Obstructive Ectopic Ureter in infants. Front Pediatr. 2017;5:208.
52. Timberlake MD, Corbett ST. Minimally invasive techniques for management of the ureterocoele and ectopic ureter: upper tract versus lower tract approach. Urol Clin North Am. 2015;42(1):61–76.
53. McLeod DJ, Alpert SA, Ural Z, Jayanthi VR. Ureteroureterostomy irrespective of ureteral size or upper pole function: a single center experience. J Pediatr Urol. 2014;10(4):616–9.

54. Chacko JK, Koyle MA, Mingin GC, et al. Ipsilateral ureteroureterostomy in the surgical management of the severely dilated ureter in ureteral duplication. J Urol. 2007;178:1689–92.
55. Christensen T, Cohen D. Ureteral Obstruction and Malformations. In Ashcraft's Paediatric Surgery, 5th ed. Eds Holcomb G and Murphy JP. 2009;6:307–15.
56. Castagnetti M, El-Ghoneimi A. Management of duplex system ureteroceles in neonates and infants. Nat Rev Urol. 2009;6:307–15.
57. Merlini E, Lelli CP. Obstructive ureterocele-an ongoing challenge. World J Urol. 2004;22(2):107–14.
58. Merguerian PA, Taenzer A, Knoerlein K, McQuiston L, Herz D. Variation in management of duplex system intravesical ureterocoeles: a survey of pediatric urologists. J Urol. 2010;184(4 Suppl):1625–30.
59. Adorisio O, Elia A, Landi L, et al. Effectiveness of primary endoscopic incision in treatment of ectopic ureterocele associated with duplex system. Urology. 2011;77:191–4.
60. Boucher A, Cloutier J, Rousseau A, Charrois R, Bolduc S. Is an initial endoscopic treatment for all ureteroceles appropriate? J Pediatr Urol. 2013;9:339–43.
61. Molitierno JA Jr, Scherz HC, Kirsch AJ. Endoscopic injection of dextranomer hyaluronic acid copolymer for the treatment of vesicoureteral reflux in duplex ureters. J Pediatr Urol. 2008;4:372–6.
62. You D, Bang JK, Shim M, Ryu DS, Kim SK. Analysis of the late outcome of laparoscopic heminephrectomy in children with duplex kidneys. BJU Int. 2010;106:250–4.
63. Lee RS, Retik AB, Borer JG, et al. Pediatric retroperitoneal laparoscopic partial nephrectomy: comparison with an age matched cohort of open surgery. J Urol. 2005;174:708.
64. Leclair MD, Vidal I, Suply E, Podevin G, Heloury Y. Retroperitoneal laparoscopic heminephrectomy in duplex kidney in infants and children: a 15-year experience. Eur Urol. 2009;56(2):385–9.
65. Garcia-Aparicio L, Krauel L, Tarrado X, Olivares M, Garcia-Nunez B, Lerena J, Suara L, Rovira J, Rodo J. Heminephroureterectomy for duplex kidney: laparoscopy versus open surgery. J Pediatr Urol. 2010;6:157–60.
66. El-Ghoneimi A, Farhat W, Bolduc S, Bagli D, McLorie G, Khoury A. Retroperitoneal laparoscopic vs open partial nephroureterectomy in children. BJU Int. 2003;91:532–5.
67. Jayram G, Roberts J, Hernandez A, Heloury Y, Manoharan S, Godbole P, LeClair M, Mushtaq I, Gundeti MS. Outcomes and fate of the remnant moiety following laparoscopic heminephrectomy for duplex kidney: a multicenter review. J Pediatr Urol. 2011;7(3):272–5.
68. Murugapoopathy V, McCusker C, Gupta IR. The pathogenesis and management of renal scarring in children with vesicoureteric reflux and pyelonephritis. Pediatr Nephrol. 2019; https://doi.org/10.1007/s00467-018-4187-9.
69. Edwards A, Peters CA. Managing vesicoureteral reflux in children: making sense of all the data. F1000Res. 2019;8:F1000 Faculty Rev-29.
70. Hoberman A, Trial Investigators RIVUR, Greenfield SP, Mattoo TK, et al. Antimicrobial prophylaxis for children with vesicoureteral reflux. N Engl J Med. 2014;370:2367–76.
71. Nagler EV, Williams G, Hodson EM, Craig JC. Interventions for primary vesicoureteric reflux. Cochrane Database Syst Rev. 2011;6:CD001532.
72. Williams G, Hodson EM, Craig JC. Interventions for primary vesicoureteric reflux. Cochrane Database Syst Rev. 2019;2:CD001532.
73. Heidenreich A, Ozgur E, Becker T, Haupt G. Surgical management of vesicoureteral reflux in pediatric patients. World J Urol. 2004;22(2):96–106.
74. Tekgül S, Riedmiller H, Hoebeke P, Kočvara R, Nijman RJ, Radmayr C, Stein R, Dogan HS. European Association of Urology. EAU guidelines on vesicoureteral reflux in children. Eur Urol. 2012;62(3):534–42.
75. Schwab CW, Wu HY, Selman H, Smith GH, Snyder HM, Canning DA. Spontaneous resolution of vesicoureteral reflux: a 15-year perspective. J Urol. 2002;168(6):2594–9.
76. Gucuk A, Burgu B, Gokce I, Mermerkaya M, Soygur T. Do antibiotic prophylaxis and/or circumcision change periurethral uropathogen colonization and urinary tract infection rates in boys with VUR? J Pediatr Urol. 2013;9(6 Pt B):1131–6.

77. Okarska-Napierała M, Wasilewska A, Kuchar E. *Urinary tract infection in children: Diagnosis, treatment, imaging—comparison of current guidelines*. J Pediatr Urol. 2017;13(6):567–73.
78. Stein R, Dogan HS, Hoebeke P, Kočvara R, Nijman RJ, Radmayr C, Tekgül S. Urinary tract infections in children: EAU/ESPU guidelines. Eur Urol. 2015;67(3):546–58.
79. National Institute for Health and Clinical Excellence NICE. Guideline on Urinary Tract Infection in Children. Urinary tract infection in under 16s: diagnosis and management. https://www.nice.org.uk/Guidance/cg54.
80. Routh JC, Bogaert GA, Kaefer M, Manzoni G, Park JM, Retik AB, Rushton HG, Snodgrass WT, Wilcox DT. Vesicoureteral reflux: current trends in diagnosis, screening, and treatment. Eur Urol. 2012;61(4):773–82.
81. Elder JS, Diaz M, Caldamone AA, Cendron M, Greenfield S, Hurwitz R, Kirsch A, Koyle MA, Pope J, Shapiro E. Endoscopic therapy for vesicoureteral reflux: a meta-analysis, I: reflux resolution and urinary tract infection. J Urol. 2006;175:716–22.
82. Sillen U, Brandstrom P, Jodal U, et al. The Swedish reflux trial in children: V. bladder dysfunction. J Urol. 2010;184:298–304.
83. Sarhan OM, Alghanbar M, Alsulaihim A, Alharbi B, Alotay A, Nakshabandi Z. Multicystic dysplastic kidney: impact of imaging modality selection on the initial management and prognosis. J Pediatr Urol. 2014;10(4):645–9.
84. Tiryaki S, Alkac AY, Serdaroglu E, Bak M, Avanoglu A, Ulman I. Involution of multicystic dysplastic kidney: is it predictable? J Pediatr Urol. 2013 Jun;9(3):344–7.
85. Psooy K, Collaboration with the Pediatric Urologists of Canada (PUC). Multicystic dysplastic kidney (MCDK) in the neonate: the role of the urologist. Can Urol Assoc J. 2016;10(1–2):18–24.

Congenital Upper Tract Anomalies: Duplication, Cystic Renal Dysplasia, Multicystic Dysplastic Kidney

10

David Chalmers

Learning Objectives

1. Explain the basic embryology of the kidneys and ureter and how that relates to pathologic conditions associated with duplication anomalies.
2. List the surgical options for managing duplication anomalies, ectopic ureteral insertion, ureterocele
3. Develop a comprehensive differential diagnosis for renal cysts in children.
4. What is the appropriate evaluation and investigations to consider for renal cysts in the pediatric population?

10.1 Introduction

A basic understanding of embryology is an important foundation for morphologic upper tract abnormalities. The embryologic development of the urinary tract occurs in several well-described stages [1]. In summary, there are three sets of nephric structures: the pronephros, mesonephros and metanephros. The pronephros is transient and regresses. The mesonephros is regulated by signals in the Wolffian duct and also regresses, although there is a functional component. The metanephros ultimately becomes the definitive kidney and development begins with the outgrowth of epithelial cells called the ureteric bud from the Wolffian duct. As the ureteric bud extends out from the mesonephric duct to reach the metanephric mesenchyme (metanephric blastema), signaling causes a critical branching cascade, which forms the elaborate collecting duct system.

D. Chalmers (✉)
Department of Urology, Maine Medical Center, S. Portland, ME, USA
e-mail: DChalmers@mmc.org

P. Godbole et al. (eds.), *Practical Pediatric Urology*,
https://doi.org/10.1007/978-3-030-54020-3_10

Reciprocal interactions between the ureteric bud and metanephric blastema explain much of the pathophysiology described within this chapter. The first branching interactions give rise to the major and minor calyces, into which the collecting ducts from the renal papillae drain. Branching problems can cause decreased kidney mass (hypoplasia) and defective structures (dysplasia). Alternatively, if the ureteric bud bifurcates or there are two distinct buds that arise from the mesonephric duct, partial or complete duplication of the kidney may result.

10.2 Renal Duplication

10.2.1 Scenario 1

A newborn infant is known antenatally to have a left duplex kidney with possible complete ureteric duplication. Postnatal VCUG is shown below (Fig. 10.1 a and b).

10.2.1.1 Question 1

What does this show and how can this be explained embryologically?

10.2.1.2 Answer 1

The VCUG shows reflux into both upper and lower moiety ureters on the left but no clubbing of the calyces. The urethra is not seen but from the limited views available, the bladder looks normal. There is suggestion of duplication on the right with reflux on the right.

Embrylogy and Anatomy

When multiple ureteric buds emerge from the developing Wolffian Duct, a variety of duplication anomalies can result, ranging from partial duplication, which may not be clinically significant, to complete duplication, representing two distinct collecting systems within the kidney and separate ureters inserting into the bladder. In >95% of cases, the anatomy follows the predictable Weigert-Meyer law [2, 3]. The upper and lower pole ureters cross prior to their respective insertions into the bladder. The lower pole moiety ureter enters the bladder at a lateral location relative to the upper pole moiety orifice. This leads to a shorter tunnel through the detrusor that is prone to reflux. The upper pole moiety ureter inserts more distally relative to the lower pole orifice, and more commonly results in an obstructive phenomenon, such as ureterocele. However, there is considerable variability in the possible pathology and it is possible for both poles to reflux, to drain normally, or for an ectopic location to obstruct. Consequently, while duplex kidneys may be normal, they are prone to dysplasia or progressive obstruction depending on the anatomy of their insertion at the level of the bladder. The more ectopic the ureteral orifice, the greater the likelihood of obstructing or refluxing pathology, and, consequently, associated dyplasia. When identified on voiding cystourethrogram, reflux into a lower pole presents in a pelvicalyceal pattern described as the "drooping lily" sign, with the lower pole calyces in a characteristic downward-deviating orientation.

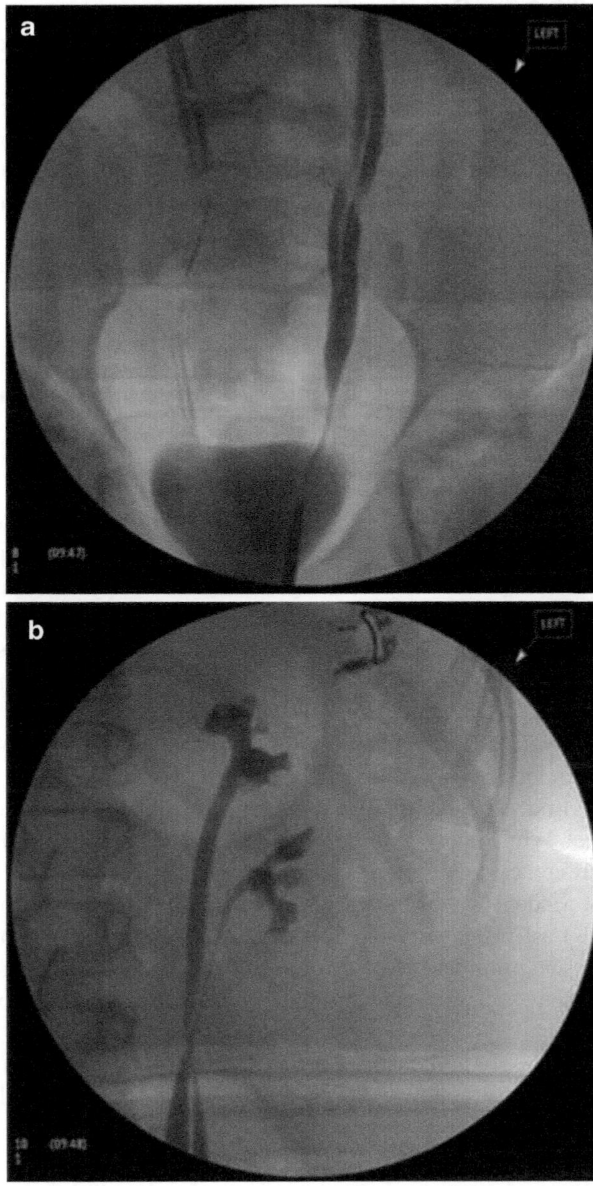

Fig. 10.1 (**a** and **b**) Select voiding cystourethrogram images of the bladder and left upper tract

Vesicoureteric Reflux in Duplex Kidneys

Due to the more lateral insertion site of the lower pole moiety orifice, reflux is a common finding, particularly in children presenting with UTI [4]. Repeated pyelonephritis in the setting of lower pole reflux may lead to a characteristic appearance of dysplasia or scarring limited to the lower moiety. It may also lead to hypertension and/or proteinuria. Pain should not be a presenting symptom of reflux.

10.2.1.3 Question 2

What would be your indications for surgical intervention in the above case?

10.2.1.4 Answer 2

Indications for surgical intervention in the setting of a refluxing duplex kidney are not different from a single system, and include prevention of recurrent UTIs, particularly febrile, and renal scarring. However, the natural history of reflux in duplex kidneys may not be as favorable. While lower grades of reflux may still resolve spontaneously, higher grades likely have a lower rate of resolution over time, which may prompt a more aggressive surgical decision [5].

10.2.1.5 Question 3

What are the surgical options if surgery is contemplated in duplex kidneys with reflux?

10.2.1.6 Answer 3

The traditional method of anti-reflux surgery for duplex systems is the common sheath reimplantation, where both the upper and lower pole moieties are mobilized and reimplanted together, regardless of the surgical technique [6]. Despite the additional degree of difficulty, success rates reportedly mirror traditional reimplantation outcomes. Of note, it is important to understand from a surgical perspective that the duplicated ureters share a common fascia as they course into the bladder, which includes a blood supply that would be compromised if separation were attempted. To avoid devascularization, the ureters should be reimplanted together, even if one of them does not reflux.

Endoscopic injection to treat reflux in duplex systems remains somewhat controversial. While many studies site a decreased success rate compared to single systems, the difference may not be statistically significant [7]. This choice likely remains very dependent on the bias of the surgeon and the shared-decision making goals of the family.

Lastly, there may be occasions when the lower pole of a duplex kidney is dyplastic and provides little function. If it continues to cause problems, while providing no benefit, a hemi-nephrectomy, either laparoscopic or open, is a reasonable option. Typically, the blood supply to a small, dyplastic pole is not robust and can be managed safely and easily. The goal is to remove as much of the associated ureter as possible, although leaving a short ureteral stump is rarely problematic [8].

10.2.1.7 Question 4

How can an ectopic ureteric insertion be explained embryologically and how can this be confirmed?

10.2.1.8 Answer 4

Ectopic Ureter in Duplex Kidneys

While ectopic ureteral insertion may occur in single system anatomy, the embryology of duplex systems encourages the upper pole moiety to insert more distally.

If the ureteral bud originates in an abnormally cranial position from the mesonephric duct, the distal ureter will migrate for a longer period along the path that the mesonephric duct follows before it is incorporated onto the bladder. If this position is too ectopic, it may not separate from the mesonephric duct at all and instead terminate in a mesonephric duct structure. In females, ectopic ureters may drain distal to the urinary sphincter into the vagina, which can result in continuous urinary incontinence. Asking parents if their girl seems to be constantly wet, or can be dry for distinct stretches of time can be revealing. Likewise, a careful examination of a girl with an ectopic ureter may identify continuous dripping of urine from the introitus. In males, a distal ectopic insertion may result in a ureter draining into a structure of the mesonephric duct, including the ejaculatory duct, seminal vesicle, vas deferens or epididymis. Although rare, the classic presentation is recurrent epididymo-orchitis.

Regardless of the patient sex, ectopic ureter leads to associated obstruction and resulting hydronephrosis. However, identifying the true orifice location can be challenging during cystoscopy or vaginoscopy. A variety of imaging studies can be used to help understand the anatomy. First, ultrasound is the most common screening tool to identify hydroureteronephrosis and perhaps an associated dysplastic appearing upper pole. However, it rarely can pinpoint the precise orifice location. Voiding cystourethrograms can be helpful, as ectopic ureters are frequently associated with reflux observed on. A ureteral orifice superior to the sphincter will demonstrate the reflux during filling, while a ureteral insertion below the sphincter commonly demonstrates reflux during the voiding phase. Lastly, CT and MRI imaging with delayed sequences may most accurately capture the precise anatomy of an ectopic insertion, however, these also represent the most time and cost intensive modalities.

10.2.1.9 Question 5

What are the management options for an ectopic ureteric insertion?

10.2.1.10 Answer 5

Ectopic ureteral insertion most commonly requires surgery. Most commonly, the associated upper pole is poorly functioning and requires upper pole hemi-nephrectomy. Similarly to the above-mentioned lower pole hemi-nephrectomy, retaining the distal ureteric stump is typically safe and may obviate the need for a more morbid complete ureterectomy [9]. In situations where there is upper pole function worth salvaging, alternatives to hemi-nephrectomy include reimplantation or uretero-ureterostomy depending on the surgeon's preference for a upper or lower tract reconstruction approach.

10.2.1.11 Question 6

What are the management options for a ureterocele associated with a duplex kidney?

10.2.1.12 Answer 6

Ureterocele in Duplex Kidneys

The risk of ureterocele is markedly higher in duplex kidneys compared to single systems, perhaps as high as 5–20% [4]. Antenatal sonography most commonly identifies hydronephrosis associated with the obstructive nature of ureteroceles, although UTI is also a possible presentation and distal ureteral stones can be observed in adult patients presenting with previously undiagnosed ureteroceles. In duplex kidneys, the ureterocele is almost always associated with the upper pole system, however, the size of the ureterocele may impact the bladder and other ureters more globally. The lower pole moiety may be obstructed by a markedly dilated upper pole ureter. Meanwhile, a cecoureterocele may obstruct the bladder outlet and affect the contralateral system as well. Finally, concurrent reflux to the ipsilateral lower pole system, and the contralateral kidney is significantly elevated [10]. It is beyond the scope of this chapter to describe all the various management options for ureterocele, and depends on the degree of obstruction, range of symptoms, and associated renal function. Options vary tremendously, from simple conservative observation, to endoscopic ureterocele puncture, to extirpative upper pole heminephrectomy, to complex reconstruction with ureterocele excision, bladder neck repair and re-implantation.

10.3 Cystic Renal Dysplasia

10.3.1 Overview

Renal cysts represent an enclosed, fluid-filled cavity that may develop in a tubular segment of the kidney. They represent an imbalance of secretory and absorptive properties of renal epithelial cells. Cystic disease may represent a wide spectrum of entities that are inheritable or sporadic, with each class representing benign and morbid conditions. Simple renal cysts, multilocular cyst (cystic nephroma), and acquired cystic renal disease represent some of the most significant sporadic conditions. Polycystic disease, Tuberous Sclerosis and von Hippel–Lindau disease are some of the most significant inheritable conditions. Finally, multicystic dysplastic kidney is a unique, non-inheritable entity.

10.3.2 Scenario 2

10.3.2.1 Question 1

This child was noted to have an incidental finding in the left kidney on a CT scan (Fig. 10.2) done for other reasons. What does this show and is the finding significant? What would be your management?

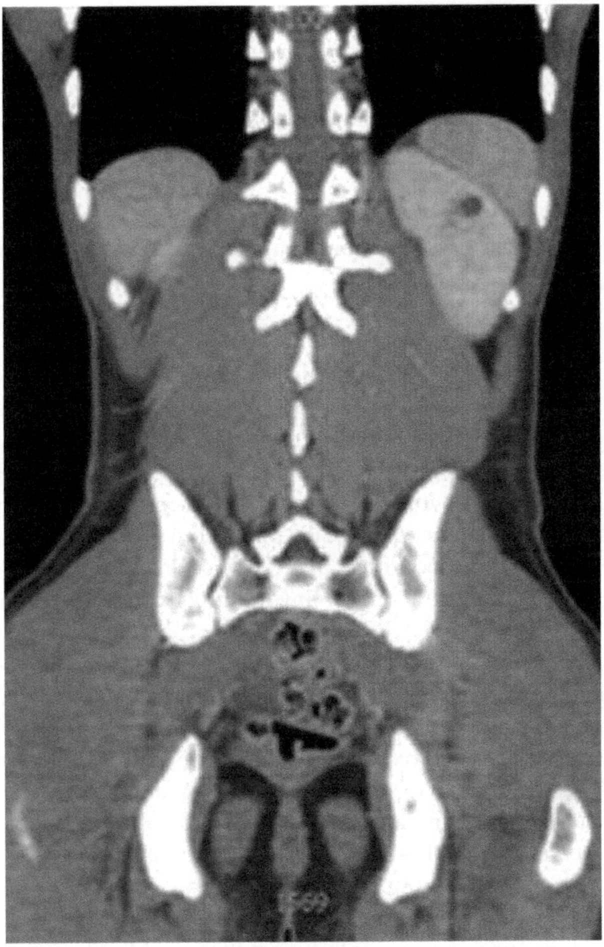

Fig. 10.2 CT scan of the abdomen and pelvis with contrast (nephrogenic phase)

10.3.2.2 Answer 1

The CT scan shows a simple renal cyst in the left kidney.

Simple Renal Cysts

Simple renal cysts are quite common in adults, but rarely found in children, thus commonly raising concern for more serious conditions. However, simple isolated renal cysts are overwhelmingly benign and are clinically insignificant. Simple renal cysts are asymptomatic and discovered incidentally by imaging. Symptoms are very rare, but could include pain from a cyst so large that there is a mass effect, or if the cyst becomes infected or hemorrhages. Observation, perhaps with serial imaging, is commonly all that is necessary, in order to rule out a developing cystic malignancy or developing polycystic kidney disease. Interventions for those complications are rarely necessary. Complex cysts include features such as internal echogenicity, non-distinct or thickened walls, septations, or solid vascular components. The Bosniak classification system, commonly used to risk stratify adult cystic lesions, can also be applied to pediatric cysts to assess concern for malignancy.

10.3.2.3 Question 2

What other cystic lesions may be found in the kidney in children?

10.3.2.4 Answer 2

Multilocular Cyst (Cystic Nephroma)

Multlocular cyst, or multilocular cystic nephroma, is considered a benign entity, although related to Wilms tumor by classification. The entity presents in a bimodal pattern of young children before 4 years of age and adults after 30 years of age. The kidney may be quite enlarged and present as a palpable mass. It is understandable that the first concern is to rule out a more serious malignancy, such as a cystic Wilms Tumor. Ultrasonography and CT scan imaging cannot rule this entity out with certainty so the treatment for any multilocular cystic lesion is nephrectomy.

Acquired Cystic Disease

Acquired renal cystic disease is defined as bilateral cyst development in the setting of end-stage renal disease. The phenomenon has been observed most commonly in adults receiving long term hemodialysis, but it is common in children as well [11]. The majority of patients are asymptomatic, however bleeding into the cysts can cause pain or hematuria, complicated by associated coagulation defects commonly seen in uremia. Furthermore, there is an increased risk of malignancy in kidneys of patients undergoing long term dialysis, including renal cell carcinoma [12, 13]. Duration of dialysis is an important risk factor for developing malignancy although not the type of renal replacement therapy. Monitoring of cyst development and cyst characterization is recommended after 3 years of dialysis. Interestingly, cysts of acquired cystic disease tend to regress after renal transplantation, but the elevated risk of malignancy may persist for many years [14].

Autosomal Dominant Polycystic Kidney Disease (ADPKD)

ADPKD is one of the most common CAKUT pathologies leading to adult dialysis or renal transplantation [15]. In contrast to the previously mentioned cystic diseases, it is inheritable. The vast majority of patients have a strong family history and the diagnosis is confirmed as renal cysts develop into adulthood. An estimated 95% of ADPDK patients will develop cysts by the third decade of life [16]. Likely complications include nephrolithiasis, UTIs/pyelonephritis, flank pain and hematuria. Associated medical problems include hypertension, hepatic and pancreatic cysts, and cerebral (Berry) aneurysms.

Well-described mutations include PKD1 and PKD2, which account for the overwhelming majority of ADPKD cases [17]. Mutations in the PKD1 gene, located on chromosome 16p13, generally lead to an earlier onset of symptoms, compared to PKD2, located on 4q13–q23. However there is significant variability both. Each gene encodes a polycystin protein, which interacts with plasma transmembrane complexes to inhibit cell proliferation [18].

In addition to numerous extrarenal medical problems, there is an increased risk of renal adenomas associated with ADPKD, similar to acquired cystic disease. However, the incidence of renal cell carcinoma is not elevated above the risk of the general population [19]. Evaluation and risk assessment for malignancy is complicated by cystic hemorrhage, proteinacious debris, and the complex architecture of the cysts. Additional management strategies are focused on delaying the onset of dialysis as long as possible. This includes aggressive blood pressure management, pain control if the cyst sizes becomes symptomatic or bleed, or even surgical cyst decortication or nephrectomy.

Autosomal Recessive Polycystic Kidney Disease (ARPKD)

ARPKD is much less common than ADPKD, about 1 in 10,000–50,000, and more commonly presents during childhood or even prenatally [20]. Prenatal sonography may identify bright, echogenic, enlarged kidneys. If there is severe bilateral disease, there is an increased chance of impaired lung development, particularly if oligohydramnios is noted [21]. Anydramnios may even be incompatible with life. Overall, about 85% of newborns surviving prenatally survive through infancy and the survival rate into the teenage years is about 70% [22]. Hypertension is the most significant associated medical problem, commonly requiring multiple medications. As the patient ages into adulthood, cysts may enlarge as seen below (Fig. 10.3) and hepatic fibrosis is an expected cormobidity related to the genetic pathophysiology.

The severity of the disease is dependent on the nature of the genetic defect. ARPKD is caused by mutations in the polycystic kidney and hepatic disease 1 gene (PKHD1), which is located on chromosome 6p21 and encodes a protein called fibrocystin [23]. Fibrocystin belongs to a class of proteins regulating cell proliferation and cellular adhesion/repulsion [24].

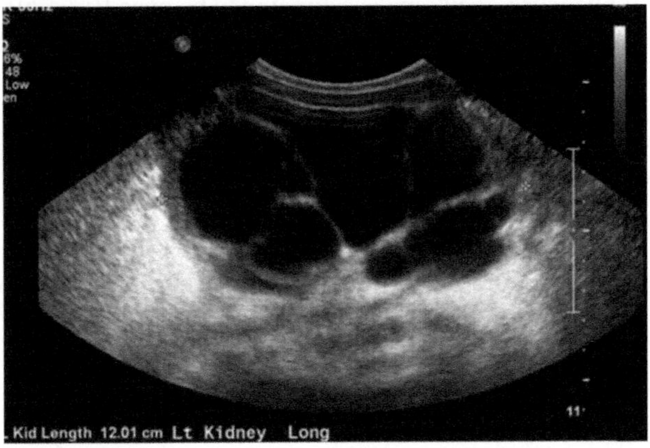

Fig. 10.3 Renal ultrasound of the left kidney, sagittal view

It is difficult to provide a prognosis for patients with ARPKD since the clinical spectrum is so diverse. However, treatment is focused on supportive pulmonary care, particularly in infancy, management of hypertension, and renal replacement and hepatic failure, including decompression of portal hypertension.

Syndromes with Renal Cysts

Tuberous sclerosis and von Hippel Lindau (VHL) are two autosomal dominant disorders most commonly encountered by pediatric urologists due to the fact that cystic dysplasia is a common feature. Tuberous sclerosis complex (TSC) is a neurocutaneous disorder characterized by the classic triad of epilepsy, mental retardation and adenoma sebaceum (angiofibromas). However, there are a variety of other major and minor criteria that now help comprise a diagnosis of TSC. Renal angiomyolipomas and renal cysts are two of those possible features. *TSC1* and *TSC2* genes are located on chromosome 9q34 and 16p13 respectively. TSC1 encodes the protein hamartin and TSC2 encodes tuberin. They are both important tumor suppressor genes part of the well described mTOR pathway [25]. Renal angiomyolipomas occur in over 50% and renal cysts develop in over 20% of patients with TSC [26]. Management of TSC renal lesions is most commonly focused on preventing hemorrhage of large angiomyolipomas. In general, sizes greater than 4 cm in diameter merit consideration for prophylactic embolization or surgical excision. Annual surveillance with ultrasonography or CT scan is a reasonable approach. A small association with renal cell carcinoma is also worth noting, although likely only about 2% [27].

VHL disease is also characterized by a spectrum of renal and extrarenal manifestations. They include angiomatous renal lesions, cerebellar hemangioblastomas, pheochromocytoma, epididymal cystadenoma, clear cell carcinoma of the kidney, and cysts of the pancreas, kidney, and epididymis. It is a rare diagnosis with a high penetrance in affected patients. The *VHL* gene is a tumor suppressor gene located on chromosome 3p25. The mean age of presentation is 35–40 years of age and most frequently presents with renal cysts [28]. They are frequently multiple and bilateral cysts. Careful surveillance is the most important job of the urologist, since the risk of clear cell renal cell carcinoma is approximately 50% in VHL patients and the risk of pheochromocytoma is estimated to be over 10% [29]. The recommended mindset is not cancer cure, but cancer control, which can be a challenging balance of surgical excision of enlarging, dangerous appearing cysts, while preserving as much renal parenchyma and adrenal gland tissue as possible.

10.3.3 Scenario 3

A 3 month old infant had an antenatal diagnosis of a possible multi cystic dysplastic right kidney. An ultrasound scan at 3 months is shown below (Fig. 10.4).

10.3.3.1 Question 1

What is the differential diagnosis?

Fig. 10.4 Renal ultrasound of the right kidney, sagittal view

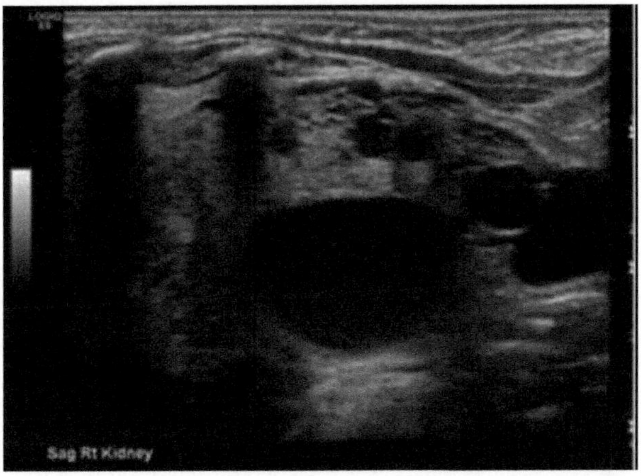

10.3.3.2 Answer 1

Differential diagnosis can include an MCDK, or a UPJ obstruction.

10.3.3.3 Question 2

What further imaging would you consider?

10.3.3.4 Answer 2

As a UPJ obstruction is being considered, A MAG 3 renogram should be considered.

10.3.3.5 Question 3

The MAG 3 renogram is shown below (Fig. 10.5)**. What does this show and what would be your diagnosis?**

10.3.3.6 Answer 3

The lack of function in the right kidney would be consistent with a right MCDK.

10.3.3.7 Question 4

What would be your subsequent management of the MCDK?

10.3.3.8 Answer 4

Multicystic Dysplastic Kidney.

Overview

MCDK represents the most common congenital cystic anomaly of the kidney, and is characterized by multiple non-communicating cysts with non-functional, minimal parenchyma. The size of the kidney may vary tremendously, from a small nubbin of tissue to a size capable of exerting a mass effect on other abdominal structures.

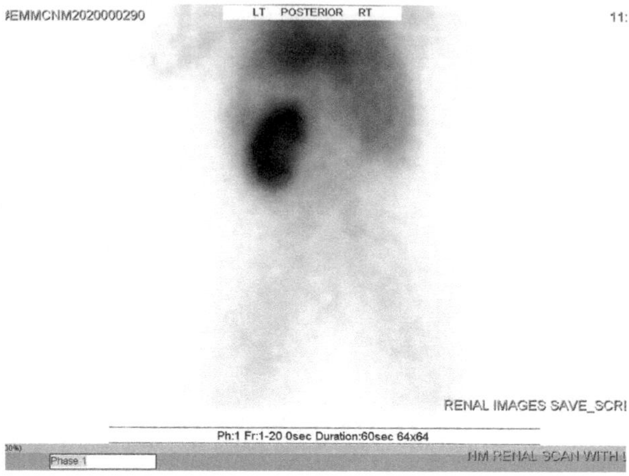

Fig. 10.5 MAG-3 study, functional/cortical phase

Unlike other cystic kidney diseases, there is not a clear etiology for MCDK. It occurs sporadically and a variety of embryologic hypotheses have been proposed:

1. MCDK represents the most extreme form of congenital obstruction, occurring early in nephrogenesis [30]
2. Abnormalities of reciprocal induction between the ureteric bud and metanephric blastema [31]

The incidence of MCKD is about 1 in 4000 and is more common in males. Although the contralateral kidney must be "normal" for the fetus to be compatible with life, there is a higher incidence of ureteropelvic junction obstruction (about 10%) and vesicoureteral reflux (about 25%) in the contralateral kidney [32, 33] Historically, a palpable mass per abdomen was the most common presentation. Today, the overwhelming majority of MCDK is discovered during antenatal ultrasonography. The hallmark appearance is a cluster of non-communicating cysts of varying sizes. In contrast, the cystic appearance of a dilated ureteropelvic junction obstruction should be a more organized appearance of smaller cysts around a larger dilated renal pelvis, and they should communicate.

MCKD should demonstrate almost no renal parenchyma. If the diagnosis is in doubt, a nuclear scan such as DMSA or MAG3 scan should confirm an absence of any function.

MCKD Management

A uniform management strategy for MCKD has not been established, however the recent trend has been towards less aggressive treatment regarding both imaging investigations, as well as surgery. First, if congenital hydronephrosis is present in the contralateral kidney, there is a greater concern for concurrent ureteropelvic junction obstruction. Ultrasongrapy and MAG3 scan can reliably distinguish obstruction vs physiologic hydronephrosis. Likewise, consideration of VCUG has been advocated to assess for contralateral vesicoureteral reflux. However, as our understanding of the natural history of reflux has evolved towards a non-surgical approach, the impetus for proactively assessing for reflux has diminished as well. Furthermore, recent studies have highlighted that the majority of reflux diagnosed by VCUG is low grade and likely to resolve spontaneously [34]. In this light, VCUG imaging in the setting of a MCDK diagnosis may be considered optional.

In the past, there has also been a concern regarding malignant transformation of MCDK due to reports of both Wilms tumor and Renal Cell Carcinoma. For this reason, prophylactic nephrectomy has been considered. However, numerous studies have demonstrated that the risk of malignancy is not increased [35, 36], including data from a large MCKD registry [37]. Similarly, the risk of other surgical indications for removal, such as hypertension, remains somewhat controversial. While there have been case reports of successful hypertension resolution following MCKD nephrectomy [38], this remains uncommon.

A final consideration regarding conservative versus surgical management for MCKD is the natural history. The majority of MCKD kidneys regress and involute over time. The MCKD registry noted an undetectable ultrasound appearance of 20 by 3 and 50% by 5 years [9]. Many urologists elect to follow MCKD with serial ultrasound imaging, as it is safe to observe a progressively decreasing size in an asymptomatic patient. The frequency and duration of this monitoring is not known and a failure to regress or failure to completely involute are relative indications for surgery.

References

1. Little MH, McMahon AP. Mammalian kidney development: principles, progress, and projections. Cold Spring Harb Perspect Biol. 2012;4:a008300.
2. Meyer R. Normal and abnormal development of the ureter in the human embryo; a mechanistic consideration. Anat Rec. 1946;96(4):355–71.
3. Whitten SM, Wilcox DT. Duplex systems. Prenat Diagn. 2001;21:952–7.
4. Bisset GS III, Strife JL. The duplex collecting system in girls with urinary tract infection: prevalence and significance. AJR Am J Roentgenol. 1987;148(3):497–500.
5. Afshar K, Papanikolaou F, Malek R, Bagli D, Pippi-Salle JL, Khoury A. Vesicoureteral reflux and complete ureteral duplication. Conservative or surgical management? J Urol. 2005;173(5):1725–7.
6. Belman AB, Filmer RB, King LR. Surgical management of duplication of the collecting system. J Urol. 1974;112(3):316–21.
7. Hensle TW, Reiley EA, Ritch C, Murphy A. The clinical utility and safety of the endoscopic treatment of vesicoureteral reflux in patients with duplex ureters. J Pediatr Urol. 2010;6(1):15–22.
8. Cain MP, Pope JC, Casale AJ, Adams MC, Keating MA, Rink RC. Natural history of refluxing distal ureteral stumps after nephrectomy and partial ureterectomy for vesicoureteral reflux. J Urol. 1998;160(3 Pt 2):1026–7.
9. De Caluwe D, Chertin B, Puri P. Fate of the retained ureteral stump after upper pole heminephrectomy in duplex kidneys. J Urol. 2002;168(2):679–80.

10. Caldamone AA, Snyder HM III, Duckett JW. Ureteroceles in children: followup of management with upper tract approach. J Urol. 1984;131(6):1130–2.
11. Hakim RM, Breyer J, Ismail N, Schulman G. Effects of dose of dialysis on morbidity and mortality. Am J Kidney Dis. 1994;23(5):661–9.
12. Resseguie LJ, Nobrega FT, Farrow GM, Timmons JW, Worobec TG. Epidemiology of renal and ureteral cancer in Rochester, Minnesota, 1950-1974, with special reference to clinical and pathologic features. Mayo Clin Proc. 1978;53(8):503–10.
13. Truong LD, Choi YJ, Shen SS, Ayala G, Amato R, Krishnan B. Renal cystic neoplasms and renal neoplasms associated with cystic renal diseases: pathogenetic and molecular links. Adv Anat Pathol. 2003;10(3):135–59. Review
14. Heinz-Peer G, Schoder M, Rand T, Mayer G, Mostbeck GH. Prevalence of acquired cystic kidney disease and tumors in native kidneys of renal transplant recipients: a prospective US study. Radiology. 1995;195(3):667–71.
15. Fick-Brosnahan GM, Tran ZV, Johnson AM, Strain JD, Gabow PA. Progression of autosomal-dominant polycystic kidney disease in children. Kidney Int. 2001;59(5):1654–62.
16. Liapis H, Winyard PJD. Cystic diseases and developmental kidney defects. In: Jennette JC, Olson JL, Schwartz MM, Silva FG, editors. Heptinstall's pathology of the kidney, vol. 2. 6th ed. Philadephia: Lippincott Williams and Wilkins; 2007. p. 1257–306.
17. Harris PC, Rossetti S. Molecular diagnostics for autosomal dominant polycystic kidney disease. Nat Rev Nephrol. 2010;6(4):197–206.
18. Wilson PD. Polycystic kidney disease: new understanding in the pathogenesis. Int J Biochem Cell Biol. 2004;36(10):1868–73.
19. Keith DS, Torres VE, King BF, Zincki H, Farrow GM. Renal cell carcinoma in autosomal dominant polycystic kidney disease. J Am Soc Nephrol. 1994;4(9):1661–9. Review
20. Zerres K, Rudnik-Schöneborn S, Steinkamm C, Becker J, Mücher G. Autosomal recessive polycystic kidney disease. J Mol Med (Berl). 1998;76(5):303–9. Review
21. Winyard P, Chitty LS. Dysplastic kidneys. Semin Fetal Neonatal Med. 2008;13(3):142–51.
22. Guay-Woodford LM, Desmond RA. Autosomal recessive polycystic kidney disease: the clinical experience in North America. Pediatrics. 2003;111(5 Pt 1):1072–80.
23. Bergmann C, Senderek J, Windelen E, Kupper F, Middeldorf I, Schneider F, Dornia C, Rudnik-Schoneborn S, Konrad M, Schmitt CP, Seeman T, Neuhaus TJ, Vester U, Kirfel J, Buttner R, Zerres K. Clinical consequences of PKHD1 mutations in 164 patients with autosomal-recessive polycystic kidney disease (ARPKD). Kidney Int. 2005;67(3):829–48.
24. Wang S, Zhang J, Nauli SM, Li X, Starremans PG, Luo Y, Roberts KA, Zhou J. Fibrocystin/polyductin, found in the same protein complex with polycystin-2, regulates calcium responses in kidney epithelia. Mol Cell Biol. 2007;27(8):3241–52.
25. Sancak O, Nellist M, Goedbloed M, Elfferich P, Wouters C, Maat-Kievit A, Zonnenberg B, Verhoef S, Halley D, van den Ouweland A. Mutational analysis of the TSC1 and TSC2 genes in a diagnostic setting: genotype--phenotype correlations and comparison of diagnostic DNA techniques in tuberous sclerosis complex. Eur J Hum Genet. 2005;13(6):731–41.
26. Chonko AM, Weiss SM, Stein JH, Ferris TF. Renal involvement in tuberous sclerosis. Am J Med. 1974;56(1):124–32.
27. Bernstein J. Renal cystic disease in the tuberous sclerosis complex. Pediatr Nephrol. 1993;7(4):490–5. Review
28. Neumann HP, Bender BU, Schultze-Seemann W, Krause T, Altehoefer C, Scheremet R, Orszagh M, Schwarzkopf G, Januszewicz A, Janetschek G, Riegler P. The kidney and von Hippel–Lindau disease: impact of molecular genetic analysis of the VHL gene for clinical management. Contrib Nephrol. 1997;122:102–8. Review
29. Levine E, Collins DL, Horton WA, Schimke RN. CT screening of the abdomen in von Hippel-Lindau disease. AJR Am J Roentgenol. 1982;139(3):505–10.
30. Tanagho EA. Surgically induced partial urinary obstruction in the fetal lamb. 3. Ureteral obstruction. Investig Urol. 1972;10(1):35–52.
31. Mackie GG, Stephens FD. Duplex kidneys: a correlation of renal dysplasia with position of the ureteral orifice. J Urol. 1975;114(2):274–80.

32. al-Khaldi N, Watson AR, Zuccollo J, Twining P, Rose DH. Outcome of antenatally detected cystic dysplastic kidney disease. Arch Dis Child. 1994;70(6):520–2.
33. Flack CE, Bellinger MF. The multicystic dysplastic kidney and contralateral vesicoureteral reflux: protection of the solitary kidney. J Urol. 1993;150(6):1873–4.
34. Calaway AC, Whittam B, Szymanski DM, Misseri R, Kaefer M, Rink RC, et al. Multicystic dysplastic kidney: is an initial voiding cystourethrogram necessary? Can J Urol. 2014;21:7510–4.
35. Beckwith JB. Wilms tumor and multicystic dysplastic kidney disease. Editorial Comment J Urol. 1997;158:2259–60.
36. Noe HN, Marshall JH, Edwards OP. Nodular renal blastema in the multicystic kidney. J Urol. 1989;142:486–8.
37. Aslam M, Watson AR, on behalf of the Trent & Anglia MCDK Study Group. Unilateral multicystic dysplastic kidney: long term outcomes. Arch Dis Child. 2006;91:820–3.
38. Snodgrass WT. Hypertension associated with multicystic dysplastic kidney in children. J Urol. 2000;164(2):472–3;discussion 473–4

Practical Pediatric Urology: An Evidence Based Approach—Vesicoureteral Reflux and Bladder Diverticulum

11

Jonathan Walker, Jacqueline Morin, Leslie Peard, and Amanda F. Saltzman

Learning Objectives

- Identify patients at risk of having vesicoureteral reflux as well as those in whom the vesicoureteral reflux is more likely to be associated with renal injury
- Describe the natural history of vesicoureteral reflux and the patient risk factors for non-resolution
- Explain the current non-surgical management options for patients with vesicoureteral reflux
- Understand the pros and cons of cystoscopic, minimally invasive, and open surgical treatment approaches to vesicoureteral reflux
- Review the current evaluation and management strategies associated with symptomatic bladder diverticula

11.1 Introduction

Vesicoureteral reflux (VUR), defined as retrograde flow of urine from the bladder into the ureters and upper urinary tract, is one of the most well-recognized entities in pediatric urology. Affecting up to 30% of all children with a urinary tract infection (UTI) [1], VUR has been linked to pyelonephritis and renal scarring, end-stage renal disease, and hypertension. Despite the long history of VUR in the medical literature, controversy remains on which patients benefit from the diagnosis and treatment of reflux. This lack of consensus is due in part to the paucity of high-quality studies as well as the heterogenous nature of the disease and study designs. Nevertheless, VUR remains an important clinical finding with potential short and

J. Walker (✉)
Erlanger Urology, University of Tennessee Chattanooga, Chattanooga, TN, USA
e-mail: Jonathan.walker@erlanger.org

J. Morin · L. Peard · A. F. Saltzman
Department of Urology, University of Kentucky, Lexington, KY, USA

P. Godbole et al. (eds.), *Practical Pediatric Urology*,
https://doi.org/10.1007/978-3-030-54020-3_11

long-term health consequences. The following case studies will highlight several common clinical scenarios encountered by the pediatric urologist, and provide an evidence-based review of the current management strategies available.

Case 1

A newborn male infant was found to have bilateral hydronephrosis on prenatal anatomy scan. Amniotic fluid levels were reportedly normal. He is currently asymptomatic and voiding spontaneously. Renal ultrasound and voiding cysto-urethrogram (VCUG) on day of life 4 are shown below:

1. **Based on his history, what are the potential diagnoses?**
2. **What does the imaging reveal?**
3. **What is the natural history associated with these findings?**

Prenatal hydronephrosis is present in up to 3% of all fetuses and is associated with several anatomic abnormalities, including, but not limited to, ureteropelvic junction obstruction, VUR, ureterovesical junction obstruction, and bladder outlet obstruction. In a male child, the major concern is that bilateral hydronephrosis may represent bladder outlet obstruction from posterior urethral valves (PUV). This postnatal renal ultrasound confirms the presence of hydronephrosis bilaterally (Fig. 11.1). Fortunately, this child's VCUG demonstrates a normal posterior urethra without evidence of PUV, but is significant for bilateral VUR (Fig. 11.2). There are five grades of vesicoureteral reflux as defined by the International Reflux Study, ranging from mild reflux of urine into the distal ureter without ureteral dilation to severe dilation and tortuosity of the ureter associated with refluxing urine into the renal pelvis and blunted renal calyceal system. This VCUG depicts bilateral grade 3 VUR based on this classification system.

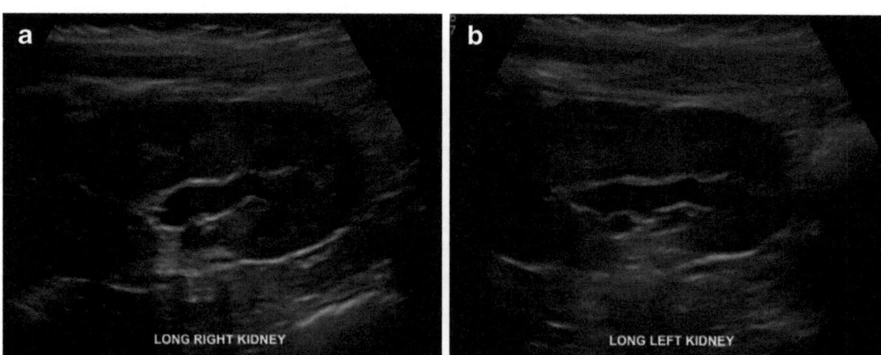

Fig. 11.1 Postnatal ultrasound images from a newborn male infant of the right (**a**) and left (**b**) kidneys in the sagittal plane. The renal parenchyma is normal in appearance. Both kidneys demonstrate splitting of the renal pelvis consistent with mild hydronephrosis that does not extend into the proximal ureter

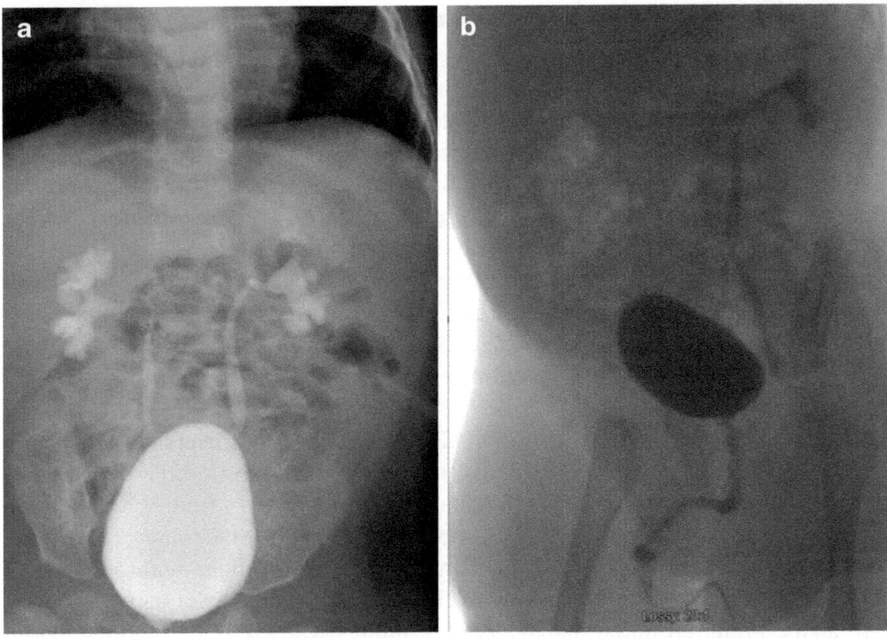

Fig. 11.2 Voiding cystourethrogram of the same male infant demonstrating bilateral, dilating vesicoureteral reflux (**a**). Voiding phase images (**b**) confirm a normal posterior urethra without evidence of posterior urethral valves

Although this child was diagnosed with VUR during the evaluation of his asymptomatic hydronephrosis, VUR is found in up to 70% of infants <1 year of age who present with a UTI [2]. VUR is more common in male infants who present with a UTI [3]; however, female infants are more likely to have UTIs in general.

Most VUR resolves spontaneously, usually within 5 years, as progressive elongation of the intravesical ureteral tunnel and stabilization of bladder dynamics naturally correct the anti-reflux mechanism. This is especially true in male children, in whom VUR is more likely to spontaneously resolve [4]. Additionally, the likelihood of resolution is inversely proportional to the initial VUR grade at the time of diagnosis with about 80% of grades I and II and 50% of grade III resolving spontaneously. Grades IV and V may have lower likelihood of spontaneous resolution, particularly if bilateral [5].

Principles of management in infants diagnosed with VUR aim at minimizing UTIs in order to allow time for spontaneous resolution while protecting renal function. Importantly, however, not all VUR is symptomatic. Patients with VUR but without a history of febrile UTIs or renal anomalies are more appropriate for conservative management.

4. **How could the risk of UTI be minimized in this currently asymptomatic male infant?**

11.1.1 Continuous Antibiotic Prophylaxis

As VUR often resolves spontaneously, many patients with VUR undergo conservative treatment initially with surveillance alone or continuous antibiotic prophylaxis (CAP). The Randomized Intervention for Children with Vesicoureteral Reflux (RIVUR) trial rigorously studied the utility of CAP in children with grades I-IV VUR who had at least one febrile or symptomatic UTI. After 2 years of follow up, the group treated with prophylactic trimethoprim-sulfamethoxazole had half the risk of UTI recurrence (hazard ratio 0.50; 95% confidence interval 0.34–0.74). In addition, CAP reduced the absolute risk of UTI recurrence by 12% compared to observation alone. Importantly however, CAP did not reduce the incidence of new renal scarring [6], although the study may not have been powered to fully evaluate this outcome.

Which patients most benefit from CAP is somewhat controversial, with many reserving CAP for symptomatic patients (i.e. those with a febrile UTI) and surgery for those who have breakthrough infections while on CAP. Both the American Urological Association (AUA) and European Association of Urology (EAU) list CAP or observation alone as management strategies for infants with grades I–II VUR without renal scarring at diagnosis. However, these organizations recommend CAP as the preferred initial management in infants who either have had a febrile urinary tract infection or who have a history of high-grade VUR [7].

11.1.2 Circumcision

The presence of foreskin has historically been cited as a risk factor for UTIs in male infants <2 years of age, and a recent meta-analysis published by Eisenburg et al. found that uncircumcised males had a much higher rate of UTIs (2.68 vs. 0.59 per 100-person years) than their circumcised counterparts. The calculated number needed to treat with circumcision in this study to prevent one UTI was 37, but dropped to 25 in males with a history of VUR [8]. As male infants with VUR are at an increased risk of developing UTIs, studies have evaluated the utility of circumcision in this population. Gücük et al.'s 2013 report demonstrated that circumcision was protective against recurrent febrile UTIs in male infants with low-grade VUR with or without simultaneous CAP [9]. As such, the AUA supports the consideration of circumcision in male infants with VUR [7].

5. **At what point should surgical intervention be considered?**

Surgery is most often considered when prophylactic antibiotics are no longer effective in preventing recurrent UTIs, if there is deterioration of renal function, if renal scarring progresses, if renal growth stunts, with complex anatomy that makes spontaneous resolution less likely, if reflux persists into older age, or if families desire surgical intervention [10]. The most common indication is breakthrough

UTIs while on CAP, although there is still no universal consensus on when surgical intervention is warranted.

Case 2
A 3-year-old female presents for evaluation after her second febrile urinary tract infection over the past year. She began potty training at age 2 and at baseline she voids 3–4 times a day with daily accidents. She has a hard bowel movement 3–4 times a week. Representative images from a renal ultrasound (RUS) and voiding cystourethrogram (VCUG) obtained by the referring provider are shown below:

1. **What are the pertinent findings on ultrasound and VCUG?**
2. **What are the key components to this patient's presentation?**
3. **What are your potential management options and are any additional tests warranted?**

Ultrasound of this patient's kidneys demonstrates normal renal parenchyma associated with mild hydronephrosis bilaterally (Fig. 11.3). The VCUG demonstrates grade 4 VUR into the left collecting system (Fig. 11.4). The patient's voiding and defecatory habits are consistent with lower urinary tract dysfunction (LUTD) and a full evaluation for this comorbid condition should be performed. Any child with VUR *and* LUTD has a higher risk of developing recurrent UTIs and renal scarring and has a lower rate of spontaneous VUR resolution [11]. Therefore, all initial treatment goals should be focused on eliminating the LUTD through healthy elimination habits, biofeedback, and supplementary medications when indicated prior to any surgical intervention. Because this patient is at such a high risk of recurrent UTI, continuous antibiotic prophylaxis (CAP) is recommended. Advanced secondary analysis of the RIVUR study identified patients with high grade reflux and

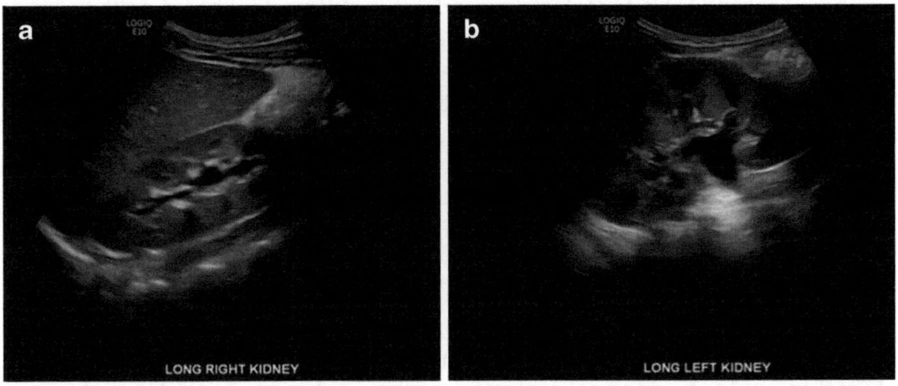

Fig. 11.3 Renal ultrasound images of a 3-year-old female with recurrent urinary tract infections. The right (**a**) and left (**b**) kidneys have mild dilation of the renal pelvis and major calyces. No obvious renal parenchymal scarring is noted

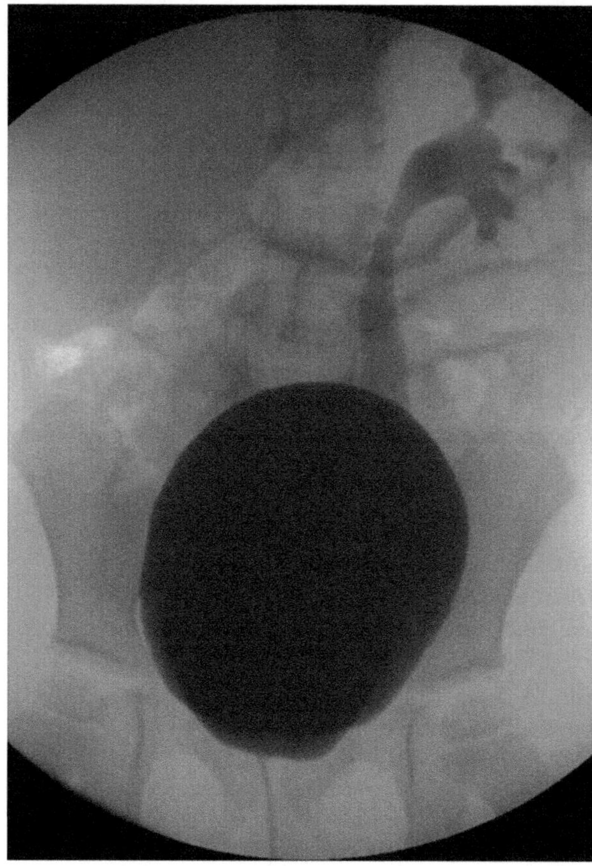

Fig. 11.4 Voiding cystourethrogram from the same female patient demonstrating high-grade vesicoureteral reflux into the left kidney that is associated with blunting of the renal calyces and tortuosity in the proximal ureter

LUTD as those who receive the most benefit from CAP in regards to reducing the number of febrile UTIs [12]. Unfortunately, it is still unclear based on the current evidence as to whether or not CAP also results in a reduction in new renal scarring. Since the evidence is not definitive, a risk-based approach to CAP is often adopted. In children who have symptomatic VUR but do not have LUTD, CAP is an option because it has not been established that CAP prevents recurrent episodes of pyelonephritis or renal scarring in this population. Likewise, patients with asymptomatic VUR without LUTD are candidates for CAP or observation alone. Patient specific considerations such as bilateral VUR, female sex, uncircumcised males, high grade VUR and LUTD should all be considered when choosing whether or not to initiate CAP. Additionally, the risk of increased antibiotic resistance seen in patients on CAP must be considered.

Since a normal renal ultrasound does not exclude the possibility of renal parenchymal injury [13], additional evaluation of the renal parenchyma for evidence of renal scarring with nuclear medicine dimercaptosuccinic acid (DMSA) or mercaptoacetyltriglycine (MAG3) imaging is also an option. Detecting the presence of renal scars in the setting of VUR is prognostically important, as renal scarring is associated with non-resolution of reflux and renal insufficiency [14, 15].

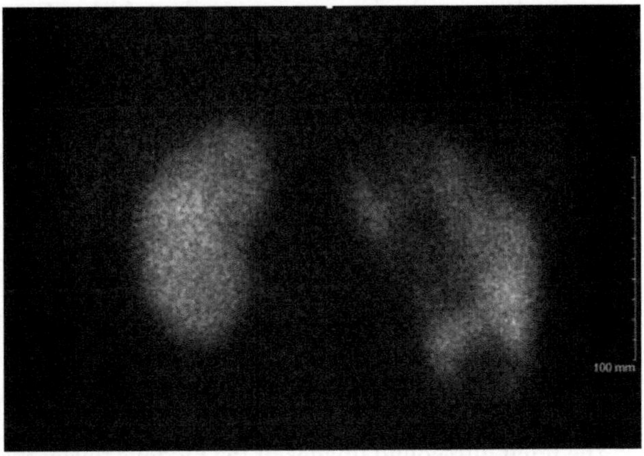

Fig. 11.5 Dimercaptosuccinic acid scan from a 3-year-old female with recurrent febrile urinary tract infections. The left kidney demonstrates areas of photopenia in the upper and lower poles consistent with renal scarring. Split renal function is 52% on the right, 48% on the left

The patient completed a DMSA scan shown below (Fig. 11.5):

DMSA images reveal evidence of left renal parenchymal damage. At this point, CAP and aggressive management of her LUTD are still appropriate prior to surgical intervention. She should be monitored closely for recurrent UTIs and/or non-resolution of her LUTD. A full repeat evaluation of her VUR should be performed once the LUTD has resolved. Conservative management is appropriate in this patient, as it is known that a large percentage of both low and high grade VUR will spontaneously resolve within 5 years of follow-up [16]. Reasons to consider surgical intervention may include breakthrough UTIs, parental preference for definitive intervention, or persistence of high grade VUR on follow-up.

4. **What are the long-term follow-up recommendations for this patient?**

Yearly height, weight, and blood pressure measurements, renal ultrasound, and urinalysis testing for early signs of proteinuria and hematuria are recommended by the AUA. Additionally, the AUA recommends a repeat diagnostic assessment for persistent VUR within 12–24 months of diagnosis [7].

Case 3

A 5-year-old female with a history of febrile UTIs and known bilateral G3 VUR without prior LUTD has been conservatively managed for the past 3 years on a trimethoprim-based antibiotic. She was doing well until the past 3 months, during which she has had two symptomatic, culture-positive UTIs, one with a fever to 39.5 °C. Both organisms have been E.coli resistant to trimethoprim.

1. **What are the next steps in evaluation of this patient?**

This patient has now had two breakthrough UTIs while on CAP, one of which was febrile. It is generally accepted that a change in management is appropriate for this patient. The first step should be a repeat, thorough evaluation for the development of LUTD. As mentioned previously, LUTD should be ruled out or aggressively treated when present, and could be the most likely cause of break-through UTIs in this patient. Simultaneously, obtaining renal ultrasound or DMSA imaging may be useful to assess for the development of new renal scarring, which could help to determine the need to abandon conservative therapy. In addition, confirming the status of her VUR (persistent, down-graded, resolved) through repeat VCUG will help to better characterize her risk profile.

On further questioning, this patient does not have any evidence of LUTD. Representative renal ultrasound and updated VCUG images are shown below:

2. **What do the renal ultrasound and VCUG images tell us about this patient's clinical risk?**
3. **What are the options to manage her VUR moving forward?**

The renal ultrasound images of the kidneys reveal that the right kidney has experienced stunted growth with areas of cortical thinning (Fig. 11.6). This patient also continues to have VUR bilaterally (Fig. 11.7). In this scenario, the patient has had a BT UTI associated with renal injury despite CAP. Based on these findings, it is appropriate to consider definitive surgical intervention, either with endoscopic therapy or ureteral reimplantation.

The choice between endoscopic management of VUR or formal ureteral reimplantation often depends on the grade of VUR involved. In a meta-analysis of over 8000 renal units with VUR treated with subuteric injection of a bulking agent, it was found that VUR resolution rates after a single injection were inversely proportional to the grade of reflux (GI–II 78.5%, GIII 72%, GIV 63%, and GV 51%). A second injection provided an additional benefit in some cases, but overall success rates were lower in those with duplicated systems (50 vs. 73%) and those with neurogenic bladders (62 vs. 74%) [17]. In one of the largest prospective, randomized studies, The Swedish Reflux Trial, dilating VUR managed with subuteric injection vs CAP vs observation alone was assessed for VUR resolution. The authors found

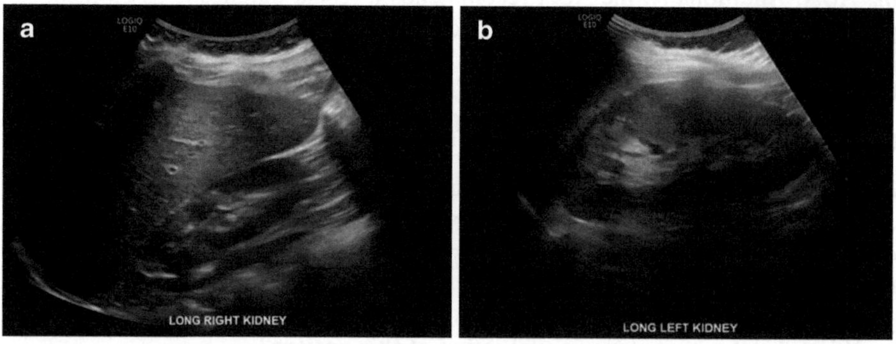

Fig. 11.6 Renal ultrasound images from a 5-year-old female with recurrent urinary tract infections and known vesicoureteral reflux. The right kidney (**a**) appears relatively smaller and has parenchymal thinning at the lower pole. The left kidney (**b**) is normal in appearance without hydronephrosis or renal scarring

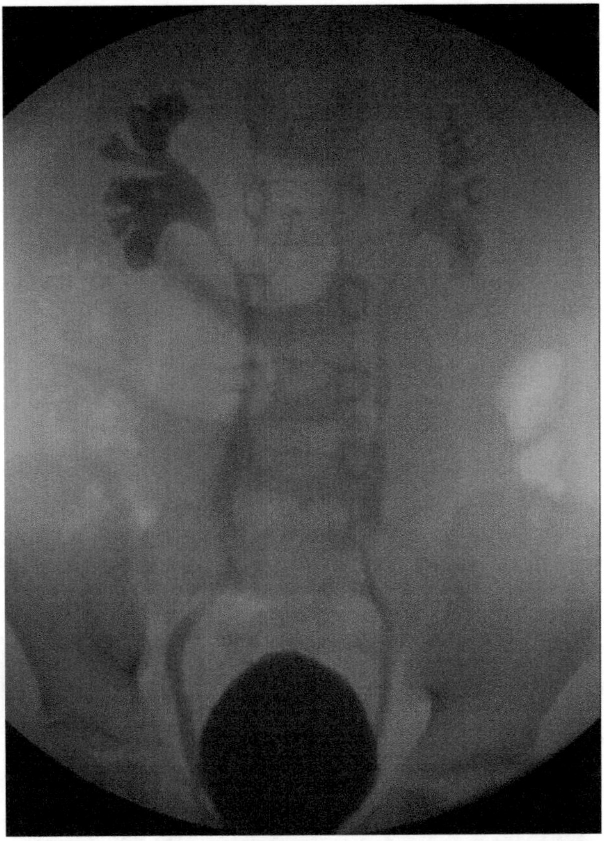

Fig. 11.7 Voiding cystourethrogram from the same 5-year-old female confirming persistent grade 3 vesicoureteral reflux on the right and grade 3 vesicoureteral reflux on the left

that resolution rates were highest in the endoscopically managed group (71%) when compared to those on CAP (39%) or surveillance (47%). However, the recurrence rate of VUR in the endoscopic group was 20% at 2 years, and new scar formation in this group was higher than those who were managed with CAP (7 vs. 0%) [18]. As such, the unknown long-term success rates after endoscopic management of VUR need further evaluation.

Open ureteral reimplantation remains the gold-standard for surgical management of VUR. There are several open surgical approaches utilized, including both intravesical and extravesical approaches, and conceptually, the goal of all of these procedures is similar: to elongate or enhance the intramural portion of the ureteral tunnel. Success rates of open surgical techniques are reported from 90 to 98% and with very low complication rates [19], although these historical numbers may be skewed by the higher percentage of low grade reflux in the study cohort.

More recently with the advances in minimally invasive surgery, laparoscopic and robot-assisted laparoscopic ureteral reimplantation (RALUR) are available as well. Several single-center and multi-center studies have compared outcomes between open and robot-assisted techniques. A meta-analysis of six studies containing over

7000 patients published by Deng et al. determined that operative times were longer, hospital stay shorter, analgesic requirement less, and short-term (90-day) complications more common in the RALUR cohort. Success rates between the two approaches were no different, but the direct cost of RALUR was significantly higher [20].

Case 4

A 9 year old male presents with hematuria, back pain, and fever to 38.7 °C. His urinalysis is consistent with a UTI. This is his third UTI in the past 6 months. After a course of culture specific antibiotics, a renal ultrasound and VCUG are obtained and are shown below:

1. **What do the ultrasound and VCUG show?**
2. **What are your options for management of this patient?**

The renal ultrasound demonstrates a normal right kidney, mild left pelviectasis, and a bladder with a large amount of echogenic debris and mild concentric wall thickening (Fig. 11.8). The VCUG has evidence of bilateral VUR that is associated with bilateral large diverticula vs ureteroceles (Fig. 11.9).

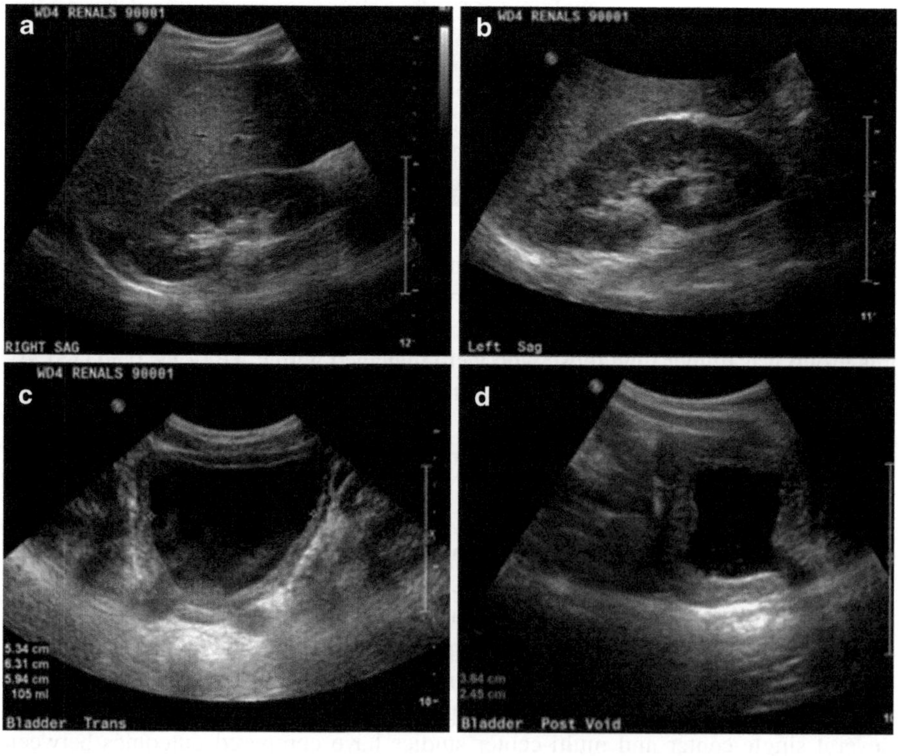

Fig. 11.8 Renal ultrasound from a 9-year-old male with recurrent urinary tract infections. The right kidney (**a**) is normal in appearance and the left kidney (**b**) demonstrates grade 1 hydronephrosis. The bladder wall appears thickened with intra-luminal debris (**c, d**)

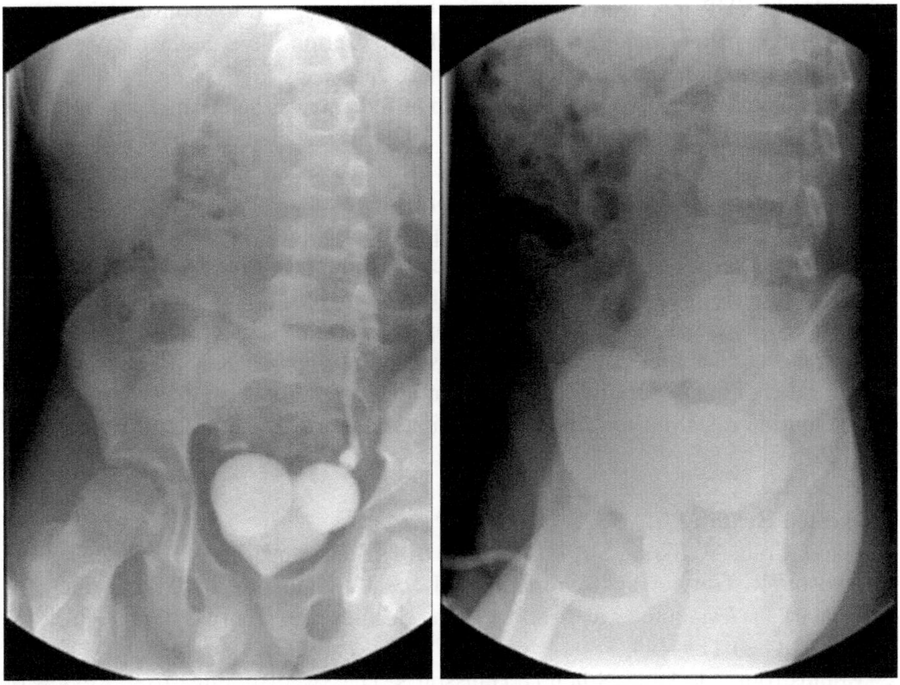

Fig. 11.9 Voiding cystourethrogram from the same male patient. There is bilateral grade 1 vesicoureteral reflux that is associated with large peri-ureteral diverticula

At this point it would be reasonable to obtain nuclear medicine imaging of the kidneys to assess for evidence of renal parenchymal damage. Additionally, proceeding with cystoscopy to delineate bladder anatomy is advisable since management would greatly differ if the anomalies seen on VCUG represented ureteroceles vs diverticula. If diverticula are present, it is important to assess the relationship between the ureterovesical junction (UVJ) and the diverticula. Cystoscopy in this patient reveals both ureteral orifices inserting into large diverticula. The bladder appears to have normal capacity without trabeculations or other sequela of dysfunctional voiding.

3. **What is your next step?**

Options at this point include observation or surgical intervention. Primary bladder diverticula are rare in children. The diverticulum represents an out-pouching of mucosa without muscular backing and is usually found in close proximity to the ureteral orifice [21]. Further, as the diverticulum enlarges over time with voiding, it can grow to incorporate the ureteral orifice. This obscures the musculature of the intramural tunnel, impacting the natural anti-reflux mechanism of the UVJ and results in VUR [22]. VUR associated with paraureteral diverticula was shown to have rates of resolution similar to VUR without paraureteral diverticula in a retrospective review by Afshar et al. [23]. Thus, in the majority of patients, the standard principles in VUR management apply, including the option for conservative management. If a patient qualifies for surgical intervention, diverticulectomy with or without ureteral reimplant is indicated in these cases.

In this older patient, surgical intervention is indicated as he has now had multiple febrile urinary tract infections. Since his VUR is associated with bilateral large diverticula that encompass the ureteral orifices, he will require bilateral ureteral reimplant with simultaneous diverticulectomy. Diverticulectomy and ureteral reimplant have been described by laparoscopic/robotic [24] and open approaches. Historically patients requiring bilateral ureteral reimplant would undergo an intravesical approach to avoid bladder denervation seen during the extravesical dissection, which often lead to high rates of post-operative urinary retention [25]. However, recent reports of nerve-sparing approaches used during RALUR have shown low overall rates of post-operative urinary retention (<10%) with no differences in urinary retention rates during unilateral vs bilateral extravesical ureteral reimplantation [26].

Suggested Reading

1. Peters Craig A., Skoog Steven J., Arant Billy S., Copp Hillary L., Elder Jack S., Hudson R. Guy, et al. Summary of the AUA Guideline on Management of Primary Vesicoureteral Reflux in Children. Journal of Urology. 2010;184(3):1134–44.
2. Brandström P, Jodal U, Sillén U, Hansson S. The Swedish reflux trial: Review of a randomized, controlled trial in children with dilating vesicoureteral reflux. Journal of Pediatric Urology. 2011;7(6):594–600.
3. The RIVUR Trial Investigators. Antimicrobial Prophylaxis for Children with Vesicoureteral Reflux. New England Journal of Medicine. 2014;370(25):2367–76.
4. Khoury AE and Bägli DJ: Vesicoureteral Reflux. In: Campbell-Walsh Urology. 11th ed. Philadelphia, PA: Elsevier 2016; pp. 3134–3172.e7.
5. Edwards A, Peters CA. Managing vesicoureteral reflux in children: making sense of all the data. F1000Res. 2019;8:29.

References

1. Sargent MA. What is the normal prevalence of vesicoureteral reflux? Pediatr Radiol. 2000;30(9):587–93.
2. Roger B, William M, John M, Irwin S. Relation of age, sex and infection to reflux: data indicating high spontaneous cure rate in pediatric patients. J Urol. 1966;95(1):27–32.
3. Hannula A, Venhola M, Renko M, Pokka T, Huttunen N-P, Uhari M. Vesicoureteral reflux in children with suspected and proven urinary tract infection. Pediatr Nephrol. 2010;25(8):1463–9.
4. Alsaywid BS, Saleh H, Deshpande A, Howman-Giles R, Smith GHH. High grade primary vesicoureteral reflux in boys: long-term results of a prospective cohort study. J Urol. 2010;184(4 Suppl):1598–603.
5. Estrada CR, Passerotti CC, Graham DA, Peters CA, Bauer SB, Diamond DA, et al. Nomograms for predicting annual resolution rate of primary vesicoureteral reflux: results from 2,462 children. J Urol. 2009;182(4):1535–41.

6. The RIVUR Trial Investigators. Antimicrobial prophylaxis for children with Vesicoureteral reflux. N Engl J Med. 2014;370(25):2367–76.
7. Peters CA, Skoog SJ, Arant BS, Copp HL, Elder JS, Hudson RG, et al. Summary of the AUA guideline on Management of Primary Vesicoureteral Reflux in children. J Urol. 2010;184(3):1134–44.
8. Eisenberg ML, Galusha D, Kennedy WA, Cullen MR. The relationship between neonatal circumcision, urinary tract infection, and health. The World Journal of Men's Health. 2018;36(3):176–82.
9. Gücük A, Burgu B, Gökçe İ, Mermerkaya M, Soygür T. Do antibiotic prophylaxis and/or circumcision change periurethral uropathogen colonization and urinary tract infection rates in boys with VUR? J Pediatr Urol. 2013;9(6, Part B):1131–6.
10. Edwards A, Peters CA. Managing vesicoureteral reflux in children: making sense of all the data. F1000Res. 2019;8:29.
11. Sillén U, Brandström P, Jodal U, Holmdahl G, Sandin A, Sjöberg I, et al. The Swedish reflux trial in children: V. bladder dysfunction. J Urol. 2010;184(1):298–304.
12. Wang ZT, Wehbi E, Alam Y, Khoury A. A reanalysis of the RIVUR trial using a risk classification system. J Urol. 2018;199(6):1608–14.
13. Scherz HC, Downs TM, Caesar R. The selective use of dimercaptosuccinic acid renal scans in children with vesicoureteral reflux. J Urol. 1994;152(2 Pt 2):628–31.
14. Nepple KG, Knudson MJ, Austin JC, Cooper CS. Abnormal renal scans and decreased early resolution of low grade Vesicoureteral reflux. J Urol. 2008;180(4, Supplement):1643–7.
15. Mor Y, Leibovitch I, Zalts R, Lotan D, Jonas P, Ramon J. Analysis of the long-term outcome of surgically corrected vesico-ureteric reflux. BJU Int. 2003;92(1):97–100.
16. Elder JS, Peters CA, Arant BS, Ewalt DH, Hawtrey CE, Hurwitz RS, et al. Pediatric Vesicoureteral reflux guidelines panel summary report on the Management of Primary Vesicoureteral Reflux in children. J Urol. 1997;157(5):1846–51.
17. Elder JS, Diaz M, Caldamone AA, Cendron M, Greenfield S, Hurwitz R, et al. Endoscopic therapy for vesicoureteral reflux: a meta-analysis. I. Reflux resolution and urinary tract infection. J Urol. 2006;175(2):716–22.
18. Holmdahl G, Brandström P, Läckgren G, Sillén U, Stokland E, Jodal U, et al. The Swedish reflux trial in children: II. Vesicoureteral reflux outcome. J Urol. 2010;184(1):280–5.
19. Duckett JW, Walker RD, Weiss R. Surgical results: international reflux study in children--United States branch. J Urol. 1992;148(5 Pt 2):1674–5.
20. Deng T, Liu B, Luo L, Duan X, Cai C, Zhao Z, et al. Robot-assisted laparoscopic versus open ureteral reimplantation for pediatric vesicoureteral reflux: a systematic review and meta-analysis. World J Urol. 2018;36(5):819–28.
21. Pieretti RV, Pieretti-Vanmarcke RV. Congenital bladder diverticula in children. J Pediatr Surg. 1999;34(3):468–73.
22. Garat JM, Angerri O, Caffaratti J, Moscatiello P, Villavicencio H. Primary congenital bladder diverticula in children. Urology. 2007;70(5):984–8.
23. Afshar K, Malek R, Bakhshi M, Papanikolaou F, Farhat W, Bagli D, et al. Should the presence of congenital Para-ureteral diverticulum affect the management of vesicoureteral reflux? J Urol. 2005;174(4, Part 2):1590–3.
24. Christman MS, Casale P. Robot-assisted bladder diverticulectomy in the pediatric population. J Endourol. 2012;26(10):1296–300.
25. Lipski BA, Mitchell ME, Burns MW. Voiding dysfunction after bilateral extravesical ureteral reimplantation. J Urol. 1998;159(3):1019–21.
26. Kawal T, Srinivasan AK, Chang J, Long C, Chu D, Shukla AR. Robotic-assisted laparoscopic ureteral re-implant (RALUR): can post-operative urinary retention be predicted? J Pediatr Urol. 2018;14(4):323.e1–5.

Lower Urinary Tract Obstruction 12

Brian T. Caldwell

Objectives

- Identify patients prenatally at risk for lower urinary tract obstruction.
- Demonstrate immediate post-natal management of patients with posterior urethral valves.
- Predict long-term renal outcomes of patients with lower urinary tract obstruction based on early renal function measurements.
- Explain the theory of Valve Bladder Syndrome and state the importance of developmental changes to bladder throughout childhood.

Case #1

A newborn boy did not void in the first 12 h of life after full-term gestational age (GA) birth. He has since voided with a marginal urine stream. Prenatal course was unremarkable and had normal imaging at 20 weeks GA. A renal/bladder ultrasound (RBUS) was obtained on day of life #1 prior to calling for consultation, which is visible below. The patient is preparing to discharge home per the NICU team at the referring hospital. He has an otherwise normal physical examination and there is no family history of urologic anomalies.

RBUS on DOL #1

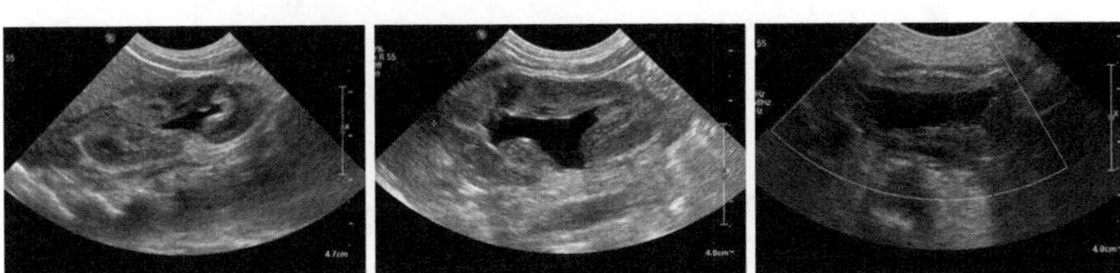

B. T. Caldwell (✉)
Department of Pediatric Urology, Children's Hospital Colorado, University of Colorado School of Medicine, Aurora, CO, USA
e-mail: brian.caldwell@childrenscolorado.org

P. Godbole et al. (eds.), *Practical Pediatric Urology*,
https://doi.org/10.1007/978-3-030-54020-3_12

Q1: What does the renal/bladder ultrasound show? What is the ideal time to obtain postnatal renal ultrasound images?

A1: Bilateral hydronephrosis with Society for Fetal Urology (SFU) grade I on the right and SFU grade II on the left. The bladder appears thickened but this is not definitive since the bladder is not well distended.

Neonates have a transient dehydration after birth due to a combination of birth stress and inadequate sustenance. The neonatal feeding volumes will rapidly expand over the first few days of life leading to increased urine production. It is recommended that RBUS be delayed until a minimum of 48–72 h of life, otherwise understaging of the hydronephrosis may occur due to relative dehydration.

Q2: Discuss what concerns arise from the clinical presentation and ultrasound imaging. What are the options for the next steps in management?

A2: In a neonatal boy who has difficulty voiding and is found to have bilateral hydronephrosis, then a lower urinary tract obstruction (LUTO) should be high on the differential diagnosis, even with low grade hydronephrosis. This is especially true with the suspicion of a thickened bladder. Because of the high cost of misdiagnosis of LUTO, a low threshold should be held for further evaluation in these cases.

In boys with bilateral hydronephrosis, if a diagnosis of LUTO is considered, then a VCUG should be obtained prior to discharge from the hospital if able [1, 2]. If VCUG is not possible, cases of severe hydronephrosis will need transfer to a location with VCUG capability. With lower grade hydronephrosis, a short interval follow up with outpatient VCUG would need to be arranged. When hydronephrosis grade is severe and there is suspicion for PUV, then an indwelling catheter is placed for bladder drainage immediately.

A VCUG was recommended prior to discharge home and was obtained.

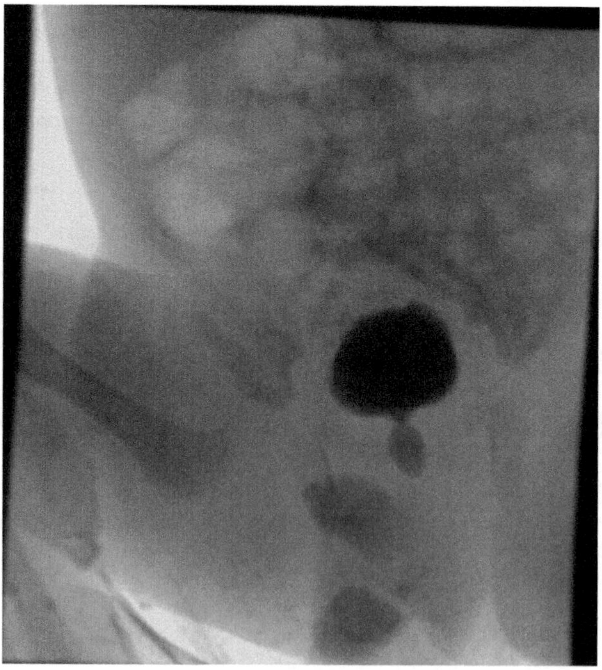

The referring facility had little experience with neonatal VCUG, therefore, no oblique views were obtained. Even with this limitation, there is clear bladder trabeculation and dilated posterior urethra consistent with posterior urethral valves (PUV).

The patient was transferred for further management with an indwelling catheter on day of life #2.

RBUS was repeated after transfer as below.

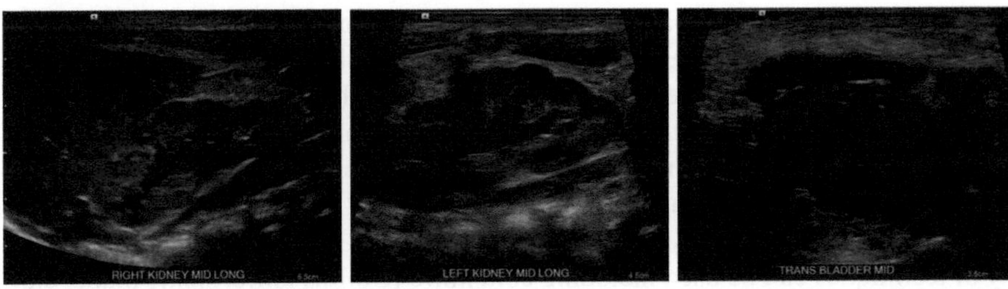

Q3: Why is persistent hydronephrosis present?

A3: Persistence of hydronephrosis after catheter drainage in PUV patients can be related to inadequate bladder decompression or due to upper urinary tract obstruction.

- A severely thickened bladder, once decompressed, can contribute to obstruction of the distal ureter as it passes through the detrusor muscle. The obstruction can be transient and improve over a few days or remain persistent, presenting a need for upper urinary track diversion.
- More commonly, the bladder will not be effectively drained, as above on RBUS, suggesting catheter malfunction or dislodgement. Because of small neonatal size, a 5fr feeding tube or 6fr catheter is often placed initially. A small size catheter can become coiled in the enlarged posterior urethra, thus, ineffectively decompressing the bladder. At times, only a 3.5fr umbilical catheter will traverse the diminutive urethra in premature infants. Bladder decompression and catheter position can be evaluated with bedside ultrasound or formal RBUS.

  Foley catheters with balloon inflated are also at risk of ineffective bladder decompression. The balloon may withdraw into the posterior urethra, effectively obstructing the catheter drainage. Additionally, balloon catheters with larger balloons have the capacity to compress the ureteral orifices leading to iatrogenic ureteral obstruction from the catheter balloon [3].

  These common catheter issues have led to some creative solutions such as using a short double-J ureteral stent to traverse the urethra. The curl at each end helps maintain the position within the bladder and at the tip of the penis. The stent can also be exchanged over a wire to help ensure proper positioning [4].

Repositioning of the catheter decompresses the bladder and resolves the hydronephrosis.

Q4: What surgical options are available to resolve the persistent obstruction?

A4:

- Cystoscopy and ablation of PUV
- Vesicostomy
- Cutaneous ureterostomy
- Nephrostomy tubes

Discussion: Choice of technique used is largely dependent on the level of the obstruction and size of the patient and/or his urethra. In this case, the patient is full term and had initial placement of 6fr foley catheter without difficulty. There are no contraindications to continued catheter drainage until the patient is large enough to proceed with cystoscopy and ablation of PUV. Ablation provides resolution of the offending obstructing agent in a minimally invasive technique. A general guideline for adequate patient size could be 3.5 kg and/or ability to accommodate an 8fr urethral catheter, since standard infant urethrotomes range between 7.5fr to 9fr. A variety of techniques can be used including cold knife (Collins knife, sickle blade, etc), electrocautery (bugbee, angled tip) or Holmium-Yag laser. Interestingly, a historic description involved blind passage of crochet hook to ablate the valves which was insulated and connected to electrocautery later [5]. More recently, usage of fogarty endarterectomy balloons have been described as well [6].

Vesicostomy is reserved for those patients that are too small to pass a catheter for effective bladder decompression or who will need catheterization for a prolonged period of time prior to ablation (severely premature patients). There were originally concerns that vesicostomy deprives the bladder of its filling and emptying cycle leading to defunctionalization of the bladder. A properly created vesicostomy will provide some cycling, which has been shown to be protective of bladder function [7].

Cutaneous ureterostomy is a technique utilized for persistent hydronephrosis due to obstruction at the ureterovesical junction (UVJ). The ureter is brought out to drain at the level of the skin, providing a low pressure drainage system. Cutaneous ureterostomy can be created as a loop, theoretically allowing some urine to pass distally into the bladder in order to promote cycling [8–10]. In addition, the distal limb can be utilized as a ureteral Mitrofanoff at the time of ureteral reimplant. Alternatively, the ureter can be ligated distally and ureter brought to the skin as an end anastomosis.

Post-Valve Ablation Follow-up at 6 weeks:

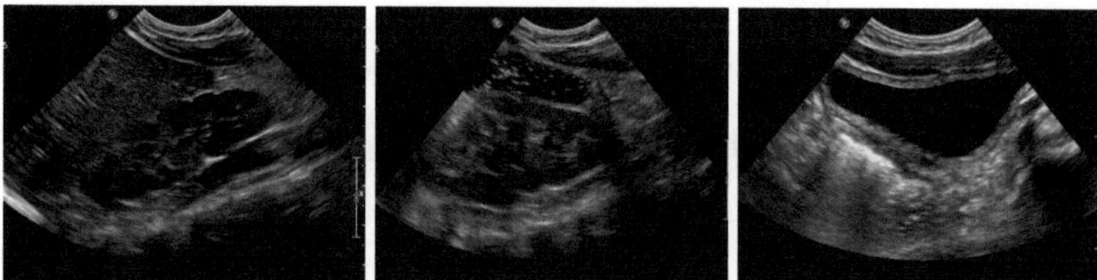

***Post-ablation VCUG compared to initial VCUG*:**

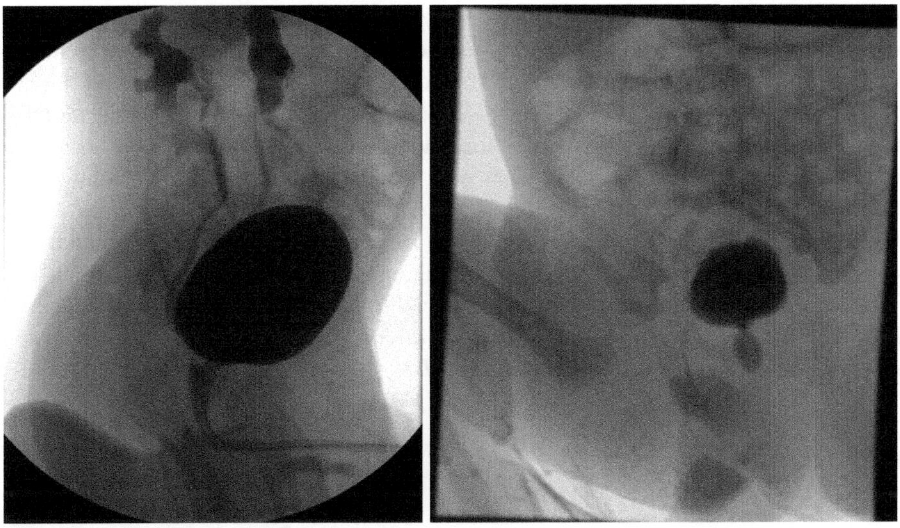

Q5: Why does the post-ablation VCUG now show vesicoureteral reflux when it did not initially? Does this mean it is worse than before?

A5: On a post-ablation VCUG, the bladder shows grade III bilateral VUR, which was not seen initially. However, the bladder is smooth-walled and the urethra now looks normal, without dilation of the posterior urethra or abrupt caliber change. The most likely explanation is that the bladder was inadequately filled on initial VCUG leading to understaging of VUR [11, 12].

Q6: What are the next steps in management for this patient post-ablation?

A6: At this point, it is vitally important to engage the family in discussion about the chronicity of the PUV disease state. Many families will feel that since the valve tissue has been ablated and the patient is visibly voiding without difficulty, then no further issues will arise. Simple observation of patients with PUV would not be prudent due to the changes that occur in the developing bladder. A classic pattern of PUV bladder dynamics progression from infancy through adolescence has been identified. During infancy a pattern of high pressure compensated voiding occurs. This high pressure often settles out during childhood to near normal pressures. By adolescence, however, detrusor myogenic failure can occur in conjunction with polyuria due to renal dysplasia. The overwhelmed bladder becomes floppy and ineffective at emptying [13]. A discussion of goals of care with the family frames the conversation about long-term care.

Knowledge of this classic development pattern should lead to long-term urologic follow-up in addition to nephrologic follow-up. Ideally, a multidisciplinary approach is utilized, which may also include psychology and nutritionist support.

Initially, adequacy of valve ablation is confirmed using either repeat VCUG or cystoscopy. The timing of this evaluation varies but will largely fall within the first 1–6 weeks after ablation. Periodic *renal ultrasound* is a mainstay of follow-up to evaluate and monitor the level of hydronephrosis in a non-invasive fashion. *VCUG* can provide ongoing information about VUR and for evaluating concerns within the urethra. VCUG seems best utilized on an as needed basis. Catheterization may be difficult in PUV patients due to sensate urethra and concomitant high bladder neck, therefore repeat cystoscopy may be necessary to assist catheter placement for VCUG or urodynamics. Uroflowometry and assessment of post-void residual provides information on voiding adequacy and simple bladder dynamics after toilet training.

Urodynamics testing (UDS) should be obtained as a baseline study over the months after valve ablation. This helps assess for bladder overactivity and provides baseline pressure measurements. Coupling UDS with video allows incorporation of information from VCUG including VUR, bladder contour and urethral anatomy. Follow-up UDS testing is approached in a variety of way by practitioners, either as an annual test or on an as needed basis using clinical or imaging changes to dictate that need [14].

UDS obtained at 6 months of age showed a smooth walled, normal capacity bladder with low filling pressures and only late loss of compliance with late overactivity. There was also resolution of the VUR.

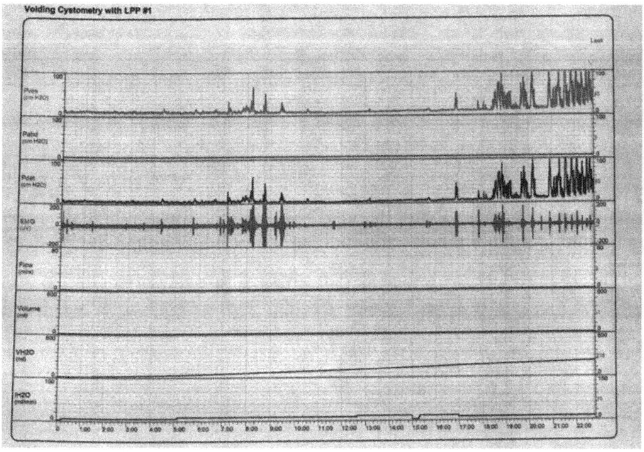

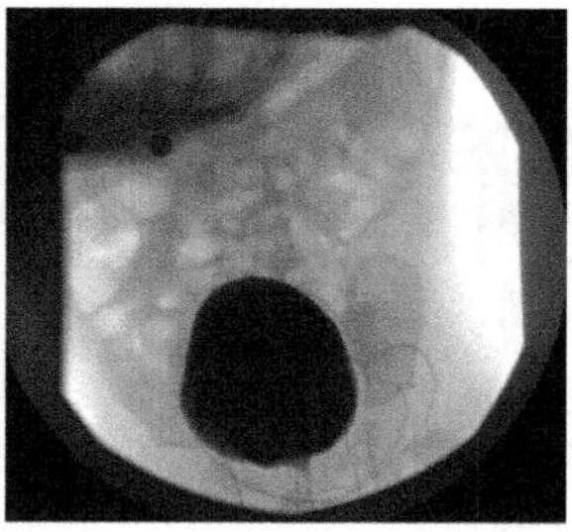

Case #2

A pregnant 31 year old female presented at 24 weeks GA for consult with the Fetal Center. She is P3G2 with no personal or family history of urologic anomalies. Her pregnancy had been uneventful until 20 week anatomy ultrasound revealed bilateral hydronephrosis with thickened bladder in a male fetus. She presented for discussion of prenatal options.

US of fetal bladder and kidneys at 24 weeks GA.

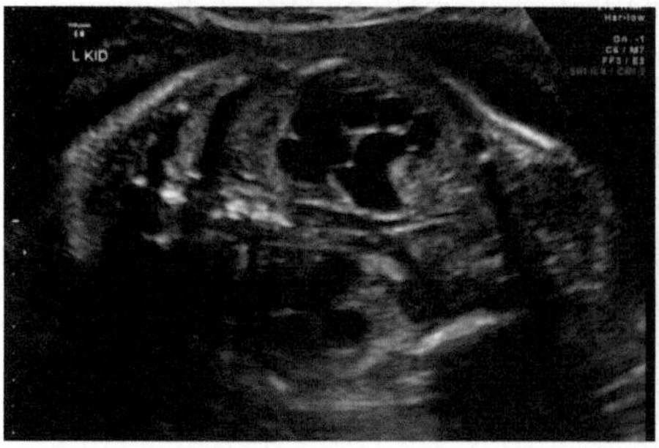

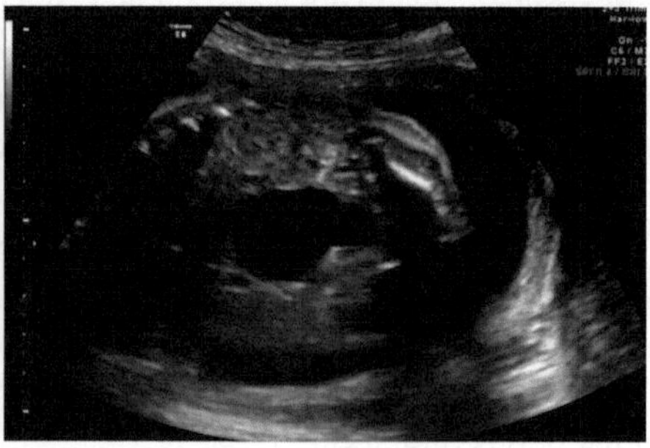

***Fetal MRI at 24 weeks GA*.**

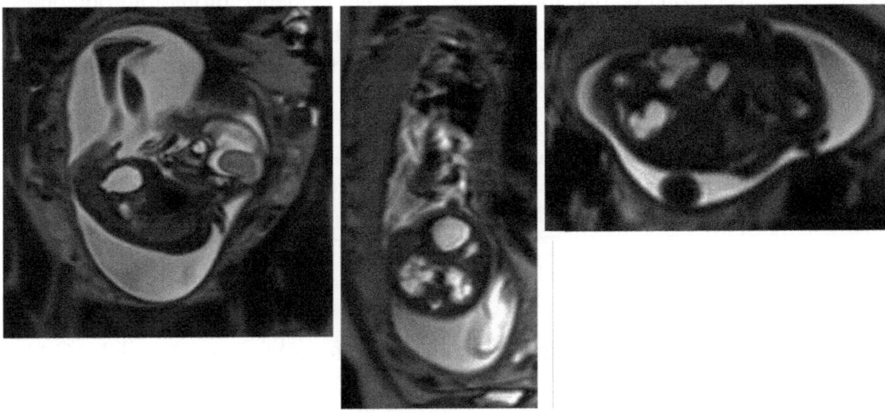

Q1: What is shown on the fetal imaging?

A1: The ultrasound demonstrates severe bilateral hydronephrosis with a classic "keyhole appearance" of dilated, thickened bladder with dilated posterior urethra. The MRI supports the ultrasound findings with enlarged bladder and dilated posterior urethra, along with bilateral severe hydronephrosis. The imaging also demonstrated normal amniotic fluid index (AFI).

Q2: Should she be offered fetal intervention for suspected posterior urethral valves? What are indications for fetal intervention and what benefits have been described?

A2: The only defined benefit of fetal intervention for LUTO is improved pulmonary outcomes due to avoidance of severe pulmonary hypoplasia. At this point, there are no convincing benefits to renal or bladder function from fetal intervention. Pulmonary hypoplasia remains the greatest cause of peninatal mortality in patients with PUV [15].

The Percutaneous vesicoamniotic shunting versus conservative management for Lower Urinary Tract Obstruction trial (PLUTO) was meant to provide prospective evaluation of prior claims about survival benefit from fetal intervention [16, 17]. The study was plagued by low enrollment and termination of pregnancy resulting in only 12 live births in each cohort. The results pointed toward a survival benefit in the shunting group at 28 days but did not reach statistical significance. At 2 years, there was very poor survival in both groups largely due to complications of pulmonary hypoplasia. Furthermore, higher levels of loss of pregnancy were thought to result from the procedures for fetal intervention leading to premature labor and early rupture of membranes [18].

Vesicoamniotic shunting has been the most commonly described technique for fetal intervention, but other, more complex techniques exist. Fetal cystoscopy and antegrade valve ablation, cutaneous ureterostomy and vesicostomy have been described. An abundance of caution should be exercised as the results of fetal surgery can lead to fetal demise in up to 40% of cases [19–21]. Fetal intervention for LUTO should be limited to experienced centers with proper resources and oversight. A multidisciplinary approach to evaluation and family counseling is mandatory in these severe cases. Additionally, due to the lack of strong evidence promoting outcomes, fetal intervention should preferentially be conducted under research protocols.

If fetal intervention is to be considered, general criteria is used for patient selection [19, 22]:

- 18–24 weeks gestational age with LUTO
- Oligohydramnios
- Dilated bladder
- Severe hydroureteronephrosis
- No renal cortical cysts
- Normal male karyotype
- Favorable prognosis based on urine electrolytes (May need serial bladder aspirations)
  - Sodium <100 mEq/l
  - Chloride <90 mEq/l
  - Osmolarity <200 mEq/l
  - 2-microglobulin <6 mg/l

This patient did not have oligohydramnios at 24 week GA evaluation, so fetal intervention was not an option. At 36 weeks GA, however, she delivered due to oligohydramnios. Images were obtained at 48 h of life.

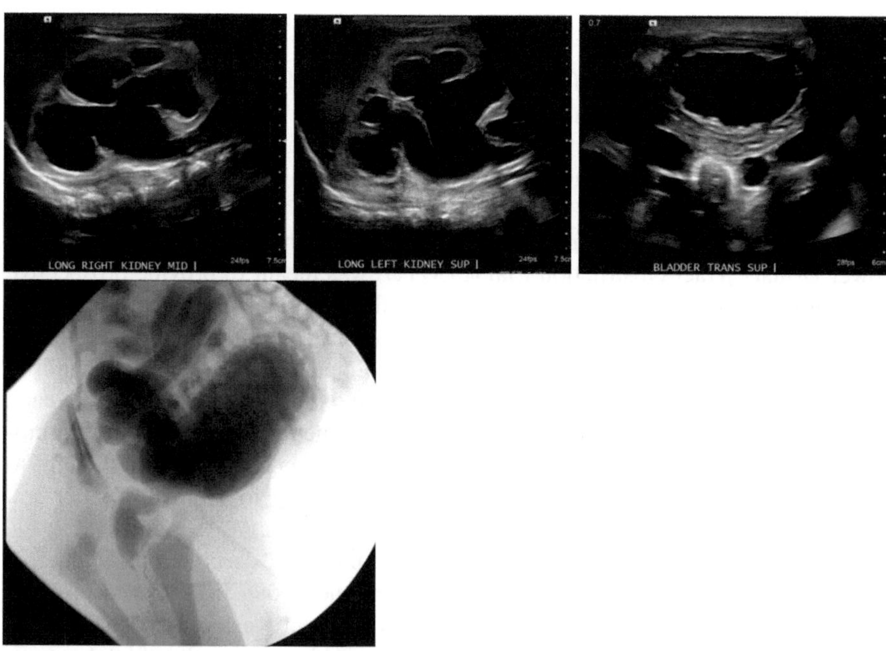

As expected based on prenatal imaging, the postnatal imaging revealed suspicion for posterior urethral valves with dilated posterior urethra, bladder trabeculation and grade V bilateral VUR on VCUG. The ultrasound also showed bilateral SFU grade IV hydronephrosis with a thickened bladder.

A catheter was placed with confirmed decompression of the bladder, however, without improvement in hydronephrosis. Creatinine continued to rise daily. Due to suspected UVJ obstructions, bilateral nephrostomy tubes were placed with antegrade nephrostograms confirming distal obstruction of the ureters at the level of the bladder.

Q3: What are the treatment options?

A3:

- Vesicostomy
- Cystoscopy and valve ablation
- Maintain nephrostomy tubes
- Cutaneous ureterostomy

12.1 Discussion

With the bladder decompressed, persistent hydroureteronephrosis and worsening creatinine, there is concern for a persistent obstruction at the ureterovesical junctions (UVJ). Direct upper tract intervention is necessary to properly drain the kidneys, therefore a cystoscopy and valve ablation or vesicostomy would not provide any improvement over urethral catheter drainage. Nephrostomy tubes can be a good short-term solution that provides adequate direct renal drainage as well as the ability to evaluate for distal obstruction, as in this case. Nephrostomy tubes are complicated by the need for periodic exchanges, risk of dislodgement/obstruction and position of the tubes in the back, which is difficult in infant patients who are most comfortable on their backs.

Cutaneous ureterostomies would provide adequate drainage into the diaper without the difficulty of tubes emanating from the back. Creating loop ureterostomies provides the potential benefits of bladder cycling if the UVJ obstruction resolves over time. It also provides the opportunity to use the distal ureteral stump as a ureteral MItrofanoff at the time of ureterostomy takedown [8–10].

Bilateral loop ureterostomies were performed at 2 weeks of life and cystoscopy performed concurrently, which confirmed posterior urethral valves.

His renal function was monitored via serum creatinine measurements throughout the first year of life as demonstrated in the following graph.

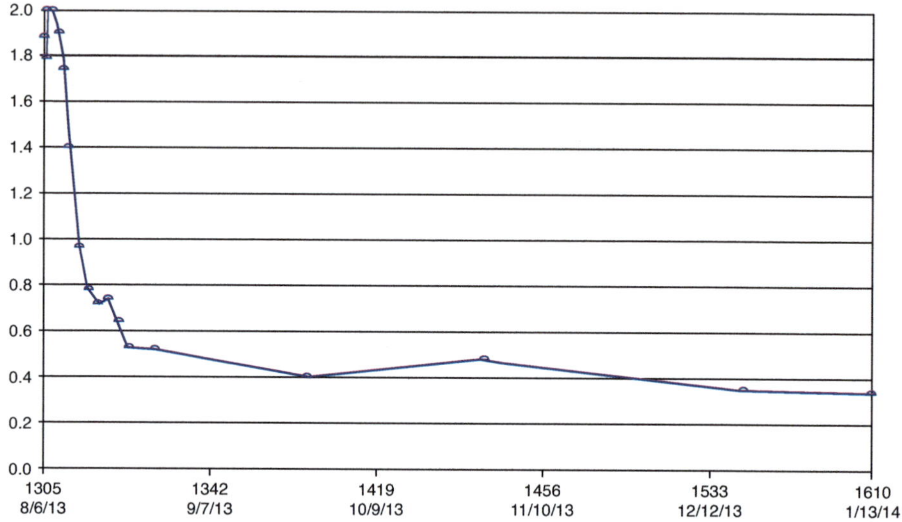

Q4: What does his nadir creatinine of 0.34 mg/dl predict about his long-term renal function?

A4: Serum creatinine is the usual method to assess early renal function in patients with PUV. After catheter drainage of the bladder, daily creatinine levels are often monitored to assess for proper trending down of the creatinine level. The levels in the first days of life correlate with maternal serum creatinine and this takes time to fully clear. Normal neonatal serum creatinine levels vary but are generally below 0.4 mg/dl. Patients with LUTO often have vastly slower clearance of maternal creatinine and thus can take weeks to achieve an initial nadir creatinine. There is usually an asymptomatic descent of the creatinine level, with initial large creatinine decrease with improvement slowing over time. If serum creatinine levels do not decrease and/or rise in the PUV neonate with confirmed catheter decompression of the bladder, then consideration should be given to intrinsic renal dysplasia or inadequate decompression of the upper urinary tracts.

For the patient above, after upper tract decompression, his creatinine achieved nadir of 0.34 mg/dl within the first year of life. Creatinine levels have long been thought to be predictive of long-term renal outcomes, and different timepoints of nadir creatinine levels have been explored. It appears that nadir level in the first year of life is most predictive of long-term renal prognosis compared to nadir at 1 month of age [23–25]. Serum creatinine level of less than 0.8 mg/dl seems predictive of a minimal risk of progression to end stage renal disease (ESRD) [23, 26].

At age 3, he underwent ablation of posterior urethral valves, bilateral ureteral reimplantation and creation of right ureteral Mitrofanoff from the stump of loop ureterostomy with continued good kidney function.

Case #3

Neonatal male born at 35 weeks GA via spontaneous vaginal delivery. He had a prenatal diagnosis of bilateral hydronephrosis and oligohydramnios that was followed in his local area with periodic ultrasounds. He had an initial void at 6 h of life and urine output of 2-3 ml/kg h afterward. Initial RBUS at 48 h revealed bilateral hydronephrosis and catheter placement was unsuccessful.

Creatinine was trended and rose precipitously:

DOL #0 = 0.8 mg/dl

DOL #1 = 1.4 mg/dl

DOL #3 = 3.27 mg/dl

Patient transferred and 3.5fr umbilical catheter placed.

RBUS with indwelling catheter and VCUG

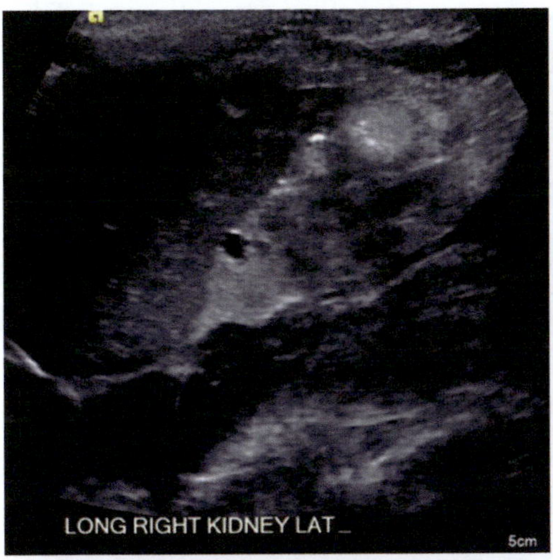

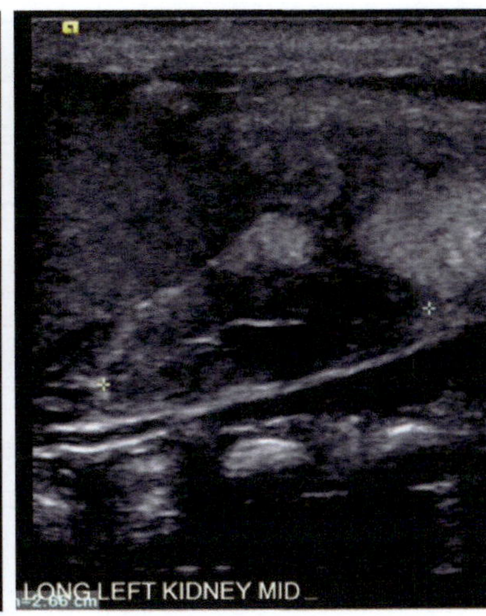

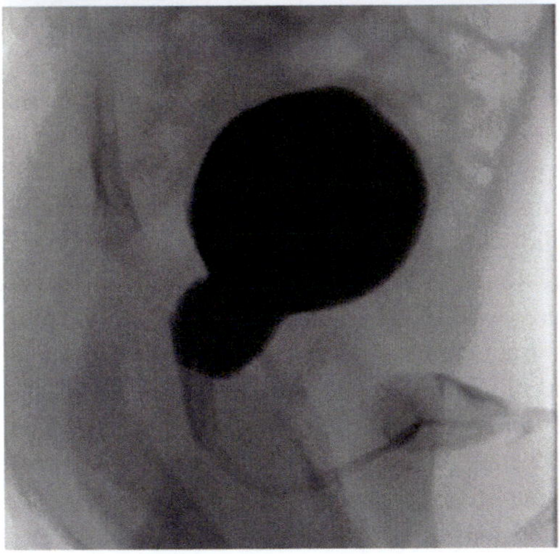

Q1: Describe the findings on RBUS and VCUG.

A1: The RBUS shows bilateral echogenic kidneys with cortical cysts and minimal hydronephrosis. VCUG demonstrated a classic "keyhole sign" with dilated bladder and posterior urethra.

Echogenic kidneys with cystic changes suggest renal dysplasia and poor prognosis for renal function. Neonatal creatinine peaked at >4 mg/dl before trending downward with catheter drainage. Nadir creatinine of 1.59 mg/dl was reached within the first 4 months of life as shown in the following graph and did not improve beyond this within the first year of life.

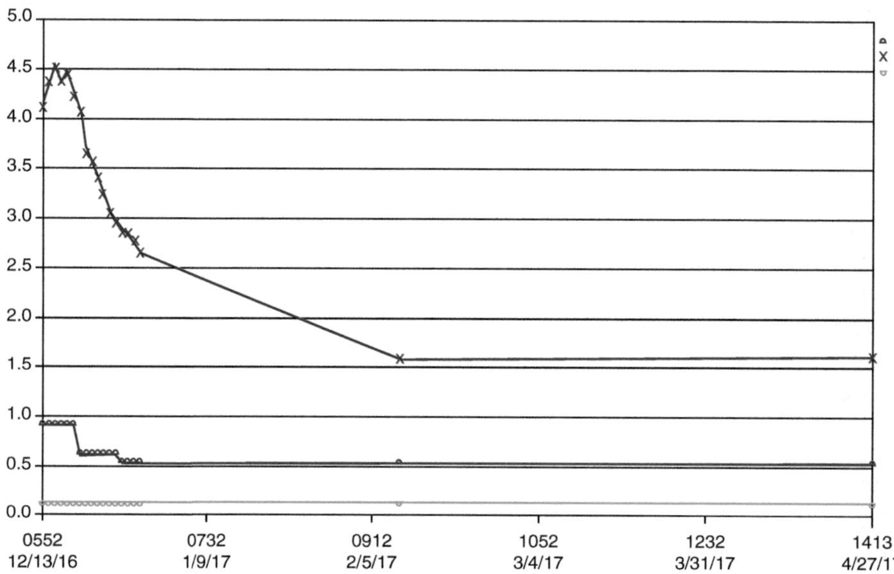

Q2: What does a nadir creatinine of 1.59 mg/dl in the first year of life predict about long-term renal function?

A2: As discussed in the previous case, the nadir creatinine in the first year of life is predictive of long-term renal outcomes. While a nadir <0.8 mg/dl is reassuring, a nadir serum creatinine >1.2 mg/dl is high risk for progression to ESRD [23, 26, 27].

Viewing the entire clinical picture, his hydronephrosis was not severe on postnatal imaging and kidneys were echogenic with cystic changes. These findings coupled with a significantly elevated creatinine are predictive of significant renal dysplasia. Sustained increased pressures within the obstructed bladder transmit pressure throughout the upper urinary tract (ureters, renal collecting system) and eventually to the renal parenchyma and glomeruli. Persistent pressure at the glomeruli may lead to structural and functional changes of the kidney [28, 29]. The hydroureteronephrosis with dilated, thickened bladder associated with PUV is illustrative of this idea. Renal dysplasia manifests as increased renal echogenicity, thinned and cystic renal parenchyma and loss of corticomedullary differentiation, which portends a poor prognosis. There is some debate about the origins of renal dysplasia in the PUV population. Classically, as described above, renal dysplasia was thought to result from prolonged pressures upon the renal units, however even with early fetal intervention and urinary tract decompression, renal function is not improved. This suggest the possibility of concurrent and separate development of renal dysplasia rather than a result of PUV [30, 31]. This patient had a surprisingly mild antenatal hydronephrosis with apparent severe renal dysplasia leading to renal failure, which supports the latter theory.

Shortly after the nadir of creatinine, his renal function deteriorated precipitously as evidenced in the following graph of creatinine over 20 months. By 1 year of age, he had progressed to end stage renal disease (ESRD) and peritoneal dialysis was started. At 20 months of age he received a living related renal transplant from his mother.

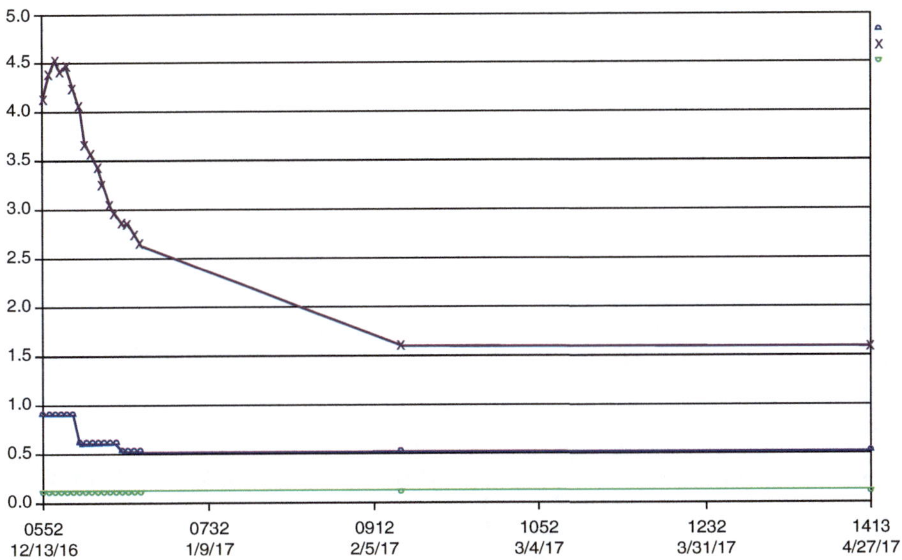

Q3: Prior to renal transplant, what evaluation needs to be completed for a patient with ablated PUV?

A3: Up to 50% of PUV patients progress to ESRD and obstructive uropathy is the second most common cause of renal transplant [32]. Patients who are candidates for renal transplantation need to undergo a multidisciplinary evaluation at baseline, but in those with ablated PUV, it is especially important that a urologist evaluate the bladder. Transplanting a kidney to drain into a hostile bladder would be irresponsible and likely lead to failure of the allograft [33].

Several aspects of bladder function need to be evaluated including bladder capacity, ability to empty and pressures generated with bladder filling, voiding and leaking. Uroflow with or without EMG and a post-void residual measurement or urodynamics can provide much of the needed information. Patients will present at a variety of ages and variety of urine outputs ranging from anuria to polyuria. In an anuric patient, the bladder can be cycled with filling and emptying prior to UDS in order to achieve a more accurate measure of the bladder capacity. In older kids, a uroflow and post-void residual should be assessed initially to evaluate urine flow rate and completeness of emptying. If the bladder is full to start, then bladder capacity may be estimated. The vast majority of post-ablation patients should undergo UDS to better assess for dangerously high bladder pressures [34, 35].

If bladder pressures are unsafe, then there are options of urinary diversion with vesicostomy or cutaneous ureterostomy. Bladder augmentation is often a last option in PUV patients but remains a reasonable one if the bladder pressures are unsafe. There is debate about the best timing of bladder augmentation in relation to renal transplant [36, 37].

Case #4

Neonatal infant born at 32 weeks gestational age secondary to spontaneous rupture of membranes. Bilateral hydronephrosis was detected late in pregnancy at 30 weeks GA. There was poor prenatal follow-up as well as in utero drug exposure.

RBUS obtained after 48 h and initial VCUG shown below. The ultrasound demonstrated right SFU grade IV hydronephrosis and left SFU grade III hydronephrosis with a thickened bladder. VCUG showed bladder trabeculation with dilated posterior urethra, abrupt caliber change and bilateral grade V VUR with left intrarenal reflux.

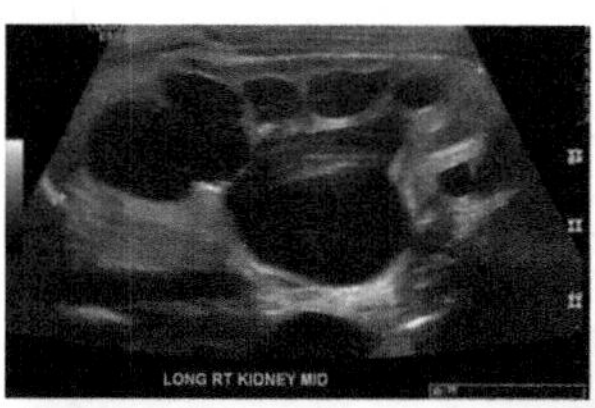

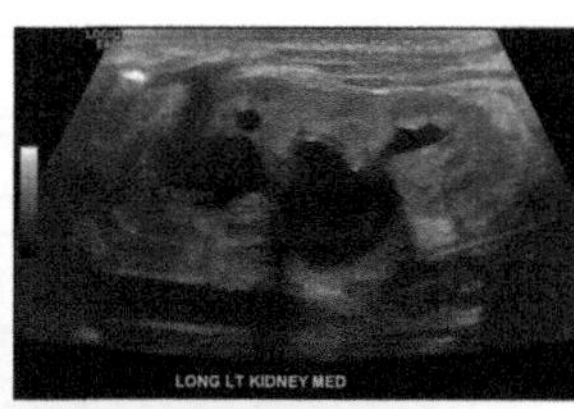

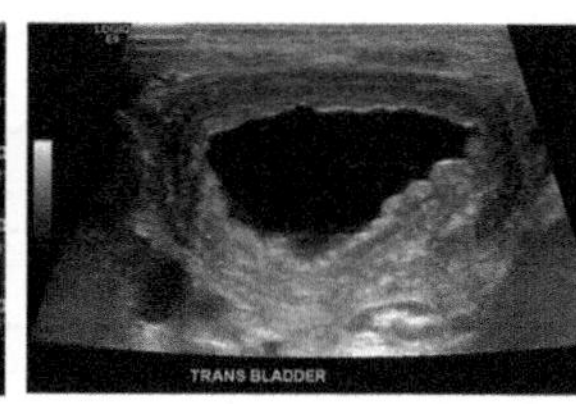

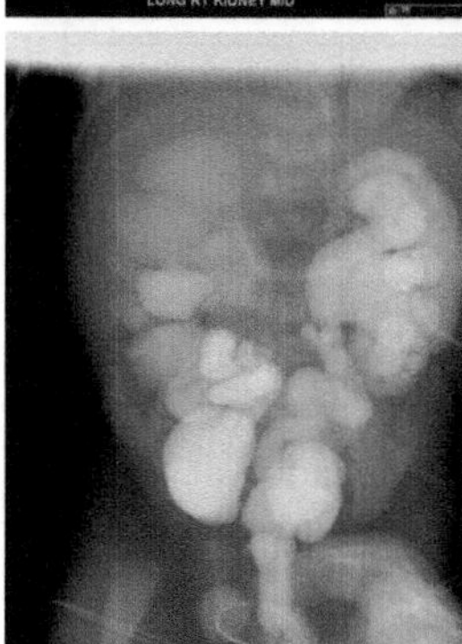
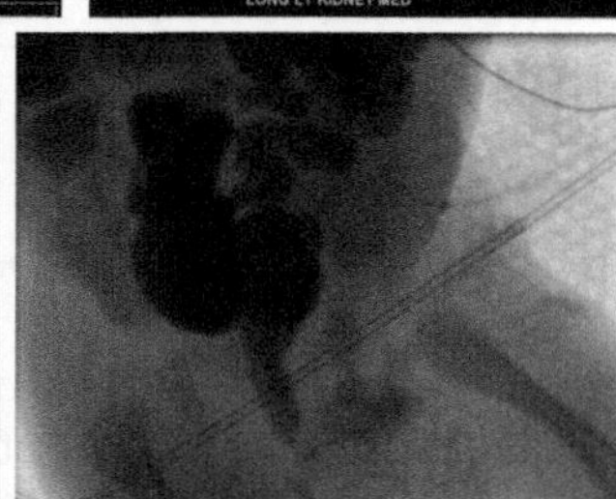

Presentation is consistent with posterior urethral valves. Because of his prematurity and small size, 5fr feeding tube was initially placed and follow-up ultrasound was obtained.

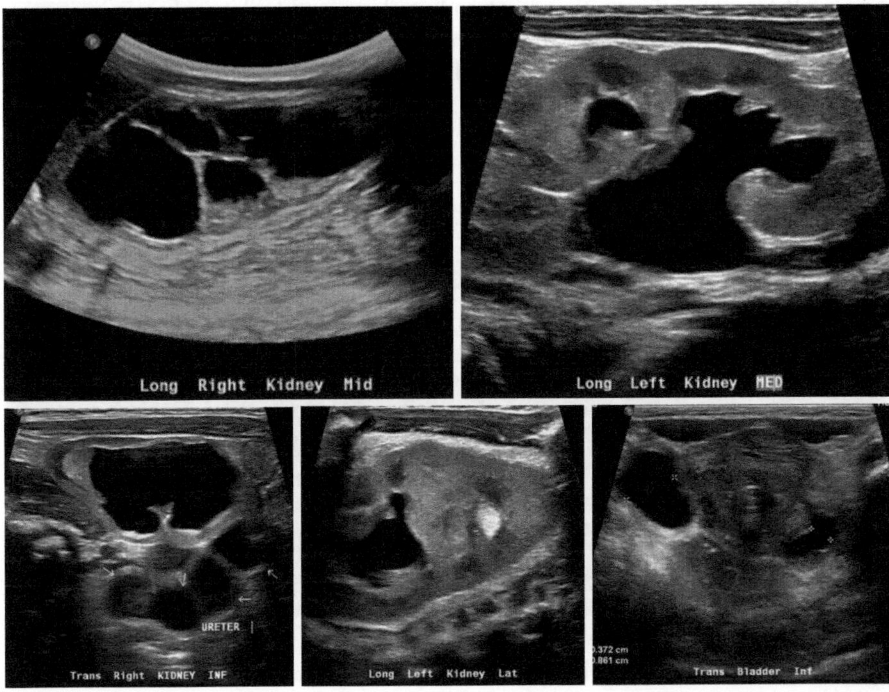

Q1: What are the concerning findings on the follow-up RBUS?
A1:

1. Hydronephrosis and hydroureter appear worse despite a decompressed bladder.
2. Echogenic focus in lower pole of left kidney. This was present on multiple images, was non-shadowing and had no twinkle artifact.

Q2: What is the most likely etiology of the echogenic focus and what further workup is needed? What is the treatment?

A2: The echogenic focus is most likely a stone or fungal ball. With no shadowing or twinkle artifact, a stone is less likely. A urine culture was obtained, which showed yeast. He was started on empiric fluconazole and had persistent fevers. Speciation confirmed the organism as candida glabrata, which was resistant to fluconazole. Amphotericin B was then initiated with periodic RBUS to follow for resolution of the fungal ball, which occurred after approximately 6 weeks. Premature infants in the NICU are at risk of fungal infections, which often have a poor prognosis and need to be treated aggressively.

Q3: With persistent hydronephrosis despite bladder decompression by catheter, what are options for treatment?

A3:

- Surveillance: Trend creatinine and periodic RBUS.
  - UVJ obstruction may occur with bladder decompression because of severe bladder wall thickening. This obstruction can be transient or persistent.

If the patient's creatinine is trending down and hydronephrosis improves, then continued monitoring is a reasonable approach.

If creatinine is rising and/or hydronephrosis does not improve or worsens, then intervention is warranted.

- Vesicostomy
- Cutaneous ureterostomy
- Percutaneous nephrostomy

After several weeks of treatment for his funguria and fungal ball, adequate growth and upsizing his catheter to 8fr, cystoscopy and valve ablation were completed. Post-ablation RBUS images are below.

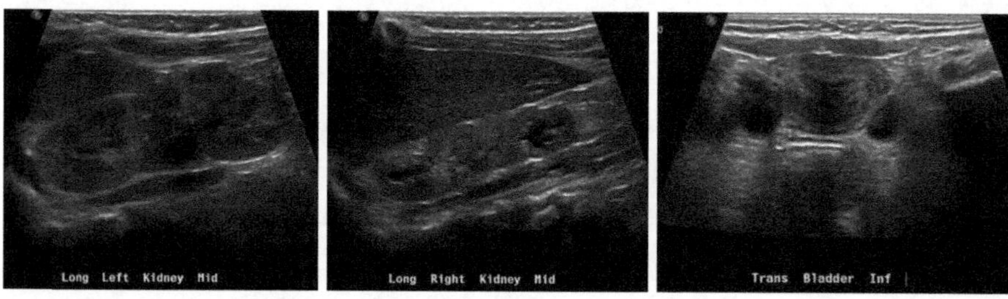

He was fully treated for his funguria and fungal ball resolved on RBUS. The patient was discharged from the hospital under the care of a foster family and further follow-up imaging was delayed till months later.

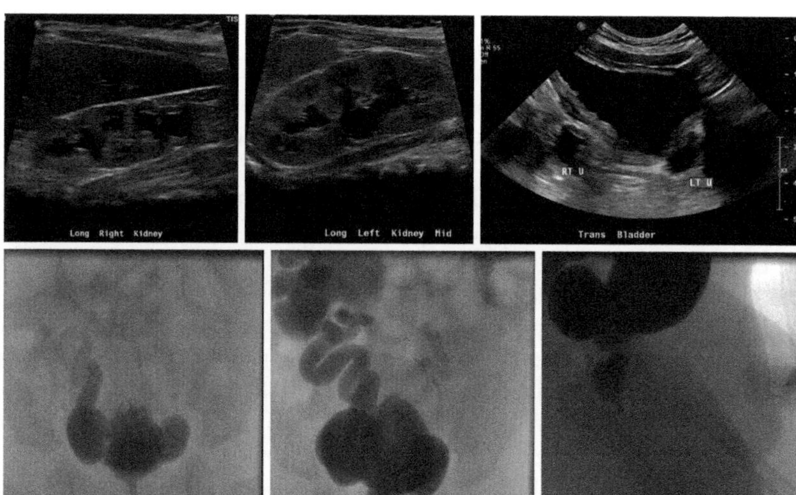

Q4: What does the imaging show?
A4:

- Bilateral grade II hydronephrosis
- Bladder trabeculation

- Bilateral periureteral diverticuli
- Right grade V VUR, grade II left VUR
- Abrupt urethral caliber change and dilated posterior urethra

Q5: What are his treatment options?

A5: There is persistent dilation of the posterior urethra and abrupt caliber change after prior cystoscopic ablation of posterior urethral valves. He also continues to show evidence of increased bladder pressures with periureteral diverticula and VUR. The cause of these persistent findings are most consistent with persistent valvular tissue, but may also represent scarring and bulbar urethral stricture. A stricture is more likely than usual in this setting because of his extensive history of fungal urinary tract infection and intrarenal fungal ball.

- Antibiotic Prophylaxis. With the high grade reflux and bladder diverticuli, antibiotic prophylaxis should be discussed and recommended if not already established.
- Cystoscopic incision of persistent posterior urethral valves versus direct visual internal urethrotomy for stricture, needs to be initiated urgently for evaluation and treatment of his urethral obstruction.

Cystoscopic evaluation revealed persistent PUV and the valves were ablated at the 5, 7, and 12 o'clock positions.

Case #5

An 8 year old boy presented to the bowel and bladder clinic with dysuria and stranguria. He embraces dysuria but denies straining, although his family details that he shakes, sweats and turns red with voiding. He was initially treated with standard bowel and bladder behavioral modification without improvement. RBUS was obtained, which did not show hydronephrosis, but the appearance of a thick-walled bladder. A VCUG was then obtained due to the concern for the thickened bladder and straining to void.

RBUS and VCUG

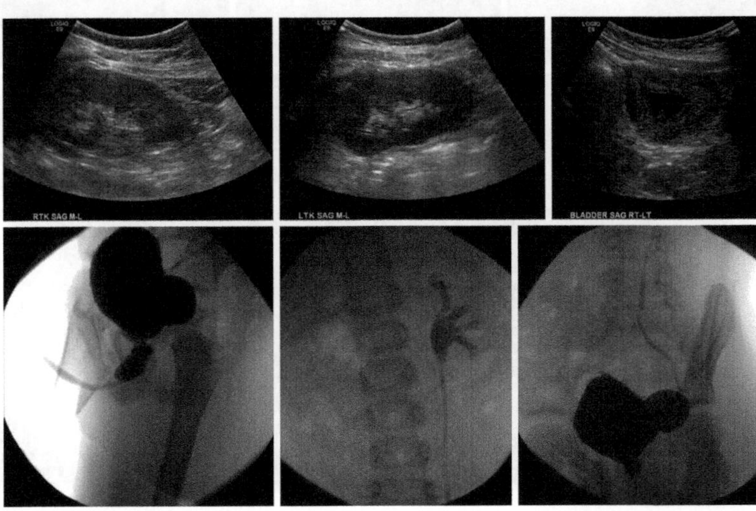

Q1: What is shown on the VCUG imaging?

A1: The VCUG shows a dilated posterior urethra and abrupt urethral caliber change with trabeculated bladder. There is also a left sided periureteral diverticulum with left SFU grade III VUR. These findings are consistent with a delayed presentation of posterior urethral valves.

Discussion: With increased sensitivity and availability of prenatal ultrasonography, it is normally assumed that a diagnosis of posterior urethral valves will be made perinatally. However, there have been several studies showing that delayed presentation and identification of PUV is common. One study indicated that 43% of PUV patients presented after 6 months of age, while another revealed that 64% of PUV patients had normal prenatal imaging. Most of the younger children presented with urinary tract infections, acute kidney injury, or difficulties with voiding [38, 39].

It has been assumed that earlier diagnosis of PUV leads to earlier intervention and thus improved renal outcomes, however, there is conflicting data related to timing of diagnosis. During the era of prenatal imaging, an overall rate of progression to ESRD has been noted at 36% of PUV patients [25]. One study saw a 41% rate of ESRD if diagnosed prior to 1 year of age, with only 15% if diagnosed after 1 year [40]. An assumption has been that later presenting children have a more mild form of obstruction, thus allowing later presentation and protecting renal function. However, several other studies have shown a significantly higher creatinine levels and worse long-term renal outcomes in patients who presented in delayed fashion [31, 41, 42]. These risks caution the practitioner to keep a high suspicion for posterior urethral valves in even older children who present with symptoms of lower urinary tract dysfunction: UTI's, incontinence, hematuria and renal insufficiency [39, 43, 44].

Cystoscopy and PUV ablation was completed. Follow-up imaging at 6 weeks is shown below.

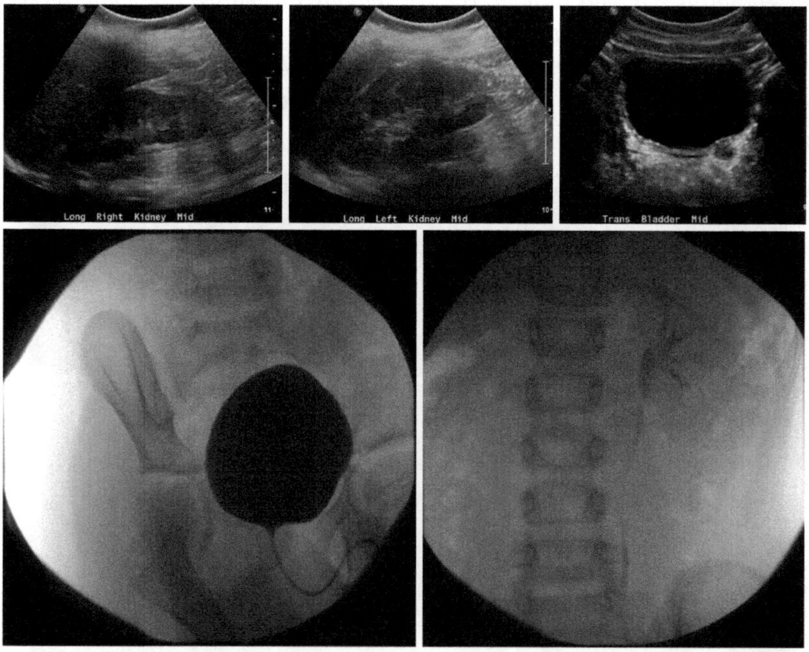

At follow-up, symptoms of dysuria had almost completely resolved. His family noted resolution of his straining symptoms of sweating and redness, but he had some persistent mild shaking associated with voiding. His renal ultrasound showed no hydronephrosis and bladder appeared less thickened. VCUG revealed a smooth-walled bladder with improvement of his left periureteral diverticulum and left VUR to SFU grade 2.

Case #6

14 year old boy with history of posterior urethral valve ablation during infancy, who now presents in adolescence with infrequent voiding and incontinence episodes after urine holding. Recently, his hydronephrosis and chronic kidney disease (CKD) have worsened, with increase from stage 2 to stage 3. He has full urethral sensation and is unable to perform clean intermittent catheterization due to discomfort.

RBUS on presentation in adolescence.

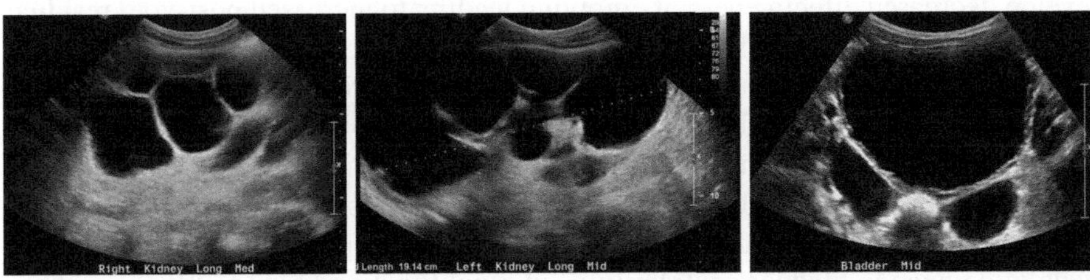

Q1: The RBUS shows SFU grade IV hydronephrosis bilaterally with bilateral hydroureter. What further workup should be performed?

A1:

- Assessment for polyuria.
  With a history of ablated posterior urethral valves he is at risk for polyuria secondary to concentrating defect from renal tubular damage (nephrogenic diabetes insipidus). This is a classic finding during the adolescent period, which contributes to the process described by Dr. Mitchell in 1982 as Valve Bladder Syndrome [29]. An analysis of his urine volume can be obtained with a simple voiding diary or a 24 h urine collection. While a 24 urine collection is more accurate, it is reliant on adherence by the patient. Knowing the extent of polyuria can help frame the results of other testing and help guide interventions such as overnight urine drainage.
- Uroflow with post-void residual (PVR).
  A uroflow provides noninvasive information about the effectiveness of detrusor contraction. Assessment of post-void residual is imperative to assess successfulness of bladder emptying and guide the addition of anticholinergic medications.
- Urodynamics testing.
  With his worsening hydronephrosis and CKD, as well as incontinence, UDS will provide needed information about bladder capacity, pressure and VUR.

- Renal scan

  If there is a suspicion for UVJ obstruction with his high grade hydronephrosis and hydroureter, then a renal scan is warranted. During testing, to specifically evaluate for upper tract obstruction, an indwelling catheter may be beneficial. This isolates evaluation of the upper urinary tracts and removes the concern for high bladder pressures inhibiting drainage.

12.2 Discussion: Valve Bladder Syndrome

Valve Bladder Syndrome has been described as a "vicious cycle" which involves three major elements in some patients with PUV: compromised bladder emptying, polyuria and high pressure transmitted to the kidneys. Initially, the PUV bladder compensates with high pressure voiding to overcome resistance, then over time can develop decreased effectiveness of emptying leading to increased post-void residual in the bladder. Coupled with polyuria from renal injury to the proximal tubules, the bladder remains under continuous stretch without effective decompression, which leads to changes in the bladder wall and decreased compliance. A bladder pressure increase ensues that is transmitted to the renal collecting system, contributing to increased hydroureteronephrosis. With voiding, the reservoir of urine stored as hydronephrosis quickly drains and fills the bladder, prompting a continuation of the cycle of damage to bladder contractility and renal function [13, 14, 29].

Overnight drainage has been shown to interrupt this cycle by providing a period of 7–12 h of bladder and upper urinary tract decompression. There is good evidence that overnight drainage improves hydroureteronephrosis, continence, rate of urinary tract infections and stabilizes renal functional impairment [28, 45].

A voiding diary revealed that he has a 24 h urine volume of 5 l.

Uroflow/PVR demonstrated a 12 ml/s flow rate with staccato pattern and 14 ml post-void residual.

UDS results:

- *Bladder Capacity 300*
- *Max filling pressure—54*

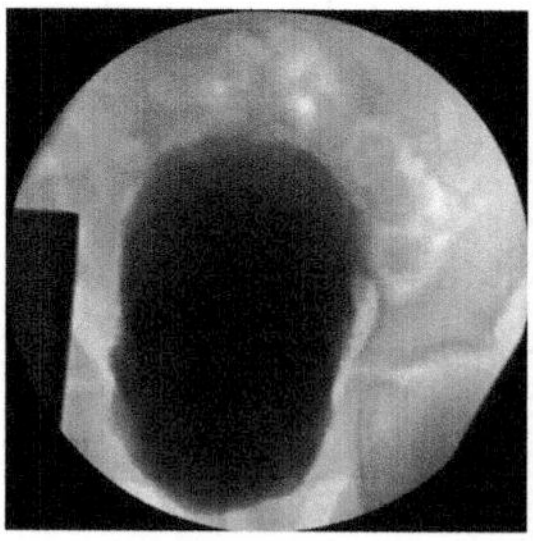

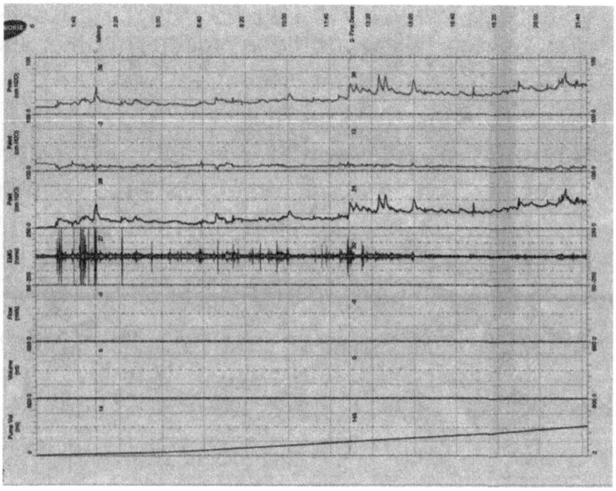

Q2: What are options for treatment?

A2: The UDS reveals a bladder capacity lower than expected for his age with a decreased compliance leading to a maximum detrusor pressure of 54 cm H_2O, which is greater than the level generally considered concerning for renal damage (40 cm H_2O). Interventions need to be focused on decreasing bladder pressure, increasing bladder capacity and improving compliance without compromising bladder emptying.

- Overnight drainage
  Placement of indwelling foley catheter during sleep allows for a period of complete bladder emptying and low pressure. Normal circadian physiology leads to overnight decrease in urine production, however, the nighttime decrease is not seen in adolescent PUV patients with polyuria due to a defect of urine concentration. Several studies have demonstrated that overnight drainage decreases the persistent hydronephrosis and hydroureter, and can improve incontinence and renal function [28, 45]. The overnight drainage is thought to provide a period of bladder decompression which interrupts the cycle of damage and remodeling that occurs with Valve Bladder Syndrome.
- Mitrofanoff
  Patients with PUV normally have sensate urethras and often an associated high bladder neck which makes urethral catheterization intolerable. A useful option is creation of an appendicovesicostomy or enterovesicostomy (Monti) using the Mitrofanoff Principle. Overnight drainage or clean intermittent catheterization can be completed without the challenge of oversensitivity, vastly improving adherence with catheterization.
- Clean Intermittent Catheterization
  Passage of a catheter to drain the bladder via urethra or Mitrofanoff during the day is largely reserved for patients who demonstrate incomplete bladder emptying or persistent findings of hydronephrosis, hydroureter and worsened renal function.
- Anticholinergic
  With low post-void residual, consideration can be given to initiation of an anticholinergic medication, which provides increased compliance and capacity of the bladder. This may be especially helpful in those patients with higher bladder pressures and those with increased incontinence. Increased compliance can lead to compromised bladder emptying, at which point cessation of the medication or CIC may be initiated [9, 46].
- Bladder augmentation
  Intestinal or ureteric augmentation of the bladder provides larger capacity and vastly increased compliance [47]. Likely because of an improved understanding of the changes that occur leading to Valve Bladder as well as earlier intervention with overnight drainage, bladder augmentation for PUV patients has been reserved for those severe patients that have been refractory to all other interventions.
- Botox
  OnabutulinumtoxinA injection to the detrusor muscle can provide longer acting increase in bladder compliance than anticholinergics, without the inva-

siveness of a bladder augmentation. Repeat administration is often necessary every 6–9 months and there is risk of urinary retention requiring catheterization. This risk must be discussed with the patient and family.

RBUS post Monti-Mitrofanoff

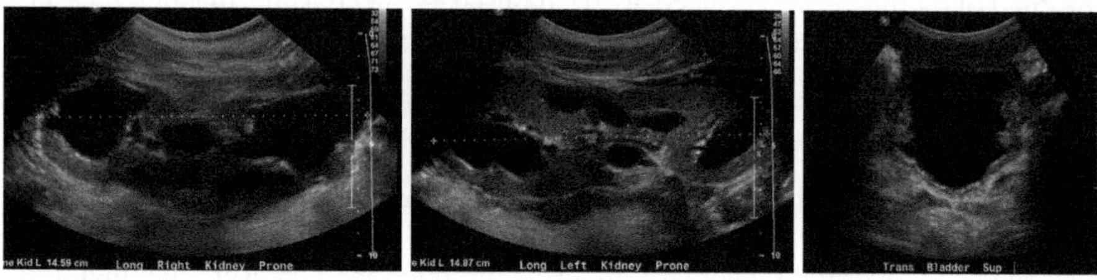

There was improvement in hydronephrosis and hydroureter post Monti-Mitrofanoff, oxybutynin and overnight drainage. CKD also improved with a return to stage 2. He voids spontaneous during the day and completes overnight drainage. He has some persistent incontinence via Mitrofanoff, especially with voiding.

Q3: What are the options to improve his incontinence?

A3: His incontinence is largely via his Mitrofanoff instead of urethra. This can signal an issue with overflow or with the Mitrofanoff channel itself.

- Strict timed voiding and double voiding for any residual urine

  Strict adherence to a voiding schedule will often improve incontinence by preventing urine overflow due to bladder overdistention. With incomplete bladder emptying, double voiding can be initiated to more fully evacuate the bladder.

- Improve Bladder Emptying

  Biofeedback. Posterior urethral valve patients are at higher risk of voiding dysfunction and studies have shown a benefit with biofeedback [48].

  Alpha adrenergic blocker. With high bladder neck and voiding dysfunction, there may be increased resistance of the bladder outlet. Alpha adrenergic blockers target receptors of the bladder neck and proximal urethra, which can lead to a decreased resistance with voiding [49].

  Initiation of CIC during the day. As discussed above, if hydronephrosis, hydroureter and worsening CKD are persistent, then escalation to daytime CIC would be warranted. If incontinence is troublesome to the patient, then CIC is also an option.

- Increase bladder compliance

  Increase anticholinergic. If anticholinergic is not at maximum dosage, then an increase may be reasonable. As discussed previously, this may improve compliance and incontinence, but worsen incomplete bladder emptying, thus necessitating CIC.

  Botox. OnabotulinumtoxinA injection to the detrusor also provides an option to further increase bladder compliance, but as discussed previously, may compromise bladder emptying and necessitate CIC.

– Revision or Bulking agent to Mitrofanoff channel
  When incontinence is persistent via Mitrofanoff despite good bladder compliance and patient adherence to bladder emptying, then intervention to the Mitrofanoff channel may improve the incontinence via the channel.

The patient was previously voiding spontaneously 2 times during the day. Initiation of strict timed voiding schedule during the day, in addition to his prior regime of overnight drainage via Monti-Mitrofanoff and oxybutynin, resolved his incontinence.

Repeat UDS results:

- *Bladder Capacity 350*
- *Max filling pressure 25*

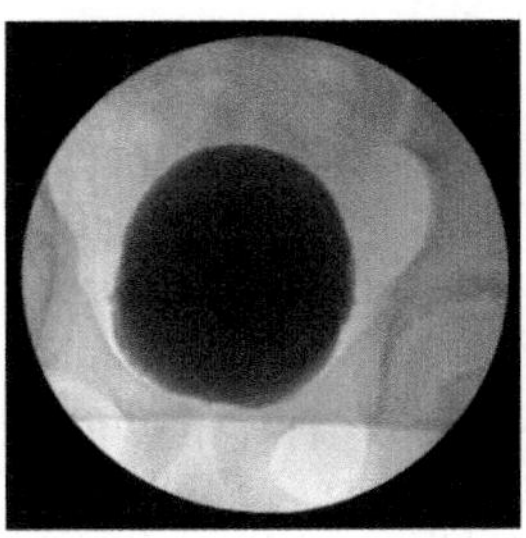

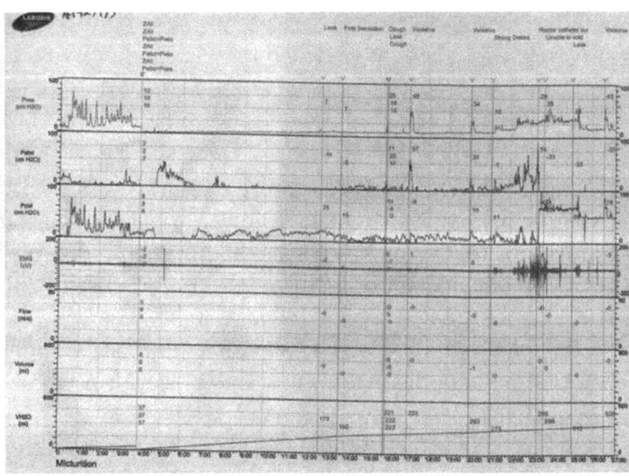

Case #7

Neonatal male born full term with prenatal diagnosis of bilateral hydronephrosis and dilated bladder but no oligohydramnios during pregnancy.

– *RBUS at 48 hours of life shown below revealed SFU grade III right and SFU grade IV left hydronephrosis with thickened bladder and hydroureter.*
– *VCUG demonstrated a trabeculated bladder but lacked distinct urethral transition point or dilated posterior urethra.*

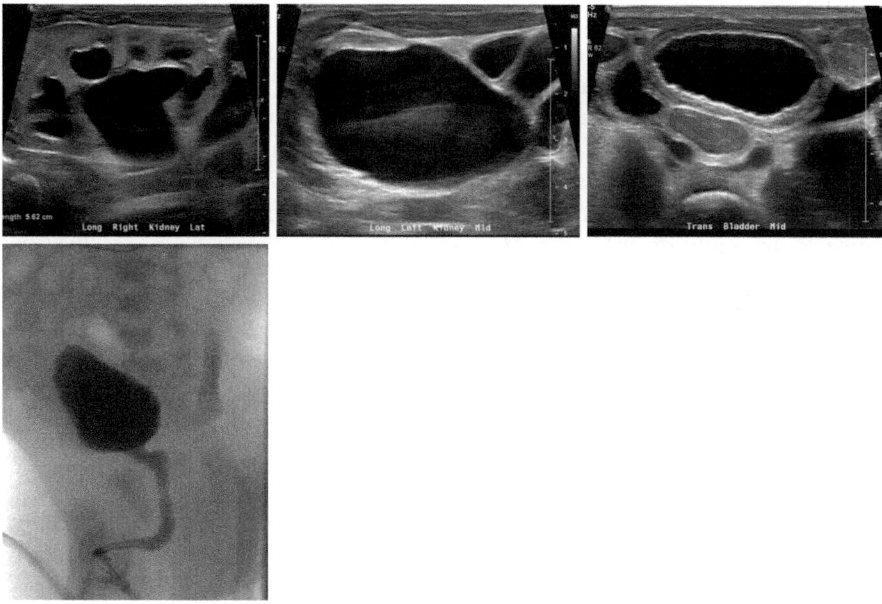

Q1: What could account for his presentation?

A1: The patient has stigmata of lower urinary tract obstruction (LUTO) without definitive obstructive pathholology noted in the urethra on VCUG. He is otherwise normal without any signs of neurologic compromise or spinal defect.

- Posterior urethral valves. Underdistention on voiding phase of single cycle VCUG may not distinctly show true posterior urethral dilation or urethral caliber change.
- Neurogenic bladder. Without clear indication of urethral anomaly, evaluation for a neurologic source of bladder dysfunction is advisable. Spine ultrasound is a good non-invasive screening tool for spinal anomalies in the neonatal period. If equivocal results, consider MRI for further workup.
- Other urethral abnormality such as anterior urethral valve, diverticulum, Cowper's gland cyst, urethral atresia

Spine ultrasound was negative for any anomalies. Cystoscopy revealed an obstructive membrane in the penile urethra that was not affiliated with any other urethral anomalies (i.e. diverticulum, bulbourethral gland abnormality). The anterior urethral valve was incised.

12.3 Discussion

Anterior urethral valves, while the most common obstruction of the anterior urethra, are approximately 30 times more rare than posterior urethral valves. Anterior urethral valves can occur anywhere along the anterior urethra, from bulbar to penile urethra. The etiology of the anterior urethral valve has been described as associated with abnormalities of the bulbourethral gland, either associated with a large urethral diverticulum or fold of the anterior urethra [50].

Presentation can vary widely from early obstruction to dysuria and UTI's. Diagnosis is confirmed with VCUG and should be differentiated from other rare obstructive processes of the anterior urethra such as Cowper's duct cyst/syringocele or urethral atresia. On VCUG, an anterior urethral valve will often show a dilated anterior urethra with signs of chronic obstruction such as high grade VUR and bladder trabeculation and/or diverticuli [51]. Treatment depends on age and size of the patient, similar to posterior urethral valves. The mainstay treatment is cystoscopy and ablation of simple anterior urethral valves. If a large diverticulum is present, then urethral reconstruction may be necessary. Premature or small infants may need supravesical drainage such as vesicostomy [52].

Similar to posterior urethral valves, patients have a high risk of developing bladder dysfunction and long-term renal function is dependent on early evidence of renal injury. Anterior urethral valves have a significantly better overall renal prognosis than PUV, with 78% having normal renal function. Regardless of the comparatively superior renal outcomes, patients need long-term follow-up to ensure continued preservation of bladder and renal function [53].

Post ablation imaging below demonstrated decompression of the entire collecting system. There was near resolution of right hydronephrosis and bilateral hydroureter with significant improvement of his left hydronephrosis. VCUG revealed a smooth-walled bladder and normal appearing urethra.

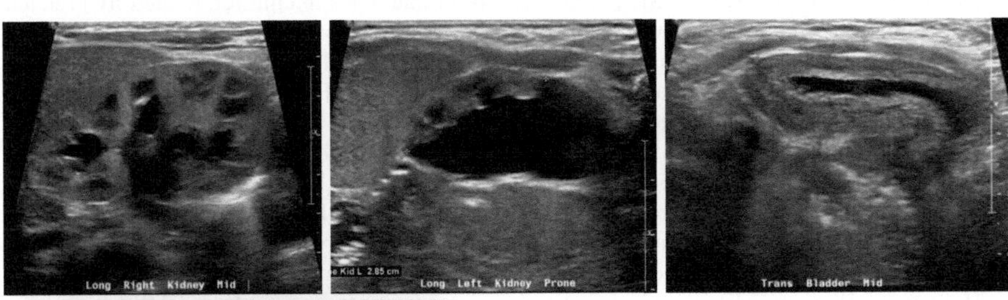

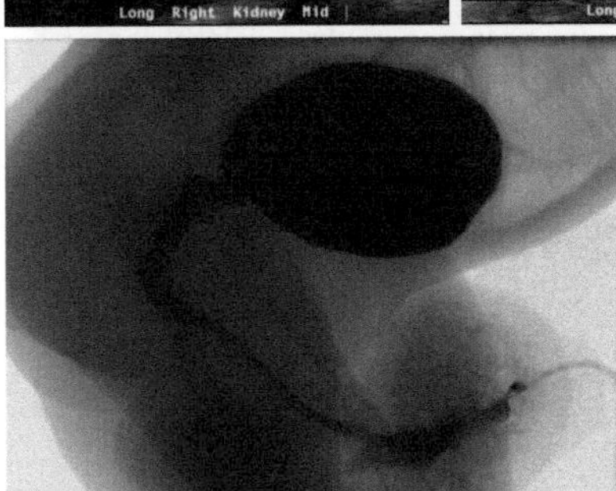

References

1. Lee RS, Cendron M, Kinnamon DD, et al. Antenatal Hydronephrosis as a predictor of postnatal outcome: a meta-analysis. Pediatrics. 2006;118:586–93.
2. St. Aubin M, Willihnganz-Lawson K, Varda BK, et al. Society for Fetal Urology Recommendations for postnatal evaluation of prenatal Hydronephrosis—will fewer voiding Cystourethrograms Lead to more urinary tract infections? J Urol. 2013;190:1456–61.
3. Jordan G, Hoover D. Inadequate decompression of the upper tracts using a Foley catheter in the valve bladder. J Urol. 1985;134:137–8.
4. Penna FJ, Bowlin P, Alyami F, et al. Novel strategy for temporary decompression of the lower urinary tract in neonates using a ureteral stent. J Urol. 2015;194:1086–90.
5. Whitaker R, Sherwood T. An improved hook for destroying posterior urethral valves. J Urol. 1986;135:531–2.
6. Soliman SM. Primary ablation of posterior urethral valves in low birth weight neonates by a visually guided Fogarty Embolectomy catheter. J Urol. 2009;181:2284–90.
7. Hutcheson JC, Cooper CS, Canning DA, et al. The use of vesicostomy as permanent urinary diversion in the child with myelomeningocele. J Urol. 2001;166(6):2351–3.
8. Pinto M, Markland C, Fraley E. Posterior urethral valves managed by cutaneous ureterostomy with subsequent ureteral reconstruction. J Urol. 1978;119:696–8.
9. Kim YH, Horowitz M, Combs AJ, et al. Management of posterior urethral valves on the basis of urodynamic findings. J Urol. 1997;158(3):1011–6.
10. Churchill B, McLorie G, Khoury A, et al. Emergency treatment and long-term follow-up of posterior urethral valves. Urol Clin N Am. 1990;17:343–60.
11. Frimberger D, Cooper CS, Ramji F, et al. Multi-institutional study comparing the height of contrast during performance of voiding Cystourethrogram in children. Urology. 2016;93:180–4.
12. Schaeffer AJ, Greenfield SP, Ivanova A, et al. Reliability of grading of vesicoureteral reflux and other findings on voiding cystourethrography. J Pediatr Urol. 2016;13(2):192–8.
13. De Gennaro M, Capitanucci ML, Mosiello G, et al. The changing urodynamic pattern from infancy to adolescence in boys with posterior urethral valves. BJU Int. 2000;85:1104–8.
14. Holmdahl G. The changing urodynamic pattern in valve bladders during infancy. J Urol. 1995;153(2):463–7.
15. Pinar H. Postmortem findings in term neonates. Semin Neonatol. 2004;9:289–302.
16. Biard J-M, Johnson MP, Carr MC, et al. Long-term outcomes in children treated by prenatal Vesicoamniotic shunting for lower urinary tract obstruction. Obstet Gynecol. 2005;106:503–8.
17. Clark T. Prenatal bladder drainage in the management of fetal lower urinary tract obstruction: a systematic review and meta-analysis. Obstet Gynecol. 2003;102:367–82.
18. Morris RK, Malin GL, Quinlan-Jones E, et al. Percutaneous vesicoamniotic shunting versus conservative management for fetal lower urinary tract obstruction (PLUTO): a randomised trial. Lancet. 2013;382:1496–506.
19. Ruano R. Fetal surgery for severe lower urinary tract obstruction. Prenat Diagn. 2011;31:667–74.
20. Quintero RA, Shukla AR, Homsy YL, et al. Successful in utero endoscopic ablation of posterior urethral valves: a new dimension in fetal urology. Urology. 2000;55:774.
21. Holmes N, Harrison MR, Baskin LS. Fetal surgery for posterior urethral valves: long-term postnatal outcomes. Pediatrics. 2001;108:e7.
22. Nicolini U, Spelzini F. Invasive assessment of fetal renal abnormalities: urinalysis, fetal blood sampling and biopsy. Prenat Diagn. 2001;21:964–9.
23. Drozdz D, Drozdz M, Gretz N, et al. Progression to end-stage renal disease in children with posterior urethral valves. Pediatr Nephrol. 1998;12:630–6.
24. Lal R, Bhatnager V, Mitra D. Long-term prognosis of renal function in boys treated for posterior urethral valves. Eur J Pediatr Surg. 1999;9:307–11.
25. Heikkilä J, Holmberg C, Kyllönen L, et al. Long-term risk of end stage renal disease in patients with posterior urethral valves. J Urol. 2011;186:2392–6.

26. DeFoor W, Clark C, Jackson E, et al. Risk factors for end stage renal disease in children with posterior urethral valves. J Urol. 2008;180:1705–8.
27. Ansari MS, Gulia A, Srivastava A, et al. Risk factors for progression to end-stage renal disease in children with posterior urethral valves. J Pediatr Urol. 2010;6:261–4.
28. Koff SA, Mutabagani KH, Jayanthi VR. The valve bladder syndrome: pathophysiology and treatment with nocturnal bladder emptying. J Urol. 2002;167(1):291–7.
29. Glassberg KI. The valve bladder syndrome: 20 years later. J Urol. 2001;166(4):1406–14.
30. Haecker F-M, Wehrmann M, Hacker H-W, et al. Renal dysplasia in children with posterior urethral valves: a primary or secondary malformation? Pediatr Surg Int. 2002;18:119–22.
31. Sarhan OM, El-Ghoneimi AA, Helmy TE, et al. Posterior urethral valves: multivariate analysis of factors affecting the final renal outcome. J Urol. 2011;185:2491–6.
32. Smith JM, Stablein DM, Munoz R, et al. Contributions of the transplant registry: the 2006 annual report of the north American Pediatric renal trials and collaborative studies (NAPRTCS). Pediatr Transplant. 2007;11:366–73.
33. Mendizábal S, Estornell F, Zamora I, et al. Renal transplantation in children with severe bladder dysfunction. J Urol. 2005;173:226–9.
34. DeFoor W, Tackett L, Minevich E, et al. Successful renal transplantation in children with posterior urethral valves. J Urol. 2003;170:2402–4.
35. Fine MS, Smith KM, Shrivastava D, et al. Posterior urethral valve treatments and outcomes in children receiving kidney transplants. J Urol. 2011;185:2507–11.
36. Rigamonti W, Capizzi A, Zacchello G, et al. Kidney transplantation into bladder augmentation or urinary diversion: long-term results. Transplantation. 2005;80:1435–40.
37. Christman MS, Canning DA, Schast AP, et al. Renal transplantation into a diverted urinary system—is it safe in children? J Urol. 2013;190:678–82.
38. Pulido JE, Furth SL, Zderic SA, et al. Renal parenchymal area and risk of ESRD in boys with posterior urethral valves. CJASN. 2014;9:499–505.
39. Engel DL, Pope JC, Adams MC, et al. Risk factors associated with chronic kidney disease in patients with posterior urethral valves without prenatal Hydronephrosis. J Urol. 2011;185:2502–6.
40. Parkhouse H, Barratt T, Dillon M, et al. Long-term outcome of boys with posterior urethral valves. Br J Urol. 1988;62:59–62.
41. El-Sherbiny MT, Hafez AT, Shokeir AA. Posterior urethral valves: does young age at diagnosis correlate with poor renal function? Urology. 2002;60(2):335–8.
42. Ziylan O, Oktar T, Ander H, et al. The impact of late presentation of posterior urethral valves on bladder and renal function. J Urol. 2006;175:1894–7.
43. Bomalaski MD, Anema JG, Coplen DE, et al. Delayed presentation of posterior urethral valves: a not so benign condition. J Urol. 1999;162:2130–2.
44. Schober JM, Dulabon LM, Woodhouse CR. Outcome of valve ablation in late-presenting posterior urethral valves. BJU Int. 2004;94:616–9.
45. Nguyen MT, Pavlock CL, Zderic SA, et al. Overnight catheter drainage in children with poorly compliant bladders improves post-obstructive diuresis and urinary incontinence. J Urol. 2005;174:1633–6.
46. Casey JT, Hagerty JA, Maizels M, et al. Early Administration of Oxybutynin Improves Bladder Function and Clinical Outcomes in Newborns with posterior urethral valves. J Urol. 2012;188:1516–20.
47. Johal NS, Hamid R, Aslam Z, et al. Ureterocystoplasty: long-term functional results. J Urol. 2008;179:2373–6.
48. Ansari MS, Srivastava A, Kapoor R, et al. Biofeedback therapy and home pelvic floor exercises for lower urinary tract dysfunction after posterior urethral valve ablation. J Urol. 2008;179:708–11.
49. Abraham MK, Nasir ARA, Sudarsanan B, et al. Role of alpha adrenergic blocker in the management of posterior urethral valves. Pediatr Surg Int. 2009;25:1113–5.
50. Paulhac P, Fourcade L, Lesaux N, et al. Anterior urethral valves and diverticula: anterior urethral valves and diverticula. BJU Int. 2003;92:506–9.

51. McLellan DL, Lebowitz RL, Mandell J, et al. Anterior urethral valves and diverticula in children: a result of ruptured Cowper's duct cyst? BJU Int. 2004;94(3):375–8.
52. Confer SD, Galati V, Frimberger D, et al. Megacystis with an anterior urethral valve: case report and review of literature. J Pediatr Urol. 2010;6:459–62.
53. Routh JC, McGee SM, Ashley RA, et al. Predicting renal outcomes in children with anterior urethral valves: a systematic review. J Urol. 2010;184:1615–9.

13 The Lower Urinary Tract

John M. Hutson

Learning Objective

- Learning objectives: enable trainees to understand the usually rare causes of urethral pathology apart from PUV.

13.1 The Lower Urinary Tract

13.1.1 Case 1

A small boy is referred to you as the mother notices a small lump adjacent to the urethral meatus on the glans, shortly after circumcision has been performed for religious indications. The lesion has the appearance of a cyst and is bluish in colour (Fig. 13.1).

Q.1.1 What is the likely diagnosis?

A. Cystic duplication of glanular urethra

Q.1.2 What is aetiology of the anomaly?

A. Probably duplication of the canalisation process that makes the glanular urethra from the endodermal strip on the ventral surface of the phallus. Canalisation of the proximal urethra occurs at 8–12 weeks under the control of circulating androgens from the testis. As the Leydig cell mass is still small at the onset of sexual differentiation the concentration of testosterone in the serum is low. Conversion of testosterone into dihydrotestesterone (DHT) by the enzyme, 5α-reductase, enables DHT to bind to androgen receptors and trigger urethral canalisation. The process

J. M. Hutson (✉)
Urology Department, Royal Children's Hospital, Melbourne, VIC, Australia

Surgical Research Unit, Murdoch Children's Research Institute, Melbourne, VIC, Australia

Department of Paediatrics, University of Melbourne, Melbourne, VIC, Australia
e-mail: John.Hutson@rch.org.au

P. Godbole et al. (eds.), *Practical Pediatric Urology*,
https://doi.org/10.1007/978-3-030-54020-3_13

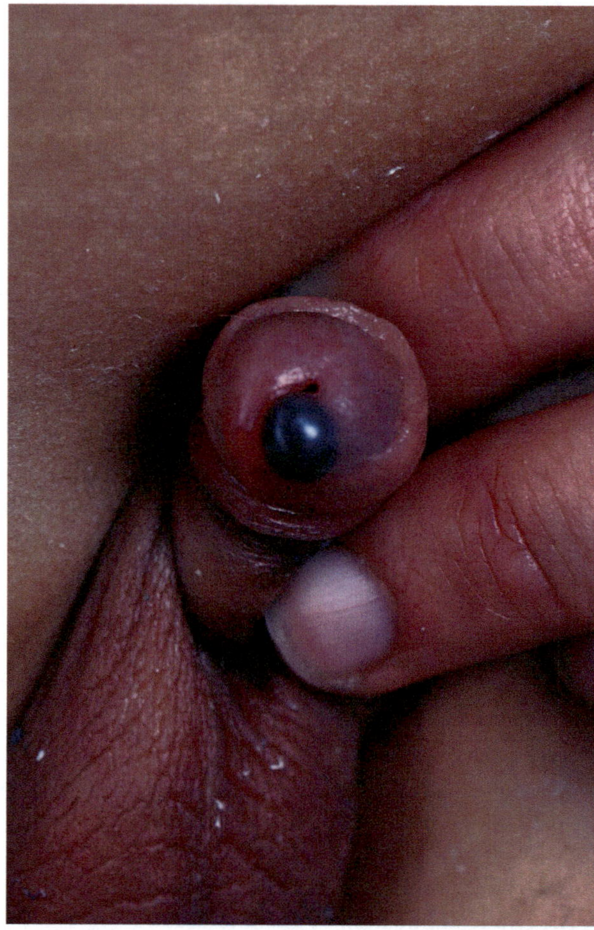

Fig. 13.1 Lateral cystic duplication of urethra filled with blood after minor trauma. (Reproduced from Pediatric diagnosis second edn, Beasley, Hutson, Stringer, Teague & King)

brings the urethral opening to the coronal groove by about 12 weeks, but canalisation of the endodermal plate on the glans occurs more slowly, so that it is not until after about 15 weeks that the urethral meatus reaches its definitive position on the tip of the glans. Minor aberration of this process may be the cause of the cystic duplication.

Q.1.3 Why was the anomaly not noticed at birth?

A. The presence of the foreskin may mask the anomaly by preventing proper examination of the glans until at time of circumcision. The blue colour is consistent with haemorrhage into the cyst after minor trauma. As the cyst is usually lined with transitional epithelium or squamous epithelium, it does not naturally fill with fluid by secretion from the lining.

13.1.2 Case 2

An infant boy presents with a tiny sinus opening on the pubic region, just above the shaft of the penis, that has exuded a few drops of purulent fluid several times. The pinhole was first noticed shortly after birth when the mother was bathing the infant, who had otherwise normal male external genitalia (Fig. 13.2).

Q.2.1 What is the likely diagnosis?

A. The anomaly is a blind-ending sinus that is a variant of urethral duplication, as the sinus usually contains transitional epithelium. The discharge is likely to be secondary to contamination with faecal flora causing low-grade sepsis in the sinus.

Q.2.2 What is the aetiology?

A. The sinus is likely to be a form fruste of duplication/epispadias, which suggests that the morphological anomalies of epispadias and dorsal urethral duplication may overlap. In this regard it is important to examine the genitalia carefully to exclude epispadias, which may show failure of the two halves of the genital tubercle

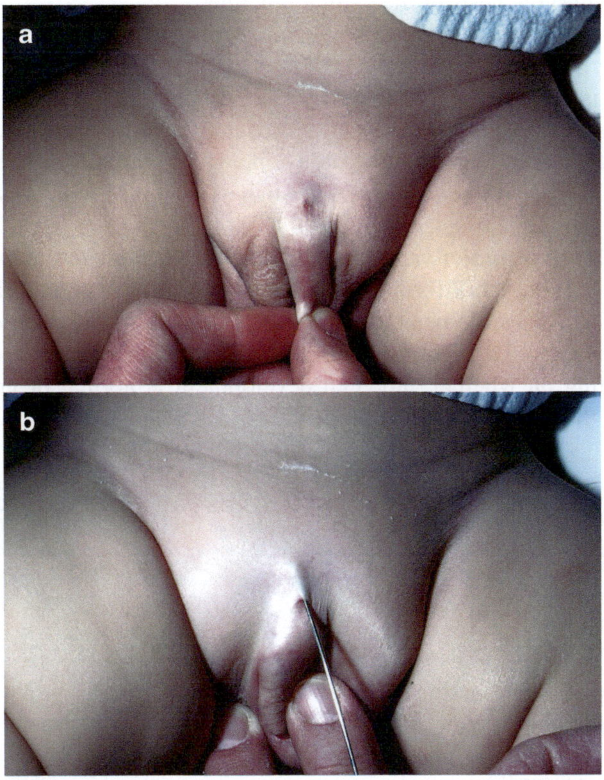

Fig. 13.2 (**a**) Congenital pre-pubic urethral sinus. (**b**) Lacrimal probe showing the sinus was about 1 cm long. (Reproduced from Pediatric diagnosis second edn, Beasley, Hutson, Stringer, Teague & King)

to fuse, leaving two hemi glans clitoris. Also it is important to check that there is no separation of the pubic symphysis.

Q.2.3 Where does this sinus go?

A. Usually it is blind-ending at the symphysis pubis, but there are reported cases of connection to the bladder neck, in which case urine may be passed through the tract.

13.1.3 Case 3

An apparently male baby presented to the neonatal ward with absence of the phallus, and an empty scrotum with no median raphe. In the perineum on the anterior rim of the anus was a small opening with pigmented skin tags around it, and from which a few drops of urine were passed (Fig. 13.3).

Q.3.1 What is the nature of the anomaly?

A. Aphallia, or penile agenesis, is presumed secondary to absence and/or loss during early embryogenesis of the genital tubercle.

Q.3.2. Is anomaly caused by androgen deficiency during sexual differentiation?

A. No, this is a non-hormonal disorder of sex development. Fusion, pigmentation and wrinkling of the scrotum shows effects of androgen between 8 and 12 weeks, but undescended testes suggest a possible deficiency of androgen in late gestation. However, the absence of the median raphe suggests a complex anomaly of morphogenesis of the genitalia affected the genital folds as well as the genital tubercle.

Q.3.3 When the genital tubercle is absent, what happens to the urethra?

A. The posterior urethra forms independently from the genital tubercle, and is usually normally present. When the genital tubercle is absent no anterior urethra can form in the male, so the urethra remains connected to the posterior cloacal structures. Depending on whether anorectal development is normal or not the urethra will open in the perineum associated with a cutaneous fistula in an anorectal

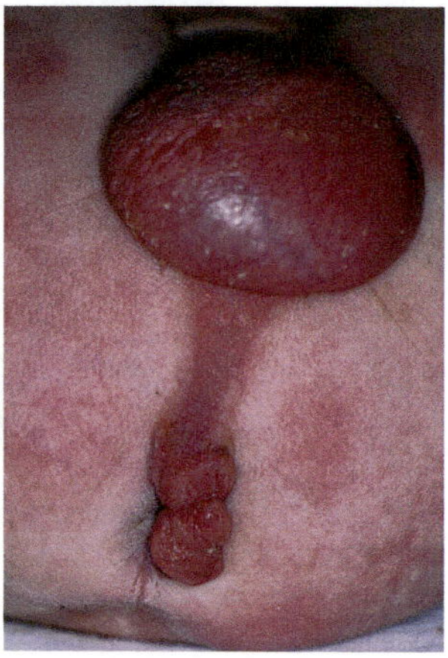

Fig. 13.3 Posterior ectopia of the penis presenting as penile agenesis. There is no phallus cranial to the scrotum which has no median raphe, but there is ectopic foreskin presenting as loose skin folds on the anterior rim of the anus. (Reproduced from Pediatric diagnosis second edn, Beasley, Hutson, Stringer, Teague & King)

malformation, or in the anterior wall of the anal canal. The skin tags represent an abortive attempt to create a foreskin [1].

Q.3.4 What does absence of the median raphe imply for prognosis?

A. In neonates with aphallia but with a normal scrotum containing a median raphe the anomaly is usually confined to the absent phallus itself, and the rest of the genitourinary system is normal. However, absence of the scrotal raphe is a marker of a more profound morphological anomaly and it is very likely that the entire urogenital tract may be abnormal, as absent scrotal raphe has a very strong association with absent or very dysplastic kidneys, so that the infant is likely to have renal failure (and may show features of Potter syndrome from oligo- or anhydramnios).

13.2 Urethral Duplication

Urethral duplication may be partial or complete. Variants include

1. Incomplete duplications presenting as cysts on the glans adjacent to the urethral meatus.
2. Short, incomplete duplications with an ectopic opening lateral or dorsal to the orthotopic urethral meatus. The second urethra many be very short, and blind-ending in the glans or extend down the shaft of the penis and into the sphincter zone of the posterior urethra.
3. Long, complete duplications may enter the bladder parallel to the orthotopic urethra or have an ectopic pathway through a deficient pubic symphysis, suggesting a relationship with an epispadiac urethra.
4. Long ectopic duplications may form an "H" fistula linking the bladder neck with the anterior rim of the anal canal.
5. Urethral duplication can be part of a caudal duplication syndrome [2].

Simple/short duplications are treated by marsupialisation or complete excision while complex/complete duplications may be not amenable to excision but might need ligation and division where they exit from the bladder. In some cases it may be impossible to tell which of the two urethral channels is the orthotopic one, but this may not matter as long as the urethral channel left behind has a continence mechanism.

13.2.1 Case 4

A 10-year-old boy presented with a recurrent stricture in the urethra and a history of recurrent sepsis in the urinary tract, which occurred whenever he had a urethral dilatation for his stricture. He had a past history of proximal hypospadias with a bifid scrotum and a unilateral impalpable undescended testis. The hypospadias had been repaired in infancy and the groin explored, but no testis was identified, and it was assumed that he had a vanishing testis. In early childhood he developed a recurrent urethral stricture at the proximal end of the neourethra, and this was treated by recurrent dilatations under GA in the local country hospital. Frequently after the dilatations he developed a urinary tract infection which often required intravenous antibiotics after signs of bacteraemia/septicaemia appeared.

Q.4.1 Why does he develop sepsis so frequently after urethral dilatation of the anterior urethral stricture?

A. The original clinical problem was thought to be hypospadias and vanishing testis, but in fact he had an undiagnosed disorder of sex development with mixed chromosomes (XO/XY) producing a streak gonad and retained hemiuterus and hemivagina on the ipsilateral side. After the hypospadias repair the increased distal urethral resistance led to progressive enlargement of the vaginal remnant. Eventually the 'utriculus' formed a large urine-storing cavity that became chronically infected with *E. coli.* The large cavity was demonstrated on urethrogram (Fig. 13.4).

Q.4.2 What is the anatomy of the vas deferens and ejaculatory duct when there is an enlarged prostatic utricle?

A. In rare cases the involution of the distal Müllerian ducts and vaginal plate are incomplete despite normally functioning hormones (AMH/DHT). In this rare circumstance it would be expected that there should be a normal verumontanum in the posterior urethra, with a small opening on the summit of the mound between the two ejaculatory ducts. Enlargement of this small cavity is rare in childhood but it occasionally presents in adults with lower urinary tract symptoms.

More frequently the 'prostatic utricle' is really a vaginal remnant in a child with a DSD, as evidenced by the ambiguity of the external genitalia. During urethroscopy a retained vaginal remnant can be identified by the absence of the verumontanum, (which indicates deficient androgenic function), and the opening is frequently lower in the posterior urethra than the normal verumonatanum. In addition, a retained

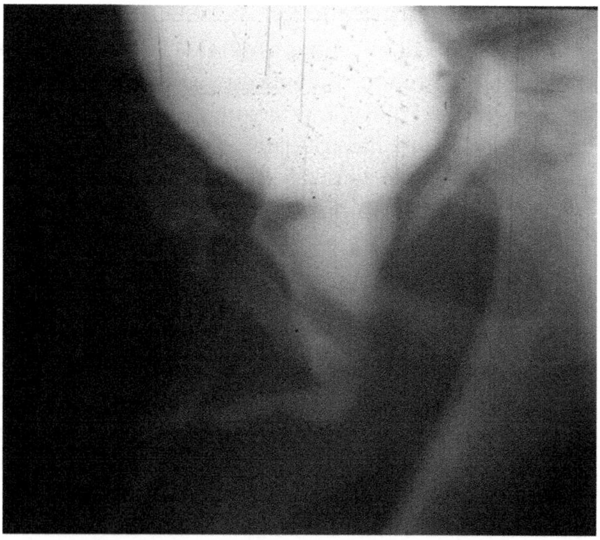

Fig. 13.4 Retrograde urethrogram showing irregular neourethra after previous hypospadias repair and a retained vaginal remnant attached to the posterior urethra

vaginal remnant often has mucusal folds obscuring the opening, which represent hymenal tissue.

Usually the vasa deferentia open into the top of the vaginal remnant on each side, and the distal Wolffian duct structures, the seminal vesicles and ejaculatory ducts, have undergone regression and are absent.

13.2.2 Case 5

A 5-year-old boy presents with a 1-year history of recurrent suprapubic pain, fever and swelling and tenderness of the right hemiscrotum. He has a past history of penoscrotal hypospadias managed successfully by a two-stage urethroplasty. At the first procedure for chordee release he had a cystoscopy,that showed a moderate-sized utriculus of about 1 cm in length. Scrotal ultrasound excludes ischaemia of the testis and shows increased blood flow in a swollen epididymis.

Q.5.1 Why is this boy developing epididymitis?

A. Epididymis is an infection of the epididymis, nearly always by spread of organisms up the vas deferens from the urinary tract, not from the blood, as blood-borne infections preferentially seed to organs with a high blood flow. Transmission of germs along the vas requires a patent lumen, which occurs only when there is circulating androgens, e.g. at 3–6 months of age at minipuberty and in puberty itself, from 13 years of age and older. In rare circumstances faecal flora can travel along the vas deferens to the epididymis when there is increased pressure in the urethra during voiding, which occurs in boys having CIC for neurogenic bladder, and after hypospadias repair. In the latter the urethroplasty increases urethral resistance, and if there is a retained utriculus, as in this boy, the utriculus may enlarge and urine (along with faecal flora) may be pushed up the vas deferens. The boy's suprapubic pain may be caused by chronic inflammation in the enlarged utriculus, as the urine-storing cavity has become colonised by faecal organisms.

Q.5.2 What treatment options are there?

A. Long-term antibiotic treatment sometimes works but risks allowing the microbiome to adapt and cause sepsis with antibiotic-resistant organisms. The retained vaginal cavity may need excision, but since the vasa drain into it this is tantamount to doing bilateral vasectomy. Nevertheless, surgical excision and/or bilateral vasectomy may prevent chronic inflammation in the epididymis which enables it to function as a normal site for sperm maturation after puberty. Fertility can then be achieved by aspiration of mature sperm from the epididymis and *in vitro* fertilisation.

13.3 Enlarged Prostatic Utricle

During development the mesonephric (Wolffian) ducts initially drain the "middle kidney", or mesonephros to the urogenital sinus [3]. Later the Müllerian ducts form as invaginations of the peritoneum covering the urogenital ridge at the cranial poles of the developing gonads. Each Müllerian duct elongates as a solid epithelial cord that canalises to form a lumen, passing caudally, following the adjacent Wolffian duct. Below the gonads the Müllerian ducts rotate around the Wolffian ducts and come in contact with each other, then as a fused, double cord migrate to the urogenital sinus between the Wolffian ducts. Contact with the urogenital sinus triggers proliferation of the epithelium to form the Müllerian tubercle. In developing females the Müllerian tubercle triggers proliferation of epithelium to form the vaginal plate, which subsequently canalises to form the vagina. By contrast, in male fetuses the circulating androgens suppress formation of the vaginal plate and anti-Mullerian hormone (AMH, also called Müllerian Inhibiting Substance, MIS) causes regression of the Müllerian ducts, leaving a small cranial remnant, the hydatid of Morgagni, and probably a small caudal remnant, the prostatic utriculus. The latter structure is short, blind-ending cavity opening onto the summit of the verumontanum between the two ejaculatory ducts [4].

The prostatic utricle is usually short, <0.5 cm, but in disorders of sex development (DSD) where androgen and AMH levels are lower than in a normal male, the cavity may be much larger, representing a persistent vagina [5].

When the cavity has canalised to form a persistent vagina, its opening in the posterior urethra is abnormally lower, near to the bulb of the urethra, and the verumontanum is absent.

The enlarged vaginal remnant may fill with urine on voiding, which can distort the urethra and lead to partial obstruction [6]. A urine-storing vagina also may become a reservoir for infected urine, leading to recurrent and/or chronic urinary sepsis. During urethral catheterisation, the catheter commonly enters the vagina rather than the bladder.

Excision of a retained vaginal remnant can be done by laparoscopy, but also sometimes by a transvescial approach as described by Monfort, and occasionally by a simple perineal approach to the bulb. In patients with a 46, XY DSD and a retained vaginal remnant the cranial ends of the Müllerian ducts are usually absent, as the dysplastic testes still make enough AMH to cause regression of the fallopian tubes and uterus. In this circumstance the Wolffian ducts usually drain into the vault of the vaginal cavity, so surgical excision of the vaginal remnant is tantamount to bilateral vasectomy.

Occasionally an enlarged prostatic utricle opens on a normal verumontanum, and in this case the cause is unlikely to be deficient androgen and AMH, but a morphological anomaly of the Müllerian tubercle and its subsequent canalisation.

13.3.1 Case 6

An adolescent boy presents with a history of acute/chronic urethritis for 6–12 months, with dysuria but only occasional malaise and fever. Urethroscopy shows a normal anterior urethra and normal posterior urethra around the verumontanum, and the bladder itself is normal, with no cystitis cystica. Around the proximal portion of the anterior urethra and bulb, however, the urethral mucosa is chronically inflamed.

Q.6.1 What is the likely diagnosis?

A. Acute/chronic infection in one or both Cowper's glands, which respond to pubertal androgen by some enlargement and secretion of mucus, which can become infected by faecal flora. Occasionally, an ultrasound scan via the perineum may show the inflamed Cowper's gland behind the bulb of the urethra.

Q.6.2. Is surgery required?

A. Only on rare occasions when an abscess may form, but usually antibiotic treatment for some weeks is sufficient to clear the infection and allow for re-establishment of function of the gland. If the duct becomes blocked by inflammatory debris the sepsis may drain spontaneously into the urethra, and create a syringocele.

13.4 Cowper's Gland Cysts and Syringoceles

Cowper's glands develop as solid paired epithelial buds in the urogenital sinus at the junction of the pelvic and perineal urethra. The buds canalise and the mucus-secreting Cowper's glands come to lie just behind the posterior urethra distal to the external sphincter. The ducts elongate with growth of the bulbar urethra and open into the anterior urethra, with two paramedian small orifices.

The Cowper's gland duct can be obstructed, which leads to a dilated proximal duct that may obstruct the urine flow in the urethra. An ectatic duct opening may obstruct micturition like a spinnaker sail: a syringocele [7, 8].

Infection in the Cowper's glands may be the cause of posterior urethritis in adolescent boys.

At cystoscopy a syringocele will appear as a defect in the ventral floor of the urethra, which may need division of its distal edge by diathermy hook or cold knife to overcome urinary obstruction.

13.4.1 Case 7

You are called to the neonatal ward to see a newborn female, as the staff report seeing a mass protruding from the introitus. Physical examination shows an otherwise normal female baby with no genital ambiguity. The vagina is partly covered by hymenal folds and there is a 1 cm diameter mass protruding from the urethral meatus. Abdominal examination as well as careful rectal examination exclude a significant space-occupying lesion in the pelvis. While you are doing the examination both urine and stool are passed, and both are normal.

Q.7.1 What is the differential diagnosis?

A. The conditions causing a mass protruding from the urethra in an infant female include (1) prolapsing ureterocele in an infant with renal duplication (2) a urethral polyp (Fig. 13.5) (3) prolapsing urethral mucosa (Fig. 13.6) or (4) a prolapsing rhabdomyosarcoma, usually arising from the bladder base (Fig. 13.7).

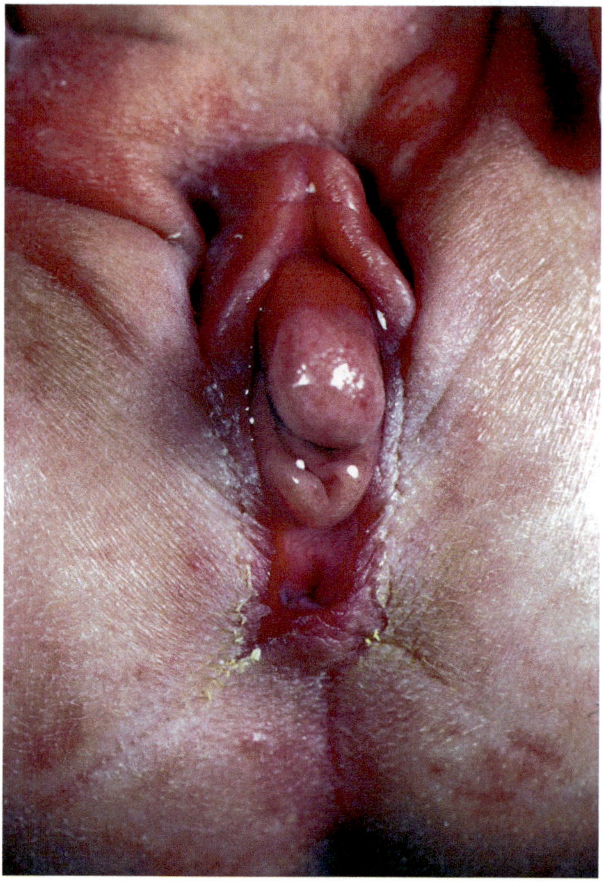

Fig. 13.5 Urethral polyp in a baby girl. (Reproduced from Pediatric diagnosis second edn, Beasley, Hutson, Stringer, Teague & King)

13.4.2 Case 8

A male toddler presents with a long history of intermittent difficulty passing urine, where sometimes he could void easily and other times he was straining and could only manage a few drops. Posterior urethral valve is suspected and an MCU is performed, that shows a filling defect in the bulbar urethra (Fig. 13.8).

Q.8.1 What is the likely diagnosis?

A. A urethral polyp is a rare cause of strangury in a boy but the intermittent feature of the symptoms suggests this is likely, as the polyp develops a long stalk secondary to the force of the urinary stream, and the polyp can flop into the bladder or urethra from its insertion at the verumontanum

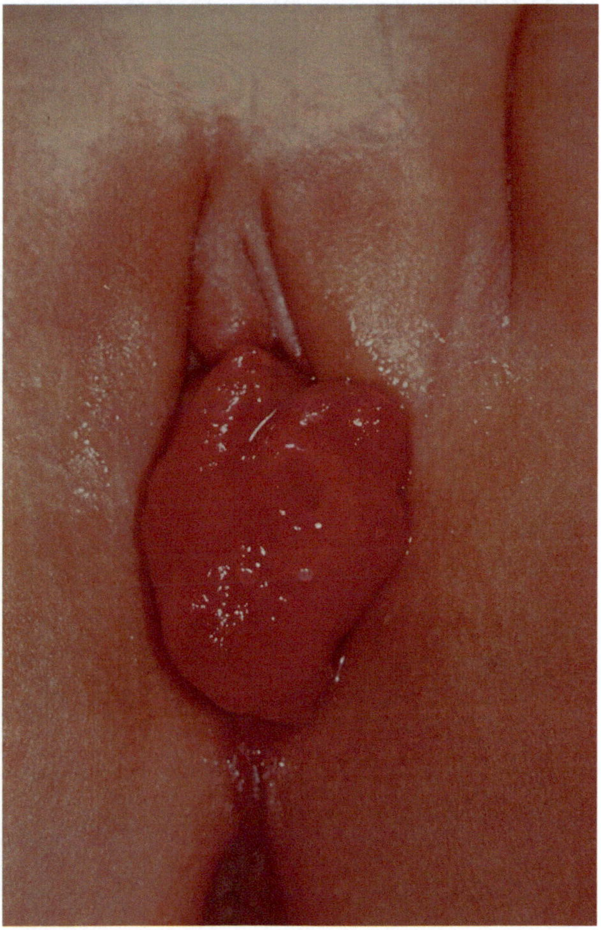

Fig. 13.6 Urethral prolapse in a small girl. (Reproduced from Pediatric diagnosis second edn, Beasley, Hutson, Stringer, Teague & King)

13.5 Verumontanum Polyp

This is a rare anomaly that is thought to be caused by abnormality of the absorption of the common stem of the Wolffian duct into the back of the urogenital sinus [3].

The polyp causes partial and intermittent obstruction of the urinary stream during voiding, and if diagnosis is delayed may lead to renal failure, similar to that seen in posterior urethral valve. The polyp acts like a ball valve in the urethra [9].

Management includes confirmation of diagnosis by MCU, where a mobile filling defect will be seen in the posterior urethra or bladder, depending on the direction of flow of the contrast.

Surgery is cystoscopy and excision of the polyp and its stalk where it arises from the verumontanum.

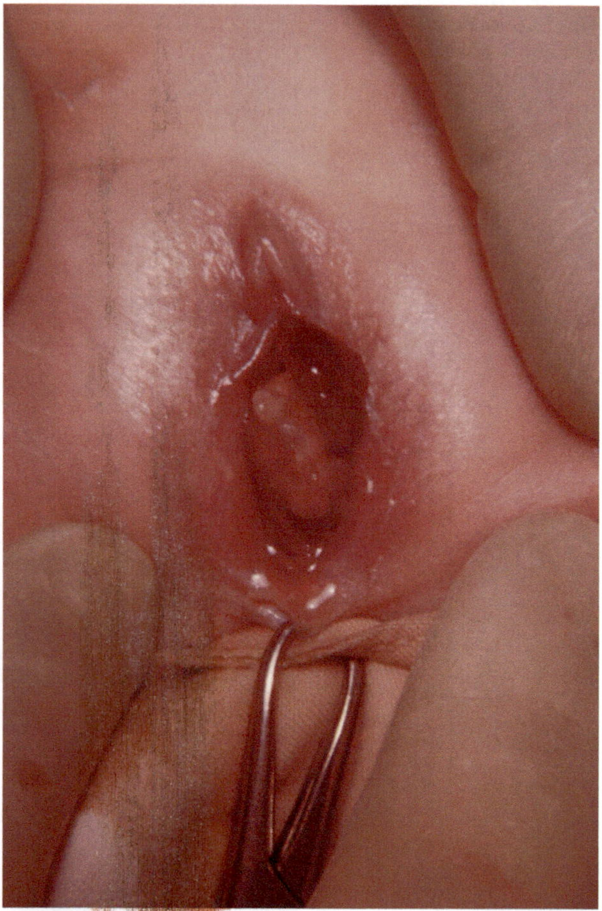

Fig. 13.7 Prolapse of a rhabdomyosarcoma of the bladder. (Reproduced from Pediatric diagnosis second edn, Beasley, Hutson, Stringer, Teague & King)

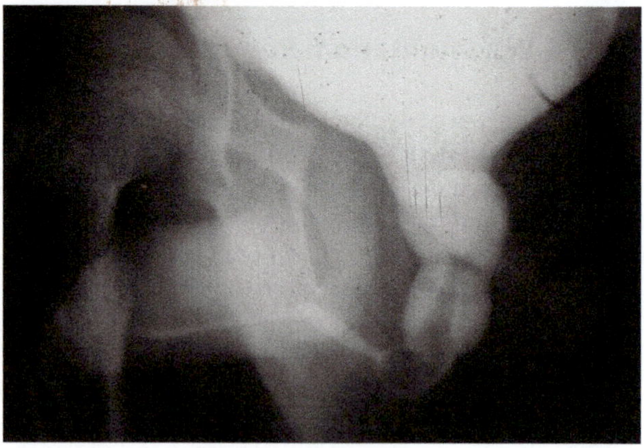

Fig. 13.8 Urethral polyp in a boy, shown on MCU. There is proximal dilatation of the posterior urethra and bladder with a narrow anterior urethra. The polyp, which is on a stalk arising from the verumontanum, is occluding the bulbar urethra. (Reproduced from Pediatric diagnosis second edn, Beasley, Hutson, Stringer, Teague & King)

Urethral polyp can also occur in the female, when the polyp usually presents as a solid lesion prolapsing from the urethral meatus. A urethral polyp in either sex must be distinguished from a rhabdomyosarcoma, which may occur in infants and even in the neonate, especially in those patients carrying the genetic anomaly causing neurofibromatosis, type 1 (NF1).

References

1. Srinivasan J, McDougall P, Hutson JM. When is 'intersex' not intersex? A case of penile agenesis demonstrates how to distinguish non-endocrine disorders in neonates with genital anomaly. J Paediatr Child Health. 2003;39(8):629–31.
2. Swaika S, Basu S, Bhadra RC, Sarkar R, Maitra SK. Caudal duplication syndrome-report of a case and review of literature. Indian J Surg. 2013;75(Suppl 1):484–7.
3. Stephens FD, Smith ED, Hutson JM. Congenital anomalies of the kidney, urinary ad genital tracts. 2nd ed. London: Martin Dunitz; 2002.
4. Ben-Meir D, Hutson JM. The anatomy of the caudal vas deferens in patients with a genital anomaly. J Pediatr Urol. 2005;1(5):349–54.
5. Kato H. Re: Male vagina is a more accurate term than prostatic utricle. Int J Urol. 2016;23(6):530.
6. le Vaillant C, Podevin G, Quere MP, Talmant C, Heloury Y, Boog G. Prenatal diagnosis of enlarged prostatic utricle by ultrasonography and magnetic resonance imaging. Ultrasound Obstet Gynecol. 2008;31(5):588–9.
7. McLellan DL, Gaston MV, Diamond DA, Lebowitz RL, Mandell J, Atala A, et al. Anterior urethral valves and diverticula in children: a result of ruptured Cowper's duct cyst? BJU Int. 2004;94(3):375–8.
8. Kajiwara M, Inoue K, Kato M, Usui A, Matsubara A, Usui T. Anterior urethral valves in children: a possible association between anterior urethral valves and Cowper's duct cyst. Int J Urol. 2007;14(2):156–60.
9. Fathi K, Azmy A, Howatson A, Carachi R. Congenital posterior urethral polyps in childhood. A case report. Eur J Pediatr Surg. 2004;14(3):215–7.

Hypospadias

14

(Glanular Hypospadias, Proximal Hypospadias, 5α Reductase Deficiency, Midshaft Hypospadias, Megameatus Intact Prepuce, Failed Hypospadias Repair)

Felicitas López Imizcoz, Elías Ramírez Velázquez, and Imran Mushtaq

Learning Objectives

- Practical aspects of diagnosis and classification of hypospadias subtypes
- To review the evidence base for preoperative hormone treatments and potential indications
- To describe the surgical decision-making based on published outcomes
- To illustrate the challenges with DSD patients and to emphasize the importance of a multidisciplinary approach
- To discuss possible treatment options in failed hypospadias repair

14.1 Glanular Hypospadias

A 6 months old boy is referred to the urology clinic by the GP for distal hypospadias (Fig. 14.1).

1. *a. How is hypospadias classified?*
   b. What type of distal hypospadias does this baby have?
2. *What is the incidence of this condition?*
3. *What is the differential diagnosis?*
4. *Do all distal hypospadias need surgical correction?*
5. *What are the surgical options?*

F. L. Imizcoz
Hospital de Pediatría Prof. Dr. Juan P. Garrahan, Buenos Aires, Argentina

E. R. Velázquez
Hospital Star Médica HIP, México City, CDMX, Mexico

I. Mushtaq (✉)
Great Ormond Street Hospital, London, UK
e-mail: imran.mushtaq@gosh.nhs.uk

P. Godbole et al. (eds.), *Practical Pediatric Urology*,
https://doi.org/10.1007/978-3-030-54020-3_14

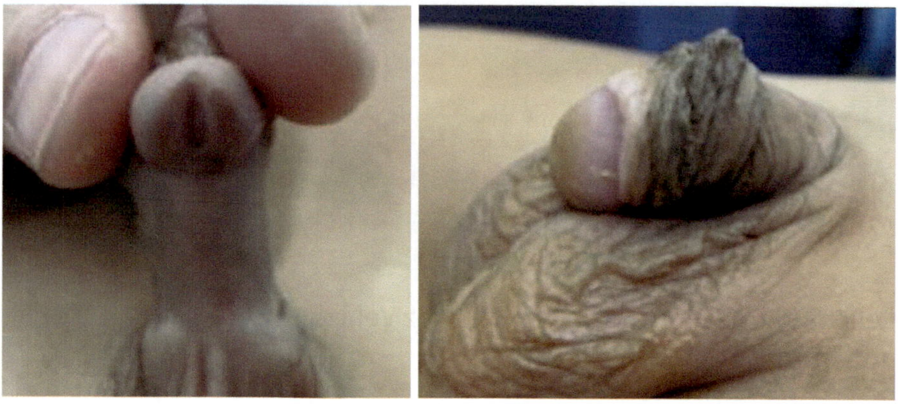

Fig. 14.1 Glanular hypospadias

1. *a.* The common classification system divides hypospadias in three different groups according to meatus position: distal-anterior hypospadias (located on the glans or distal shaft of the penis), intermediate-middle hypospadias (penile) and proximal-posterior (penoscrotal, scrotal and perineal) [1]. However, after skin release during surgery, the pathology might be different and a reclassification may need to be done. The position of the meatus alone is therefore not a reliable indicator of hypospadias severity as far as the choice of an appropriate surgical procedure is concerned [1, 2]. Several aspects should be considered such as: level of division of the corpus spongiosum, the degree of hypoplasia of the tissues forming the ventral surface, degree of curvature, urethral plate quality, penile size, glans size and shape and preputial skin availability [2]. The EUA Guidelines (2018) on Pediatric Urology suggest an alternative classification based on severity of the problem: mild hypospadias (glanular or penile isolated hypospadias without associated chordee, micropenis or scrotal anomaly); and severe hypospadias (penoscrotal, perineal hypospadias with associated chordee and scrotal anomalies) [1].

   b. This baby has a glanular hypospadias. Clinical examination alone is sufficient for the diagnosis. The clinical findings include:
   - Glanular meatus, above and distal to the coronal sulcus.
   - Good glans size and groove.
   - Hooded foreskin, deficient ventrally.
   - No curvature (chordee).
   - Both testes fully descended.
2. In newborn males, hypospadias is the second most common congenital anomaly after undescended testis [3]. Over the last 25 years, a significant increase in the incidence of hypospadias has been found which may simply reflect a more frequent or early diagnosis of minor forms of hypospadias over time, or an increasing tendency to report them to congenital-anomaly registries [4]. According to

the last EUROCAT registry-based study (from 2001 to 2010) the total prevalence of hypospadias in Europe is 18.6 new cases out of 10,000 births (5.1–36.8). The mean worldwide prevalence varies from 34.2 in North America, 5.2 in South America, 0.6–69 in Asia, 5.9 in Africa and 17.1–34.8 in Australia [1].

3. The differential diagnosis includes other forms of distal hypospadias. This is the most common type and represent 65% of all cases of hypospadias [1, 5]. They include four distinct forms: glanular 15%, coronal 50%, sub coronal 30% (distal shaft of the penis) and a fourth type mega meatus with intact prepuce (MIP) which represents 5% [5, 6].
4. The primary goal of hypospadias repair is to achieve both cosmetic and functional normality [7]. In theory therefore, penile curvature must be corrected and a neo-urethra of an adequate size with opening on the tip of the glans formed, with adequate skin coverage of the penile shaft [8]. Ironically, the very distal forms of hypospadias, are sometimes the most challenging in terms of the decision-making process, because cosmesis is often the only real indication for surgery [7]. Meatal stenosis, a ventrally deflected urine stream and parent preference are the most usual indications for surgical correction of glanular hypospadias. Increasing dissatisfaction with urethroplasty techniques, such as the Snodgrass repair, have led to many surgeons preferring more minimal procedures (circumcision, chordee correction, meatoplasty) that have minimal complications but an equal patient and parent satisfaction.

   According to a survey conducted by the European association of urology including pediatric urologists, pediatric surgeons, urologists, and plastic surgeons in 68 countries, 78% opted for a surgical management on distal hypospadias and only 12% for non-surgical approach [9]. Although the majority of pediatric urologists choose a surgical correction for distal hypospadias, conservative management is still a valid option considering there is not always functional compromise in these group of patients. Parents should be fully informed about all the different management options.
5. For children with glanular hypospadias, the need for surgery and the surgical technique to be used remain controversial. Techniques described include meatal advancement and glanuloplasty (MAGPI) [9], meatal mobilization and glanuloplasty (MMGPI) [5], glanular approximation procedure (GAP) [6], a simple modified circumcision and meatoplasty, tubularized incised plate procedure (TIP) and Mathieu flap technique. Case selection is a crucial factor influencing the complication rate. For example, the MAGPI technique is one of the most common operation for glanular and coronal hypospadias repair. Ventral glanular tilt, meatal retraction (seen in up to 22%) [10] and splaying of the urinary stream can result from performing a MAGPI in a patient with non-compliant urethra with deep grooved glans [8]. Whatever technique is used, one should expect a predictable outcome with complication rates below 10% in distal hypospadias (fistula, meatal stenosis, dehiscence, recurrent ventral curvature, and haematoma) [1].

14.2 Proximal Hypospadias

A male infant is born at 33 weeks' gestation (IVF twin pregnancy). He attends the clinic at the age of 3 months because his parents are concerned that he urinates from the base of a small penis. Both testes are palpable on the scrotum (Fig. 14.2).

1. *What is the most likely diagnosis?*
2. *What other clinical features are mandatory to examine in a boy with this diagnosis?*
3. *What are the risk factors for this condition?*
4. *Is hormone therapy recommended in this case?*
5. *What are the surgical options for this condition?*

1. The most likely diagnosis is proximal-posterior penoscrotal hypospadias.
2. The diagnostic evaluation, apart from the hypospadias clinical features, includes an assessment of associated anomalies, which are:
   - cryptorchidism (in up to 10% of cases of hypospadias);
   - patent processus vaginalis or inguinal hernia (in 9–15%) [1].

   Severe hypospadias with unilaterally or bilaterally impalpable testes, or with ambiguous genitalia, requires a complete genetic and endocrine work-up immediately after birth to exclude a disorder of sex development (DSD), especially congenital adrenal hyperplasia [1].
1. Risk factors associated with hypospadias can be genetic, placental and/or environmental (Level of Evidence: 2b) [1, 11]. In the case of this infant, prematurity, low weight at birth together with in vitro fertilization (IVF) would be identified

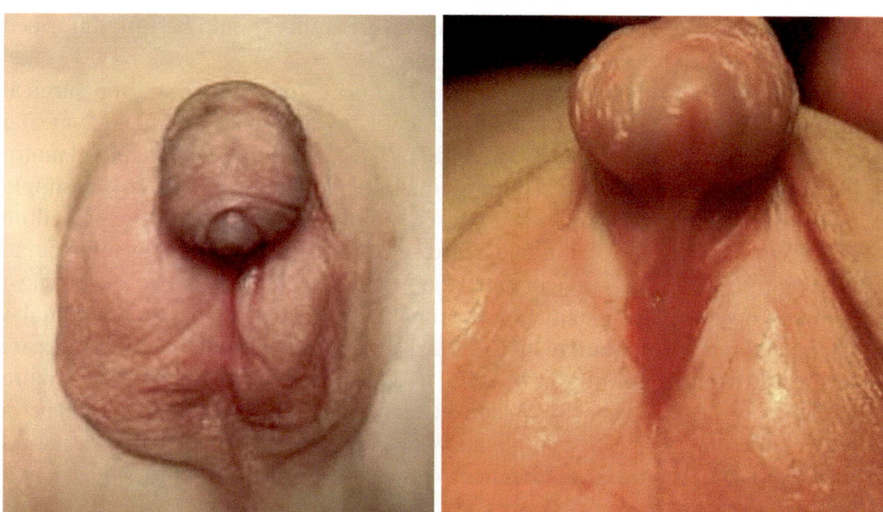

Fig. 14.2 Proximal-posterior hypospadias

as risk factors to his condition. IVF is associated to a five-fold increased risk of hypospadias, which may be related to maternal progesterone administration [12]. Parents should be counseled about this risk as well as the possibility that 7% of other family members may also be affected [1]. Interactions between genetic and environmental factors may help explain non-replication in genetic studies of hypospadias. The use of oral contraceptives prior to pregnancy has not been associated with an increased risk of hypospadias in offspring, but their use after conception increases the risk of middle and posterior hypospadias [1].

2. Pre-operative hormonal treatment may be recommended in this case due to small penile and glans size. Therapy options are local or parenteral application of testosterone, dihydrotestosterone or beta-chorionic gonadotropin. It use is limited to small appearing penis, reduced glans circumference or reduced urethral plate because it was reported to lead to significant enlargement of the glans and shaft of the penis (Level of Evidence: 1b) [13, 14]. According to expert opinion, a small penis is defined as penile length <25 mm during the first year of life and a glans with a diameter <14 mm [15].

   Moderate quality evidence from three randomized controlled studies demonstrated significantly lower rates of urethrocutaneous fistulae and reoperation rates in patients who received pre-operative hormonal treatment [16].

   Side effects such as changes in child's behavior, increased genital pigmentation, appearance of pubic hair, penile skin irritation and redness, increased erections and peri-operative bleeding have been reported, but no persistent side effects related to hormonal stimulation have been reported in the literature. There is also no evidence about possible effects on bone maturation [16–18].

3. Surgical options for this infant include either one stage repair versus a two stage repair. Considering the short urethral plate, the severe ventral curvature (more than 45°) and the proximal division of corpora spongiosum, this infant is most likely to require a two-stage repair. The decision making should be taken after assessment of the length and quality of the urethral plate and the degree of chordee once the penis has been degloved [1].

   Previously reported series of single-stage repairs for proximal defects have reported high complication rates of 20–50% [19]. Regardless of convincing results recently published [20], in the survey conducted by the European association of urology, the TIP repair in the correction of proximal hypospadias is not widely used and around 43.3–76.6% prefer a two-stage repair for these complex cases [9]. The two-stage procedure has become more popular due to lower risk of chordee recurrence and more robust long term favorable outcome [1].

   Two stage procedures include two-stage preputial flaps (Byars or Dennis Brown) or two-stage preputial graft repair (Bracka). According to Cuckow et al. [21], in a cohort of 208 pediatric patients who underwent two-stage Bracka procedure using free grafts (preputial, buccal or retro auricular), cosmetic and functional result were considered excellent in 90% of patients, good in 3.7% and 6.3% required reoperation. Complications after the second stage were: urethrocutaneous fistulae (3.4%), meatal stenosis (1.4%), and three partial glans dehiscence (1.4%).

14.3 DSD (5α Reductase Deficiency)

A new-born baby, with no antenatal history, is in NICU for respiratory distress. The neonatal team is concerned with the sex assignment due to the genital appearance, which are ambiguous with severe penoscrotal transposition, a small phallus, perineal-scrotal hypospadias, bifid scrotum and two perineal openings (Fig. 14.3). Both gonads are palpable in the genital folds.

1. *How are these group of disorders named?*
2. *How should this patient be managed?*
3. *What is the most likely diagnosis and what are the differential diagnosis?*
4. *When is the best timing for surgical repair? Is hormone therapy indicated in this case?*

1. These disorders, formerly called 'intersex disorders', are characterized by a presentation in which there is a discordance between chromosomal, gonadal, or anatomical sex [1]. They were renamed in 2005 as "disorders of sex development" (DSD), by the European Society for Paediatric Endocrinology and the Lawson Wilkins Pediatric Endocrinology Society in a document known as the Chicago Consensus Statement [22]. However, in a recent publication, Gorduza et al. suggest a new terminology to avoid the confusion and distress the terms 'disorder' or 'sex' may cause [23]. The term "anomalies of gonadal/genital development" (AGD) was proposed to outline the current surgical approach to these very distinct conditions and address the many current controversies regarding each of them. AGD can be divided into five main groups: virilized 46 XX, unvirilized 46 XY, chromosomic mosaicism or chimerism (essentially the mixed gonadal dysgenesis 45 XO/46 XY and 46 XX/46 XY), ovotesticular 46 XX and heterogeneous category including cloacal exstrophy, aphallia and some complex cloacal anomalies.
2. This baby should be referred to a DSD multidisciplinary team, comprising geneticists, pediatric urologist, gynaecologists, endocrinologists, psychologists and biochemists. The challenge during the neonatal period is to use the information available to make the most appropriate choice in order to select a gender concor-

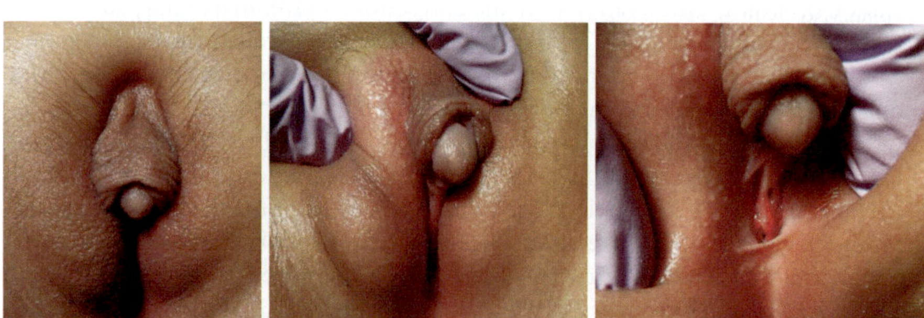

Fig. 14.3 Desorder of sex development (DSD)

dant with the individual identity of the child (which is invisible during this period), the social identity (which is the way the 'society' looks at the individual and the only tangible identity approachable after birth) and the behavioral identity, which is not yet apparent [24]. The situation should be explained to the caregivers fully and kindly. Registering the birth and naming the baby should be delayed as long as necessary [1].

A careful physical examination is mandatory evaluating pigmentation of genital and areolar area, hypospadias or urogenital sinus, size of phallus, palpable and/or symmetrical gonads and blood pressure [1]. If it is possible to palpate a gonad, it is almost certainly a testis; this clinical finding therefore virtually excludes 46XX DSD [1]. The following laboratory investigations are needed for the initial assessment: karyotype, plasma 17-hydroxyprogesterone assay and plasma electrolytes. Abdominal ultrasound to evaluate the presence of Müllerian duct structures is also recommended [1].

3. Laboratory results exclude congenital adrenal hyperplasia (CAH), which is the most frequently occurring DSD. Karyotype result is 46 XY. Abdominal US revealed no Mullerian structures. Endocrine evaluation detected elevated mean plasma testosterone but low dihydrotestosterone (DHT) levels. After hCG stimulation, the testosterone-to-DHT ratio increased to greater than 20:1. According to these results, this baby's most likely diagnosis is a 5-α-Reductase type 2 deficiency. The diagnosis is confirmed by sequencing the entire 5α-reductase type 2 *(SRD5A2)* gene [25]. It is a rare autosomal recessive sex-limited condition resulting in the inability to convert testosterone to the more physiologically active DHT. Wide range of genital ambiguity can manifest at birth and pronounced masculinization at puberty.

Differential diagnosis includes other apparent female DSD with clitoral hypertrophy, such as CAH or other under virilized 46 XY such as partial androgen insensitivity syndrome (PAIS). Genetic studies will exclude 46XX or chromosomal mosaicism. Furthermore, endocrine evaluation is crucial to determine exact entity.

4. In reference to the consensus statement [22], it is clear that the timing of surgery is nowadays much more controversial. The rationale for early surgery includes: beneficial effects of oestrogens on infant tissue; minimizing family anxiety; mitigating the risks of stigmatization and gender-identity confusion [26]. However, adverse outcomes have led to recommendations to delay unnecessary surgery to an age when the patient can give informed consent. Surgery that alters appearance is not urgent [1].

   In this case, where male assignment has been done early in life, treatment includes hormone and surgical correction of severe hypospadias. Knowing that 5-α-Reductase type 2 deficiency patients will have an acceptable physiological virilization during puberty, deferring hypospadias reconstruction may be advantageous. Although the recommended age for surgical correction of hypospadias is 6–18 (24) months [1], there is a view that this group should be the exception and hypospadias repair should be delayed until post puberty.

14.4 Midshaft Hypospadias

A year-old male infant is referred to the urology service by the GP for hypospadias. On clinical examination both testes are in the scrotum, there is some degree of chordee with a midshaft meatus and hooded foreskin. The glans is small and has no groove (Fig. 14.4).

1. What is the incidence of midshaft hypospadias?
2. Are all midshaft hypospadias treated in the same way?
3. a. What are the surgical options for this case?
   b. Is a graft needed?
4. How is the follow up of hypospadias patients?

1. Midshaft hypospadias is the least common variety, accounts for 10% of hypospadias [7].
2. Midshaft hypospadias should be reassessed after the shaft has been degloved and the degree of chordee is measured [1]. The level of division of the corpus spongiosum is the main determinant of the severity of hypospadias, as the urethral segment sitting proximal to the meatus is usually hypoplastic and deficient of spongiosum. Only then can the appropriate urethroplasty technique be chosen for each case in particular, not being able to universalize one technique [2]. Caregivers should be correctly informed about the different options before the surgery takes place.
3. a. During this baby's surgery, after shaft is degloved, mild chordee (<30°) is evident, and the urethral plate is adequate to be preserved. Chordee is corrected with a dorsal plication. Assessment of the urethral plate is crucial to determine whether it can be closed without a midline incision (Thiersch-Duplay), if a

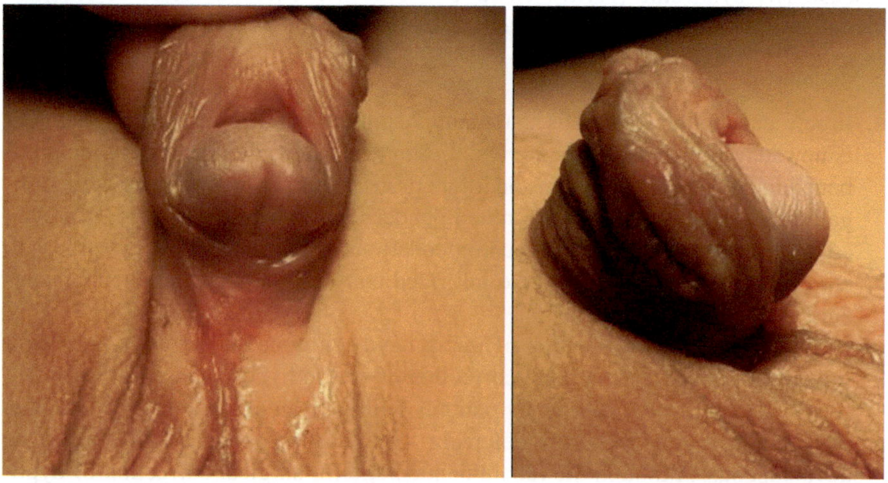

Fig. 14.4 Midshaft hypospadias

medial deep dorsal incision is required (Snodgrass TIP procedure), or if augmentation is necessary (onlay flap, Snodgraft procedure). However, this assessment is somewhat subjective [2, 15]. Mouriquand believes that length, width and thickness define the quality of the urethral plate and therefore need to be taken into account in decision making [15]. Ru W et al. highlights the value of the ratio between the urethral plate and the glans width for objectivity and accuracy in urethral plate evaluation, which in turn serves as an independent factor influencing outcomes in tubularized incised plate repair [27]. According to Seleim et al., in a recent prospective evaluation of 104 preservable narrow plate primary hypospadias repair (<8 mm), 4 mm width is the lower limit of clinical relevance that defines poor urethral plate [28].

b. In this case, an augmenting graft should be considered as a good option. In the presence of a narrow, shallow, inelastic urethral plate and conical small glans, a more substantial augmentation is required, rather than just incising the plate [7]. This can apply to distal hypospadias, but more particularly to severe penile forms where the application of an extended Snodgrass procedure may generate concerns for the long-term outcome [7]. The onlay preputial island flap, described by Duckett, is a good option. However, the more recent Snodgraft procedure could also be considered. The resulting meatus is wide and slit like. The excellent take of graft material enables a satisfactory urethra to be recessed back into the glans [29]. The Snodgraft procedure has been also utilized in redo hypospadias repair and specifically BXO cases [7].

5. EUA Guidelines strongly recommend long-term follow-up to detect urethral stricture, voiding dysfunctions, recurrent penile curvature, ejaculation dysfunction and patient satisfaction [1]. However, urethral performance after reconstruction is still difficult to assessed. Most often surgeons only rely upon the parent's or the patient's views, or the observation of the urine stream is not done in optimal conditions. Urine flow studies are not reliable as most patients who received urethral surgery have long-lasting dyssynergic voiding and because the urodynamic profile of the reconstructed urethra is abnormal even without significant urethral stricture [7]. This explains why most urine flow studies after hypospadias surgery have a flat profile despite satisfactory urethroplasty [15]. Although peak flow rates and uroflow curve rates have unclear meaning, Snodgrass recommends urethroscopy when there is a flat tracing with a flow rate less than 5 cc/s, and/or in patients with obstructive voiding symptoms [15]. The use of validated objective scoring systems to assist in evaluating the functional and cosmetic outcome should be developed [1].

14.5 Mega-Meatus Intact Prepuce (MIP)

A 2-year old boy is referred to the clinic because parents notice a wide meatus proximal to the coronal sulcus with splayed urinary stream and normal retractable prepuce (Fig. 14.5).

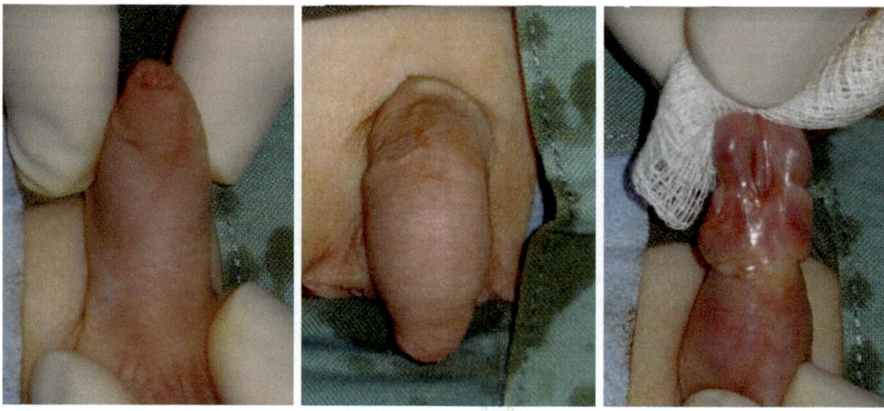

Fig. 14.5 Megameatus intact prepuce (MIP)

1. What is the most likely diagnosis?
2. What are the clinical features that characterizes this entity?
3. How is the diagnosis done? Is it the same as other type of hypospadias?
4. What is the incidence of this condition?
5. What are the different modalities of treatment?

1. The most likely diagnosis is megameatus with intact prepuce.
2. MIP is a unique anatomical variant of hypospadias characterized by a deep glanular groove, a large meatus and an intact prepuce that completely covers the glans [30].
3. Diagnosis and management of MIP can be particularly challenging [31]. Typical hypospadias diagnosis is usually straightforward, identified at birth or even antenatally [32]. However, in MIP cases, the diagnosis is often delayed either late in life in non-circumcised boys at the time of retraction of the prepuce or at the time of neonatal circumcision [30]. It was once hypothesized that the cause of the glans defect was previous surgery, however it is now understood that this is a urethral formation defect [32, 33].

   There are several differences between MIP and typical distal hypospadias. In MIP, by definition, there is a completely formed prepuce with a patulous meatus, no chordee and the frenulum is usually absent [34]. Fahmy et al. identified 15 cases of MIP, in a cohort of 12,518 boys, concluding that any deviation from normal penile medial raphe (deviation, hyperpigmentation, prominent or bifurcation) should raise suspicion about presence of MIP, with a sensitivity of 80%, a specificity 99.8% and positive predictive value of 24.4% [32].
4. The MIP is a rare variant of glanular hypospadias first described by Juskiewenski et al. in 1983 [35]. The reported prevalence is 1 of 10,000 patients, which represents an incidence of 3–6.8% of all hypospadias although its true incidence is unknown given the fact that a number of patients with MIP may not be identified [32, 36].

5. Patients diagnosed with MIP variant of hypospadias should be referred to a pediatric urologist before age 6 months [36]. Surgical repair could be offered, between the age of 6–18 months, for those patients with a large fish mouth or blunderbuss appearing meatus that opens close or at the coronal margin. When the caliber of the urethral meatus is minor, the location is close to the tip of the glans with good urinary stream, surgical repair may not be necessary [36].

   Several anatomical considerations should be taken into account during MIP reconstruction surgery. In general, the urethral plate is often irregular and may extend laterally to the level of the coronal margin making the dissection more difficult. If the lateral extent of the urethra is not recognized, injury can occur at the time of repair, making reconstruction more problematic [36].

   Numerous techniques have been described, starting by Duckett and Keating in 1989 who being dissatisfied with the results of the MAGPI and peri meatal-based flap procedure, described the "pyramid procedure" [37]. Yet another technique designed to overcome the challenges of a wide, deep glanular groove and a noncompliant fish mouth procedure is the glans approximation procedure (GAP) [6]. Tubularized incised plate urethroplasty and modified Thiersch-Duplay tubularization of the urethral plate are other techniques with excellent cosmetic and functional results [36, 38]. Cedron adapted the principle of the Mathieu procedure to the repair of MIP with the advantage of an improved visualization of the urethra during dissection and also providing healthy vascularized coverage to the reconstructed urethra [36].

   Reported complications of surgical treatment are: 0–9% rate of urethra cutaneous fistula and 0–18% rate of meatal stenosis [36, 39].

14.6 Failed Hypospadias Repair

A 12-year old boy attends with his parents to the urology clinic. They are concerned about the cosmetic appearance of his penis after three surgical procedures in another centre. He is having curved erections, and has to urinate siting down on the toilet because the urine stream flows downwards. He describes abdominal straining during micturition. On clinical examinations there is firm scar tissue in the ventral aspect of the shaft, with a narrow distal penile meatus (Fig. 14.6).

1. How should this patient be managed?
2. When is the best timing for surgery?
3. What are the surgical options in this case?
4. What grafts are there available when prepuce is absent?

1. This patient is a case of failed hypospadias repair. This group includes patients with persisting functional complications after previous hypospadias repair, that present either as recurrent stricture, urethrocutaneous fistula, glans dehiscence, urethral dehiscence, chordee, or glans deformity. In a series of 100 redo hypo-

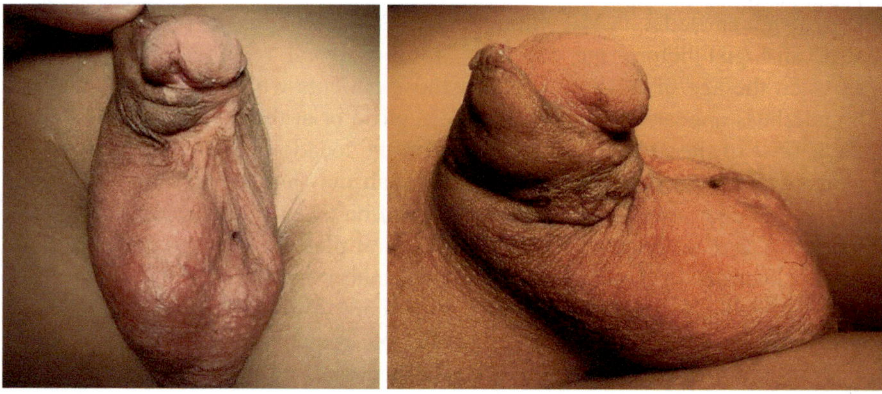

Fig. 14.6 Failed hypospadias repair

spadias surgery, BXO was found as one of the most important yet often unrecognized causes of late hypospadias failures [7].

Failed hypospadias is a complex and challenging issue [40]. Preoperative uroflowmetry and post voiding US are important to asses for any bladder or upper urinary tract compromise. The assesment should begin with a diagnostic cystoscopy to evaluate the neo-urethra and the severity of any stricture.

2. In this case, at least minimal intervention should be done as soon as possible to treat outlet obstruction. Suprapubic line or even perineal urethrostostomy should be considered as transient solution if the patient is not psychologically ready for a major reconstruction.

   Once the obstruction has been dealt with, there is controversy on the age at which to operate as well as the technique to be used. These group of patients are usually older and therefore the patient himself should play an essential role in the decision making.
3. There are no clear guidelines for the management of these types of patients [1]. Single stage repair of redo cases usually is not possible due to the lack of vascularized tissues to reconstruct the urethra, provide good skin cover and an interposing tissue layer [41]. Hence, failed hypospadias merit two-staged grafted urethroplasty [41]. Planning the surgery in a staged fashion gives the surgeon the opportunity to remove the non-vascularized tissues, address the curvature and lay down a vascularized tissue usually a graft to be utilized in a second stage for urethral reconstruction. It has been reported an overall success rate of 72% using staged graft repair [41].
4. Grafts are commonly taken from either genital or non-genital sites like inner preputial graft if the child is not circumcised, buccal mucosa graft and post auricular skin graft. Following the principles published by Cuckow et al., in the case of not having enough foreskin in proximal hypospadias, alternatives are posterior auricular Wolfe graft and / or oral mucosa [19].

However, up to 12% of patients will need a revision of the first stage because of graft retraction. Leslie et al. [42], in retrospective study on 30 children with prior failed repairs reported induration and thickening in the graft after the first stage that in their experience affected the incidence of complications in a significant way. This may support the use of corticoid betamethasone cream beginning 4 weeks after healing of the graft and thereafter for at least 6 months to prevent the occurrence of hypertrophy and induration.

References

1. *EAU Guidelines*. Edn. Presented at the EAU Annual Congress Copenhagen 2018. ISBN 978–94–92671-01-1.
2. Mouriquand P, Gorduza D, Noche ME, Targnion A. Long-term outcome of hypospadias surgery: current dilemas. Curr Opin Urol. 2011;21:465–9.
3. Bouty A, Ayers KL, Pask A, Heloury Y, Sinclair AH. The genetic and environmental factors underlying hypospadias. Sex Dev. 2015;9:239–59.
4. Dolk H. Rise in prevalence of hypospadias. Lancet. 1998;351:770.
5. Moradi M, Kazemzadeh B, Hood B, Rezaee H, Kaseb K. Meatal mobilization and Glanuloplasty: A viable option for coronal and glanular hypospadias repair. Urology. 2016;94:204–7.
6. Zaontz MR, Dean GE. Glandular hypospadias repair. Urol Clin North Am. 2002;29(2):291–298, V–VI.
7. Manzoni G, Bracka A, Palminteri, Marrocco G. Hypospadias surgery: when, what and by whom? BJU Int. 2004;94:1188–95.
8. Belman AB. Hypospadias and chordee. In: Belman AB, King LR, Kramer SA, editors. Clinical Pediatric Urology. London: Martin Dunitz; 2002.
9. Springer A, Krois W, Horcher E. Trends in hypospadias surgery: results of a worldwide survey. Eur Urol. 2011;60(6):1184–9.
10. Unluer ES, Miroglu C, Ozturk R. Long-term follow up results of the MAGPI (meatal advancement and glanuloplasty) operations in distal hypospadias. Int Urol Nephrol. 1991;23(6):581–7.
11. Morera AM, et al. A study of risk factors for hypospadias in the Rhone-Alpes region (France). J Pediatr Urol. 2006;2:169.
12. Silver RI, Rodriguez R, Chang TS, Gearhart JP. In vitro fertilization is associated with an increased risk of hypospadias. J Urol. 1999;161(6):1954–7.
13. Netto JM, et al. Hormone therapy in hypospadias surgery: a systematic review. J Pediatr Urol. 2013;9:971.
14. Malik RD, et al. Survey of pediatric urologists on the preoperative use of testosterone in the surgical correction of hypospadias. J Pediatr Urol. 2014;10(5):840–3.
15. Snodgrass W, Macedo A, Hoebeke P, Mouriquand P. Hypospadias dilemmas: A round table. J Pediatr Urol. 2011;7:145–57.
16. Chua ME, et al. Preoperative hormonal stimulation effect on hypospadias repair complications: Meta-analysis of observational versus randomized controlled studies. J Pediatr Urol. 2017;13:470.
17. Kaya C, et al. The role of pre-operative androgen stimulation in hypospadias surgery. Transl Androl Urol. 2014;3:340.
18. Wright I, et al. Effect of preoperative hormonal stimulation on postoperative complication rates after proximal hypospadias repair: a systematic review. J Urol. 2013;190:652.
19. Johal N, Nitkunan T, O'Malley K, Cuckow P. The Two-Stage Repair for Severe Primary Hypospadias. E Urol. 2000;50:366–71.

20. Snodgrass W, Bush N. Tubularized incised plate proximal hypospadias repair: continued evolution and extended applications. J Pediatr Urol. 2011;7:2–9.
21. Pfistermüller K, Manoharan S, Desai D, Cuckow P. Two-stage hypospadias repair with a free graft for severe primary and revision hypospadias: A single surgeon's experience with long-term follow-up. J Pediatr Urol. 2017;13(1):35.e1–7.
22. Lee PA, et al. Consensus statement on management of intersex disorders. International Consensus Conference on Intersex. Pediatrics. 2006;118:488.
23. Gorduza D, Quigley C, Caldamone A, Mouriquand P. Surgery of Anomalies of gonadal and genital Development in the "Post-Truth Era". Urol Clin N Am. 2018;45:659–69.
24. Vidal I, Gorduza DB, Haraux E, et al. Surgical options in disorders of sex development with ambiguous genitalia. Best Pract Res Clin Endocrinol Metab. 2010;24:311–24.
25. Wein AJ, Kavoussi LR, Partin AW, Peters CA. Campbell-Walsh Urology. 11th ed. Philadelphia, PA: Elsevier; 2016.
26. Bergman JE, et al. Epidemiology of hypospadias in Europe: a registry-based study. World J Urol. 2015;33:2159.
27. Ru W, Shen J, Tang D, Xu S, Wu D, Tao C, Chen G, Gao L, Wang X, Shen Y. Width proportion of the urethral plate to the glans can serve as an appraisal index of the urethral plate in hypospadias repair. Int J Urol. 2018;25(7):649–53.
28. Seleim HM, et al. Comprehensive evaluation of grafting the preservable plates with consideration of native plate width at primary hypospadias surgery. J Pediatr Urol. 2019; https://doi.org/10.1016/j.jpurol.2019.05.002.
29. Kolon TF, Gonzales ET Jr. The dorsal inlay graft for hypospadias repair. J Urol. 2000;163:1941–3.
30. Bhat A, Bhat M, Singh V. Results of tubularized urethral plate urethroplasty in Megameatus Intact Prepuce. Indian J Urol. 2017;33:315–8.
31. Marco C, Bulotta AL, Varetti C, et al. Ambiguous external genitalia due to defect of 5-α-reductase in seven Iraqi patients: prevalence of a novel mutation. Gene. 2013;526:490–3.
32. Fahmy M, et al. Othman D. Penile Median Raphe Anomalies as an Indicator of Megameatus Intact Prepuce Anomaly in Children Undergoing Routine Circumcision. Urology. 2018;121:164–7.
33. Peretz D, Westreich M. Pseudo-iatrogenic hypospadias: the megameatus intact-prepuce hypospadias variant. Plast Reconstr Surg. 2003;111(3):1182–5.
34. Elbatarny A, Shehata S, Ismail K. Megameatus intact prepuce variety of hypospadias: tips for repair using the modified glanular approximation procedure. Ann Pediatr Surg. 2011;7(2):1687–37.
35. Juskiewenski S, et al. Treatment of anterior hypospadias. (Balanoplasty). J Urol (Paris). 1983;89(2):153–6.
36. Cendron M. The Megameatus, Intact Prepuce Variant of Hypospadias: Use of the Inframeatal Vascularized Flap for Surgical correction. Front Pediatr. 2018;6:55.
37. Duckett J, Keating M. Technical challenge of the megameatus inctact prepuce hypospadias variant: the pyramid procedure. J Urol. 1989;141:1407–9.
38. Faasse MA, et al. Repair of megameatus: A modified approach. J Pediatr Urol. 2015; https://doi.org/10.1016/j.jpurol.2015.01.003.
39. Snodgrass WT, Khavari R. Prior circumcision does not complicate repair of hypospadias with an intact prepuce. J Urol. 2006;176:296–8.
40. Kulkarni S, Joglekar O, Alkandari M, Pankaj J. Redo hypospadias surgery: current and novel techniques. Res Repo Urol. 2018;10:117–26.
41. Badawy H, et al. Staged Repair of Redo and Crippled Hypospadias: Analysis of Outcome and Complications. J Pediatr Urol. 2019;15(2):151-1–151-10.
42. Leslie B, Lorenzo AJ, Figueroa V, Moore K, Farhat WA, Bägli DJ. Pippi Salle JL. Critical outcome analysis of staged buccal mucosa graft urethroplasty for prior failed hypospadias repair in children. J Urol. 2011;185(3):1077–82.

Bladder Exstrophy 15

Chapter in Book "Practical Pediatric Urology—An Evidence Based Approach"

Sébastien Faraj and Marc-David Leclair

Learning Objectives

- Provide appropriate prenatal counselling
- Understand differences in possible neonatal management strategies
- Manage urethral complications after closure of bladder exstrophy

15.1 Case 1

A couple is seen in clinic with a prenatally possible classical bladder exstrophy diagnosed. The ultrasonography performed at 24 WG shows absent bladder on repeated examinations, low insertion of the umbilical cord.

Q1. What do you tell them?

A1. Classical bladder exstrophy is a rare malformation, with an incidence of approximately 1:46.000 birth [1]. The absence of visualization of the bladder is the strongest sign in favor of this diagnosis, together with low insertion of the umbilical cord [2], and spreading of the pubic bone ossification points [3]. The main messages to emphasize at the time of the first prenatal consultation are:

1. The surgical management can follow different approaches [4], but all require possible multiple surgeries during life (childhood and adulthood) with subsequent follow-up by pediatric urologist, nephrologist and gynaecologist [5].
2. Urinary continence is a major concern, and several reconstructive attempts may be necessary. It is accepted that at least 80% of these children will achieve dryness [6, 7], but only a minority will achieve physiological continence and voiding per-urethra.

S. Faraj · M.-D. Leclair (✉)
Paediatric Surgery and Urology Department, NANTES University Children Hospital, Centre Hospitalier Universitaire de Nantes, Nantes Cedex, France
e-mail: mdleclair@chu-nantes.fr

P. Godbole et al. (eds.), *Practical Pediatric Urology*,
https://doi.org/10.1007/978-3-030-54020-3_15

3. Overall survival is excellent [6–10].
4. Neonatal referral of the child to an expert centre should be considered.
5. Termination of the pregnancy may be an option, in some countries, especially for boys whose genital prognosis remain poor. It may be a great help to ascertain fetal gender by non invasive methods (detection of circulating SRY sequence in maternal boy) [11] before undertaking any further discussions.

At birth, you see a malformation similar to the two examples below (Figs. 15.1 and 15.2).

Q2. How can you describe the different elements of these bladder exstrophy patients?

A2. Classical bladder exstrophy gathers several anomalies [12]:

1. bladder template is open. Here we can see a small/good sized bladder template [13] with/without bladder polyps [14].
2. the urethra is wide open along the dorsal aspect, forming an epispadias, always present in classical bladder exstrophy [15]. In some cases, epispadias can be isolated and state as a complete malformation.

Fig. 15.1 Large bladder, normal mucosa

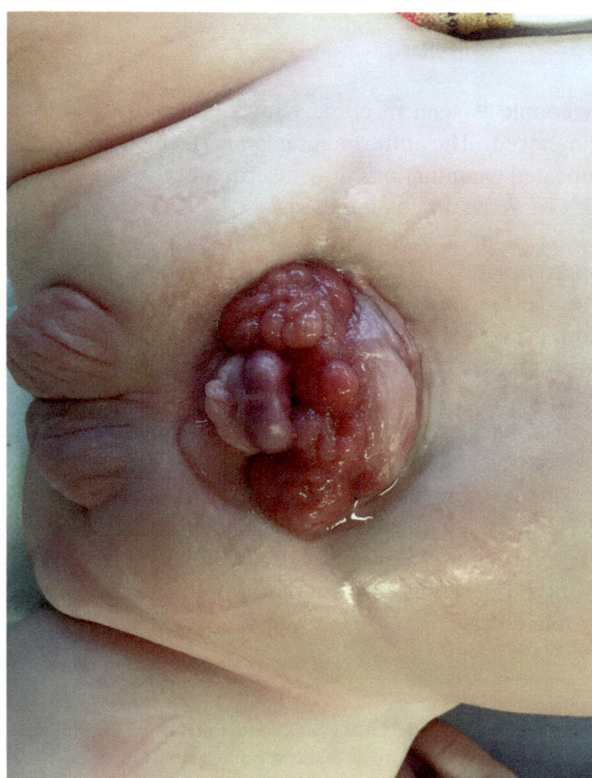

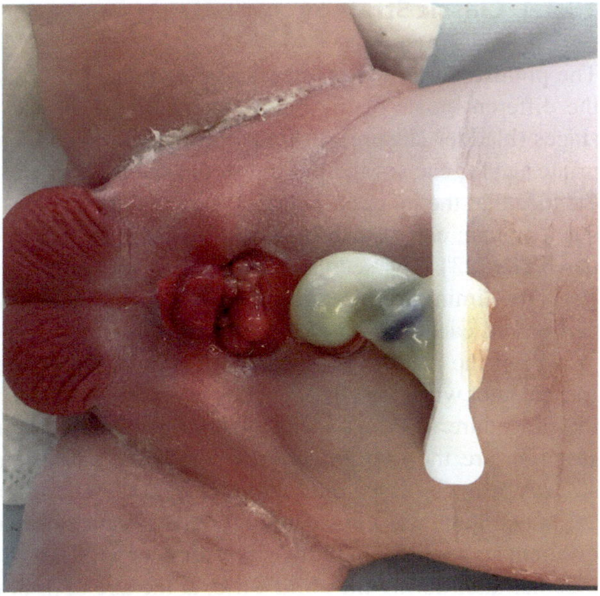

Fig. 15.2 Small bladder template, multiple polypoid formations

3. pubic bones are separated with a wide diastasis. This examination detail can be the only visible particularity found in very distal epispadias.
4. length of the penis is always a short [16], because of the attachment of the corpora cavernosa on a distracted pubic bones, associated with dorsal curvature [17].

Q3. What do you do at birth?

A3. At birth, there are some important things to do:

1. Explanation of the malformation to the parents, on their newborn.
2. Refer the child to an expert center [18], or make contact with it to determine timing and stages of the surgical strategy
3. Protection of the bladder template can be advised using silicon non adherent silicon dressings, if a delayed strategy is chosen.
4. Minimal imaging workup studies can be performed: pelvic X-ray, renal ultrasound, and ultrasound of the spinal cord

Q4. What are the different possibilities of management of classical bladder exstrophy?

A4. Surgical management of classic bladder exstrophy is still challenging for pediatric and urologic surgeons interested in this complex pathology. The strategy has constantly been renewed [4] since the first work in the early twentieth century [19–21].

15.1.1 Classic Strategy

The philosophy of the modern staged repair [4, 22] was to allow achievement of the different goals of the management of the classic bladder exstrophy in three stages (bladder closure, penile reconstruction, continence procedure) at an appropriate age for each of them. First step is the bladder closure performed at birth with the idea that the more early the closure is done the less complications on the bladder template; early closure avoids the need for pelvic osteotomy in a majority of newborns [23]. The second step consists on reconstruction of the male genitalia [24]. The timing of this step was also under debate and was through history done earlier and earlier to be perform during the first year of life, participating to the growth of the bladder [24]. The third step is the management of continence, performed later when the child reaches psychological and physical favorable status for the procedure to be a success. Ureteric reimplantation and bladder neck reconstruction are the two procedures performed at this time [25]. Each step of this strategy was discussed and modified by numbers of team operating exstrophy [7, 22] but strategy was considered effective precisely because of the separation of the different stages [26]. In the Warsaw approach [27], the last two steps are performed together later during the child's life, at the age of 4–8, in the selected cases of satisfying bladder growth.

15.1.2 Complete Primary Repair of Exstrophy

Another approach of the classic bladder exstrophy was popularized by Mitchell [28], consisting in a complete primary repair of exstrophy. In this strategy, a complete penile disassembly of the urethral plate and the corporeal bodies is performed with total reconstruction at the same time of the bladder neck reconstruction and the bladder closure [6]. The idea is to avoid multiple surgeries and so avoid multiple general anesthesia by performing all the needed steps in one stage [29]. Two supplementary advantages were linked to this strategy: a theoretical improved growth of the bladder [30] because of the earlier reconstruction of the voiding channel with early resistance and a theoretical better position of the final bladder inside the pelvis [6]. However, the feasibility of such a long/complex procedure during the haemodynamically unstable neonatal period, and subsequent potential vascular risks, led multiple center to avoid this strategy [26].

15.1.3 The Kelly Procedure

J.H. Kelly described in 1975 a novel approach [31, 32] aiming at anatomical reconstruction of the urogenital complex [33]. The objective is to detach and use all skeletal muscular structures of the pelvic floor, attached in bladder exstrophy patients on the abnormal pelvic girdle, and reconstruction on the midline at the supposed best location for continence. The idea is to create passive resistances with existent muscular structures [34]. This reconstruction is enables after a radical soft tissue mobilization, which is performed during a second stage at the age of 3–6 months, after an initial bladder closure at birth. In theory, the radical soft tissue mobilization, by its complete detachment of the corpora from the inferior rami [35], allows lengthening of the penis but may also require creation of a hypospadiac meatus to optimize length gain [9].

15.1.4 The Delayed Bladder Closure Approach

All these strategies included a neonatal bladder closure, associated or not to the other goals of exstrophy management, which are reconstruction of genitalia and reconstruction of bladder neck to reach a continence status. Alongside these questionings about the different stages and the possible combinations of them, several teams began to delay the bladder closure step [18]. It has been suggested that delaying the bladder closure had finally not so negative consequences on the bladder template as previously thought [36, 37]. In several countries throughout the world, with limited access to high-level pediatric surgical facilities [38], many children reach the age of 5–10 with a bladder template left untouched, some of them still being eligible for delayed bladder closure. W. Rösch and coworkers showed the limited and reversible morphological and histological changes observed on the bladder mucosa in delayed closure patients series [39].

Additional advantages to elicit a delayed bladder closure strategy include:

1. Potential improvement of mother-child bond building, when the newborn is discharged home soon after birth.
2. Avoiding neonatal catabolism that occurs during the first days of life (wound healing), and renal function immaturity, respiratory and haemodynamic instability period of the newborn, to take advantage of a more favourable window some weeks later.
3. planification, organization of the surgery [40], and possibly referral to an expert center or involvement of other paediatric urologists with expertise in bladder exstrophy reconstruction [41].

15.1.5 The Nantes Approach

The Nantes Approach [10] is a strategy combining delayed closure, and Kelly RSTM, resulting in a one-stage procedure, performed at the age of 2 months. In this global approach, both parents are seen during pregnancy to provide information on the malformation and its management. Protection of the bladder plate is advised using non adherent silicon dressing, and peripheral skin care around the plate protected with ointment cream. Closure is performed during the third month of life, combined with RSTM and Kelly reconstruction of the bladder, bladder-neck, and epispadias [10].

Q5. In this particular case, a delayed closure is planned. What are the advices regarding wound care.

A5. Dressings protecting the bladder mucosa from mechanical aggression can be advised. These dressings can be done with using non adherent silicon interface dressing placed on the bladder template. A formula based on paraffin oil, silicon, and lanolin oil can be used to protect the peripheral skin around the plate. No specific risk of infection justifies local/systemic antibioprophylaxis.

15.2 Case 2

A 7 year old boy with bladder exstrophy closed at birth has recently moved from a remote country. Parents described no dry period longer than 30 min with the necessity for the child to wear diapers permanently. There was no infection but the continence situation was more and more difficult to accept with impact on his scholar life, especially during elementary school. On the clinical examination, there is one supra pubic scar and meatus still is in epispadiac position. There is indeed urine leakage through the urethra.

Q1. What do you do for further exploration?

A1. The objective is to evaluate all the aspect of the bladder exstrophy complex to choose the adequate procedure for this boy.

First, the **kidneys** and renal function must be analyzed, by performing at least a renal ultrasound and serum creatinin [42].

The **bladder assessment** requires a combination of cystogram, endoscopy, some urodynamic evaluation [43]. This can be achieved under general anesthesia, first by slow filling of the bladder with physiologic serum, measuring the rise in filling pressure. The advantage of general anesthesia is to combine endoscopy, urethrocystogram (with a balloon blocked in the bladder neck), filling-pressure assessment, and occasionally, placement of a suprapubic catheter to allow formal urodynamic studies. During the bladder endoscopy, position of ureteral meatus and presence or not of bladder augmentation has to be noticed. The urethra would be also evaluated at this time.

The presence of **bladder outlet resistances** can be more difficult to appreciate in these cases. Interrogation on timing of urinal leakage takes an important place in this evaluation. Examination under general anesthesia and urodynamic evaluation permit also to better understand the status of the child.

The goal of all these evaluations is to understand the mechanism of the incontinence situation, which is the result of a complex balance between bladder function and pressure and infravesical resistances. One must obtain an evaluation of maximum and functional bladder capacity, end-filling bladder pressure, and sphincteric resistances [44].

The urodynamic evaluation of the bladder function revealed a small bladder with poor capacity evaluated at about 70 ml at the age of 7. At this volume, intravesical pressure was very high inducing a poor compliance of 5. Renal evaluation showed bilateral good parenchymal aspect, normal function, and no hydro-uretero-nephrosis.

Q2. What management do you propose to perform in this boy?

A2. The surgical management aims to achieve social continence, not jeopardizing the renal function.

The surgical plan could include an association of:

1. **bladder augmentation** [45] **with continent Mitrofanoff appendiceal cystostomy** [46]: the bladder capacity is insufficient, because of absence of infravesical resistances resulting in poor bladder growth. Augmentation can be performed with ileal or sigmoid patch. A continent derivation must be performed at the same time to allow acceptable bladder emptying.
2. **urethro-cervicocystoplasty**: the objective is to avoid urine incontinence through urethra. Multiple procedures exist, as variant of Young-Dees procedure [47]. None of them will allow physiological voiding, and one may accept obstructive bladder outlet resistances to achieve social dryness [48]. It is therefore mandatory that continence bladder neck reconstruction in this context be associated with some form of continent diversion (Mitrofanoff) [46].
3. **epispadias reconstruction by Cantwell Ransley procedure** [49, 50]: the goal is to have a well cosmetic aspect of the penis. The functional part of the urethra is in this case at a second level because of the presence of the continent channel. The Kelly radical softtissue mobilization [9] in this situation allows anatomical reconstruction of the penis with maximal length gain.

In this case, a sigmoid patch was used for bladder augmentation and a Young Dees cervicocystoplasty procedure was realized. The Mitrofanoff cystostomy was positioned at the umbilicus. Urethra was reconstructed following a Cantwell Ransley procedure.

Q3. Do you perform ureteral reimplant and how do you perform it?

A3. Ureteral reimplant in bladder exstrophy patients has to be considered as an adjunct to bladder outlet procedures [25], to minimize the risks of high pressure voiding when voiding per urethra is a viable option [29]. Another situation may be the need to displace the ureteral orifices hindering adequate bladder neck tailoring. In the present case, and as a matter of principles, vesico-ureteric reimplantation is not always necessary, especially when performing bladder augmentation for a low-pressure catheterizable reservoir. Several open bladder techniques can be used, and the classic cranial reimplantation described by R. Jeffs [51] is the one that best adapt to natural orientation of the ureters and the need for lengthening the bladder neck. The Gil-Vernet trigonoplasty is an alternative [52], with probably very low success rates.

Finally, in bladder exstrophy children with non augmented native bladder, one may take into consideration the potential negative impact of high grade reflux on bladder growth, prompting to early reimplantation at the time or soon after bladder closure [25, 42].

Q4. Do you perform supplementary osteotomy?

A4. The objective of pelvic osteotomy in the bladder exstrophy patient is to allow a tension-free closure, increasing the chances of good healing. Through history of bladder exstrophy management, multiple ways of performing it were described, like innominate or posterior osteotomies [53–55]. The choice of doing it depends on multiple various facts [56], which can be all discussed for each case:

1. at birth, natural plasticity of all tissues and especially the bone allow closure without osteotomy [23]. Osteotomy can be discussed to minimize the tension during the postoperative period, which is also done by the immobilization of the child (plastercast or other management).
2. in the delayed bladder closure, osteotomy is sometimes needed to allow the pubis approximation and so minimize the tension during the postoperative period. This is the same for older child for whom we want to perform supplementary surgery as the mitrofanoff procedure or cervicoplasty.

It must be accepted that whether an osteotomy has been performed or not, the pubic diastasis will eventually re-enlarge, despite any methods of immobilization. This indicates that osteotomy should be considered as a help for closure during the operative and for a help to minimize post operative tension but not as an anatomical reconstruction of the pelvis [8].

The Kelly procedure in its very essence allows a tension free midline position of all the structures of interest by detaching them from the bones [33]. At least, the continence results of this technique are independent of pelvic bone reconstruction. However, in a delayed and combined approach with the Kelly repair, it may be safer to secure abdominal closure with some form of osteotomy [10].

15.3 Case 3

A boy with classic bladder exstrophy is followed-up after neonatal bladder closure and staged reconstruction. At the age of 3y.o, he presents with recurrent febrile UTIs. An examination under anesthesia is performed and reveals a urethral stenosis.

Q1. How can you manage these types of urethral stenosis in boys with classical bladder exstrophy?

A1. Urethral stenosis is a common complication after classical bladder exstrophy closure and epispadias reconstruction. It can be observed at the level of the neomeatus when transposed in hypospadias position, or along the distal urethra. It can be explained by ischemia occurring during the urethral reconstruction [57] and so is likely more frequent after radical soft tissue mobilization or CPRE, due to extensive dissection.

The management of urethral stricture can be performed using:

- **smooth dilatation** performed under local or general anesthesia with upgrading catheter.

- **dilatation using high-pressure balloon** under general anesthesia. Sessions can be repeated after a few weeks to increase the chance of success.
- **endoscopic urethrotomy** is rarely possible to perform, because of the short length of the urethra in such children.
- **redo-urethroplasty** can be achieve but still is difficult to perform in boys with a high risk of recurrence of the stricture. In girls, a meatoplasty can be tried under general anesthesia but can also be followed by recurrence stenosis.

In this case, dilatations were performed under general anesthesia followed by dilatations with balloon catheter. Infections continued to occur during 2 years with multiple hospitalizations. Bladder endoscopy showed some bladder trabeculations with a quite good capacity. A new examination under general anesthesia was carried out and showed a recurrence of the urethral stenosis leading to this obstructive situation.

Q2. What can you propose to this boy in this obstructive situation?

A2. The outlet obstruction and high voiding pressures obviously puts at risk the upper-tracts. Incomplete bladder emptying triggers recurrent infections and bladder stone formation. Clean intermittent catheterization seems mandatory to avoid further bladder and renal deterioration.

CIC through native/reconstructed urethra seems difficult, but is worth to try, with dedicated clinical nurses in a specialized setting. Creation of a continent catheterizable channel (appendico-vesicostomy following the Mitrofanoff procedure) is an alternative in case of failure of urethral CIC, allowing adequate bladder emptying without pain [46].

Q3. Do you perform a supplementary procedure on the bladder neck during the mitrofanoff procedure?

A3. Two main problems need to be addressed when undertaking this reconstruction:

- the urodynamic characteristics of the reservoir during the filling phase need to be assessed by formal cystomanometry, to ensure the need for bladder augmentation in case of small or poorly compliant reservoir.
- the efficiency of bladder outlet mechanisms, to clarify whether infra-vesical resistances need to be reinforced at the same time of Mitrofanoff creation ± bladder augmentation.

Different procedures can be performed at the same time of the appendicovesicostomy on the bladder neck:

- **cervical injection of bulking agent**, which can be done when the bladder is open and repeated by endoscopic injections if needed [58].
- **redo-cervicoplasty** following a Young-Dees procedure or one of the modified techniques. This procedure can be done only in bladder with good capacity because of utilization of part of the bladder and is difficult to perform because of the lack of smoothness of the tissues surrounding the bladder neck.

- **closure of the bladder neck** [59] can be performed even in little bladder. This procedure states as a radical procedure, which can be difficult to accept by the family. This is still a good choice to avoid urine leakage with a simplest procedure than a bladder neck reconstruction.

It is also possible to choose not to perform any bladder neck procedure, counting on the urethral stricture to prevent from leaks. In this situation, injection of bulking agent by endoscopy could be done eventually if necessary.

In this case, a bladder neck reconstruction and ileocystoplasty were performed at the same time than the Mitrofanoff channel, allowing the patient to achieve dryness without infection.

At the age of 14, he is reported to show behavioral and psycho-social difficulties, and deterioration of scholar attendance. The genital aspect seems to represent his biggest concern.

Q4. What are the possibilities?

A4. It has been well documented that puberty and early adulthood represent a difficult transitional period for exstrophy patients [42, 60], with major psychological consequences. Most urological problems of early childhood are usually resolved at this age, and sexological questioning comes into foreground [61]. Initiating the transition of care toward a multidisciplinary adult team is extremely important [62]. Among sexological concerns, having a short penis often states as the main problem in exstrophic boys reaching adult age [63]. It can be a personal wondering because of a poor body self-image, or a demand motivated by the presence of a partner and the ask for having intercourses. Sufficient length for a penis should allow efficient penetrations without difficulties and without pain. Residual dorsal curvature and scars on an intrincally short penis may aggravate the penetrations difficulties. Surgical possibilities to lengthen the penis are usually not able to make it longer of more than a few centimeters [64], and in some cases, phalloplasty will be the only option. It should be performed only in highly specialized centers, after thorough urologic, plastic, and psychological preoperative assessment.

References

1. Cervellione RM, et al. Prospective study on the incidence of bladder/cloacal exstrophy and epispadias in Europe. J Pediatr Urol. 2015;11(6):337.e1–6.
2. Featherstone NC, Cuckow PM. Spiral rotational flap for the creation of a new umbilicus in bladder exstrophy. J Pediatr Urol. 2015;11(2):96–7.
3. Tourchi A, Inouye BM, Di Carlo HN, Young E, Ko J, Gearhart JP. New advances in the pathophysiologic and radiologic basis of the exstrophy spectrum. J Pediatr Urol. 2014;10(2):212–8.
4. Purves JT. Modern approaches in primary exstrophy closure. Semin Pediatr Surg. 2011;20(2):79–84.
5. Inouye BM, et al. How to close classic bladder exstrophy: are subspecialty training and technique important? J Pediatr Urol. 2018;14(5):426.e1–6.
6. Shnorhavorian M, Grady RW, Andersen A, Joyner BD, Mitchell ME. Long-term Followup of complete primary repair of Exstrophy: the Seattle experience. J Urol. 2008;180(4S):1615–20.

7. Dickson AP. The Management of Bladder Exstrophy: the Manchester experience. J Pediatr Surg. 2014;49(2):244–50.
8. Leclair MD, et al. One-stage combined delayed bladder closure with Kelly radical soft-tissue mobilization in bladder exstrophy: preliminary results. J Pediatr Urol. 2018;14(6):558–64.
9. Kazachkova N, Gontar J, Verlinsky O, Ilyin I. Successful early fetal sex determination using cell-free fetal DNA isolated from maternal capillary blood: a pilot study. Eur J Obstet Gynecol Reprod Biol X. 2019;3:100038.
10. Ebert A-K, Reutter H, Ludwig M, Rösch WH. The Exstrophy-epispadias complex. Orphanet J Rare Dis. 2009;4:23.
11. Lee BR, Perlman EJ, Gearhart JP. Evaluation of smooth muscle and collagen subtypes in normal newborns and those with bladder exstrophy. J Urol. 1996;156(6):2034–6.
12. Jayman J, Tourchi A, Shabaninia M, Maruf M, DiCarlo H, Gearhart JP. The surgical Management of Bladder Polyps in the setting of Exstrophy Epispadias complex. Urology. 2017;109:171–4.
13. Maruf M, et al. Variant presentations of the Exstrophy-Epispadias complex: a 40-year experience. Urology. 2019;125:184–90.
14. Reynaud N, et al. Male sexuality, fertility, and urinary continence in bladder Exstrophy-Epispadias complex. J Sex Med. 2018;15(3):314–23.
15. Stec AA. Embryology and bony and pelvic floor anatomy in the bladder exstrophy-epispadias complex. Semin Pediatr Surg. 2011;20(2):66–70.
16. Ahn JJ, Shnorhavorian M, Katz C, Goldin AB, Merguerian PA. Early versus delayed closure of bladder exstrophy: a National Surgical Quality Improvement Program Pediatric analysis. J Pediatr Urol. 2018;14(1):27.e1–5.
17. Wilhelmi OJ. Exstrophy of the bladder with Pyelographic follow-up. J Urol. 1948;59(6):1108–20.
18. Higgins CC. Exstrophy of the bladder: review of 70 cases**read at annual meeting, American Association of Genito-Urinary Surgeons, White Sulphur Springs, W. Va., may 10, 1949. J Urol. 1950;63(5):852–7.
19. Purves JT, Baird AD, Gearhart JP. The modern staged repair of bladder exstrophy in the female: a contemporary series. J Pediatr Urol. 2008;4(2):150–3.
20. Inouye BM, et al. Newborn exstrophy closure without osteotomy: is there a role? J Pediatr Urol. 2016;12(1):51.e1–4.
21. Kufner M, Gearhart JP, Mathews R. Impact of epispadias repair on bladder growth in boys with classic bladder exstrophy. J Pediatr Urol. 2010;6(6):578–81.
22. Tourchi A, et al. Ureteral Reimplantation before bladder neck reconstruction in modern staged repair of Exstrophy patients: indications and outcomes. Urology. 2015;85(4):905–8.
23. Chua ME, et al. Modified staged repair of bladder exstrophy: a strategy to prevent penile ischemia while maintaining advantage of the complete primary repair of bladder exstrophy. J Pediatr Urol. 2019;15(1):63.e1–7.
24. Baka-Jakubiak M. Combined bladder neck, urethral and penile reconstruction in boys with the exstrophy-epispadias complex. BJU Int. 2000;86(4):513–8.
25. Mitchell ME, Bagli DJ. Complete penile disassembly for Epispadias repair: the Mitchell technique. J Urol. 1996;155(1):300–4.
26. Borer JG, et al. Early outcome following complete primary repair of bladder exstrophy in the newborn. J Urol. 2005;174(4 Part 2):1674–9.
27. Borer JG, et al. Bladder growth and development after complete primary repair of bladder exstrophy in the newborn with comparison to staged approach. J Urol. 2005;174(4 Part 2):1553–8.
28. Kelley JH, Eraklis AJ. A procedure for lengthening the phallus in boys with exstrophy of the bladder. J Pediatr Surg. 1971;6(5):645–9.
29. Kelly JH. Vesical exstrophy: repair using radical mobilisation of soft tissues. Pediatr Surg Int. 1995;10(5):298–304.
30. Leclair M-D, Villemagne T, Faraj S, Suply E. The radical soft-tissue mobilization (Kelly repair) for bladder exstrophy. J Pediatr Urol. 2015;11(6):364–5.

31. Varma KK, Mammen A, Kolar Venkatesh SK. Mobilization of pelvic musculature and its effect on continence in classical bladder exstrophy: a single-center experience of 38 exstrophy repairs. J Pediatr Urol. 2015;11(2):87.e1–5.
32. Ben-Chaim J, et al. Kelly procedure for exstrophy or epispadias patients: anatomical description of the pudendal neurovasculature. J Pediatr Urol. 2016;12(3):173.e1–6.
33. Jarzebowski AC, McMullin ND, Grover SR, Southwell BR, Hutson JM. The Kelly technique of bladder Exstrophy repair: continence, Cosmesis and pelvic organ prolapse outcomes. J Urol. 2009;182(4S):1802–6.
34. Ferrara F, Dickson AP, Fishwick J, Vashisht R, Khan T, Cervellione RM. Delayed exstrophy repair (DER) does not compromise initial bladder development. J Pediatr Urol. 2014;10(3):506–10.
35. Baradaran N, Cervellione RM, Stec AA, Gearhart JP. Delayed primary repair of bladder Exstrophy: ultimate effect on growth. J Urol. 2012;188(6):2336–42.
36. Wiersma R. Overview of bladder exstrophy: a third world perspective. J Pediatr Surg. 2008;43(8):1520–3.
37. Rösch W, Christl A, Strauss B, Schrott KM, Neuhuber WL. Comparison of preoperative innervation pattern and postreconstructive urodynamics in the exstrophy-epispadias complex. Urol Int. 1997;59(1):6–15.
38. Borer JG, Vasquez E, Canning DA, Kryger JV, Mitchell ME. An initial report of a novel multi-institutional bladder Exstrophy consortium: a collaboration focused on primary surgery and subsequent care. J Urol. 2015;193(5S):1802–7.
39. Ellison JS, Ahn J, Shnorhavorian M, Grady R, Merguerian PA. Long-term fate of the upper tracts following complete primary repair of bladder exstrophy. J Pediatr Urol. 2017;13(4):394.e1–6.
40. Baradaran N, Cervellione RM, Orosco R, Trock BJ, Mathews RI, Gearhart JP. Effect of failed initial closure on bladder growth in children with bladder Exstrophy. J Urol. 2011;186(4):1450–4.
41. Diamond DA, et al. Normal urodynamics in patients with bladder exstrophy: are they achievable? J Urol. 1999;162(3 Pt 1):841–4; discussion 844–845,.
42. Puri A, Mishra K, Sikdar S, Unni KES, Jain AK. Vesical preservation in patients with late bladder Exstrophy referral: histological insights into functional outcome. J Urol. 2014;192(4):1208–14.
43. Mitrofanoff P. Trans-appendicular continent cystostomy in the management of the neurogenic bladder. Chir Pediatr. 1980;21(4):297–305.
44. Donnahoo KK, Rink RC, Cain MP, Casale AJ. The Young-Dees-Leadbetter bladder neck repair for neurogenic incontinence. J Urol. 1999;161(6):1946–9.
45. Mouriquand PDE, et al. Long-term results of bladder neck reconstruction for incontinence in children with classical bladder exstrophy or incontinent epispadias. BJU Int. 2003;92(9):997–1001; discussion 1002,.
46. Gearhart JP, Leonard MP, Burgers JK, Jeffs RD. The Cantwell-Ransley technique for repair of epispadias. J Urol. 1992;148(3):851–4.
47. Diamond DA, Ransley PG. Male epispadias. J Urol. 1995;154(6):2150–5.
48. Canning DA, Gearhart JP, Peppas DS, Jeffs RD. The cephalotrigonal reimplant in bladder neck reconstruction for patients with exstrophy or epispadias. J Urol. 1993;150(1):156–8.
49. Gil-Vernet JM. A new technique for surgical correction of vesicoureteral reflux. J Urol. 1984;131(3):456–8.
50. Tomaszewski R, Pethe K, Koszutski T. Salter pelvic osteotomy in operative treatment in patients with bladder extrophy. Chir Narzadow Ruchu Ortop Pol. 2010;75(2):126–8.
51. Sponseller PD, Gearhart JP, Jeffs RD. Anterior innominate osteotomies for failure or late closure of bladder exstrophy. J Urol. 1991;146(1):137–40.
52. Mushtaq I, et al. Primary bladder Exstrophy closure in neonates: challenging the traditions. J Urol. 2014;191(1):193–8.
53. Zaman M, et al. Impact of pelvic immobilization techniques on the outcomes of primary and secondary closures of classic bladder exstrophy. J Pediatr Urol. 2019;15(4):382-e1.

54. Cervellione RM, Husmann DA, Bivalacqua TJ, Sponseller PD, Gearhart JP. Penile ischemic injury in the exstrophy/epispadias spectrum: new insights and possible mechanisms. J Pediatr Urol. 2010;6(5):450–6.
55. Burki T, Hamid R, Ransley PG, Mushtaq I, Duffy PG. Injectable polydimethylsiloxane for treating incontinence in children with the exstrophy-epispadias complex: long-term results. BJU Int. 2006;98(4):849–53.
56. Hernandez-Martin S, et al. Bladder neck closure in children: long-term results and consequences. Eur J Pediatr Surg Off J Austrian Assoc Pediatr Surg Al Z Kinderchir. 2015;25(1):100–4.
57. Diseth TH, Bjordal R, Schultz A, Stange M, Emblem R. Somatic function, mental health and psychosocial functioning in 22 adolescents with bladder exstrophy and epispadias. J Urol. 1998;159(5):1684–9; discussion 1689–1690,.
58. Ebert AK, Bals-Pratsch M, Seifert B, Reutter H, Rösch WH. Genital and reproductive function in males after functional reconstruction of the exstrophy-epispadias complex--long-term results. Urology. 2008;72(3):566–9; discussion 569-570,.
59. Ebert A, Scheuering S, Schott G, Roesch WH. Psychosocial and psychosexual development in childhood and adolescence within the exstrophy-epispadias complex. J Urol. 2005;174(3):1094–8.
60. Silver RI, Yang A, Ben-Chaim J, Jeffs RD, Gearhart JP. Penile length in adulthood after exstrophy reconstruction. J Urol. 1997;157(3):999–1003.
61. Morrison SD, Shakir A, Vyas KS, Kirby J, Crane CN, Lee GK. Phalloplasty: a review of techniques and outcomes. Plast Reconstr Surg. 2016;138(3):594–615.
62. Schaefer AA, Sakaguchi S. Exstrophy of the bladder: report of two patients operated upon at two months of age. J Pediatr. 1945;26(5):492–500.
63. Borer JG, et al. Short-term outcomes of the multi-institutional bladder exstrophy consortium: successes and complications in the first two years of collaboration. J Pediatr Urol. 2017;13(3):275.e1–6.
64. Schmidt AH, Keenen TL, Tank ES, Bird CB, Beals RK. Pelvic osteotomy for bladder exstrophy. J Pediatr Orthop. 1993;13(2):214–9.

Genitalia: Undescended Testis, Acute Scrotum, Buried Penis

16

Diboro Kanabolo and Mohan S. Gundeti

Learning Objectives: At the End of the Chapter, the Reader Should Be Able To

1. Understand the common presentations, aberrant mechanisms, and conditions associated with UPJ obstruction.
2. Provide a differential diagnosis, initial workup, and optimal management timeline of patient presenting with an acute scrotum.
3. Describe definition, etiology, and management of buried penis.
4. Delineate clinical manifestations, workup, and management of Ureteropelvic junction obstruction.

16.1 Genitalia: Undescended Testis, Non-Palpable (2 Figures Required)

Scenario 1: An ex-38-week gestation, 16-month-old male Caucasian child is referred to your clinic with an undescended left testis. Your physical exam is significant for orthotopic right testis, though left is nonpalpable in both the inguinal region and scrotum. Inspection of the scrotum does not reveal erythema or edema, with the epididymis on right shown to be present on palpation. No palpable masses are seen in the inguinal region. Scrotal ultrasound (US) confirms undescended testis on the

Book Chapter for: Practical Pediatric Urology: An Evidence Based Approach.

D. Kanabolo
University of Washington, Department of Urology, Seattle, WA, USA

M. S. Gundeti (✉)
Department of Surgery, Section of Urology, University of Chicago Medicine and Comer Children's Hospital, Chicago, IL, USA
e-mail: mgundeti@surgery.bsd.uchicago.edu

P. Godbole et al. (eds.), *Practical Pediatric Urology*,
https://doi.org/10.1007/978-3-030-54020-3_16

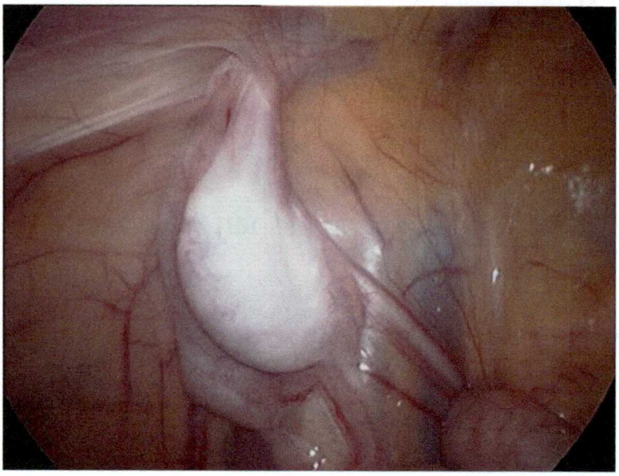

Fig. 16.1 Undescended left testes, non-palpable, located within the abdomen with Laparoscopy

left (unable to locate). Right epididymis and testis show no signs of pathology. Metabolic panel significant for creatinine of 0.68 mg/dl suggesting no abnormalities in kidney function. Informed consent is obtained from caregivers, and patient undergoes two-stage left orchiopexy. Intra-abdominal testes is seen on laparoscopy (Fig. 16.1). Patient does well with normal intra-scrotal testes post-orchiopexy [1].

Question 1: Please describe the aberrant mechanisms of development in this child.

The etiology of cryptorchidism, or non-palpable undescended testes is somewhat controversial. Some suggest the condition is due to blunting of the gonadotropin surge seen during development [2, 3]. Some others suggest that hypoandrogenism may be a cause. A genetic component may be suggested, as undescended testis is associated with a 6–10% fraternal, and 4% paternal concordance [4].

Question 2: Can this patient be managed non-surgically?

In the 2014 American Urological Association (AUA) consensus statement for the management of undescended testis, treatment of unilateral or bilateral undescended testis using hormonal therapy, such as human chorionic gonadotropin (hCG) or Luteinizing Hormone Releasing Hormone (LHRH) is not recommended. This is due to the decreased response rates and lack of long-term efficacy. Orchiopexy is generally the gold standard for undescended testis, whenever possible [5].

Question 3: What is the theoretical harm to this patient by treating conservatively?

In patients with undescended testis, there is increased risk of testicular germ cell tumors, in particular seminoma or carcinoma in situ, likely due in part to multinucleation of cells from impaired spermatogenesis. In children under age 12, the relative risk is 2–3, increasing to 2–6 when repaired after age 12 [6, 7].

Question 4: Is there a role for US in the diagnosis of cryptorchidism?

A Canadian retrospective study published in *Pediatrics* in 2015 provided evidence that US correctly approximates physical exam findings in only 54% of undescended testes cases. The study also showed that definitive surgical management is delayed on average by 3 months with the use of co-incident scrotal US. The 2014 AUA guidelines provide a Grade B recommendation against the use of ultrasound in cryptorchidism, as it rarely changes management of the condition. Thus, it is often routine clinical practice not to perform the imaging in nonpalpable testis, as it does not often add to clinical management. Laparoscopy under general anesthesia will allow localization and orchiopexy in one or two stages, based on location. However, there may be role in those with comorbid conditions not amenable to general anesthesia. The decision is to be made based on location of testis to prevent future malignancy (i.e. intrabdominal, higher risk vs. Inguinal) and consideration of pros and cons of surgery.

16.2 Genitalia: Undescended Testis, Palpable

Scenario 2: An ex-36-week gestation, 5-year-old male African American child is referred to your clinic with an undescended left testis. Inspection of the scrotum reveals no (is it what you menat to say?) erythema or edema. Your physical exam is significant for orthotopic right testis, with left palpable in the inguinal region. Metabolic panel significant for creatinine of 0.88 mg/dl suggesting no abnormalities in kidney function. The testis is able to be moved from its location in the external inguinal ring down to the scrotum, remaining there for 2 min before beginning to rise to the level of the inguinal ring. The patient's caregiver is reassured that the patient may be managed conservatively, with follow up annually.

Question 1: What is the general phenomenon seen in this case known as?

This is a case of retractile testes, due to an overactive cremaster muscle on the left side. The cremaster reflex is at its strongest for boys between the age of 2 and 7. The testis may be manually replaced into the scrotal position and remains there temporarily [8, 9].

Question 2: What is meant by "conservative management" for this patient?

The AUA recommends that providers assess the position of the testicle at least annually to ensure there is no further ascent into the inguinal canal. The condition is considered a normal variant in pre-adolescence. Hence, the patient must be followed with at least annual physical exam and palpation by the urologist until descent is noted, usually around puberty. Measures for continued home monitoring by parents are additionally helpful, such as assessment after a warm shower. Descended testes help in confirming the retractility of the testis. Some pediatric urologists may recommend more immediate follow up if testes fail to descend with warmth.

Question 3: In the event of no descent in the case above, or in the patient without retractile testes, what is the appropriate management?

Surgery is recommended due to the elevated risk of testicular cancer (Fig. 16.2). If the testicle is palpable, an inguinal or scrotal incision is made with due respect to the anatomic location of the testis. Either approach is effective for providing satisfactory access to the high riding testis [10].

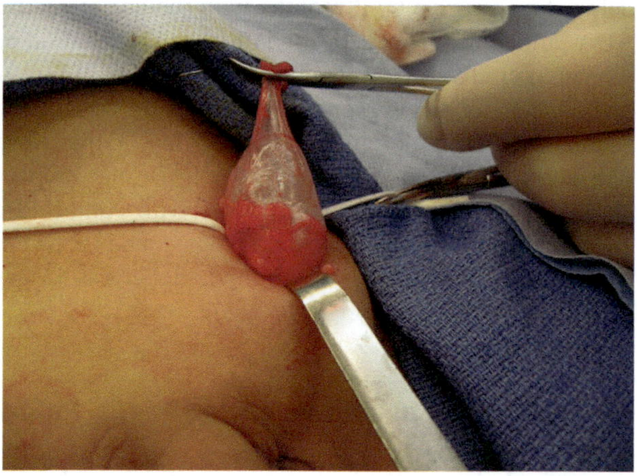

Fig. 16.2 Palpable inguinal testes within the hernial sac delivered through low transverse abdominal incision

16.3 Genitalia: Undescended Testis, with Hernia

Scenario 3: An ex-39-week gestation, 11-year-old boy was presented to the emergency room with a 10-day history of swelling of the right inguinoscrotal region, of slow evolution. 36 h prior to presentation, his pain became acute. The patient had no history of hernia or abdominal abnormality. He was afebrile, without abdominal pain, and reported no nausea or vomiting. His past medical history was negative. Past surgical history was positive for acute appendicitis at age 13. Family history is negative. The examination revealed a soft abdomen with bulging inguinal region. Right hemiscrotum was distended, tense, and fluctuant but non-trans illuminant (Fig. 16.3). With valsalva maneuver, bulge grows in size, causing some pain in the right hemiscrotum. Of note, the right testis is not palpable due to edema of scrotum. The left testis was confirmed to be in the left scrotum and without apparent abnormalities. Complete blood count showed hemoglobin and a hematocrit level of 13.1 g/dl and 35.7%, respectively, and a white blood cell (WBC) count of 12, 240/μl with 75% neutrophils [11].

Question 1: Is sonography useful or indicated for the patient at this stage?

While Doppler ultrasound may be a useful test for this patient, as literature has shown its diagnostic accuracy, history and physical exam is necessary to confirm the diagnosis of hernia [12, 13]. Immediate exploratory surgery is necessary if the patient's signs and symptoms are concerning for an acute abdomen or scrotum. If the physician's interpretation of the history and physical exam is equivocal, doppler is able to differentiate between surgical emergency and other causes of scrotal pain in 84% of children [14]. Color component may be of use because it allows for the characterization of blood flow and may differentiate flow originating in intratesticular versus scrotal wall regions. Surgery is immediately recommended in any scenario in which flow is found to be diminished or absent to testis [15].

Question 2: What is the role for computed tomography (CT) scan in this scenario?

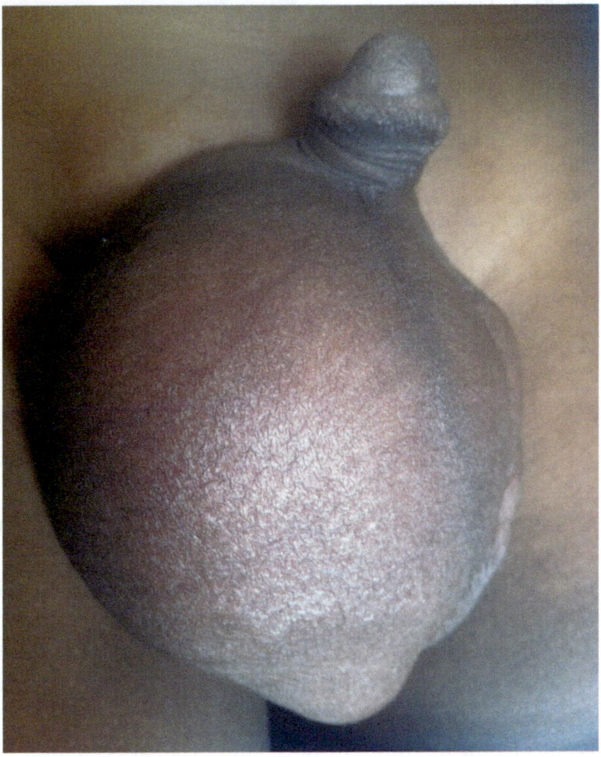

Fig. 16.3 Dense, enlarged right hemiscrotum with inguinal bulge on right indicative of incarcerated hernia

If there is concern for clinically occult groin hernia, as seen by sonography, one may opt to pursue non-contrast computed tomographic imaging methods. 1 study assessing 158 consecutive patients over 5 years with groin or lower abdominal pain showed a positive predictive value detection rate of 92%, and negative predictive value of 96% for the patients with occult groin hernia (n = 54). However, CT has been deemed by the European Hernia society as being without 'significant role' in inguinal hernia diagnosis, despite a sensitivity of 79–83% and a specificity of between 67 and 83% [16–18].

Scenario continued: Surgical exploration of the right inguinal region was begun. Surgery proceeded with a transinguinal approach. The right inguinal canal was opened through skin crease incision. After opening the herniated peritoneal sac, 12 ml of fluid was cleared out. After further exploration, a partial component of omentum was found, but most of this component was normal (Fig. 16.4). Of note, the testis was found to be normal. The omentum affected was resected and the remaining higher portions were reduced back into the peritoneal cavity. The right testis was able to return to the scrotum after omentum resection and reduction. A high ligation herniotomy was performed, with complete resolution of symptoms at 2-months postoperatively.

Question 3: How immediate should this boy's surgery have been performed? Describe the risks and benefits of an immediate vs delayed approach.

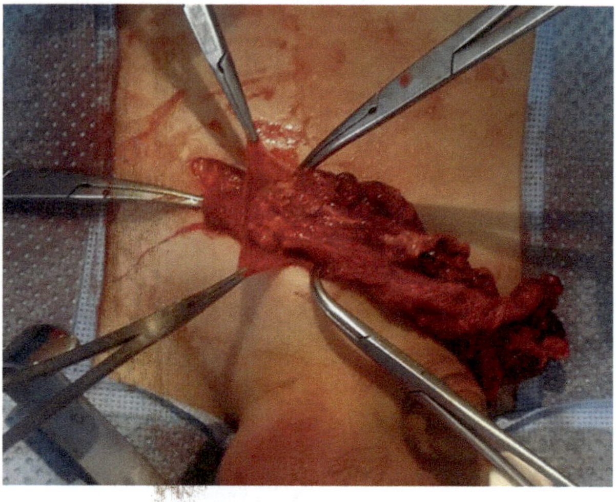

Fig. 16.4 Omentum incarcerated in inguinal bernia with a segmental infarct. (Reprinted with permission from "Unusual cause of acute scrotum in children: a case report" by Idrissa, Oukhouya, Tazi, Mahmoudi, Elmadi, Khattala, and Bouabdallah. Journal of Surgical Case Reports. 2017)

Immediate repair of an inguinal hernia, whether direct or indirect, reduces the risk of recurrent incarceration. This benefit is counterbalanced by the risk of swelling and inflammation, resulting in a more technically challenging procedure due to distortion of anatomical landmarks. These combine to create an elevated risk of direct herniation as a complication [17–19]. This risk is avoided with delayed repair. However, a delay in incarcerated hernia repair, as defined by 0.5–120 days from initial incarcerated hernia discovery, is associated with a 16–35 percent risk of recurrent incarceration. Many pediatric surgeons opt to hospitalize the patient and wait 24–48 h to allow the involved tissues to return to a closer approximation of their normal texture [19–21]. When the hernia is detected incidentally, without previous incarceration, many pediatric surgeons advocate for an elective repair.

16.4 Acute Scrotum—Appendix Testes

Scenario 4: A 13-year-old male presents to the ED with sudden testicular pain awakening him during the night. He had intermittent left scrotal pain for approximately 16 h prior to examination. Mild erythema is noted on the left hemiscrotum, and mild point tenderness is elicited between the upper testicular pole and epididymis. Patients left scrotal sac appears to have a hypoechoic center with an echogenic rim on US. Normal testicular flow is noted bilaterally. Color doppler in left epididymis shows possible increased flow but is inconclusive [22].

Question 1: What may be most concerning in this case?

While acute or sub-acute scrotal pain in the adolescent male can produce diagnostic concern, the primary consideration is for testicular torsion, as misdiagnosis can be disastrous and irreversible, leading to ischemia and loss of the testis. Other items to consider include torsion of the testicular appendage, epididymitis in a sexually active male, orchitis, and tumor. Multiple consecutive case series have provided evidence that testicular appendix torsion is the second most common cause of acute scrotum, following testicular torsion [23, 24].

Question 2: What features inherent to the testicular appendix facilitated this patient's presentation?

Testicular appendix torsion is represented by persistent vestigial remnants of Mullerian and mesonephric duct systems. Most cases arise in children between ages seven and fourteen, with a mean age of diagnosis at 10 years. The appendix testis is located at the anterosuperior portion of the testis (Fig. 16.5) and is predisposed to torsion due to its pedunculated shape [12].

Question 3: If this patient had presented immediately, how might you manage this patient?

While in the immediate presentation phase, patients may have considerable pain. This should be addressed with the appropriate analgesics. The physical examination includes assessment for blue dot sign (gangrenous appendix). Patients will be assessed for the presence of a cremasteric reflex, traditionally absent in testicular torsion, but present in this case. Sonography shows evidence of testicle adjacent to a hypoechoic mass (appendix) surrounded by color Doppler showing an area of perfusion. Given this, the patient can continue to be managed supportively, with analgesics, bed rest, and scrotal support. Pain usually resolves within 5–10 days, with surgery reserved only for pain in persistent cases [13–15]. It cannot be overstated that this diagnosis, if equivocal on history and physical and/or US, should be confirmed with surgical exploration of the scrotum to rule out testicular torsion. In the present scenario, however, the patient was re-evaluated 1 week later and is found to no longer have pain.

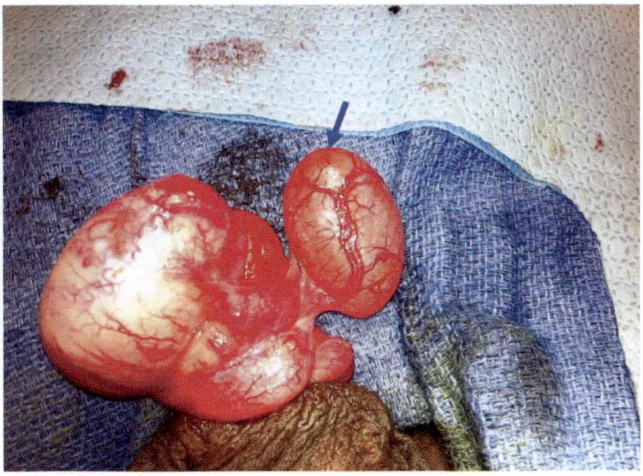

Fig. 16.5 exploration of testicular appendage torsion. Hyperemic component of testicular appendage

16.5 Acute Scrotum-Nonvascular—Epididymo-Orchitis

Scenario 5: A 17-year-old male with a history of sexual activity with 2 female partners in the last 1 year and presents to a community clinic at which you volunteer with a 4-day history of one-sided testicular pain. He also complains of intermittent white discharge from the penis. When asked, he reports that he does not use barrier protection. He also reports pain with urination. Physical exam reveals a swollen right testicle with substantial induration. Urinalysis reveals positive leukocyte esterase, negative nitrites, and 23 wbc/hpf. He is prescribed antibiotics for epididymitis.

Question 1: What tests for this condition allow us to rule out an emergency?

If there is low suspicion for testicular torsion, Doppler US for blood circulation in the spermatic cord may be assessed. The test has a sensitivity for detection of torsion of 89%, and specificity of 91.3% (Fig. 16.6) [13, 14].

Question 2: What is the appropriate diagnostic workup in this scenario?

Given high rates of co-infection, the gonorrhea-chlamydia nucleic acid amplification test (NAAT) of the urine is needed for definitive diagnosis. Additionally, 98% of symptomatic gonorrhea infections may be found by the presence of gram negative diplococci on gram stain [19]. Urinalysis may also be conducted to assess for leukocyte esterase and nitrate. The leukocyte esterase, a test of WBC activity is positive, with 10 or more cells/hpf. Nitrites, a metabolite induced by increased nitrate reductase activity are negative in Neisseria gonorrhea infection [25–27].

Question 3: Is there any surgical management indicated in this case?

No surgical exploration is indicated. Antibiotics directed against both N. Gonorrhea and Chlamydia are first line in the management of sexually active

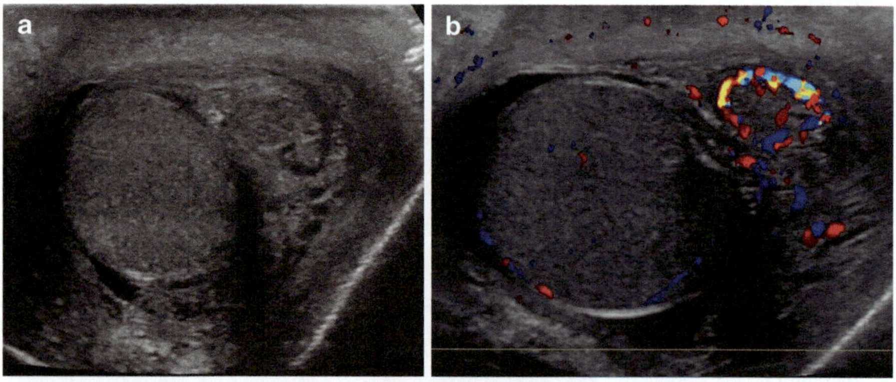

Fig. 16.6 Appearance of epididymo-orchitis (**a**) Gray-scale image showing minimal-reflective areas in upper pole of testis. Extra-testicular fluid and epididymis distortion are seen. (**b**) Doppler image provides evidence of increased blood flow. (Reprinted with permission from "Clinical and Imaging Features of Testicular Torsion: Role of Ultrasound: Review" by Sidhu. Clinical Radiology. 1999, 54, 343–352)

patients under age 35 with high suspicion for epididymitis or orchitis [26, 27]. In addition to surgical management, proper sexually transmitted disease (STD) counselling and education must be provided for this patient.

16.6 Acute Scrotum-Vascular—Testicular Torsion

Scenario 6: A 16-year-old male is referred for sudden, severe, right groin pain of 4 h duration. Patient denies any urethral discharge or urinary symptoms. Physical examination is negative for pain relief with gentle lifting of the testis, and cremasteric reflex is not present. Physical exam shows a (approximately 12 ml volume) tender, elevated right testis. The patient is immediately taken to the operating room for surgical exploration. During surgery, he is found to have a viable left testis and hyperemic right testis with a Bell-Clapper deformity. Bilateral 3-point orchiopexy is performed [28].

Question 1: Is there a need for USS scan in this scenario?

If immediately available, Color Doppler Ultrasound will conform the diagnosis. However, because time is of the essence here no unnecessary time should be wasted in confirmation of the diagnosis. If resources are not available and clinical diagnosis is confirmatory, immediate surgical exploration is a must, ideally within 6 h to salvage the testis.

Question 2: What is meant by a Bell-Clapper deformity? How may it relate to risk of testicular torsion?

Failure of the normal testis to be anchored posteriorly to the epididymis is the term for bell-clapper (Fig. 16.7). The term is analogous to the clapper inside of a bell because it allows for the testis to swing freely, rotating inside the tunica vaginalis of the scrotum. The incidence of bell-clapper in autopsy series is roughly 12%. The Bell-Clapper deformity accounts for up to 90% of testicular torsion cases [29].

Question 3: How is testicular size and position impacted by testicular torsion?

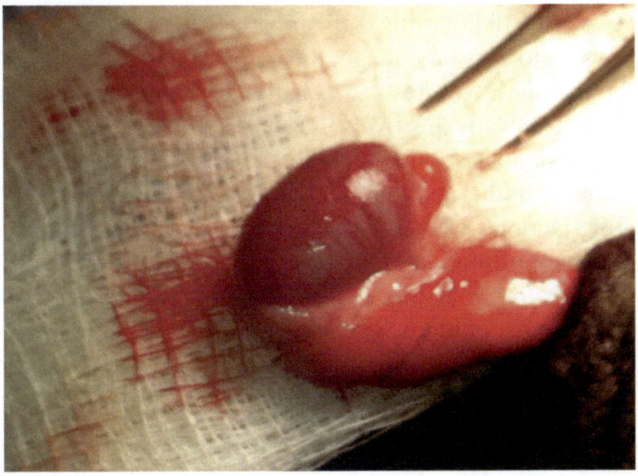

Fig. 16.7 Normal testicular investment with tunica vaginalis parietal lamina (TVPL) attached to a large portion of epididymis. The TVPL attaches to a small portion of the epididymis, but the tail of the epididymis is free

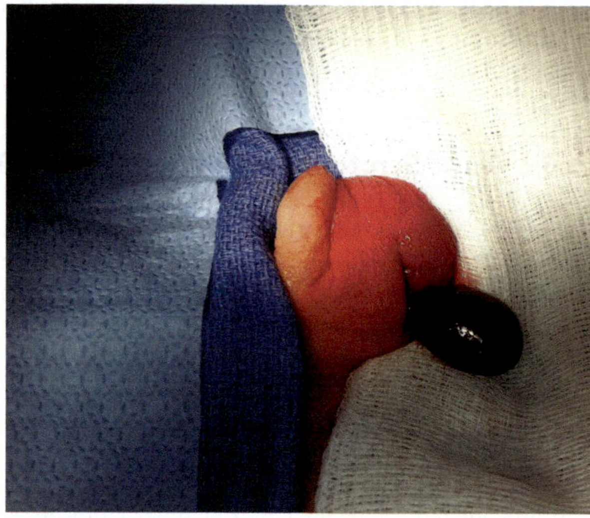

Fig. 16.8 Non-viable, necrotic testes—torsion

In patients with torsion, the spermatic cord becomes shortened as it continues to twist, causing it to rise higher in the testicle. The testis is then seen as higher with comparison to the contralateral testis, a specific finding—especially for left sided torsion, in which the testicle lays in a more dependent position. Additionally, due to venous congestion from the testicular vein, the testis begins to swell. Therefore, the normal 3–5 cm in length, 2–4 cm in width testicle may seem larger in the initial period (under approximately 6 h). After this, testicular atrophy occurs if vascular supply is unrestored beyond 6 h (Fig. 16.8) [30].

Question 4: What features of the case allow you to consider the diagnosis of testicular torsion instead of epididymo-orchitis (the presumed diagnosis in the original case)?

Acute epididymo-orchitis, an inflammation of the testis and epididymis may be due to sterile inflammation, or infection, resulting in pain for a period of less than 6 weeks. Epididymitis is the most frequent etiology of intrascrotal inflammation. In boys up to 13 years of age, the incidence is 1.2 per 1000. In testicular torsion one of the hallmark features is a negative cremasteric reflex (sensitivity and specificity of 96 and 88%, respectively). The absence of this reflex is more likely to lead to a diagnosis of testicular torsion [31]. Prehn's sign (pain relief with elevation of the testis) is traditionally associated with epididymitis, but the finding is highly unreliable. Doppler US for blood circulation in the spermatic cord has a sensitivity for detection of torsion of 89%, and specificity of 91.3% (Fig. 16.9) [13, 14].

Question 5: If this patient's timeline from symptom to presentation had been 36 h, how should this have changed management?

With delayed presentation, it is reasonable and common practice to proceed with an exploratory surgery. The benefit of this is twofold: first, it is important to rule out the possibility of a viable testis, though unlikely; secondly, one must be sure to pin the contralateral testis, given the reasonably high risk of torsion (approximately 40%) [14].

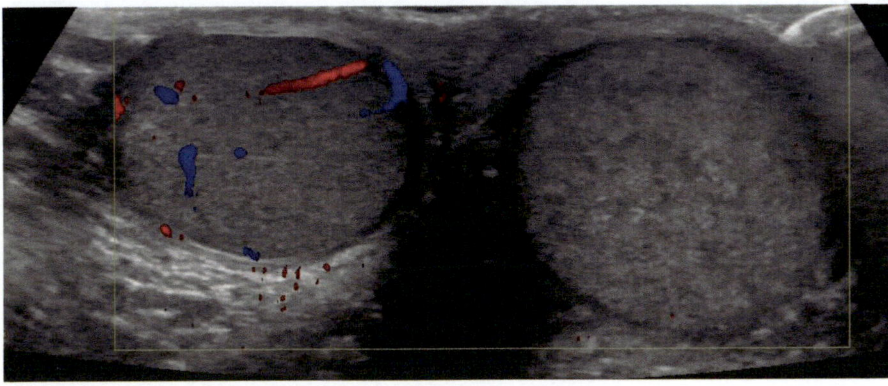

Fig. 16.9 USS showing left sided testicular torsion

16.7 Buried Penis-Acquired

Scenario 7: An ex 37-week gestation, 10-year-old male was referred because his mother is concerned about the appearance of his penile shaft in combination with "peeing on himself". On examination, you find an obese (BMI >95 percentile), uncircumcised child, Tanner Stage 1, with a prominent mons pubis. 2 cm of the penis is visible (Fig. 16.10), though suprapubic fat pad palpation shows evidence of a penile length that is within normal physiologic limits. Due to the likely absence of benefit from surgery, the patient and mother are instructed about the importance of lifestyle modification for the management of his condition. The patient and mother agree to adhere to your instructions. At follow up over the next several years, patient proceeds from Tanner stage 1 up to 3, followed by increasing protuberance of the penis [32].

Question 1: What is the strict definition of a buried penis? How does this definition differ from that of micropenis?

The buried penis is a diagnosis carried by patients in whom a penis of normal size can be appreciated (stretched penile length of 4.4 ± 0.6, 5.8 ± 0.8 and 7.2 ± 1.6 cm at birth, age 5, and age 11, respectively). Micropenis is a disorder of the Hypothalamic-Pituitary-Adrenal (HPA) axis in which the penis length is 2.5 standard deviations less than that of the normal child [33].

Question 2: What is the etiology of acquired buried penis?

The buried penis in childhood is due to two unique etiologies. In this particular scenario, the buried penis is from abundant adipose tissue on the anterior abdominal wall in older children. As a consequence, it is possible to recognize the condition prenatally. This results in poor fixation of the penile skin at the penile base, with excessive suprapubic adipose weight causing further symptomatic distress [34].

Question 3: Does timeline for surgery matter?

Buried penis is widely considered as a challenging condition to manage in both pediatric and adult populations [34]. Many surgeons decide to delay surgery

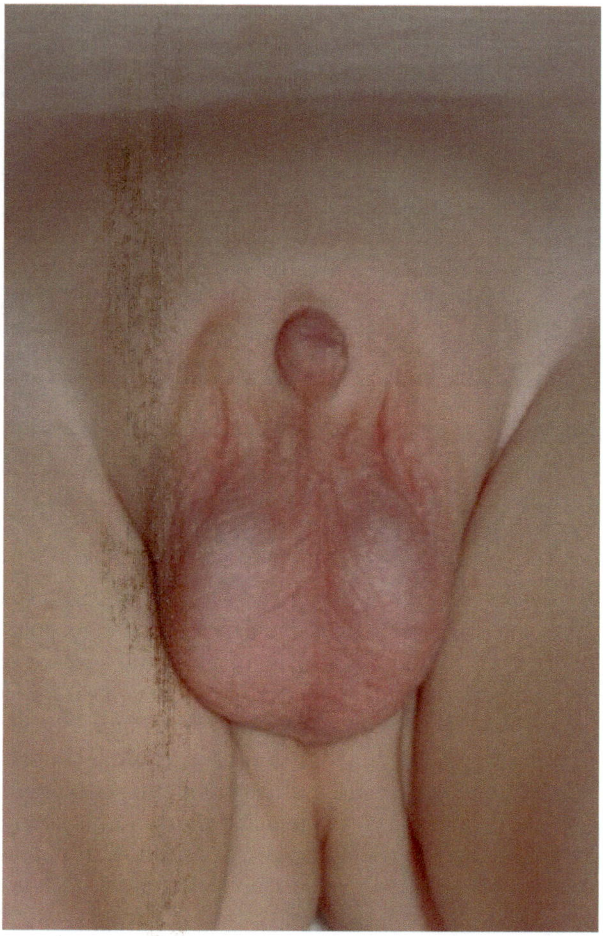

Fig. 16.10 Obesity induced acquired buried penis. (Reprinted with permission from "Buried Penis: Evaluation of Outcomes in Children and Adults, Modification of a Unified Treatment Algorithm, and Review of the Literature" by King, Tahir, Ramanathan, and Siddiqui is licensed under CC BY 3.0)

(Fig. 16.11) up to years in extreme cases, in the hopes of providing an improved prognosis for obese patients. A considerable concern is for prevention of obesity-related anesthesia complications. A further reason for the delay in surgical intervention is for the determination of the effect that skin shrinkage may have on the hidden penis. Children are often referred primarily on the basis of cosmesis. It is thought that children with the condition have a 57% chance of spontaneous resolution, with a large proportion of children in the spontaneous resolution group under age 3 [35]. After age 3, many urologists indicate that primary reason for repair should take into consideration the ability to void while standing during the toilet training period. Failure to do so, especially in the uncircumcised, delays proper hygiene, and leads to an increased rate of urinary tract infection (UTI). Though the authros preference is mainly focuss on diet and obesity has the surgery has poor outcomes.

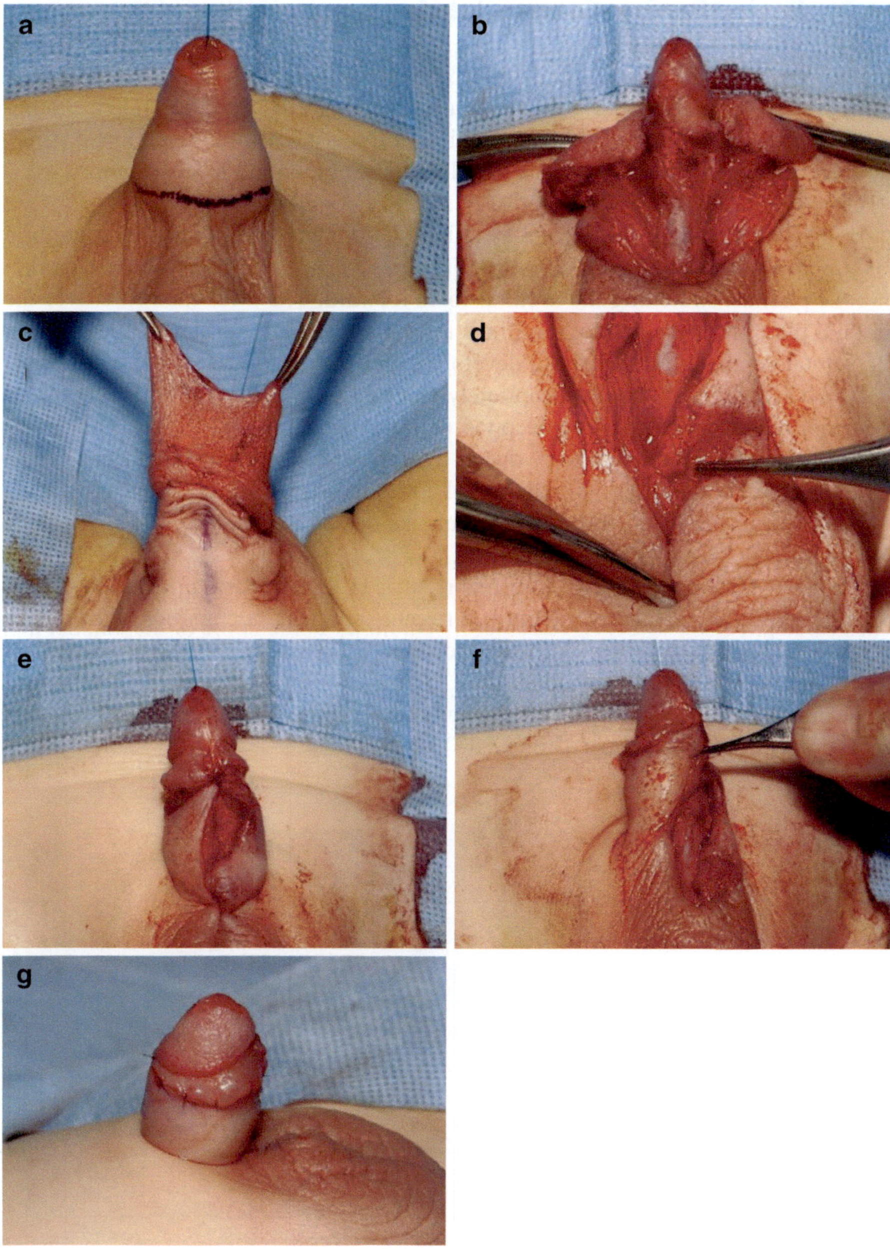

Fig. 16.11 **a-g** Anatomical repair of buried penis

16.8 Buried Penis—Congenital Megaprepuce

Scenario 8: A 12-month-old boy is referred with a 9-month history of gross penile swelling and an inability to void spontaneously (Fig. 16.12). The child's mother enables him to void with manual expression of the urine from the ballooned penis. No evidence of inflammation in the glandular or preputial tissue was found.

Question 1: What is the etiology of this child's condition?

In normal gestation, the scrotal swellings appear bilaterally about the urethral folds in the sixth week of development. The genital tubercle begins its elongation into the phallus, stretching the urethral folds forward. The folds then fuse over the urethral plate, with the scrotal swellings migrating caudally until they meet across the scrotal septum. If all of these developmental planes fail to separate appropriately, the scrotum may be inappropriately elevated in the groin, and the corpora of the penis may be tethered to the deep fascia of the pubic region [36, 37]. The condition has also been postulated to be due to dysgenesis of the dartos fascia in infancy, resulting in inelastic tissue with abnormal adhesions to the proximal portion of the corpus cavernosum [34]. Abnormalities may be detected prenatally.

Question 2: Surgical management?

Unless the patient presents with recurrent UTI and voiding into the megaprepuce, surgery is indicated. Many different surgical techniques have been described.,the author prefers anatomical repair as described in (BJUI 1999 Smulders et al) Still, many authors agree that initial routine circumcision is not recommended in the management of children with the condition, as it removes portions of foreskin necessary for penile coverage (Fig. 16.13) [38].

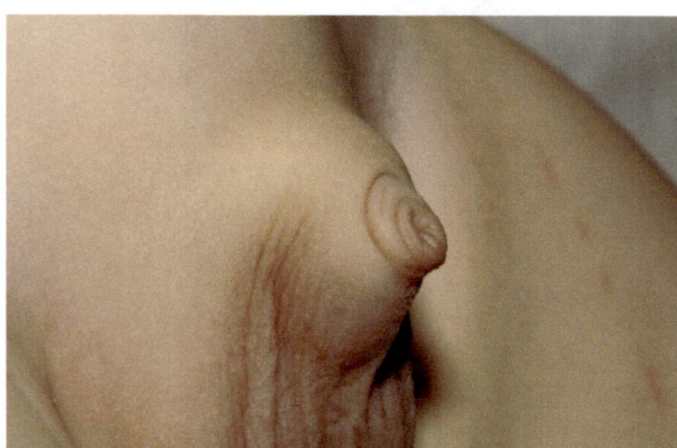

Fig. 16.12 Congenital megaprepuce, prior to repair

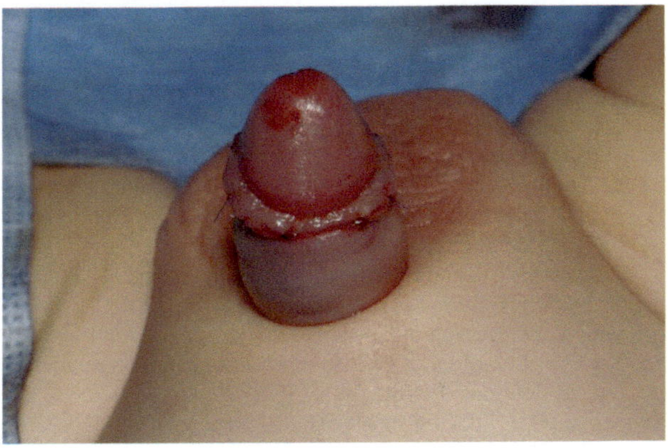

Fig. 16.13 Congenital megaprepuce, after repair

16.8.1 Scenario 1

16.8.2 Scenario 2

16.8.3 Scenario 3

Scenario 4

16.8.4 Scenario 5

16.8.5 Scenario 6

16.8.6 Scenario 7-Acquired

16.8.7 Scenario 8-Congenital

Acknowledgments The authors would like to acknowledge Dr. Kate Feinstein, Professor of Radiology and Surgery, Section Chief, Pediatric Radiology at the University of Chicago for her contribution with image collection.

References

1. Yu YD, Hong YK. A case of cryptorchidism with Ipsilateral congenital unilateral absence of the vas deferens and contralateral renal agenesis. Case Rep Urol. 2016;2016
2. Huff DS, Hadžiselimovič F, Snyder HM, Blyth B, Duckett JW. Early postnatal testicular maldevelopment in cryptorchidism. J Urol. 1991;146(2):624–6.
3. Pierik FH, Deddens JA, Burdorf A, Keizer-Schrama SM, Jong FH, Weber RF. The hypothalamus-pituitary-testis axis in boys during the first six months of life: a comparison of cryptorchidism and hypospadias cases with controls. Int J Androl. 2009;32(5):453–61.
4. Schnack TH, Zdravkovic S, Myrup C, Westergaard T, Wohlfahrt J, Melbye M. Familial aggregation of cryptorchidism—a nationwide cohort study. Am J Epidemiol. 2008;167(12):1453–7.
5. Schlegel PN, Shin D, Goldstein M. Urogenital anomalies in men with congenital absence of the vas deferens. J Urol. 1996;155(5):1644–8.
6. Wood HM, Elder JS. Cryptorchidism and testicularcancer: separating fact from fiction. J Urol. 2009;181:452–61.
7. Lee MM, Misra M, Donahoe PK, MacLaughlin DT. MIS/AMH in the assessment of cryptorchidism and intersex conditions. Mol Cell Endocrinol. 2003;211(1–2):91–8.
8. Kolon TF, Herndon CA, Baker LA, Baskin LS, Baxter CG, Cheng EY, Diaz M, Lee PA, Seashore CJ, Tasian GE, Barthold JS. Evaluation and treatment of cryptorchidism: AUA guideline. J Urol. 2014;192(2):337–45.
9. Healthwise. Reviewers Pope J, Anderson P. Retractile testes. University of Michigan Health. Rev 2011 Apr 1. Accessed 2018 March 01. http://www.uofmhealth.org/health-library/rt1127.
10. Eltayeb AA. Single high scrotal incision orchidopexy for unilateral palpable testis: a randomised controlled study. Afr J Paediatr Surg. 2014;11(2):143.
11. Idrissa S, Oukhouya MA, Tazi M, Mahmoudi A, Elmadi A, Khattala K, Bouabdallah Y. Unusual cause of acute scrotum in children: a case report. Journal of surgical case reports. 2017;1(9):rjx172.
12. Fisher R, Walker J. The acute paediatric scrotum. Br J Hosp Med. 1994;51(6):290–2.
13. Edelsberg JS, Surh YS. The acute scrotum. Emerg Med Clin North Am. 1988;6(3):521–46.
14. Pillai SB, Besner GE. Pediatric testicular problems. Pediatr Clin. 1998;45(4):813–30.
15. Flanigan RC, Dekernion JB, Persky L. Acute scrotal pain and swelling in children: a surgical emergency. Urology. 1981;17(1):51–3.
16. Simons MP, Aufenacker T, Bay-Nielsen M, Bouillot JL, Campanelli G, Conze J, De Lange D, Fortelny R, Heikkinen T, Kingsnorth A, Kukleta J. European Hernia Society guidelines on the treatment of inguinal hernia in adult patients.
17. Højer AM, Rygaard H, Jess P. CT in the diagnosis of abdominal wall hernias: a preliminary study. Eur Radiol. 1997;7(9):1416–8.
18. Steinau G, Treutner KH, Feeken G, Schumpelick V. Recurrent inguinal hernias in infants and children. World J Surg. 1995;19(2):303–6.
19. Stylianos S, Jacir NN, Harris BH. Incarceration of inguinal hernia in infants prior to elective repair. J Pediatr Surg. 1993;28(4):582–3.
20. Gahukamble DB, Khamage AS. Early versus delayed repair of reduced incarcerated inguinal hernias in the pediatric population. J Pediatr Surg. 1996;31(9):1218–20.
21. Galejs LE. Diagnosis and treatment of the acute scrotum. Am Fam Physician. 1999;59(4):817–24.
22. Cohen HL, Shapiro MA, Haller JO, Glassberg K. Torsion of the testicular appendage. Sonographic diagnosis. J Ultrasound Med. 1992;11(3):81–3.
23. Anderson P, Giacomantonio J. The acutely painful scrotum in children: review of 113 consecutive cases. Can Med Assoc J. 1985;132(10):1153.
24. Hornak M, Bárdos JA. Diagnostic and therapeutic problems of acute scrotum. Czech Med. 1986;9(1):29–33.

25. Asgari SA, Mokhtari G, Falahatkar S, Mansour-Ghanaei M, Roshani A, Zare A, Zamani M, Khosropanah I, Salehi M. Diagnostic accuracy of C-reactive protein and erythrocyte sedimentation rate in patients with acute scrotum. Urol J. 2009;3(2):103–7.
26. Waller DG, editor. Sexually transmitted infections, HIV & AIDS E-book: key articles from the medicine journal: Elsevier Health Sciences; 2016.
27. Gaydos CA, et al. Comparison of three nucleic acid amplification tests for detection of chlamydia trachomatis in urine specimens. J Clin Microbiol. 2004;42(7):3041–5.
28. Khan F, Muoka O, Watson GM. Bell clapper testis, torsion, and detorsion: a case report. Case Rep Urol. 2011;2011
29. Ringdahl E, Teague L. Testicular torsion. Am Fam Physician. 2006;15(74(10)):1739–43.
30. Hebert SC, Chong WK, Deurdulian C. Essentials of scrotal ultrasound: a review of frequently encountered abnormalities. Appl Radiol. 2012;41(9):7.
31. Schmitz D, Safranek S. How useful is a physical exam in diagnosing testicular torsion?. Clin Inquiries, 2009 (MU). 2009.
32. Bergeson PS, Hopkin RJ, Bailey RB, MCGill LC, Piatt JP. The inconspicuous penis. Pediatrics. 1993;92(6):794–9.
33. Lee JH, Ji YH, Lee SK, Hwang HH, Ryu DS, Kim KS, Choo HS, Park S, Moon KH, Cheon SH, Park S. Change in penile length in children: preliminary study. Korean J Urol. 2012;53(12):870–4.
34. King IC, Tahir A, Ramanathan C, Siddiqui H. Buried penis: evaluation of outcomes in children and adults, modification of a unified treatment algorithm, and review of the literature. ISRN urology. 2013;29:2013.
35. Radhakrishnan J, Razzaq A, Manickam K. Concealed penis. Pediatr Surg Int. 2002;18(8):668–72.
36. Sadler TW. Langman's medical embryology. Philadelphia, PA: Lippincott Williams & Wilkins; 2011.
37. Smeulders N, Wilcox DT, Cuckow PM. The buried penis–an anatomical approach. BJU Int. 2000;86(4):523–6.
38. Podestá ML, Podestá M Jr. Megaprepuce reconstruction: a single center experience. Front Pediatr. 2018;6:64.

Inguinal Hernia, Hydrocele, Varicocele, Spermatocele and Abdomino-Scrotal Hydrocele

17

Neetu Kumar and Imran Mushtaq

Learning Objectives

1. To differentiate between the common groin/scrotal conditions that present in the paediatric age group.
2. To recognize the emergency/urgent vs elective cases and to deal with it appropriately.
3. To understand the investigation pathway to assist with the differential diagnosis.
4. To keep updated with current management options of groin/scrotal conditions.
5. To understand the nuances associated with difficult scenarios in groin/scrotal pathologies.

17.1 Inguinal Hernia

Baby boy born at 32 weeks' gestation is on NICU. He is now 4 weeks old and the neonatal doctor has noted a lump in the left groin. It is reducible.

- **Q1. What is the most likely diagnosis?**
- **Q2. What is the incidence of this condition?**
- **Q3. What clinical findings help differentiate it from other conditions?**
- **Q4. When is the best time to operate?**

A1. The most likely diagnosis is an inguinal hernia.

A2. Inguinal hernia in children is a common presentation to the paediatric urologist. The incidence of an inguinal hernia in a term neonate is 3–5%. This increases to 10–30% with the degree of prematurity [1–3]. It is nearly 5 times more prevalent in boys, the right-side hernias being twice as common as the left side ones. 15%

N. Kumar · I. Mushtaq (✉)
Great Ormond Street Hospital, London, UK
e-mail: neetu.kumar@gosh.nhs.uk; imran.mushtaq@gosh.nhs.uk

P. Godbole et al. (eds.), *Practical Pediatric Urology*,
https://doi.org/10.1007/978-3-030-54020-3_17

occur bilaterally [4]. Conditions that increase the risk of inguinal herniae include cystic fibrosis, hydrocephalus, peritoneal dialysis, abdominal wall defects connective tissue disorders (Ehlers Danlos syndrome) mucopolysaccharidosis (Hunter or Hurlers syndrome), ascites, cryptorchidism, congenital hip dislocation and myelomeningocele.

A3. An inguinal hernia in a child is usually an indirect hernia. The aetiology is the persistence of the patent processes vaginalis (PPV) after birth, which allows peritoneal contents like bowel and omentum to come through to present as a lump in the groin. Most parents will give a history of a bulge in the groin especially after straining or crying.

On clinical examination, positive 'silk glove sign' (thickened PPV in the cord) is palpated. One may feel the testis separately from the lump but cannot get above the swelling (difference from hydrocele). This lump is reducible. Large hernia may extend into the scrotum in boys. Ultrasonography may demonstrate a PPV with peritoneal contents through it but radiological investigations are not commonly used.

A4. Timing of surgery plays a key role in decision making in children. Most surgeons would prefer to repair the hernia in premature infants once they are ready to discharge from the neonatal unit [5]. Infants under the age of 6 months are operated on the next available operating list. Asymptomatic children over the age of 1 year can be operated electively. Parents are advised about the risk of incarceration and the signs and symptoms to watch for during the waiting time till surgery.

9-month-old boy is brought to the Accident and emergency department by his parents with a red tender lump in the right groin, which is irreducible.

- **Q1. What is the diagnosis?**
- **Q2. What are the risks/ complications of this condition?**
- **Q3. What is the management strategy for this patient?**
- **Q4. What are the advantages and disadvantages of open vs laparoscopic technique of repair?**

A1. This patient has an incarcerated right inguinal hernia.

A2. The complications of incarceration and bowel obstruction along with compression of cord structure is possible. Torsion and ischemia of the ovary (in females) is also known to complicate the inguinal hernia.

A3. In emergency cases of incarceration, every attempt should be made to reduce the hernia as soon as possible. In infants <3 months of age that have required manual reduction, the inguinal herniotomy should be done before discharge as these have a 15% reincarceration incidence with delayed repair after 5 days [5, 6]. In older children, the procedure can be done electively. However, in an irreducible inguinal hernia the patient should be taken to theatres for reduction and inspection of the hernial contents followed by the inguinal herniotomy.

A4. The incidence of incarceration of inguinal hernia ranges between 6 and 18%. It is much higher in infants with the risk increasing up to 30% [7]. Surgery is therefore an indication to all children presenting with an inguinal hernia. The traditional open inguinal approach still remains popular amongst Paediatric Urologists. The PPV is separated from the vas and vessels, high ligation with absorbable sutures (up to the deep ring) and divided. The risks following this procedure are low (<1%) but the potential injury to the vas and vessels remains, including wound infection, haematoma, testicular atrophy and recurrence of hernia.

Laparoscopic inguinal hernia repair has been in practice since 1993, first described by Montupet. The initial description has been of an intracorporeal repair consisting of a purse string suture in the peritoneum at the level of the internal ring [8]. Since then various modifications and variations have been introduced [9]. It can be an intracorporeal or extracorporeal/percutaneous. There is insufficient evidence to support one technique from the other [10]. The benefits of laparoscopic approach vs the traditional open technique includes visualisation of contralateral open ring, improved cosmesis and post-operative pain. However, with every laparoscopic procedure increase in length of operative timing, cost and introduction of pneumoperitoneum in small infants still remains the potential disadvantages.

Many surgeons advocate the advantage of laparoscopic approach in the oedematous groin following an episode of incarceration with subsequent manual reduction. It allows inspection of the hernial contents, viability of bowel and avoids the risk of damage to the vas and vessels, which in the open inguinal technique can prove be very challenging and associated with increased morbidity and complications.

Laparoscopy has over the years evolved with fine instruments and sophisticated technical details. It definitely has its benefits in bilateral inguinal hernia repairs, visualising uncommon conditions like direct or femoral hernia and reducing the occurrence of metachronous contralateral hernia. However, the evidence does not show either approach to be superior from one another [11]. Parents should be made aware of both techniques with advantages and disadvantages of each.

17.2 Hydrocele

2-year-old boy is seen in Accident and Emergency Department. He had a viral upper respiratory tract illness and 2 days later they have noticed a swelling in the scrotum.

- **Q1. What is the differential diagnosis of a swelling in the scrotum in a 2-year old presenting to the Accident & Emergency Department?**
- **Q2. What is the usual presentation and clinical examination findings of this condition?**
- **Q3. How common is this condition? Is it a congenital problem?**
- **Q4. What is the best management approach?**
- **Q5. Name some other types of hydrocele.**

A1. The differential diagnosis of an acute scrotum would include torsion of the testis, torsion of hydatid cyst of Morgagni, inguinal hernia, hydrocele and idiopathic scrotal oedema.

A2. Most boys will present with a scrotal swelling usually noticed by the parents. It may precede a viral infection. In girls, there is a groin lump. Some parents of the toddlers give a good history of it being small first thing in the morning and noticeably bigger at the end of the day suggesting a communicating hydrocele. Non-communicating hydroceles are not as common and usually occur in older boys.

It is a painless swelling and, in most cases, the underlying testis can be felt separately. In the tense hydroceles, the testes are difficult to palpate. The ability to get above the irreducible swelling distinguishes it from an inguinal hernia. Transillumination test is positive but not a reliable test in children as the incarcerated bowel may also transilluminate. Clinical examination is enough to make a diagnosis. In some cases of doubt, ultrasonography is a reliable investigation.

A3. Hydrocele is a collection of peritoneal fluid within the tunica vaginalis testis. It is the result of persistence of the processus vaginalis, allowing fluid to communicate to the scrotum via the patent processus vaginalis (PPV). It is a common cause of swelling in the scrotum and occurs in 2–5% of boys, usually before the age of 5 years [12]. It is uncommon in girls and when present is called Hydrocele of the canal of Nuck.

Hydroceles can be classified as congenital or acquired. The acquired or secondary causes may be due to infection, trauma, torsion, tumour, or iatrogenic like following varicocele surgery. Children with indwelling ventriculo-peritoneal shunts or peritoneal dialysis have increased intraperitoneal fluid which may exacerbate a hydrocele.

A4. PPV ligation is a common procedure performed by the Paediatric Urologist. However, the surgical indications unlike that of inguinal hernia is age dependent. In a recent UK survey, most paediatric surgeons/urologists would manage hydroceles conservatively for the first 2 years of life and offer surgery if it persists beyond the age of 2–3 years [13]. However, a significant number of surgeons deferred it until 4 years and offered surgical intervention prior to the child starting school.

Surgery is performed as a day case via a groin incision, with separation of the PPV from the vas and vessels and high ligation with an absorbable suture. Laparoscopic repairs similar to inguinal hernias with aspiration of the scrotal fluid is also practised.

A5. Encysted hydrocele occurs when the fluid gets trapped within its layers during the natural closure of the processus vaginalis. Meconium hydrocele is a neonatal condition secondary to the gastrointestinal perforation leading to meconium staining of the hydrocele fluid. Non-communicating hydroceles in older boys can be approached via the scrotum and a Lord procedure (excision of excess of processus vaginalis) [13, 14] or a Jaboulay procedure (marsupialisation of the free edge of tunica vaginalis) is performed. Recurrent hydrocele is rare. Ultrasound is performed to exclude a recurrent inguinal hernia and these children may need re exploration of the groin combined with the scrotal approach.

17.3 Varicocele

15-year boy is referred to the urology clinic with 4-month history of dull ache in the left testis.

- **Q1. What is the differential diagnosis?**
- **Q2. What clinical findings and investigations are key to the diagnosis?**
- **Q3. What is the pathophysiology of this condition?**
- **Q4. What are the indications for a surgical intervention?**
- **Q5. What are the different modalities of treatment?**
- **Q6. What is the effect on fertility?**

A1. The differential diagnosis should always exclude torsion of the testis with careful history and clinical examination. The others include inguinal hernia, hydrocele, epididymal cyst and varicocele.

A2. The majority of boys and young adult men present with a painless scrotal swelling. At times however, there may be a dull ache or dragging sensation, exacerbated by exercise or in hot weather conditions.

On examination, the dilated veins are palpated like a 'bag of worms'. It is imperative that the genitalia are examined in both standing and lying down positions to confirm disappearance of the dilated veins in supine position. The clinical grading system of Dublin and Amelar was recently expanded by the World Health Organisation (WHO) to include an additional 'subclinical' grade 0.

- Grade 0: Subclinical, detected on ultrasound only.
  - Grade 1: Palpable on Valsalva's manoeuvre
  - Grade 2: Palpable (not visible) without Valsalva's manoeuvre
  - Grade 3: Visible, negating the need for palpation

Testicular size or volume should also be assessed as baseline during the physical examination. This is useful for assessing size and volume discrepancy between the two sides to direct further follow up. Various methods such as Prader orchidometer, Rochester (Takihara) orchidometer, rulers and callipers have been used to evaluate the testicular size and volume. Lambert's formula is widely used for calculating the testis volume (in millilitres) when applying a two-dimensional measuring system. As described by Lambert, the volume is calculated by multiplication of width x length x depth in centimetres by a constant usually 0.71 [15].

Ultrasonography is now increasing being used to confirm the diagnosis and accurately document the testicular size. Ultrasound is a more reliable method as compared to an orchidometer as there are less inter-observer differences with the imaging modality [15, 16].

It is to be noted that right sided varicoceles are rare. Varicocele in a young child is equally rare. An abdominal ultrasound is recommended to rule out neoplasms such as Wilms tumour in very young children as a varicocele may be a secondary finding in such cases due to venous congestion.

A3. Varicocele is described as an abnormal enlargement of the pampiniform venous plexus that drains blood from the testis. The prevalence in children and adolescents is estimated to be between 10 and 15% [17] and it is uncommon in boys under 10 years of age [18].

The pampiniform plexus drains mainly into the testicular vein which drains further into the inferior vena cava on the right and into the renal vein on the left. The testicular vein draining into the left forms an approximately 90-degree angle that leads to the left renal vein being easily compressed between the adjacent superior mesenteric artery and the aorta, thus resulting in impeded venous drainage from the left testis, described as the nutcracker effect [18, 19]. This anatomical difference between the right and the left venous drainage can explain the predominant left sided varicocele formation.

A4. In the year 2016, The European Urology Pediatric Guidelines made the following recommendations with regards criteria for varicocele treatment in children and adolescents: varicocele associated with low testicular volume, presence of an additional testicular condition with affected fertility, varicoceles that are bilateral and palpable, abnormal sperm quality in older adolescents with varicoceles, or symptomatic varicoceles- irrespective of the grade of the varicocele. Regular follow up with clinical examination and ultrasound to measure the testicular size is recommended.

Of note, in a study by Cervellione et al., 28% of their subclinical varicocele cohort progressed on to a clinically detectable varicocele at 4 year follow up, and 67% remained unchanged [20].

A5. Varicoceles can be treated by various techniques. The basic principle of treatment is to interrupt the venous return through the internal spermatic vein. Angiographic occlusion of the internal spermatic veins can be performed by retrograde or antegrade injection of a sclerosing agent. This technique is considered as lymphatic and internal artery sparing technique, which in turn prevents hydrocele formation. Failure rate varies between 5 and 20% [21].

Surgical approach may either be an inguinal approach (Ivanissevich), the high approach (Paloma) or the microsurgical approach. The microsurgical repair technique is considered to have fewer complications and lower recurrence rates of all but does require extensive microsurgical training.

The Paloma technique is widely adopted in clinical practice. It is an open surgical approach with access achieved proximally on the spermatic vessels.

Laparoscopic varicocelectomy follows the same principles as the Paloma procedure. Its advantages include early post-operative recovery, better optic magnification and cosmesis, though the success rates are reported to be similar to the open procedure.

Published meta-analysis in children show that results after laparoscopic technique are similar to open with recurrence rates of 8.6 and 4.7% respectively and post-operative hydrocele rate of 6.7 and 7.1% respectively. Laparoscopic lymphatic sparing approach has a lower incidence of hydrocele (4.3 vs. 17.6%) but higher incidence of recurrence (3.5 vs. 2.2%) than the Paloma procedure [21, 22]. There is low level of evidence in support of radiological or surgical intervention for varicoceles in children and adolescents to improve testicular volume or sperm concentration [23].

A6. There is a normal 10% size variation between the two testes [24]. Studies by Diamond et al. showed that relative testicular size discrepancy greater than 10% in Tanner stage 5 adolescents is associated with decreased sperm concentration and total sperm count [25]. Further, sperm abnormality was greater for volume differences in excess of 20% between the two sides [25, 26]. Also to note, small ipsilateral testis has shown that corrective surgery may result in catch up growth in 80% of those testes [27]. The cause and relationship between varicocele and fertility is not fully clear or understood. Studies have shown that the prevalence of varicocele is 20–40% in men seeking investigations for fertility reasons [27–29]. However, only 15–20% of men with varicocele require treatment for infertility, suggesting that most men with varicocele do not report any adverse fertility issues [30]. This fact is important to emphasise during counselling of adolescent boys and their parents and post pubertal boys should be offered semen analysis to confirm appropriate sperm count and motility as baseline.

17.4 Abdomino-Scrotal Hydrocele

6-month-old boy is referred to the clinic with a large inguinal scrotal lump. He is asymptomatic.

- **Q1. What is the differential diagnosis?**
- **Q2. What clinical examination and radiological investigations help with the diagnosis?**
- **Q3. Is this a congenital abnormality? What is the pathophysiology of this condition?**
- **Q4. (a) What are the indications for surgical management?**
  (b) What is the surgical approach?

A1. The differential diagnosis includes inguinal scrotal hernia, lymphatic malformation and Abdomino-Scrotal Hydrocele (ASH).

A2. On clinical examination, a combination of a scrotal swelling with an abdominal swelling just above the inguinal ligament, ASH should be suspected. The cross fluctuant between the tense hydrocele and abdominal mass is the 'Springing back ball' sign [31]. A cough impulse may be present. It can be partially reduced or emptied on lying supine. Trans-illumination test is positive. Ultrasound is diagnostic. Contrast enhanced compute tomography or magnetic resonance imaging are useful investigations to demonstrate the extension of the hydrocele. Other commonly associated pathologies that occurs in nearly 20% of cases include ipsilateral or contralateral cryptorchidism, contralateral inguinal hernia or simple hydrocele [32].

A3. Abdomino-scrotal hydrocele (ASH) is a rare congenital abnormality of the processes vaginalis. It is characterised by a fluid filled mass in the inguinal scrotal area with a hidden, often deep intra-abdominal component that communicates in an hour glass fashion through the inguinal canal. The incidence is between 1.25 and 3.1% of all hydroceles noted in infancy [32, 33]. The incidence of ASH increasing with the expanding use of Ultrasonography. Bilateral ASH is rare.

There is only one sonographic report of prenatal detection [34]. The first paediatric case was reported by Syme, though the term ASH was termed by Bickel in 1919. Dupuytren described it a 'hydrocele en bisac' in 1834. The aetiology is unclear. Many theories are postulated including the valve theory, diverticulum theory and displacement as per Laplace's theory [35]. The most popular and accepted theory is that of Dupuytren's which suggests that excessive intracystic pressure causes cephalad extension of the scrotal swelling through the deep inguinal ring [35].

A4 (a) Recent Systematic review (Doudt et al) showed there were no cases of complete spontaneous resolution [32]. The potential for compressive or secondary effects like lower extremity oedema, hydronephrosis, torsion, haemorrhage, infection and the tangible chance of malignant transformation are indications for surgical intervention [31, 32].

(b) Various surgical approaches have been described in the literature. The inguinal approach is the most common, however given individual presentations combined inguinal+ extra peritoneal, combined inguinal+ scrotal approach is also described. A standard inguinal skin crease incision and the external oblique fascia and muscles are opened. The inguinal component of ASH is exposed. The tense hydrocele makes it difficult to separate it from the surrounding stricture. Aspiration of fluid from the scrotum rather than the inguinal area facilitates the procedure [32]. A patch of tunica vaginalis can be left attached to the spermatic cord structures when the hydrocele is associated with a thickened wall as separation of vas and vessels will be difficult and results in bleeding. The key principle is to excise the abdominal and scrotal component. The PPV is not always seen. Pre-operative clinical grading (simple and complex with further subclasses) has been proposed that may support differentiation of severity of the associated cumulative risks [32, 36].

17.5 Spermatocele

15-year-old boy is referred to the Urology clinic. The GP had arranged an ultrasound of the scrotum for another pathology and it showed a 1 cm extra testicular cystic structure. The patient is asymptomatic.

- **Q1. What is the differential diagnosis?**
- **Q2. What is the difference between the two diagnoses?**
- **Q3. (a) What are the typical clinical findings?**
  (b) What are the characteristic features seen on ultrasound to help with the diagnosis?
- **Q4. How should this patient be managed?**
- **Q5. What is the effect on fertility with surgical intervention?**

A1. The differential diagnosis includes Epididymal cyst or a Spermatocele.

A2. Spermatocele or spermatic cyst is a fluid-filled sac within the epididymis. It is a common type of extra testicular cyst and represents cystic dilatation of the tubules of the efferent ductules in the head of the epididymis. They sometimes can develop in varying locations from the testicle to locations along the course of vas deferens [37]. These are benign cysts and similar to epididymal cysts. The difference being the spermatocele contains fluid and sperm cells. Spermatoceles are not common in children but when they occur, they usually present around puberty.

A3. (a) Spermatoceles present with a painless lump felt just above and separate to the testicle. It is usually small in size ranging from a few mm to 2 cm, however large lesions up to 8 cm have been reported. Transillumination may be possible to differentiate it from solid lesions [37, 38].

(b) Ultrasound shows typical appearances of spermatocele. MRI is therefore not indicated. These cystic lesions show no arterial or venous blood flow within them on colour Doppler [38]. It appears as a unilocular or a multilocular hypoechoic cystic lesion. They may show low level echogenic internal echoes due to proteinaceous fluid containing dead sperms [38, 39].

A4. Small cysts are best left alone. Large asymptomatic cysts can be regularly followed up. The cyst if become symptomatic and causes discomfort or is increasing in size should be considered for removal [40]. Spermatocelectomy or excision of the cyst under general anaesthetic is performed in young boys. Aspiration of the fluid followed by injection of sclerosing agent (99.5% alcohol, phenol, 5% ethanolamine) is an alternative to surgery [41].

A5. The surgical procedure itself does not improve fertility. Sclerosing agents should be used with caution in reproductive-aged men for the risk of inducing chemical epididymitis which further may cause epididymal damage and possible future infertility.

References

1. Harper RG, Garcia A, Sia C. Inguinal hernia: a common problem of premature infants weighing 1,000 grams or less at birth. Pediatrics. 1975;56:112–5.
2. Kumar VHS, Clive J, Rosenkrantz TS, Bourque MD, Hussain N. Inguinal hernia in preterm infants (≤32-week gestation). Pediatr Surg Int. 2002;18:147–52.
3. Grosfeld JL. Current concepts in inguinal hernia in infants and children. World J Surg. 1989;13:506–15.
4. Six thousand three hundred sixty-one pediatric inguinal hernias: a 35-year review. In: Paperpile. https://paperpile.com/app/p/65f11b78-2cb5-0c7a-9594-0c05d5a7c824. Accessed 18 Mar 2019.
5. Groff DB. Inguinal hernias in premature infants operated on before discharge from the neonatal intensive care unit. Arch Surg. 1985;120:962.
6. Koivusalo A, Pakarinen MP, Rintala RJ. Laparoscopic herniorrhaphy after manual reduction of incarcerated inguinal hernia. Surg Endosc. 2007;21:2147–9.
7. Parelkar SV, Oak S, Gupta R, Sanghvi B, Shimoga PH, Kaltari D, Prakash A, Shekhar R, Gupta A, Bachani M. Laparoscopic inguinal hernia repair in the pediatric age group—experience with 437 children. J Pediatr Surg. 2010;45:789–92.

8. Esposito C, St. Peter SD, Escolino M, Juang D, Settimi A, Holcomb GW. Laparoscopic versus open inguinal hernia repair in pediatric patients: a systematic review. Journal of Laparoendoscopic & Advanced Surgical Techniques. 2014;24:811–8.
9. Ostlie DJ, Ponsky TA. Technical options of the laparoscopic pediatric inguinal hernia repair. Journal of Laparoendoscopic & Advanced Surgical Techniques. 2014;24:194–8.
10. Esposito C, Escolino M, Farina A, Settimi A. Two decades of history of laparoscopic pediatric inguinal hernia repair. J Laparoendosc Adv Surg Tech A. 2014;24:669–70.
11. Esposito C, Escolino M, Turrà F, Roberti A, Cerulo M, Farina A, Caiazzo S, Cortese G, Servillo G, Settimi A. Current concepts in the management of inguinal hernia and hydrocele in pediatric patients in laparoscopic era. Semin Pediatr Surg. 2016;25:232–40.
12. Madden N (2008) Testis, hydrocoele and varicocoele. Essen Paediatr Urol, 2nd ed, p 247–263.
13. Jobson M, Hall NJ. Current practice regarding timing of patent processus vaginalis ligation for idiopathic hydrocele in young boys: a survey of UK surgeons. Pediatr Surg Int. 2017;33:677–81.
14. Koutsoumis G, Patoulias I, Kaselas C. Primary new-onset hydroceles presenting in late childhood and pre-adolescent patients resemble the adult type hydrocele pathology. J Pediatr Surg. 2014;49:1656–8.
15. Paltiel HJ, Diamond DA, Di Canzio J, Zurakowski D, Borer JG, Atala A. Testicular volume: comparison of orchidometer and US measurements in dogs. Radiology. 2002;222:114–9.
16. Diamond DA, Paltiel HJ, DiCanzio J, Zurakowski D, Bauer SB, Atala A, Ephraim PL, Grant R, Retik AB. Comparative assessment of pediatric testicular volume: orchidometer versus ultrasound. J Urol. 2000:1111–4.
17. Meacham RB, Townsend RR, Rademacher D, Drose JA. The incidence of varicoceles in the general population when evaluated by physical examination, gray scale sonography and color Doppler sonography. J Urol. 1994;151:1535–8.
18. Akbay E, Çayan S, Doruk E, Duce MN, Bozlu M. The prevalence of varicocele and varicocele-related testicular atrophy in Turkish children and adolescents. BJU Int. 2000;86:490–3.
19. Stassen CM, Weil EH, Janevski BK. Left renal vein compression syndrome ("nutcracker phenomenon"). Rofo. 1989;150:708–10.
20. Cervellione RM, Corroppolo M, Bianchi A. Subclinical Varicocele in the pediatric age group. J Urol. 2008;179:717–9.
21. Clarke SA, Agrawal M, Reidy J. Percutaneous transfemoral testicular vein embolisation in the treatment of childhood varicocoele. Pediatr Radiol. 2001;31:515–7.
22. Borruto FA, Impellizzeri P, Antonuccio P, Finocchiaro A, Scalfari G, Arena F, Esposito C, Romeo C. Laparoscopic vs open varicocelectomy in children and adolescents: review of the recent literature and meta-analysis. J Pediatr Surg. 2010;45:2464–9.
23. Locke JA, Noparast M, Afshar K. Treatment of varicocele in children and adolescents: a systematic review and meta-analysis of randomized controlled trials. J Pediatr Urol. 2017;13:437–45.
24. Zachmann M, Prader A, Kind HP, Häfliger H, Budliger H. Testicular volume during adolescence. Cross-sectional and longitudinal studies. Helv Paediatr Acta. 1974;29:61–72.
25. Diamond DA, Zurakowski D, Bauer SB, Borer JG, Peters CA, Cilento BG Jr, Paltiel HJ, Rosoklija I, Retik AB. Relationship of varicocele grade and testicular hypotrophy to semen parameters in adolescents. J Urol. 2007;178:1584–8.
26. Kurtz MP, Zurakowski D, Rosoklija I, Bauer SB, Borer JG, Johnson KL, Migliozzi M, Diamond DA. Semen parameters in adolescents with Varicocele: association with testis volume differential and Total testis volume. J Urol. 2015;193:1843–7.
27. Costabile RA, Skoog S, Radowich M. Testicular volume assessment in the adolescent with a varicocele. J Urol. 1992;147:1348–50.
28. Organization WH, World Health Organization. The influence of varicocele on parameters of fertility in a large group of men presenting to infertility clinics**Supported by the Special Programme of Research, Development, and Research Training in Human Reproduction, World Health Organization, Geneva, Switzerland. Fertil Steril. 1992;57:1289–93.
29. Bogaert G, van den Heijkant M, Albersen M. Varicocele in children and adolescents: a challenge for diagnosis and treatment indications. Eur Urol Suppl. 2017;16:171–6.

30. Skoog SJ, Roberts KP, Goldstein M, Pryor JL. The adolescent Varicocele: What's new with an old problem in young patients? Pediatrics. 1997;100:112–27.
31. Wlochynski T, Wassermann J, Generowicz Z. Abdominoscrotal hydrocele in childhood. J Pediatr Surg. 1993;28:248–50.
32. Doudt AD, Kehoe JE, Ignacio RC, Christman MS. Abdominoscrotal hydrocele: a systematic review. J Pediatr Surg. 2016;51:1561–4.
33. Avolio L, Chiari G, Caputo MA, Bragheri R. Abdominoscrotal hydrocele in childhood: is it really a rare entity? Urology. 2000;56:1047–9.
34. Sasidharan P, Crankson S, Ahmed S. Fetal abdominoscrotal hydrocele. Am J Obstet Gynecol. 1991;165:1353–5.
35. Kamble PM, Deshpande AA, Thapar VB, Das K. Large abdominoscrotal hydrocele: uncommon surgical entity. Int J Surg Case Rep. 2015;15:140–2.
36. Gadelkareem RA. Abdominoscrotal hydrocele: a systematic review and proposed clinical grading. Afr J Urol. 2018;24:83–92.
37. Rioja J, Sánchez-Margallo FM, Usón J, Rioja LA. Adult hydrocele and spermatocele. BJU Int. 2011;107:1852–64.
38. Tartar VM, Trambert MA, Balsara ZN, Mattrey RF. Tubular ectasia of the testicle: sonographic and MR imaging appearance. Am J Roentgenol. 1993;160:539–42.
39. Jain N, Chauhan U, Sethi S, Goel V, Puri SK. Tubular Ectasia of rete testis with Spermatocele. J Clin Diagn Res. 2015;9:TJ03–4.
40. Gray CL, Powell CR, Amling CL. Outcomes for surgical Management of Orchalgia in patients with identifiable intrascrotal lesions. Eur Urol. 2001;39:455–9.
41. Shan CJ, Lucon AM, Pagani R, Srougi M. Sclerotherapy of hydroceles and spermatoceles with alcohol: results and effects on the semen analysis. Int Braz J Urol. 2011;37:307–13.

Urolithiasis

18

Sajid Sultan, Sadaf Aba Umer, and Bashir Ahmed

Learning Objectives

1. To understand the diagnostic techniques used to evaluate urinary tract stone disease in children
2. To understand the various minimally invasive approaches used to manage paediatric urinary stone disease including PCNL, ESWL, URS etc.
3. To understand the indications and the rationale for the use of the various interventional techniques in paediatric urinary stone disease

18.1 Preamble

Urolithiasis is a common but mysterious and a very complex pathology known to mankind from at least 3000 B.C. and has many facets. This chapter will focus on the surgical management of urolithiasis in children.

It will attempt to cover some common and some not so common presentations of paediatric urolithiasis which are presented in the form of case scenarios with their representative imaging and laboratory findings. There will be some pertinent questions to be asked related to the case scenarios and the answers will guide the decision making process for management. In addition, trouble shooting, problem solving and weighing the pros and cons of various treatment modalities will be addressed.

First of all, a brief review of the imaging modalities which may be used, and some technical aspects of the techniques employed to remove the stone(s) are necessary.

Chapter in Book "Practical Pediatric Urology – An Evidence Based Approach"

S. Sultan (✉) · S. A. Umer · B. Ahmed
Philip G. Ransley Department of Paediatric Urology, Sindh Institute of Urology and Transplantation (SIUT), Karachi, Pakistan

P. Godbole et al. (eds.), *Practical Pediatric Urology*,
https://doi.org/10.1007/978-3-030-54020-3_18

18.2 Imaging

18.2.1 Ultrasonography (USG)

Ultrasonography (USG) of the kidneys, ureters and bladder is the primary imaging modality used to evaluate patients and can provide information about the size and location (except in the mid ureter) of the stones. At the same time it provides information about renal size, cortical thickness and echogenicity, hydronephrosis and hydroureter. Scanning with a full bladder can help in picking up distal ureteric stones, vesical calculi and associated vesical and distal ureteric abnormalities if present.

18.2.2 X-Ray

A plain X-ray KUB can pick up radiopaque stones, associated bony abnormalities and faecal loading. This information may be pertinent to future decision making.

USG and X-ray KUB may be sufficient imaging in 80–90% of cases [1].

18.2.3 Intravenous Urogram (IVU)

Intravenous Urogram (IVU) may be performed in selected cases to delineate the pelvicalyceal anatomy especially where CT scan is not available or requires general anaesthesia. However it is cumbersome and bowel gas shadows in children obscure key information at times.

18.2.4 Non-Contrast Computed Tomography (NCCT)

Non-Contrast Computed Tomography (NCCT) is to be recommended judiciously keeping in mind not only its radiation hazards but also that in babies and small children it may require general anaesthesia. However, it is helpful in providing more precise information about the size and location of the stone and especially for identifying mid ureteric stones. Therefore it is the first choice of imaging in suspected ureteric colic. It allows measurement of the density of the stone which is recorded in Hounsfield units, its fragility and composition especially to differentiate between calcium and non-calcium stones. It also provides information about the associated pathology and any surrounding inflammatory process by looking at the fat stranding. Another advantage of NCCT is the ability to assess the spatial relationship of the kidney relative to the stone and that of the kidney in relation to the adjacent peritoneal and retroperitoneal structures. Retro renal colon which is not evident on USG has been reported although in less than 1% of all patients [2].

- **Hounsfield Units (HU)** It is a quantitative scale to measure and characterise relative radio densities/radiation attenuation in different tissues determined by

CT. Distilled water at standard temperature and pressure (STP) is defined as 0 HU, the radio density of air is defined as −1000 HU [3]. Urinary calculi present with a wide range of attenuation values. Urate stones are <500 HU, Mixed stones (Urate + calcium) are 500–900 HU and calcium stones are >1000 HU [1].

18.2.5 Contrast Computed Tomography (Urogram)

It is advised only in selected cases of urolithiasis with very large stone burdens, atypical pelvicalyceal systems or renal anomalies such as malrotation, ectopic or crossed fused kidneys in order to document their complex vascular and urinary tract anatomy.

18.2.6 Dimercaptosuccinic acid (DMSA) Scintigraphy

It is advised to look for differential renal function and presence of scarring, especially in cases where there is renal size disparity, reduced cortex, altered echotexture, large stone burden and repeated UTI. It serves as a baseline prior to intervention.

18.3 Treatment Modalities

18.3.1 Open Surgery

Anatrophic Nephrolithotomy, Pyelolithotomy, Ureterolithotomy and Cystolithotomy for stones in kidneys, ureters, and bladder are rarely performed these days but may be the treatment of choice in <10% of cases which are those with a very large stone burden, anatomical abnormalities, sepsis or severe renal dysfunction [4].

18.3.2 Minimally Invasive Surgery (MIS)

The majority (>90%) of stones in the urinary tract in children are being managed today by MIS [4, 5] which includes the following.

18.4 Renal Stones

18.4.1 Extra Corporeal Shockwave Lithotripsy (ESWL)

Its outcome depends on the age, size, location, stone composition and the type of machine available. It is operator dependent. Certain nomograms have been developed which can predict the outcome of ESWL [6, 7]. In children it is performed under general anaesthesia in almost all cases in order to avoid the patient's apprehension, pain and movement. Therefore, ESWL has a limited role in the management of paediatric urolithiasis. To avoid repeated anaesthesia and to allay the concerns of renal damage in the developing kidney, ESWL is mostly reserved for 6–15 mm stones in the kidneys [1, 4, 8–10].

18.4.2 Retrograde Intra Renal Surgery (RIRS)

RIRS has developed as a result of the advancement in sophisticated, miniaturised, actively deflectable, flexible ureterorenoscopes (FLURS), incorporating high power Holmium:YAG lasers and intra-corporeal grasping devices. RIRS is gaining popularity as it carries a high possibility of achieving complete stone clearance in a single session especially for renal stones up to 2 cm [11–14].

The ureterorenosope is introduced through the natural route thus the urologists find the learning curve relatively less difficult as compared to renal puncture techniques. RIRS is more invasive than ESWL but considered less invasive than PCNL [15–19]. RIRS could be a good option in cases with a coexisting bleeding diathesis.

RIRS in most cases requires the placement of a 9/11FG Ureteric Access Sheath (UAS). This is placed to allow the flexible ureterorenoscope (FLURS) to be removed and reintroduced repeatedly in order to allow the stone fragments and dust to clear and maintain good vision. The UAS allows irrigation fluid to flow easily and so maintain a low intrarenal pressure thereby decreasing the chances of pyelovenous and pyelolymphatic backflow. This decreases the chances of developing sepsis. However the use of UAS requires active dilatation of the ureterovesical junction/ureteric orifice which carries the risk of traumatic damage and vesicoureteric reflux [20] or passive dilatation by pre-stenting for 3–4 weeks which requires additional anaesthesia. In most of these cases post-operative stenting is advisable [14, 16, 21]. UAS can also lead to ureteric injury ranging from minor mucosal damage to major lacerations, stricture and avulsion [17].

There are controversies in the RIRS results which need to be understood. The majority of the series of RIRS in children which document the outcome from a single session do not take into consideration the anaesthesia session for pre-stenting to provide passive ureteral dilatation. Similarly, the majority of cases require postoperative stenting especially where an UAS was used and so many of them require another anaesthesia session for stent removal. Therefore, the outcome of RIRS in these patients is really that of a staged procedure requiring 2–3 general anaesthesia and not a genuine single session. The majority of RIRS series, especially where the results are compared with PCNL, are biased by the fact that the children treated by RIRS are somewhat older and the stone burden generally less than the PCNL groups [16, 18, 22–24].

In addition, FLURS is a very costly treatment option as the endoscopes are very costly and fragile. Several studies have highlighted the fact that the flexible scope undergoes wear and tear and requires major repair after 14–32 RIRS sessions. Even apportioning the high initial cost of the instrument, the maintenance and repair costs over each session of RIRS still makes it a highly expensive treatment option [25, 26].

18.4.3 Percutaneous Nephrolithotomy (PCNL)

Classical PCNL in children required a 30FG Amplatz sheath and employed a 24FG Nephroscope which had the advantage of achieving very high (>90%) clearance rates in a single session but was not easily applicable in small children and risked renal damage or excessive bleeding requiring blood transfusion. Miniaturisation has led to the development of the 'Miniperc' and its derivatives so that the sheath size can be reduced to 14FG or less and single puncture composite needles with integrated optics at 4.8FG avoid the need for any tract dilatation (Microperc) [9, 27]. The Microperc instruments are costly and meant to be disposable.

In parallel, the stone disintegration modalities have become smaller and more effective. Ultrasonic disintegration can effectively be used with Nephroscopes ≥18FG. The Pneumatic lithoclast can be used with scopes down to 10FG (Mini Perc). Ho:YAG Laser fibres can be used even with flexible nephroscopes and 4.8FG Microperc needles. Laser technology is advancing rapidly and allows the stone to be converted to dust which exits via the irrigation channel.

By careful selection of approach and technology the majority of renal stones can now be dealt with successfully by Mini or Microperc techniques [9]. There are certain limitations of Microperc. Firstly, vision gets compromised more quickly with the slightest bleeding and stone dust and secondly stone fragments may migrate and can become inaccessible.

Our preferred indications for PCNL are stone sizes of 1.5 cm or more, previous open surgery, failed ESWL, or stones where more than two sessions of ESWL would be required. Active or untreated UTIs, sepsis and bleeding diathesis are a few of the contraindications which should be mentioned. Spinal deformity such as scoliosis and kyphosis can affect the choice of procedure and should be elucidated prior to surgery.

PCNL is carried out under general anaesthesia, either in the conventional prone position or more recently, supine. Pre-operative considerations should include negative urine culture, prophylactic antibiotics, proper draping and the availability of isotonic irrigation fluid at body temperature.

The puncture site is chosen on the basis of the stone location, bulk, and pelvicalyceal anatomy. We prefer subcostal posterior-superior calyceal punctures when suitable, as this gives access to the majority of the calyces with little torque on the kidney, and also allows access to the pelviureteric junction and lower calyces in the case of stone migration. In certain situations, the supracostal approach can also be utilised with marginal risks of hydropneumothorax which can also be avoided in experienced hands [1, 4, 28].

18.4.4 Endoscopic Combined Intra Renal Surgery (ECIRS)

This is a combined procedure where both RIRS and PCNL are performed simultaneously by two surgeons together. It may be performed either in the supine or prone positions. ECIRS is usually recommended for complete clearance of a large stone bulk, such as a staghorn calculus and for multiple stones located in difficult anatomical positions. Such complex stones cannot be cleared either by RIRS or PCNL alone in a single session. It also reduces the operating time. The most appropriate renal puncture and the PCNL tract can be acquired with the assistance of ureterorenoscopy and especially if combined with ultrasound [29]. There is still limited data on the outcomes of ECIRS in children [30, 31].

18.4.5 Laparoscopic/Robotic Surgery

Development of laparoscopy and subsequently robotic surgery are other means to avoid open surgery. It may be an option if the expertise and facilities are available. It may be performed through transperitoneal or retroperitoneal approaches. However, because of relatively higher morbidity and longer hospitalization, a laparoscopic or robotic approach for stone removal should be considered only if the results with ESWL or other endoscopic approaches are expected to be poor. In certain cases a laparoscopic or robotic approach is considered to be a reasonable option. Situations such as pyeloplasty with pyelolithotomy, stones in poorly functioning polar areas or non-functioning kidneys. In pelvic kidneys with a large stone burden laparoscopy can be employed to reflect overlying bowel thus facilitating percutaneous stone removal or possibly laraoscopic pelolithotomy. It must be recognised that such procedures can be technically demanding if they are to be performed with minimum morbidity and therefore require a skilled Laparoscopic / Robotic surgeon. Case series have been published with stone free rates ranging from 28 to 91% [2, 32, 33].

18.5 Ureteric Stones

Ureterorenoscopy (URS) with a Holmium-YAG laser (LL) and Pneumatic Lithoclast (PL) is the mainstay of treatment for ureteric stones. Semi-rigid URS of size 4.5/6, 6/7.5, and 8/9.8 FG are used depending on the age and anatomy of the patient, the size of the stone and considering the technical requirements. The semi-rigid URS are more durable, can access the whole ureter even as far as the PCS and have better visibility, faster irrigation flow, and larger working channels. In contrast, the ability of the scope to bend is limited and, especially with large psoas muscles, access to the upper ureter may be difficult in comparison with a flexible ureterorenoscope (FLURS). The deflectable tip of the flexible 'scopes is more suitable for a tortuous ureter and for upper ureteric stones which can easily migrate into the kidney. The flexible 'scope can follow them and retrograde intrarenal surgery may be possible in the same session. The flexible ureteroscope permits only lasertripsy. FLURS is costly and fragile therefore the treatment is lot more expensive than with semirigid scopes.

Lower ureteric stones can be managed by semirigid ureterorenoscopes by employing the pneumatic lithoclast or Ho:YAG lasertripsy. The outcome in terms of stone clearance and complication rates are excellent and comparable, whereas PL is significantly cheap as compared to LL. PL can only be used through 6/7.5FG scopes and above while LL can be used with small 'scopes (4.5/6 FG) which is an advantage for infants and small children [1, 4, 34].

18.6 Vesical Stones

Most vesical stones can be managed endoscopically via the urethra using a cystolithoclast (PUCL), for stones up to 2 cm in size. The percutaneous cystolithoclast (PCCL) is required for stones greater than 2 cm and up to 3.5 cm [1, 4, 35].

18.7 Endoscopic Intra Corporeal Lithotripsy (EIL) Disintegration Technologies

As has already been noted in passing, various types of devices are available. Each device has certain unique properties that make it more suitable for a particular application. Manufacturers claims may contain elements of bias and therefore a thorough and impartial evaluation is important in order to be able to select the most appropriate device in any particular situation.

Four stone disintegration technologies are available for intra corporeal lithotripsy during endoscopic management of urolithiasis [2, 36].

18.7.1 Electro Hydraulic Lithotripsy (EHL)

Although EHL is the least costly and can be used even with flexible 'scopes. However it is relatively the most traumatic intra-corporeal lithotripsy and seldom used now.

18.7.2 Ballistic Lithotripsy (Pneumatic Lithoclast)

It provides a durable, reusable, safe and a cost-effective means for stone fragmentation. It may be especially advantageous when large and hard stones are encountered. Disadvantages could be a higher rate of stone repulsion and it can only be used with rigid scopes.

18.7.3 Ultrasonic Lithotripsy

It is safe and although it may cause mucosal stripping it does not create deeper perforations. For effective stone disintegration it requires relatively larger scopes with a 4.5FG working channel to accommodate the hollow probe. It works best with standard PCNL for a large stone burden. It is less effective than pneumatic lithoclast for hard stones.

18.7.4 Combination Devices

A Pneumatic lithoclast combined with an ultrasonic beam aims to combine the advantages of both techniques. The superior fragmentation ability of the pneumatic component is complemented by the simultaneous evacuation of the fragments via the hollow ultrasonic probe.

18.7.5 Holmium YAG Laser (Ho:YAG)

This has brought great versatility to EIL by allowing safe fragmentation in the entire urinary tract. The laser output (power) can be adjusted by modulating the laser characteristics of energy (PE) and frequency (Fr). There are various generations of laser machines ranging from low power ($\leq$20 watts) to high power (120 watts). The later machines allow for much more adjustment in PE and Fr thus allowing the stone to be disintegrated into fragments (high PE, low Fr) or converted into dust/powder (low PE, high Fr). The fragments can be removed by baskets and dust/powder exits with the irrigation fluid without the need for retrieval devices [37, 38].

18.8 Case 1

A 3 year old girl suffering from abdominal pain with normal renal function, negative urine culture and normal right kidney on USG.

What are the findings on USG of left kidney and X-ray KUB?

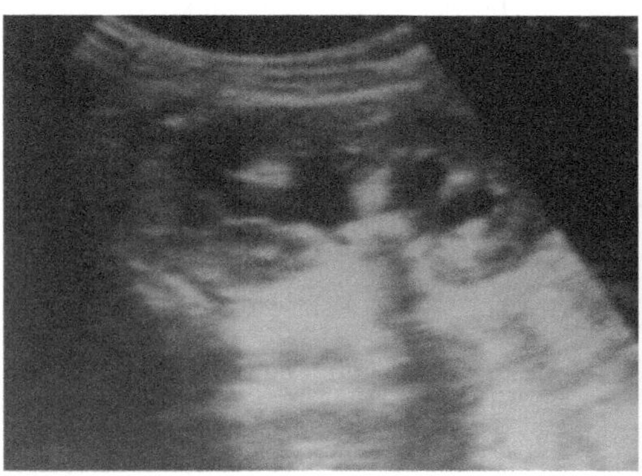

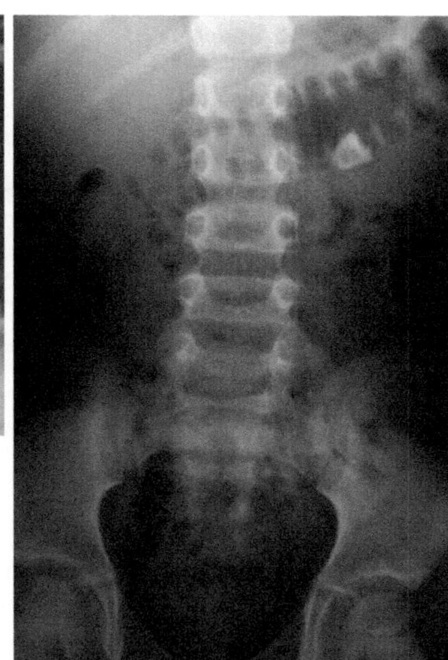

A 1. Left kidney shows renal pelvic stone of 1.6 cm with mild hydronephrosis and good cortex. X-ray KUB shows radiopaque stone in the left renal area.

Q 2. What are the possible surgical options in this case? Discuss the Pros and Cons to justify the preferred option?

A 2. All options including open pyelolithotomy, laparoscopic pyelolithotomy, ESWL, RIRS and all variations of PCNL are applicable and possible in this case. Therefore, the decision making, counselling and consent should be undertaken on the basis of the facilities and expertise available.

Open Pyelolithotomy can be an option only if no other facility or expertise is available, as it carries comparatively high morbidity of a large incision, scar, pain and prolonged hospital stay. Similarly laparoscopic/robotic pyelolithotomy requires facilities and expertise which may not be available. Even if available this also causes relatively more morbidity than some other MIS options. The main problem is the risk of stone or fragment migration into a calyx which converts the case into more complex surgery.

ESWL considered to be the least invasive of all, however it will also require general anaesthesia in a 3 years old. As per the nomogram the risk of failure after single session in this case is about 50% [6] and chances of complete clearance in one session are only 40% and may require up to 4 sessions for the complete clearance [7]. At the same time it carries the risk of steinstrasse, leading to an unpredictable hospital stay or emergency room visit and added procedures such as URS with or without JJ stent. As it is a radiopaque stone on X-ray, it is likely to be a dense stone such as calcium oxalate monohydrate (COM) and thus difficult to fragment on ESWL. If it has an infective (struvite) stone component then any residual fragment is even more likely to lead to stone regrowth and recurrence.

RIRS is a recommended treatment modality for renal stones ≤2 cm [11]. Therefore it may be an attractive option to treat this stone and carries a good probability of clearance as compared to ESWL [15, 39]. As shown by Alsagheer et al. [39] in comparable group of patients the stone free rate after one session of RIRS is higher (81.4%) than ESWL (53.3%) with comparable rates of complications. In this series, all patients (100%) in the RIRS group were pre-stented for 2–4 weeks requiring another anaesthesia session. Similarly, this being a 3 years old girl, RIRS would require UAS and pre and post procedure stenting [23, 24]. At the same time RIRS is relatively the most costly treatment option [25, 26].

PCNL offers the highest (>90%) chance of complete stone clearance in a single session. Mini PCNL is relatively more invasive than RIRS and risks blood transfusion in <10% of the cases. It may be performed with a working sheath between 12–16 FG. and a reusable rigid scope between 10–12 FG. with the help of either pneumatic lithoclast or Ho:YAG laser thus making it the cost effective treatment option. Micro PCNL, although less invasive than Mini PCNL, requires disposable equipment which is costly. Comparative studies between RIRS, Mini and Micro PCNL have shown higher stone free rates with Micro and Mini PCNL [23, 24, 28].

18.9 Case 2

A 6 year old girl with a 1.4 cm stone in the lower calyx of solitary left kidney as shown on USG and X-ray KUB. The right kidney is congenitally absent. Renal function is normal.

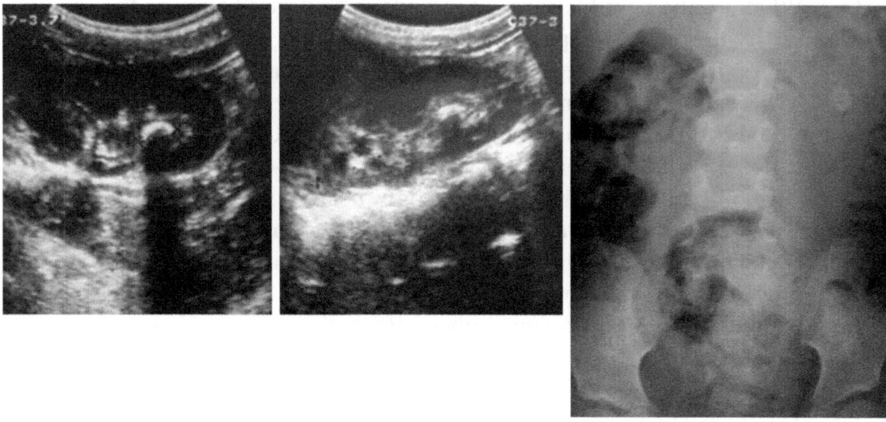

Q 1. Do you recommend any further radiological imaging for this patient and why?

A 1. I would recommend contrast imaging with either IVU or, preferably, contrast CT urogram in order to look especially at the lower calyceal anatomy; infundibular length, infundibular width and infundibulo-pelvic angle, the presence of diverticula and to determine the density of the stone in Hounsfield unit (HU). This information will help in decision making and opting for the right choice of procedure.

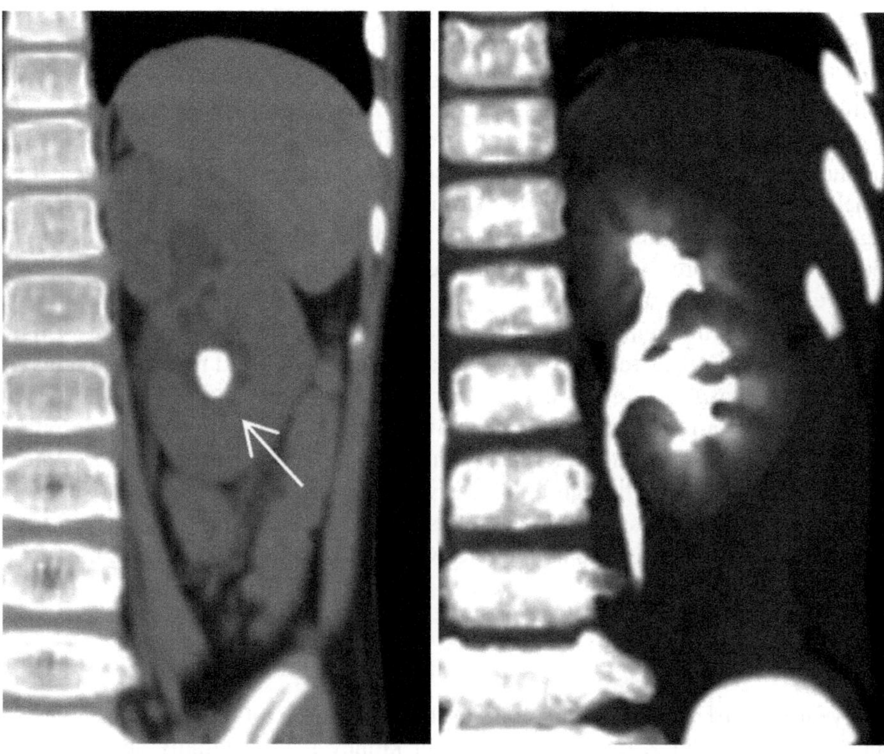

This image of CT urogram shows normal size left kidney with single dense (1070 HU) stone of 1.4 cm in a lower calyx. The pelvicalyceal anatomy has bifid pelvis with the long upper pole infundibulum. The lower pole calyces have short, wide infundibula with an obtuse infundibulopelvic angle (Favourable anatomy).

Q 2. What are the possible surgical options?

A 2.

I. **ESWL** A lower calyceal stone has a poor clearance rate compared with the same size and composition of stone presenting elsewhere in the pelvicalyceal system [9, 10]. However clearance of a lower calyceal stone can be achieved with an increased number of treatment sessions. A 1.4 cm lower calyceal stone has about 75% risk of failure in single session [6] and up to 91% chance of clearance in 4 sessions [7]. Shockwave lithotripsy outcome for the lower calyceal stone varies with lower pole anatomy. The study of Khan et al. in adults showed that that lower infundibular length and width are significant anatomical factors in determining stone clearance following ESWL treatment and these should be assessed before planning the treatment for lower calyceal stones [40]. Tan et al. showed that infundibulopelvic angle and infundibular length significantly affected the stone-free rates with ESWL for inferior calyceal stones in children [41]. In this case, as shown in the CT urogram the infundibulopelvic angle is obtuse and lower pole infundibulum is wide and short therefore the anatomy is favourable and ESWL can be considered as a treatment option. However a radiopaque stone with HU of 1070 is dense and less able to be fragmented with ESWL. In view of the solitary kidney and considering the risks of steinstrasse and obstruction it would require pre-placement of a JJ stent.

II. **RIRS (FLURS)** is relatively difficult when treating lower calyceal stone because of limited maneuverability and significant discomfort for the surgeon. The newer flexible 'scopes allow for acute deflection to negotiate lower calyceal anatomy. One of the techniques could be to move the stone from the lower calyx into the pelvis or upper calyx with the help of a basket and then to pulverise the stone [18]. The other option could be to pulverise the stone in situ (lower calyx) with the use of high power laser in dusting mode to avoid any larger fragment (>2 mm) and the use of a basket for fragment retrieval.

   Several studies have shown high success rate of RIRS for <2 cm renal stone including lower calyx. Majority of these cases require pre-stenting, UAS and post-stenting thus converting it into a staged procedure with two or more anaesthesia sessions [22–24]. Considering the high cost of treatment and possibility of staged procedure, RIRS in this case is not our most preferred option.

III. **PCNL**: Mini PCNL is a valid option with an expected stone clearance rate of >90%. A less invasive option but requiring considerable experience and expertise could be direct puncture into the relevant lower calyx using the Microperc technique with direct vision using the all seeing needle. This avoids the need for any tract dilatation and the stone may be disintegrated into dust using a high power laser on the dusting setting.

   This 6 year old girl with a dense (1070 HU) lower calyceal stone in a solitary kidney stands the best chance of being stone free in a single session with

PCNL. Though relatively more invasive but most cost effective. Mini PCNL would be our preferred choice in this case.

18.10 Case 3

A 6 year old girl presented with a high grade fever and painful urination. Urine examination revealed pyuria and a positive culture with E.Coli. Hematology showed leukocytosis. There was a history of similar episodes twice in the last 3 months. USG KUB showed right kidney full of stones (staghorn stones) in the pelvicalyceal system. The cortical thickness and echotexture is normal. The contralateral kidney and urinary bladder is normal.

Q 1.How will you manage the patient initially?

A 1. This patient will be treated preferably with the intravenous antibiotic according to the sensitivity.

Q 2. What does this X-ray show?

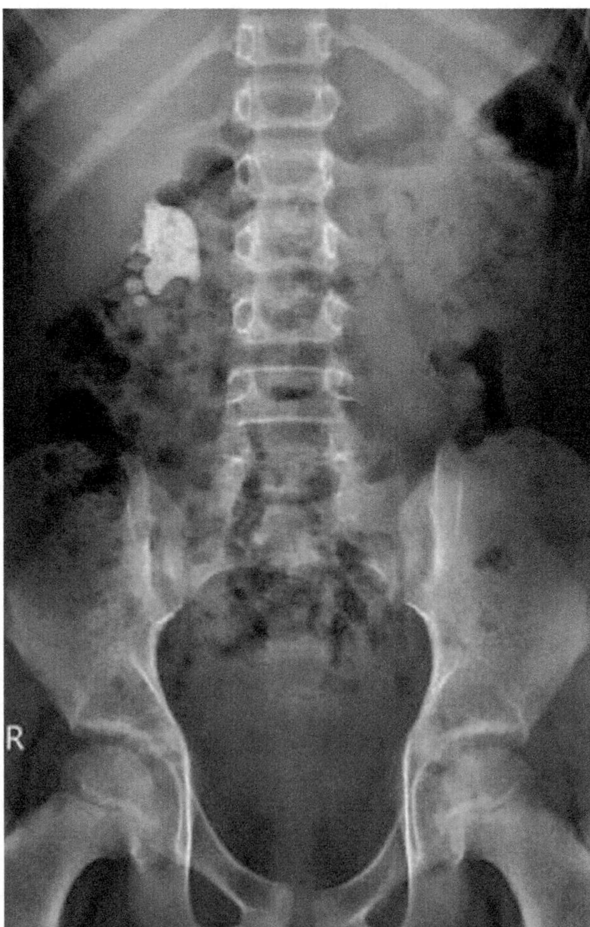

A 2. X-ray KUB shows radiopaque shadow suggestive of staghorn stone in right kidney.

Q 3. What further radiological investigations may be helpful (needed) in this patient to plan surgical management?

A 3.

A. Dimercaptosuccinic acid (DMSA) renal scan
B. Non contrast computed tomography (NCCT)

Q 4. What do these images show?

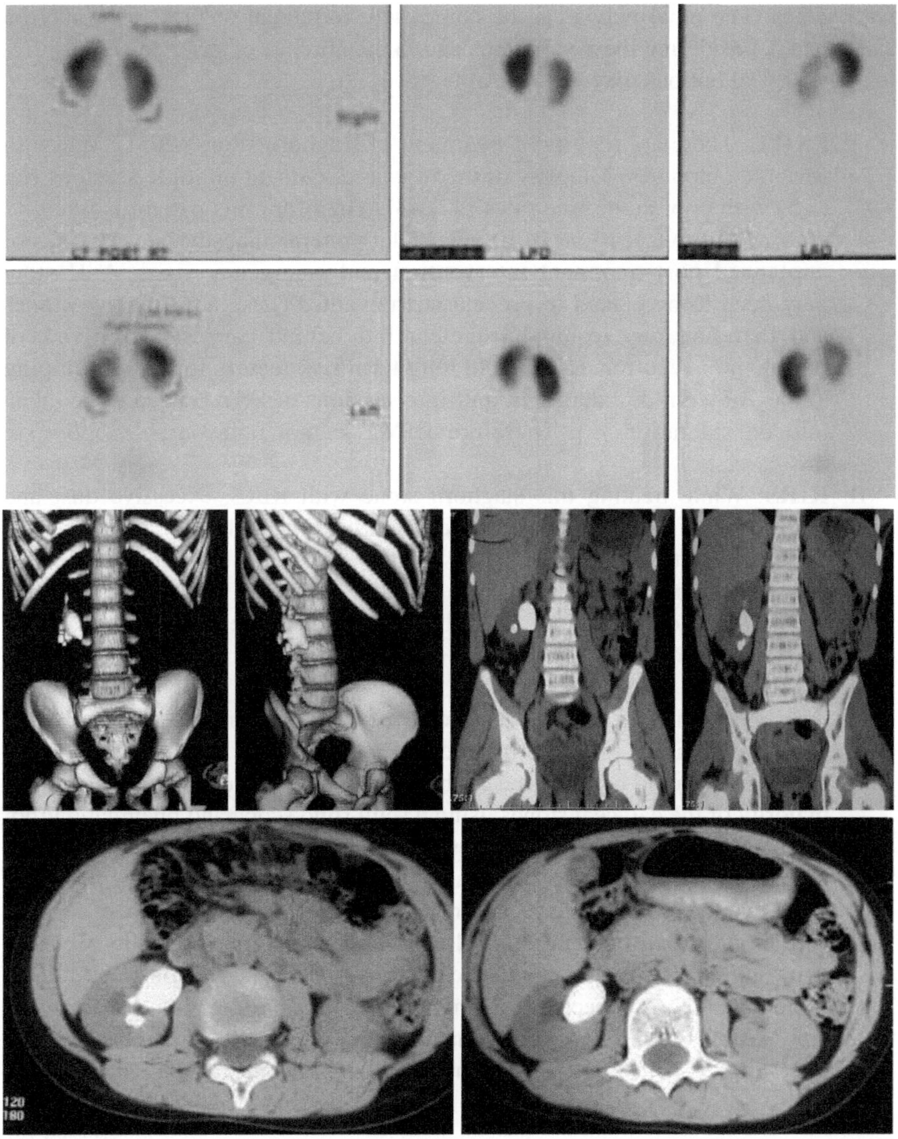

- DMSA of this patient reveal a differential function of 45% for the right kidney with cortical scarring at upper pole.
- Non contrast computed tomography (NCCT)—Shows staghorn calculus measures 5.7 × 4.0 cm (1234 HU), completely occupying the renal pelvis which is partly extra renal and mostly intrarenal. The stone has branches which extend into all the major calyces and multiple minor calyces of the lower pole.

Q 4. What surgical options are available?

A 4. The staghorn calculus has many forms and at times the term can be used rather loosely. The staghorn calculus can vary from a stone in the renal pelvis extending into two calyces to an extensively branching pelvicalyceal system packed with stones. The renal pelvis can be completely intrarenal or most of it may be extrarenal. Considering these variations and in the absence of strict guidelines, following surgical options may be applicable.

I. **ESWL**: There are reports of treatment of staghorn stone with ESWL with variable outcomes. Majority of the reports document multiple sessions (up to 5) with poor stone free rates [42, 43]. Therefore this patient is likely to require multiple sessions of ESWL under general anaesthesia with risks of unplanned post treatment intervention and emergency visits. A JJ stent may need to be placed to prevent such events. These are infective stones and therefore any residual fragment left behind carries a high risk of regrowth or recurrence. Possible long term risk factors for the developing kidney of a child undergoing multiple sessions of ESWL need to be taken into consideration [2]. Therefore ESWL is not a favourable option in this case.

II. **RIRS**: While treating this staghorn stone with RIRS, excessive dust and blurred vision will lead to prolonged operating time and a high risk of sepsis. It also necessitates the use of UAS with its own inherent risks and the need for pre-stenting and post-stenting.

    As it is likely to require multiple sessions therefore RIRS alone is not a preferred option.

III. **PCNL** would be our first choice in this staghorn stone. By using the smaller instruments of Mini PCNL the majority of complications including bleeding can be minimised. Considering the complexity of the stone an upper pole access tract would be preferred enabling clearance of the pelvic stone and the majority of the calyceal stones using a semi rigid scope and pneumatic lithoclast or Ho:YAG laser [44]. However some inaccessible calyces will require the use of a flexible nephroscope and Ho:YAG laser. There may be a need of more than one or multiple access tracts with some additional risks of complications including bleeding and blood transfusion. The possibility of more than one PCNL session cannot be excluded. However, a stone free rate of more than 90% is expected in a single PCNL session.

IV. **Endoscopic Combined intrarenal surgery (ECIRS):** This requires two operating surgeons; one performing RIRS and the other PCNL and provides a high possibility of complete stone clearance in a single session. It is in effect an adjunct to PCNL in order to minimise the number of access tracts which would be required if PCNL was used as monotherapy. Similarly it can avoid the need for multiple anaesthesia sessions compared with RIRS or PCNL used alone. However there is a limited data on ECIRS being used to treat staghorn stone in small children [30, 31]. We will prefer ECIRS when PCNL alone would require multiple tracts or repeat sessions and where RIRS can be performed without prestenting in the same session so that we can avoid both a second anaesthesia session and multiple tracts.

V. **Sandwich therapy**: A combined approach, primarily a PCNL followed by ESWL for residual calculi is a recommended option for staghorn calculus [45]. Improvements in PCNL and RIRS equipment, techniques and skills and ECIRS have reduced the need for additional ESWL. As mentioned above our preferred option will be to make this patient stone free in single session with PCNL or ECIRS however any unintended residual fragments ≤1.0 cm will be managed by ESWL (Sandwich therapy).

VI. **Laparoscopic/ Robotic assisted Pyelo/nephrolithotomy and combined pyeloscopy:** It must be recognized that such procedures can be technically challenging and require a skilled laparoscopic/robotic surgeon. However there are reports with stone free rates ranging from 28 to 91% [2, 32, 33].

VII. **Open combined endoscopic pyelolithotomy**: The major stone bulk in the extrarenal pelvis is easily removed with an open, extended (Gil-Vernet) Pyelolithotomy. Following this, those branches of the stone which are in the peripheral calyces can be approached and visualized with the help of an endoscope/ miniscope and fragmented with the pneumatic lithoclast or Ho:YAG laser. Fragments may be retrieved with grasping forceps or a basket.

VIII. **Anatrophic nephrolithotomy**: It is an option which is more invasive and with high morbidity. Although it carries the highest chance of complete stone clearance in a single surgery and has been the standard treatment in the past. In this case it may be replaced by more modern techniques.

With the treatment armamentarium available at present and weighing the pros and cons, our preferred option in this case would be PCNL as monotherapy. There is more than 90% chance of complete stone clearance in a single session with the minimum morbidity.

18.11 Case 4

A 12 year old girl presented with history of recurrent left flank colicky pain requiring parenteral analgesia. She has normal renal functions, negative urine culture and normal right kidney on USG. The Images given below shows X-ray KUB, USG of left kidney and urinary bladder.

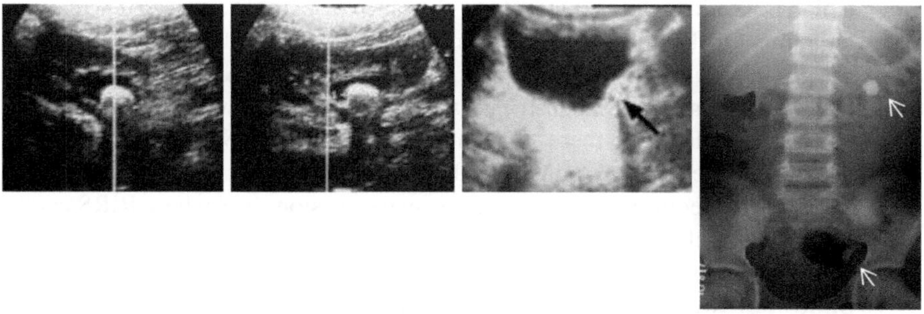

Q 1. What are the findings?

A 1. USG shows Mild hydronephrosis, renal pelvic stone. 1.2 cm, distal ureteric stone 7 mm with hydroureter and normal urinary bladder. X-ray KUB shows radiopaque shadows in left renal and distal ureteric region.

Q 2. What are the possible surgical options?

A 2.

I. URS + RIRS
II. URS + PCNL (supine or prone)
III. URS + ESWL (later)

Discussion: As she is suffering with colicky pain and the distal ureteric stone is causing obstruction, she requires early surgical intervention.

The distal ureteric stone can be dealt with using either a rigid or flexible ureterorenoscopy (but preferably rigid) under general anaesthesia and using the pneumatic lithoclast or Ho:YAG laser. If the ureteric stone is cleared quickly then one can try to proceed for RIRS or PCNL in the same session.

RIRS would be performed preferably with a flexible ureterorenoscope (FLURS). As she is a 12 years old girl and the ureter is already dilated above the stone, FLURS may be performed without UAS or an access sheath may be placed without prestenting. It may be possible to completely clear both ureteric and renal stones in one session.

PCNL: Once the ureteric stone is cleared in reasonable time the other option could be to proceed directly to Mini/Micro PCNL preferably in the supine position [46] or the patient may be turned prone. Simultaneous PCNL is a little more invasive but can provide complete stone clearance in a single session.

However if the ureteric stone has taken longer time and or UAS is difficult to place without UVJ dilatation, then one can leave a JJ stent in place and return on a second occasion for the renal calculus by RIRS, PCNL or ESWL.

ESWL: It is the least invasive of all other options. However each session will be performed under General anaesthesia or sedoanalgesia (as she is 12 years). The stone bulk is 1.2 cm it is possible that multiple sessions will be required for stone free status [6, 7].

18.12 Case 5

An 8 year old boy presented with 1.0 cm radiopaque stone in the right distal ureter with mild urinary frequency and urgency.

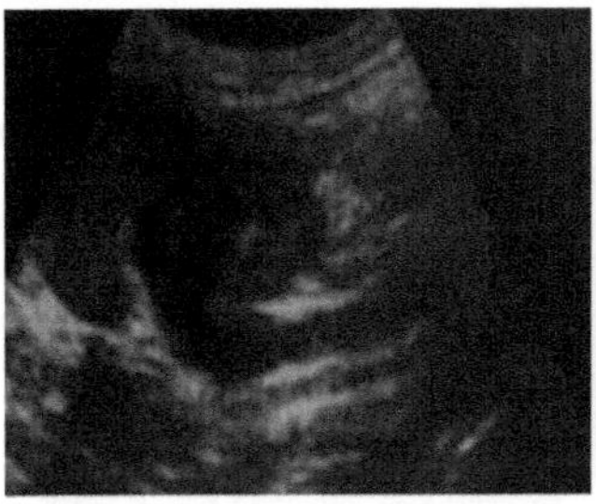

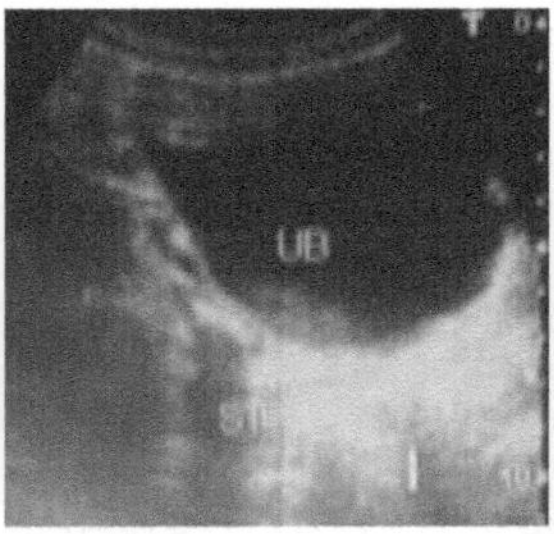

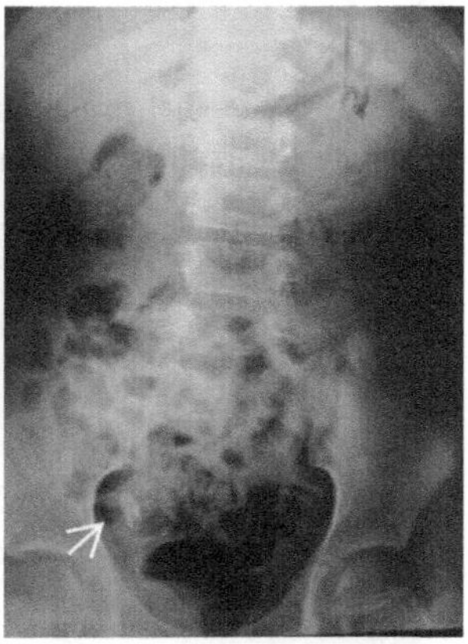

Q 1. What is the role of Medical expulsive therapy (MET) in ureteric stones?

A 1. There is abundance of alpha adrenergic receptors in ureteric smooth muscles especially in the distal third. Alpha adrenergic blocker inhibits basal smooth muscle tone with no effect on tonic propulsive contraction. Several studies have shown the effectiveness of alpha blocker as medical expulsion therapy for distal ureteric stone but in some studies no added advantage of MET have been observed [47].

Q 1. What are the chances of spontaneous passage of this stone?

A 1. Lower ureteric stones of 0.4–0.5 cm have a >90% chances of spontaneous passage. However 10 mm distal ureteric stone has very little chance of spontaneous passage and being a male has the added risk of the stone getting stuck in the urethra or at the external urethral meatus.

Q 3. What is the role of ESWL in this patient?

A 3. ESWL would need to be performed under GA and the stone may be difficult to localize. The results are unpredictable and there is relatively less chance of complete stone clearance than with URS.

Q 4. What is the best treatment option available for this patient?

Ureterorenoscopy and stone fragmentation with pneumatic lithoclast or Ho:YAG laser is the best treatment option with >90% chances of complete stone clearance in a single session.

Q 5. When is open surgery indicated for a lower ureteric stone?

A 5.

I. High risk patient precluding multiple anaesthesia.
II. Anatomical condition of the ureter that prevents positioning of ureterorenoscope (often a reimplanted ureter).
III. Cases where transurethral instrumentation is not possible or advisable e.g. patients with an urethral stricture or bladder neck reconstruction.

IV. Difficulties in patient positioning for Ureterorenoscopy.
V. If it is associated with VUJO then open ureterolithotomy and ureteroneocystostomy is recommended.

18.13 Case 6

A 10 year old girl presents with a history of repeated abdominal pain and dysuria and with the following radiological investigations (IVU, NCCT, DMSA).

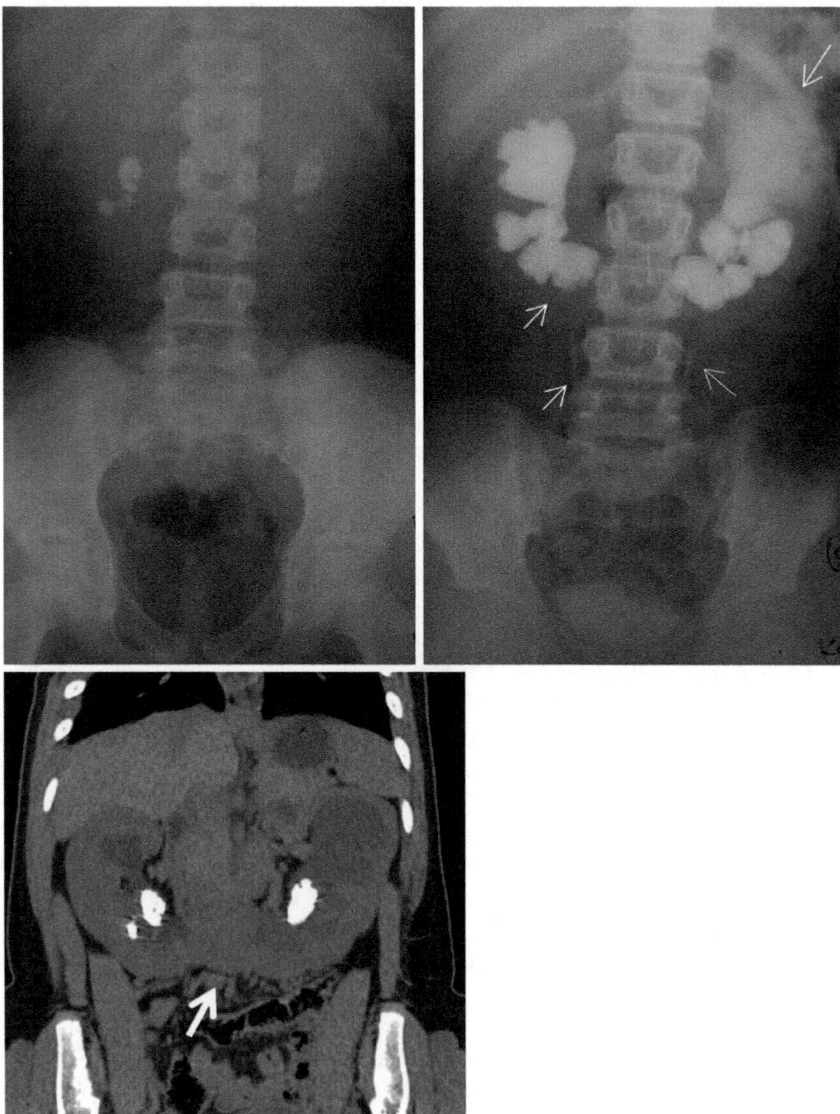

Q 1. What are the findings?

IVU: The scout image shows bilateral radiopaque shadows in renal areas.

The contrast image shows a horseshoe kidney (HSK) with the characteristic feature of medially directed lower poles and the lower calyces are medial to the ureters. There are bilateral obstructing stones in the renal pelves with dilated pelvicalyceal systems and more substantial dilatation of the left upper calyx.

NCCT: The lower poles of both moieties are medially placed and fused with each other in the midline. The right moiety shows an obstructing calculus of 1.9 × 0.9 cm in the pelvis and an additional stone 1.3 × 0.7 cm in the lower calyx. The left moiety has an obstructing stone in the pelvis measuring 2.4 × 1.2 cm causing moderate hydronephrosis and another stone of 0.8 × 0.5 cm in the lower calyx.

Q 2. Does a DMSA scan provide added information in this case?

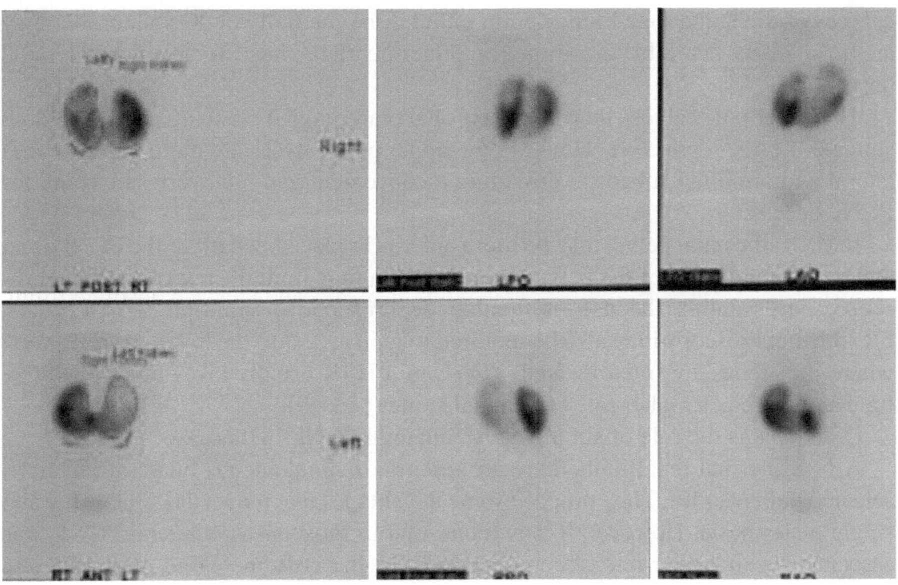

A 2. Yes. As shown on the image the right moiety shows good tracer uptake (64%) and is well outlined whereas left moiety shows reduced uptake (36%) and is faintly outlined particularly at the upper pole which correlates with the IVU and NCCT images of reduced parenchyma at the upper pole.

Q 3. What are the principles of managing bilateral renal stones?

A 3. Bilateral renal stones reflect an aggressive disease. In this case, being a horseshoe kidney, anatomy and urinary stasis appear to be the predominating factors. However especially in children the metabolic/genetic, dietary, environmental, hereditary /familial risks factors should be taken into consideration. Therefore a thorough risk factor analysis should be performed and preventive measures to be advised.

For surgical management a minimally invasive procedure is generally recommended in children on account of the high risk of recurrence in bilateral renal stones.

The treatment option to be decided as per the stone burden, location, pelvicalyceal anatomy, renal status and function of each renal unit.

Q 4. What is your preferred treatment option in this case?

A 4. Bilateral PCNL

Q 5. What specific anatomical considerations are relevant while performing PCNL in a horseshoe kidney?

A 5. In considering a horseshoe kidney the orientation of the collecting systems and the abnormal blood supply should be taken into account. Along with the normal renal arteries they often have accessory and aberrant polar and isthmus arteries. An important observation is that all blood vessels except some to the isthmus enter the kidney from the ventromedial aspect. The dorsal arteries to the isthmus are protected by the spine therefore a renal access tract on the dorsal or dorsolateral aspect will be away from the major renal vessels. Because most of the calyces of the horse shoe kidney point either dorsomedially or dorsolaterally, they are in a more favorable position for puncture than those in the normal renal unit [2].

The lower pole calyces lie within a coronal plane angled medially and are seldom suitable for direct puncture. However the upper pole calyces are more posterior and lateral and are often subcostal providing a convenient and relatively safe route for PCNL access.

In HSK, the renal pelvis may be more anteriorly placed, length of the PCNL tract and or the angulation of the pelvicalyceal system may limit the use of rigid nephroscope, necessitating the use of flexible nephroscope or multiple access tracts. Flexible nephroscopy may also be required to gain access to the lower medial calyx, where the stones are often located. PCNL in a HSK usually takes more operative time and there is a higher rate of residual stones [48, 49].

Q 6. What is the role of simultaneous bilateral PCNL in this case?

A 6. In normal renal units there are reports of simultaneous bilateral PCNL in selected patients [50]. They propose some advantages like reduced hospital stay and single anaesthesia. However, it was found that in most cases, bilateral PCNL was associated with higher rate of complications, higher cost, increased morbidity and delayed convalescence as compared to unilateral PCNL one at a time [51].

Taking all the evidence together, a simultaneous bilateral approach should be selected only in cases with a small stone burden with non-complex anatomy. In any event the second side should be done only if the first side is completed in a short time with no significant bleeding.

Considering the complex anatomy and stone burden bilateral simultaneous PCNL is not an option in this case.

Q 7. What are the other treatment options?

A 7.

I. ESWL
II. RIRS
III. Laparoscopic pyelolithotomy

Discussion

ESWL: The horse shoe kidneys are fused at the lower poles of two moities accross the midline. There is high insertion of the ureteropelvic junction and the ureters pass over the isthmus anteriorly which results in restricted urinary drainage and long drainage time. Thus there may be poor clearance of stone even after an optimal calculus fragmentation. Therefore the stone free rates in these patients require multiple ESWL sessions and clearance rate are even lower than with normal kidneys. The residual fragments associated with the stasis and higher risk of infection predisposes to early recurrence. It is therefore not really a suitable option in this case [52, 53].

RIRS: Apart from the usual limitations of RIRS with a large stone burden in the paediatric age group with normal kidneys, there are some additional problems related to horseshoe kidneys. The pelvis of the horseshoe kidney is flatter than that of normal kidneys and the intrarenal space is narrower which increases the difficulty of deflecting and steering the URS inside the kidney. The acutely angled entrance of calyces to the renal pelvis causes difficulty in reaching renal stones located in the lower pole. Even with the newer generation FLURS the limitation of deflection and working angle means that at times it is not possible to relocate a lower calyceal stone into a more favourable location. Fragments of lower pole stones do not pass with ease and stones in this location were found to be a statistically significant factor for failure of RIRS in HSK [54]. In HSK the FLURS needs to stay in extreme deflective status for relatively long periods and this increases the risk of damage and repair cost. The horseshoe kidney is lower than normal with shorter ureteric length and the use of UAS risks more damage to the renal pelvis and ureter. There is limited data of use of RIRS in horse shoe kidney in children [54, 55]. Therefore RIRS in this case is not a favourable option.

Laparoscopic/Robotic assisted pyelolithotomy: such a procedure in this case will be technically challenging and require a skilled laparoscopic/ robotic surgeon. Calyceal stone removal may require use of flexible nephroscope and high power Ho:YAG laser through the laparoscopic port. It can be a favourable procedure in cases associated with pelviureteric junction obstruction requiring pyeloplasty as well [56].

18.14 Case 7

An 11 year old boy presented with the complaint of suprapubic pain. On evaluation he was found to have normal right kidney but the left kidney was ectopic in the pelvis above the urinary bladder as visualized on USG. The left ectopic pelvic kidney was hydronephrotic with an obstructing stone in the renal pelvis and another small stone in a calyx. X-ray abdomen shows radiopaque stones in the pelvis.

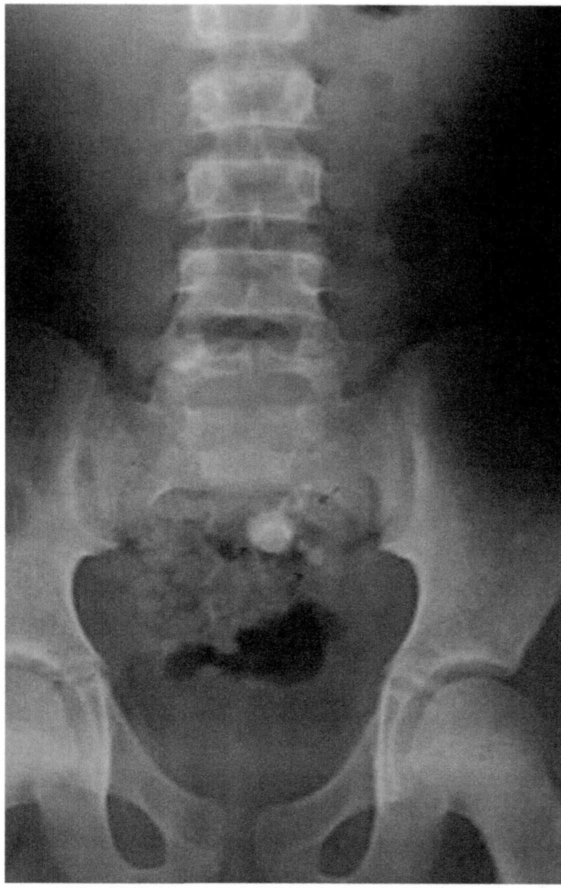

Q 1. What further radiological investigation would you like to perform in this case?

A.

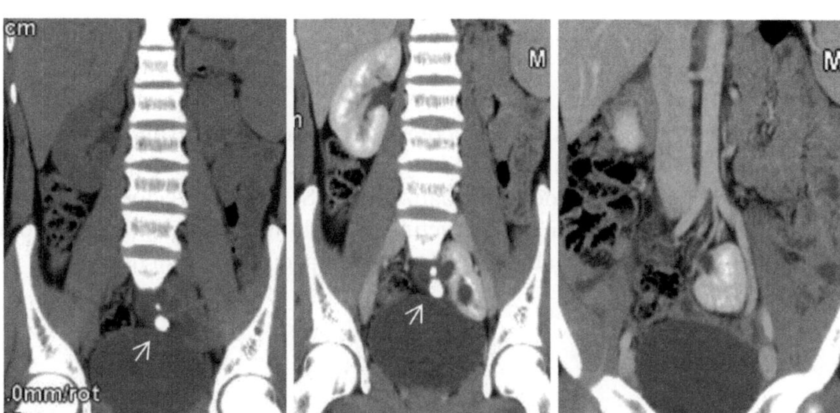

I. **Contrast Computed Tomography (Urogram):** To document vascular and urinary tract anatomy. Right kidney normally located with normal contrast excretion. Left kidney is seen in the region of the left hemipelvis measuring 8.0 cm and is malrotated. A partially obstructing stone is seen in the pelvis measuring 1.9 cm causing mild to moderate hydronephrosis. Another non obstructing stone is seen in a calyx. Normal parenchymal enhancement with normal contrast excretion.

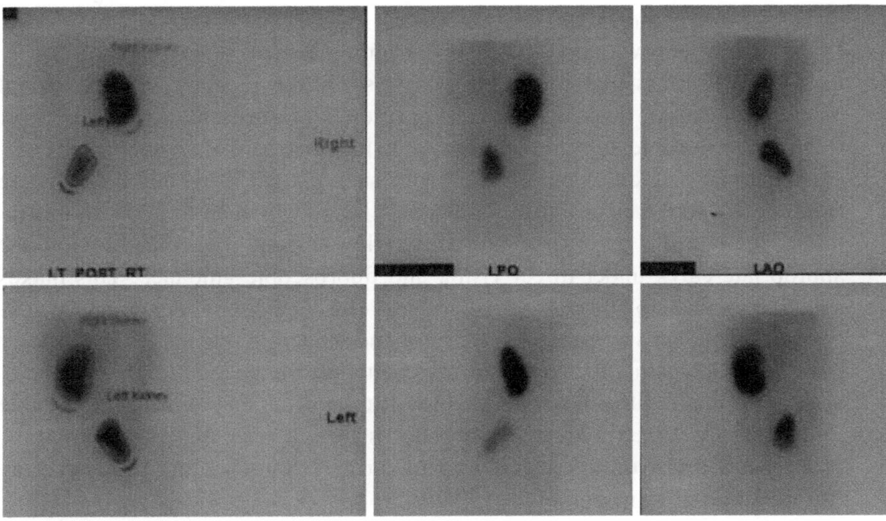

II. **Dimercaptosuccinic acid (DMSA) Scintigraphy**: For more accurate evaluation of differential renal function. As the image shows the right kidney is normal in position and function (73%). The left kidney is present in the pelvic region and has reduced tracer uptake by the cortical tissue (27%) (Note that anterior imaging is necessary for more accurate differentials in such cases).

Q 2. What are the available surgical options?

A 2. The abnormal insertion of the ureter, rotation anomalies and different localisation of the kidney make the management of calculi in an ectopic kidney much more challenging for the paediatric urologist. Renal lithiasis in the pelvic kidney can be managed by means of open surgery, extracorporeal shock wave lithotripsy (ESWL), percutaneous nephrolithotomy (PCNL), laparoscopic assisted PCNL, and retrograde intrarenal surgery (RIRS). Classically urolithiasis in the pelvic kidney has been managed by open surgery. Considering the increased morbidity of large incision, scar and postoperative pain and the advent of MIS has encouraged surgeons to utilise the other options.

I. **ESWL** in a pelvic kidney is complicated due to surrounding bone and bowel thus makes it more difficult to localize the stone. The presence of hydronephrosis, high insertion of ureter and accompanying impaired mobility significantly hamper the clearance of stone fragments [57]. In this patient considering the stone burden and location, ESWL is likely to be less effective and with chances of multiple sessions under anaesthesia. Therefore risk of high failure rate or incomplete clearance.

II. **RIRS** has been attempted to avoid renal puncture. Most of the time it becomes technically difficult to negotiate the ureter and pelvicalyceal system of an ectopic malrotated kidney. This results in treatment failure especially with large stone burden such as in this case. In this abnormal urinary tract using an UAS makes it more complex and less attractive.

III. **PCNL**: In patients with pelvic kidney conventional ultrasound and fluoroscopic guided PCNL is associated with increased risks of bowel injury, intraabdominal bleeding and urine leak owing to the presence of surrounding bowel loops, mesenteric blood vessels and unpredictable blood supply of an abnormally oriented ectopic pelvic kidney [2]. Hence for such patient Eshghi et al. [58] were the first to describe laparoscopic assisted PCNL in which preliminary mobilisation of the bowel is performed in order to allow for safe renal puncture into the appropriate calyx under direct vision and fluoroscopic guidance. This makes sure that there is no bowel or vascular injury during the renal puncture. The use of Mini PCNL adds a further safety factor and reduces blood loss. A high power laser with the dusting technique ensures better clearance than fragmentation or use of pneumatic lithoclast as it become cumbersome and at times impossible to remove the stone fragments from inaccessible calyces. A nephrostomy tube and an abdominal drain are required for urinary drainage and to handle any extravasation of urine and blood [59, 60].

Our preferred approach in this case would be a laparoscopic assisted mini PCNL utilizing a high power laser through rigid and flexible neprohoscopes.

References

1. Sultan S. Urolithiasis. In: Lima M, Manzoni G, editors. Pediatric urology: contemporary strategies from fetal life to adolescence. Milan: Springer; 2015. p. 365–78.
2. Maltaga BR, Krambeck AE, Lingeman JE. Surgical management of upper urinary tract calculi. In: Wein AJ, Kavoussi LR, Partin AW, Peters CA, editors. Campbell-Walsh urology. 11th ed. Amsterdam: Elsevier; 2015. p. 1260–90.
3. Hounsfield GN. Computed medical imaging. Med Phys. 1980;7(4):283–90.
4. Rizvi SA, Sultan S, Zafar MN, Ahmed B, Umer SA, Naqvi SA. Paediatric urolithiasis in emerging economies. Int J Sur. 2016;36:705–12.
5. Sarica K, Sahin C. Contemporary minimally invasive surgical Management of Urinary Stones in children. Eur Uro Supp. 2017;16(1):2–7.
6. Dogan HS, Altan M, Citamak B, Bozaci AC, Karabulut E, Tekgul S. A new nomogram for prediction of outcome of pediatric shock-wave lithotripsy. J Pediatr Urol. 2015;11(2):84e1–6.
7. Onal B, Tansu N, Demirkesen O, Yalcin V, Huang L, Nguyen HT, et al. Nomogram and scoring system for predicting stone-free status after extracorporeal shock wave lithotripsy in children with urolithiasis. BJU Int. 2013;111(2):344–52.
8. Özgür BC, Irkilata L, Ekici M, Hoşcan MB, Sarici H, Yücetürk CN, et al. Pediatric extracorporeal shock wave lithotripsy: multi-institutional results. Urologia. 2016;83(2):83–6.

9. Silay MS, Ellison JS, Tailly T, Caione P. Update on urinary stones in children: current and future concepts in surgical treatment and shockwave lithotripsy. Eur Urol Focus. 2017;3(2–3):164–71.
10. Alsagheer G, Abdel-Kader MS, Hasan AM, Mahmoud O, Mohamed O, Fathi A, et al. Extracorporeal shock wave lithotripsy (ESWL) monotherapy in children: predictors of successful outcome. J Pediatr Urol. 2017;13(5):515e1–5.
11. Gamal WM, Hussein MM, El Nisr Rashed AD, Mmdouh A, Fawzy F. Pediatric retrograde intrarenal surgery for renal stones< 2 cm in solitary kidney. Indian J Urol. 2016;32(4):296–300.
12. Li J, Xiao J, Han T, Tian Y, Wang W, Du Y. Flexible ureteroscopic lithotripsy for the treatment of upper urinary tract calculi in infants. Exp Biol Med. 2017;242(2):153–9.
13. Rob S, Jones P, Pietropaolo A, Griffin S, Somani BK. Ureteroscopy for stone disease in paediatric population is safe and effective in medium-volume and high-volume Centres: evidence from a systematic review. Curr Urol Rep. 2017;18(12):92.
14. Xiao J, Wang X, Li J, Wang M, Han T, Zhang C, et al. Treatment of upper urinary tract stones with flexible ureteroscopy in children. Can Urol Assoc J. 2018;30(13(3)):E78.
15. Freton L, Peyronnet B, Arnaud A, Tondut L, Hascoet J, Pradere B, et al. Extracorporeal shockwave lithotripsy versus flexible ureteroscopy for the management of upper tract urinary stones in children. J Endourol. 2017;31(1):1–6.
16. Pelit ES, Atis G, Kati B, Akin Y, Çiftçi H, Culpan M, et al. Comparison of mini-percutaneous nephrolithotomy and retrograde intrarenal surgery in preschool-aged children. Urology. 2017;101:21–5.
17. Komori M, Izaki H, Daizumoto K, Tsuda M, Kusuhara Y, Mori H, et al. Complications of flexible ureteroscopic treatment for renal and ureteral calculi during the learning curve. Urol Int. 2015;95(1):26–32.
18. Baş O, Dede O, Aydogmus Y, Utangaç M, Yikilmaz TN, Damar E, et al. Comparison of retrograde intrarenal surgery and micro-percutaneous nephrolithotomy in moderately sized pediatric kidney stones. J Endourol. 2016;30(7):765–70.
19. Saad KS, Youssif ME, Hamdy SA, Fahmy A, Hanno AG, El-Nahas AR. Percutaneous nephrolithotomy vs retrograde intrarenal surgery for large renal stones in pediatric patients: a randomized controlled trial. J Urol. 2015;194(6):1716–20.
20. Resorlu B, Sancak EB, Resorlu M, Gulpinar MT, Adam G, Akbas A, Ozdemir H. Retrograde intrarenal surgery in pediatric patients. W J Neph. 2014;3(4):193–7.
21. Berrettini A, Boeri L, Montanari E, Mogiatti M, Acquati P, De Lorenzis E, et al. Retrograde intrarenal surgery using ureteral access sheaths is a safe and effective treatment for renal stones in children weighing< 20 kg. J Pediatr Urol. 2018;14(1):59–e1.
22. Sen H, Seckiner I, Bayrak O, Dogan K, Erturhan S. A comparison of micro-PERC and retrograde intrarenal surgery results in pediatric patients with renal stones. J Pediatr Urol. 2017;13(6):619e1–5.
23. Lu P, Song R, Yu Y, Yang J, Qi K, Tao R, et al. Clinical efficacy of percutaneous nephrolithotomy versus retrograde intrarenal surgery for pediatric kidney urolithiasis: a PRISMA-compliant article. Medicine. 2017;96(43):e8346.
24. Chen Y, Deng T, Duan X, Zhu W, Zeng G. Percutaneous nephrolithotomy versus retrograde intrarenal surgery for pediatric patients with upper urinary stones: a systematic review and meta-analysis. Urolithiasis. 2018;24:1–1.
25. Legemate JD, Kamphuis GM, Freund JE, Baard J, Zanetti SP, Catellani M, et al. Durability of flexible Ureteroscopes: a prospective evaluation of longevity, the factors that affect it, and damage mechanisms. Eur Urol Focus. 2018;5(6):1105–11.
26. Kramolowsky E, McDowell Z, Moore B, Booth B, Wood N. Cost analysis of flexible ureteroscope repairs: evaluation of 655 procedures in a community-based practice. J Endourol. 2016;30(3):254–6.
27. Zeng G, Zhu W, Lam W. Miniaturised percutaneous nephrolithotomy: its role in the treatment of urolithiasis and our experience. Asian J Urol. 2018;5(4):295–302.
28. Pelit ES, Kati B, Çanakci C, Sağir S, Çiftçi H. Outcomes of miniaturized percutaneous nephrolitotomy in infants: single Centre experience. Int Bra J Urol. 2017;43(5):932–8.

29. Ng FC, Yam WL, Lim TY, Teo JK, Ng KK, Lim SK. Ultrasound-guided percutaneous nephrolithotomy: advantages and limitations. Investig Clin Urol. 2017;58(5):346–52.
30. Taguchi K, Hamamoto S, Okada A, Mizuno K, Tozawa K, Hayashi Y, et al. First case report of staghorn calculi successfully removed by mini-endoscopic combined intrarenal surgery in a 2-year-old boy. Int J Urol. 2015;22(10):978–80.
31. Li J, Wang W, Du Y, Tian Y. Combined use of flexible ureteroscopic lithotripsy with micro-percutaneous nephrolithotomy in pediatric multiple kidney stones. J Pediatr Urol. 2018;14(3):281.e1–6.
32. Kirac M, Ergin G, Kibar Y, Köprü B, Biri H. The efficacy of Ureteroscopy without fluoroscopy for ureteral and renal stones in pediatric patients. J Endourol. 2018;32(2):100–5.
33. Khosa AS, Hussain M. Safety and efficacy of transurethral pneumatic lithotripsy for bladder calculi in children. J Pak Med Assoc. 2012;62(12):1297–300.
34. Alken P. Intracorporeal lithotripsy. Urolithiasis. 2017;7.
35. Santiago JE, Hollander AB, Soni SD, Link RE, Mayer WA. To dust or not to dust: a systematic review of ureteroscopic laser lithotripsy techniques. Curr Urol Rep. 2017;18(4):32.
36. Kronenberg P, Somani B. Advances in lasers for the treatment of stones—a systematic review. Curr Urol Rep. 2018;19(6):45.
37. Alsagheer GA, Mohamed O, Abdel-Kader MS, Hasan AM, Razek MA, Fathi A, et al. Extracorporeal shock wave lithotripsy (ESWL) versus flexible ureteroscopy (F-URS) for management of renal stone burden less than 2 cm in children: a randomized comparative study. Afr J Urol. 2018;24(2):120–5.
38. Khan M, Lal M, Kash DP, Hussain M, Rizvi S. Anatomical factors predicting lower calyceal stone clearance after extracorporeal shockwave lithotripsy. Afr J Urol. 2016;22(2):96–100.
39. Tan MÖ, Karaoğlan Ü, Şen I, Deniz N, Bozkırlı I. The impact of radiological anatomy in clearance of lower calyceal stones after shock wave lithotripsy in paediatric patients. Eur Urol. 2003;43(2):188–93.
40. Hammad FT, Kaya M, Kazim E. Pediatric extracorporeal shockwave lithotripsy: its efficiency at various locations in the upper tract. J Endourol. 2009;23(2):229–36.
41. Horuz R, Sarica K. The management of staghorn calculi in children. Arab J Urol. 2012;10(3):330–5.
42. Bujons A, Millán F, Centeno C, Emiliani E, Martín FS, Angerri O, et al. Mini-percutaneous nephrolithotomy with high-power holmium YAG laser in pediatric patients with staghorn and complex calculi. J Pediatr Urol. 2016;12(4):253e1–5.
43. Ponsky LE, Streem SB. "Sandwich" therapy for the treatment of complex renal stones. Braz J Urol. 2000;26:18–23.
44. Agrawal V, Bajaj J, Acharya H, Chanchalani R, Raina VK, Sharma D. Laparoscopic management of pediatric renal and ureteric stones. J Pediatr Urol. 2013;9(2):230–3.
45. Landa-Juárez S, Rivera-Pereira BM, Castillo-Fernández AM. Management of Pediatric Urolithiasis Using a combination of laparoscopic lithotomy and Pyeloscopy. J Laparoendosc Adv Surg Tech. 2018;28(6):766–9.
46. Caione P, De Dominicis M, Collura G, Matarazzo E, Nappo SG, Capozza N, et al. Microperc for pediatric nephrolithiasis: technique in Valdivia-modified position. Eur J Pediatr Sur. 2015;25(01):94–9.
47. Elgalaly H, Eliwa A, Seleem M, Salem E, Omran M, Shello H, et al. Silodosin in the treatment of distal ureteric stones in children: a prospective, randomised, placebo-controlled study. Arab J Urol. 2017;15(3):194–8.
48. Raj GV, Auge BK, Weizer AZ, Denstedt JD, Watterson JD, Beiko DT, et al. Percutaneous management of calculi within horseshoe kidneys. J Urol. 2003;170(1):48–51.
49. Osther PJ, Razvi H, Liatsikos E, Averch T, Crisci A, Garcia JL, et al. Percutaneous nephrolithotomy among patients with renal anomalies: patient characteristics and outcomes; a subgroup analysis of the clinical research office of the endourological society global percutaneous nephrolithotomy study. J Endourol. 2011;25(10):1627–32.
50. Guven S, Ozturk A, Arslan M, Istanbulluoglu O, Piskin M, Kilinc M. Simultaneous bilateral percutaneous nephrolithotomy in children: no need to delay. J Endourol. 2011;25(3):437–40.

51. Kadlec AO, Greco KA, Fridirici ZC, Hart ST, Vellos TG, Turk TM. Comparison of complication rates for unilateral and bilateral percutaneous nephrolithotomy (PCNL) using a modified Clavien grading system. BJU Int. 2013;111(4b):E243–8.
52. Viola D, Anagnostou T, Thompson TJ, Smith G, Moussa SA, Tolley DA. Sixteen years of experience with stone management in horseshoe kidneys. Urol Int. 2007;78(3):214–8.
53. Blackburne AT, Rivera ME, Gettman MT, Patterson DE, Krambeck AE. Endoscopic management of urolithiasis in the horseshoe kidney. Urology. 2016 Apr 1;90:45–9.
54. Atis G, Resorlu B, Gurbuz C, Arikan O, Ozyuvali E, Unsal A, et al. Retrograde intrarenal surgery in patients with horseshoe kidneys. Urolithiasis. 2013;41(1):79–83.
55. Ding J, Huang Y, Gu S, Chen Y, Peng J, Bai Q, et al. Flexible ureteroscopic management of horseshoe kidney renal calculi. Int Braz J Urol. 2015;41(4):683–9.
56. Symons SJ, Ramachandran A, Kurien A, Baiysha R, Desai MR. Urolithiasis in the horseshoe kidney: a single-Centre experience. BJU Int. 2008;102(11):1676–80.
57. Cinman NM, Okeke Z, Smith AD. Pelvic kidney: associated diseases and treatment. J Endourol. 2007;21(8):836–42.
58. Eshghi AM, Roth JS, Smith AD. Percutaneous transperitoneal approach to a pelvic kidney for endourological removal of staghorn calculus. J Urol. 1985;134(3):525–7.
59. Aquil S, Rana M, Zaidi Z. Laparoscopic assisted percutaneous nephrolithotomy (PCNL) in ectopic pelvic kidney. JPMA. 2006;56(8):381–3.
60. D'souza N, Verma A, Rai A. Laparoscopic-assisted mini percutaneous nephrolithotomy in the ectopic pelvic kidney: outcomes with the laser dusting technique. Urol ann. 2016;8(1):87–90.

Urologic Tumors

19

Patrick J. Hensley and Amanda F. Saltzman

Here Are Our Objectives

1. Describe the approach, staging and treatment of renal tumors in children, including Wilms tumor, renal cell carcinoma and other more rare kidney tumors.
2. Describe the workup, staging and treatment of testis tumors in both pre and post-pubertal males.
3. Describe the approach to diagnosis, stage, group and risk assignment, and management of rhabdomyosarcoma of the genitourinary tract.
4. Describe the approach to diagnosis and common treatments for children with bladder tumors.
5. Describe common predisposition syndrome of malignancy of the genitourinary tract in children.
6. Describe common late effects of treatment for genitourinary tumors in children and how to mitigate these upfront when possible.

19.1 Part 1: Kidney Tumors

19.1.1 Wilms Tumor

Wilms Tumor (WT), or nephroblastoma, accounts for 85% of all pediatric renal tumors, with approximately 500 new cases annually in the United States (Table 19.1) [1]. Patients are typically diagnosed between ages 3–5 years, and 95% of cases are diagnosed in children <10 years of age. African-Americans have the highest predisposition to the development of WT, and Asians appear to have the lowest risk [2].

Multiple genetic syndromes may predispose children to WT, including Denys Drash, Beckwith-Weideman, and Frasier Syndrome [2]. This predisposition is

P. J. Hensley · A. F. Saltzman (✉)
Department of Urology, University of Kentucky, Lexington, KY, USA
e-mail: amanda.saltzman@uky.edu

P. Godbole et al. (eds.), *Practical Pediatric Urology*,
https://doi.org/10.1007/978-3-030-54020-3_19

Table 19.1 Incidence of pediatric renal tumors

Histology	Frequency (%)
WT	85
CMN	5
RCC	4
CCSK	4
RTK	2

Adapted from Denes 2013

highest (98%) in WT-aniridia (WAGR) syndrome, which involves the presence and/or development of WT, aniridia, genital abnormalities and mental retardation. Patients with predisposition syndromes and bilateral tumors typically present at earlier ages than those without. The involved gene *WT1*, located on the short arm of chromosome 11 (11p), is a tumor suppressor encoding a transcription factor involved in embryologic genitourinary development. Homozygous mutations of *WT1* or coding regions nearby result in the development of WT with high penetrance. Studies suggest that screening patients with predisposition syndromes may result in diagnosis at an earlier stage, but this data is unclear. While formal recommendations on screening high risk children remain inconclusive, abdominal ultrasonography every 3–6 months for the first 7–10 years of life has generally been adopted [3].

Patients typically present with a spectrum a palpable abdominal mass, hematuria, hypertension and/or abdominal pain. The initial imaging modality of choice for a patient with a suspected intra-abdominal mass is abdominal ultrasound which is capable of guiding further cross-sectional imaging [4]. For patients with a solid renal mass on ultrasound, staging CT of the chest, abdomen and pelvis with intravenous (iv) contrast in a single setting or CT chest and MRI of the abdomen and pelvis with iv contrast is indicated. MRI is the initial imaging modality of choice for bilateral tumors (5–10% of cases) to reduce radiation exposure given anticipated future use of repeated cross-sectional imaging in current treatment protocols. Laboratory studies should include complete blood count, liver function panel, basic metabolic panel, urinalysis and coagulation studies as 4–8% of patients with WT develop acquired von Willebrand disease [2].

Pre-operative clinical staging and decisions have significant impacts on treatment strategies, as outlined in Table 19.2. There exists competing diagnosis and treatment strategies among two international cooperative working groups. The Children's Oncology Group (COG), responsible for treatment guidelines, tumor registries and clinical trials for renal masses in North America, advocate upfront surgery with the interpretation of primary unaltered pathology guiding further treatment. The Société Internationale d'Oncologie Pédiatrique (SIOP), the European equivalent to COG, alternatively advocates for neoadjuvant chemotherapy for all patients with a solid renal mass followed by surgery and then histologic evaluation to guide subsequent therapy [2]. The remainder of this chapter will focus on the COG guidelines. It is essential to establish early multidisciplinary care with medical oncologists familiar with ongoing protocols.

Table 19.2 Therapy and clinical outcomes by Wilms tumor stage

Stage	Incidence (%)	Criteria	Therapy (FH)[a,b]	4-year survival (%FH–%UH)
I	40–45	Confined to kidney Negative margin No nodal involvement	Radical nephrectomy with LN sampling[c] + VA	83–99
II	20	Spread beyond kidney Negative margins No nodal involvement	Radical nephrectomy with LN sampling[c] + VA	81–98
III	20–25	Peritoneal implants Positive margin Preoperative biopsy Preoperative chemotherapy Intraoperative tumor rupture Nodal involvement	Radical nephrectomy with LN sampling[c] + VAD + abdominal XRT	72–94
IV	10	Metastatic disease	Radical nephrectomy with LN sampling[c] + VAD + abdominal and chest XRT	38–86
V	5	Bilateral tumors	VA + nephron-sparring surgery with LN sampling	55–87

VA vincristine + actinomycin, VAD vincristine + actinomycin + doxorubicin, *XRT* external beam radiation, *FH* favorable histology, *UH* unfavorable histology

[a]Chemotherapeutic agent only, not regimen

[b]With UH, use doxorubicin and XRT earlier with lower stages and 5 drug chemotherapy if diffuse UH

[c]Preoperative chemo only indicated with unresectable primary tumor/abdominal disease

The initial treatment of unilateral, non-syndromic WT is open radical nephrectomy with regional lymphadenectomy. Notably, pre-operative renal mass biopsy confers a clinical stage III designation and has adjuvant therapy treatment implications (Table 19.2). Biopsy is rarely indicated or used in COG protocols due to this potential upstaging. Neoadjuvant chemotherapy may be considered in locally-advanced, unresectable tumors or those with overwhelming pulmonary or hepatic metastases impairing normal function, based on surgeon judgement. Nephron-sparing surgery (NSS, partial nephrectomy) is reserved for patients with solitary kidneys, bilateral (stage V) or syndromic tumors and is often preceded by neoadjuvant chemotherapy in attempts to improve feasibility of NSS (Fig. 19.1).

Due to poor sensitivity of cross sectional imaging to estimate the local extent of disease, emphasis is placed on intra-operative findings to adequately stage the patient. Ureteral tumor extension occurs in up to 5% of patients with WT, thus any

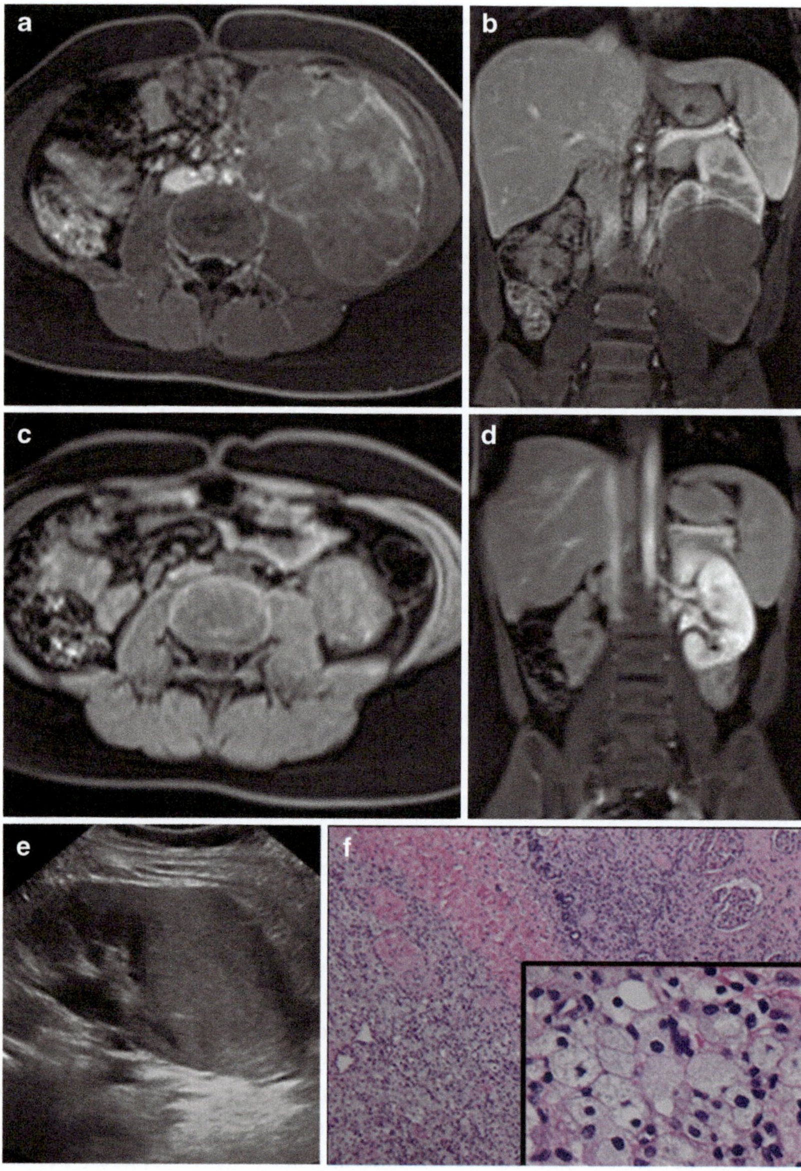

Fig. 19.1 Recurrent Wilms tumor in a solitary kidney of an 11 year-old female. At age 6, the patient presented with stage V disease and underwent neoadjuvant chemotherapy followed by right radical nephrectomy and left partial nephrectomy. She developed an 11 cm left lower pole recurrence confirmed on MRI (T2-weighted, A-axial, B-coronal). After neoadjuvant VAD chemotherapy, the tumor measured 5 cm (T2-weighted MRI, C-axial, D-coronal; E-renal ultrasound). She underwent open left partial nephrectomy. Pathology showed benign histiocytic proliferation and scarring (F-H&E section 100× magnification, insert 1000×). (**a**) T2 weighted MRI, axial at diagnosis. (**b**) T2 weighted MRI, coronal at diagnosis. (**c**) T2 weighted MRI, axial after neoadjuvant chemotherapy. (**d**) T2 weighted MRI, coronal after neoadjuvant chemotherapy. (**e**) renal US, after neoadjuvant chemotherapy. (**f**) H&E section, 100× magnification, insert 1000× magnification

patient with gross hematuria should undergo cystoscopy with retrograde pyelography at the time of extirpative surgery to ensure en-block tumor excision without spillage [2]. As with pre-operative renal mass biopsy, non-contiguous intraabdominal tumor implants or intra-operative tumor spillage confers clinical stage III disease. All of these situations have each been independently associated with poor survival [2]. Standard treatment for all stages of favorable histology WT are outlined in Table 19.2.

The most significant histologic factor implicated in prognosis and treatment strategy is the finding of anaplasia in poorly differentiated tumors [2]. Loss of heterozygosity for both chromosomes 1p and 16q is associated with increased risk of relapse and cancer-specific mortality and mandates more aggressive adjuvant chemotherapy, when identified [2].

Improvements in surgical technique and optimization of chemoradiation protocols have imparted survival advantages exceeding 90% (Table 19.2). Due to favorable long-term outcomes, recent efforts have focused on mitigating long term morbidity from treatment, including CKD as well as secondary malignancies, cardiac toxicity and infertility [2].

19.1.2 Renal Cell Carcinoma

Renal cell carcinoma (RCC) comprises nearly 4% of pediatric renal masses and is the second most common malignant tumor in children. The median age at presentation is 12.9 years, and RCC is the most common renal mass in children >12 years [2, 5]. There does not appear to be a gender or racial predilection. Multiple gene mutations have been associated with predisposition syndromes for sub-types of RCC (Table 19.3). While most adult tumors are identified incidentally, pediatric RCCs commonly present with a palpable abdominal mass or gross hematuria.

Staging and grading systems are the same as those used for adult tumors (Table 19.4). Like protocols adopted for WT, complete staging involves CT chest and cross-sectional abdominopelvic imaging (CT or MRI). Laboratory evaluation incudes complete blood count, comprehensive metabolic panel and urinalysis. While NSS and minimally invasive approaches for adult RCC have well characterized roles and are stressed in recent guidelines, their role in pediatric RCC is less clear. These limitations likely are derived from empiric use of WT COG protocols emphasizing open, radical nephrectomy for initial diagnosis and staging for pediatric masses prior to definitive diagnosis. Additionally, this histologic subtype of RCC is different from adult RCC, and thus, lymph node metastases is often underrecognized in pre-operative staging imaging (sensitivity 57%) yet identified in 48% of clinical stage T1 tumors. As such, lymph node sampling is strongly encouraged in patients <40 years of age with a renal mass suspicious for malignancy for both diagnostic and therapeutic reasons [2].

Unlike adult tumors where clear cell RCC predominates (75–88%), the most common histologic subtype in children is translocation RCC, accounting for nearly half of all cases. Translocation tumors are characterized by activating mutations in

Table 19.3 Genetic syndromes associated with RCC

Genetic predisposition syndrome	Gene	Presentation
Von Hippel Lindau	*VHL* (3p)	Clear cell RCC Retinal and CNS hemangioblastomas Pheochromocytomas Pancreatic cysts/tumors Epididymal cystadenomas
Tuberous sclerosis	*TSC1* or *TSC2*	AMLs Clear cell RCC Seizures Mental retardation Facial angiofibromas Hamartomas
Hereditary papillary RCC	*MET*	Low grade type 1 papillary RCC
Birt-Hogg-Dubé	*FLCN*	Chromophobe RCC Fibrofolliculomas Lung cysts and blebs
Hereditary Leiomyomatosis and RCC	*FH*	High grade type 2 papillary RCC Uterine fibroids at young age
Succinate dehydrogenase RCC	*SDH*	Different RCCs Paragangliomas Pheochromocytomas

Table 19.4 American joint committee on cancer (AJCC) TNM staging for renal cell carcinoma (seventh Edition)

Primary tumor (pT)	
T1a	Tumor confined to kidney, <4 cm
T1b	Tumor confined to kidney, ≥4 cm but <7 cm
T2a	Tumor confined to kidney, ≥7 cm but <10 cm
T2b	Tumor confined to kidney, ≥10 cm
T3a	Tumor extends grossly into renal vein or its segmental branches, or tumor invades perirenal and/or renal sinus fat but not beyond Gerota's fascia
T3b	Spread to infra-diaphragmatic IVC
T3c	Spread to supra-diaphragmatic IVC or IVC wall invasion
T4	Involvement of ipsilateral adrenal gland or invades beyond Gerota's fascia
Nodal stage	
N0	No nodal involvement
N1	Metastatic involvement of regional LN
Metastasis stage	
M0	No distant metastases
M1	Distant metastases
Stage groupings	
Stage I	T1 N0 M0
Stage II	T2 N0 M0
Stage III	T3 or N1 with M0
Stage IV	T4 or M1

TFE3 on Xp11.2, resulting in constitutive tyrosine kinase activity and downstream mammalian target of Rapamycin (mTOR) pathway activation with resultant unregulated proliferation (a common pathway for RCC development). These tumors confer aggressive phenotypes and are associated with locally advanced or metastatic disease in 63% of children [2].

A recent National Cancer Database study attributed a 5-year overall survival of 71–100% for patients with organ confined disease (pT1–3), 55% for patients with nodal involvement and 8% for patients with metastatic disease [6]. While traditional targeted therapies (tyrosine kinase and mTOR inhibitors) may be utilized in children with advanced disease or adverse histopathologic characteristics, data are limited on their use in the adjuvant setting for pediatric RCC. The only reported cases of survival in widely metastatic translocation RCC involve complete surgical resection (primary tumor, regional lymph nodes, and metastatic lesions).

19.1.3 Other Pediatric Renal Tumors

19.1.3.1 Clear Cell Sarcoma of the Kidney

Clear cell sarcoma of the kidney (CCSK) occurs predominantly in children between 1 and 4 years of age with a 2:1 male predominance [1]. There are no known familial predisposition syndromes or cases of bilateral CCSK. Patients typically present with a palpable abdominal mass, although 15–60% of children present with pain related to skeletal metastases. Imaging and laboratory studies for staging purposes are similar to those of RCC and WT and mass characteristics on CT are indistinguishable from WT.

Treatment consists of radical nephrectomy with regional lymph node sampling. Adjuvant therapy is commonly instituted and includes radiation and chemotherapy (vincristine, doxorubicin, cyclophosphamide and etoposide) [7]. The 5-year overall survival is 85–90% despite a high relapse rate in the first 3 years after treatment, especially in younger patients. While bone metastases are classically attributed to metastatic CCSK, advances in treatment have resulted in metastasis and late recurrences most commonly in the brain [2]. Close follow up and surveillance is prudent.

19.1.3.2 Rhabdoid Tumor of the Kidney

Rhabdoid tumor of the kidney (RTK) is a rare, aggressive pediatric renal tumor with 80% of cases occurring in children <2 years of age [1]. The majority of these patients exhibit germline mutations in *INI-1* on chromosome 22. While hematuria is the predominant presenting symptom, symptomatic metastases can occur in up to 80% of cases [1]. Staging imaging is the same as the other pediatric renal tumors, but also includes central nervous system imaging given the predilection of RTK to metastasize there. Brain MRI is indicated, especially in children <1 year of age, given the high risk of metastatic disease to the brain [2]. Radical nephrectomy with lymphadenectomy is the primary treatment modality as RTK is highly resistant to chemotherapy and radiation [1]. Overall 4-year survival ranges between 20 and 36 months, with younger patients exhibiting worse survival than older patients. CNS involvement is nearly universally fatal.

19.1.3.3 Congenital Mesoblastic Nephroma

Congenital mesoblastic nephroma (CMN) is the most common renal tumor in infants <6 months of age, making CMN the presumed diagnosis for a solid renal mass in this age group [1]. CMN is thought to be derived from an abnormal proliferation of nephrogenic mesenchyme during the neonatal period. It is often diagnosed prenatally on ultrasound and is associated with polyhydramnios and preterm birth [2]. Ultrasound findings characteristically include large, partially cystic masses confined to the kidney. Although originally described as a benign tumor, CT scan of the chest, abdomen and pelvis should complete staging as there have been cases reported of recurrent and/or metastatic disease. Radical nephrectomy is considered both diagnostic and therapeutic. Lymph node sampling is indicated for accurate staging and since a diagnosis of WT or RCC cannot be excluded. Prognosis is generally good, especially with surgery within the first 6 months of life. While a follow up regimen has not been established, serial abdominal ultrasonography for 2 years has generally been advised.

19.1.3.4 Renal Medullary Carcinoma

Renal medullary carcinoma is an extremely aggressive RCC variant presenting in patients with sickle cell trait or disease, and thus there is a strong African-American predominance [1]. The majority of patients present with gross hematuria and/or abdominal/flank pain. Over 90% of patients present with advanced disease. Complete cross-sectional staging imaging is necessary. Radical nephrectomy is the primary treatment modality as medullary carcinoma is unresponsive to chemoradiation. The tumor is, unfortunately, nearly universally fatal, with average survival between 4 and 16 months.

19.1.3.5 Angiomyolipoma

Angiomyolipoma (AML) derives its name from its three characteristic histologic components: blood vessels, muscle and adipose. These vascular tumors are commonly seen in patients with Tuberous Sclerosis and often present with spontaneous retroperitoneal hemorrhage. Similar to treatment strategies employed in adult AML, annual monitoring with ultrasonography or MRI for size and stability is prudent. Efforts should be directed towards nephron-sparring management, including selective arterial embolization, especially in patients with Tuberous Sclerosis who are prone to multifocal, recurrent tumors. These patients are at increased risk of developing RCC [2].

19.1.3.6 MCN/CPDN/WT Spectrum

Multilocular cystic nephroma (MCN) and cystic partially differentiated nephroblastoma (CPDN) represent a clinicopathologic spectrum of kidney tumors that are often indistinguishable from cystic WT in clinical presentation and radiological appearance. These tumors commonly present in patients <2 years of age (in contrast to WT with highest incidence between ages 3 and 5 years). Surgical excision and histologic findings confirm the diagnosis, and radical nephrectomy is considered curative. If nephron-sparring approaches are undertaken, frozen section analysis to confirm negative margins is indicated [2].

MCN is classically a tumor with well-defined cysts with septae, and are classified as CPDN if poorly differentiated tissue or blastemal cells are found in the septae by pathology. Cystic WT exhibits more solid strictures between the cysts with stromal, mesenchymal or epithelial components. MCN and stage I CPDN are considered benign lesions managed with surveillance only. Patients with stage II CPDN are treated with vincristine and actinomycin, similar to stage I–II WT. Cystic WT are treated based on stage-dependent WT guidelines (Table 19.2).

19.2 Part 2: Testis Tumors

19.2.1 Introduction

Prepubertal testis tumors vary significantly from adult testis tumors in pathologic distribution, malignant potential and prognosis. Primary testicular tumors in children and adolescents are rare, with an estimated incidence is 0.5–2 per 100,000 children and accounting for 1–2% of all pediatric solid tumors. Pediatric testis tumors have a bimodal age distribution with peaks within the first 4 years of life and again around age 15 years [8].

Classification of pediatric tumors mirrors that of adults, with tumors divided into seminoma, non-seminomatous germ cell tumors (GCT), sex cord-stromal tumors (Sertoli cell, Leydig cell, granulosa cell tumors), mixed germ cell/sex cord tumors, secondary testicular tumors and parastesticular masses. GCT primarily arise from the gonads, but may involve any site along the migration path of primordial germ cells to the genital ridge, including the pineal gland, mediastinum, peritoneum, and sacrum. While up to 60% of adult tumors exhibit mixed histologic subtypes, pediatric tumors more commonly comprised only one subtype [8]. Testicular GCT are the most common malignancy in males between 15 and 35 years and account for 20% of all malignancies in this age category and 98% of all testicular tumors overall, making this a very important disease to pediatric urologists.

Well defined predisposing risk factors for testicular cancer include personal history of cryptorchidism as well has personal or family history of testicular cancer. Patients with cryptorchidism exhibit a fourfold increased risk of developing GCT, with an estimated 10% of cases linked to history of undescended testis. This risk is mitigated by prepubertal orchiopexy, but the risk does not return to baseline. Additionally, high levels of maternal estrogens, high and low birth weights, neonatal jaundice, and disorders of sexual development (DSD) have been implicated in the development of testicular GCT. While the majority of prepubertal GCTs are sporadic, chromosome 12p polyploidy, deletions in 1p and 6q, as well as abnormalities in chromosomes 2 and 3p have been described.

19.2.2 Evaluation

Nearly 90% of testis tumors present as painless testicular masses, and less commonly masses are identified on ultrasound obtained for scrotal pain or infection.

Hydrocele can accompany testis masses in 15–20% of cases, thus hydroceles should be investigated with ultrasonography [8]. Clinical history should focus on identifying risk factors (cryptorchidism, family history, etc.) and should elucidate pubertal status as well as the presence or absence of virilization indicative of hormone secreting tumors. Physical examination should attempt to determine the origination of the lesion (testicular, parastesticular, epididymis, spermatic cord) as well as closely evaluate the contralateral testicle. Complete physical examination should involve chest auscultation and assessment for supraclavicular lymphadenopathy.

Clinical suspicion or abnormal examination findings should prompt scrotal ultrasonography, which is characterized by nearly 100% sensitivity for detecting intrascrotal masses [8]. Scrotal ultrasound has poor specificity to differentiate benign and malignant testicular lesions. However, there are key radiographic features that hint at common testicular tumors: seminomas are homogenous and hypoechoic, yok sac tumors are hypervascular, heterogeneous masses, and teratomas exhibit marked heterogeneity owing to cystic/solid tissue components (Fig. 19.2).

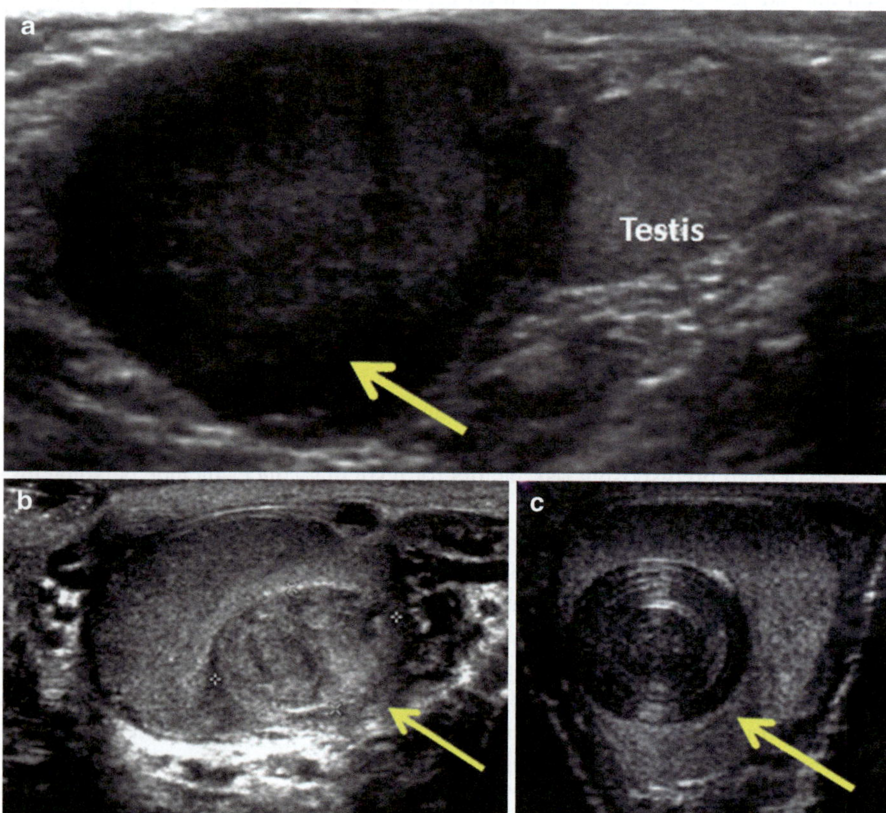

Fig. 19.2 Ultrasound characteristics of testicular masses. (**a**) US of paratesticular mass. (**b**) US showing intra-testicular mass suspicious for GCT. (**c**) US showing classic onion-skin appearance of epidermoid cyst

Prior to any medical or surgical intervention, serum tumor markers must be evaluated to guide clinical staging and further imaging. Human chorionic gonadotropin-β (hCG) is rarely elevated in prepubertal tumors but can be elevated in both seminomatous and non-seminomatous GCTs in adults. α-fetoprotein (AFP) has diagnostic, staging and surveillance utility in children and is elevated in 92% of yolk sac tumors. Resulting from physiologic fetal yolk sac persistence, gastrointestinal and hepatic production of AFP, interpretation of levels in children <1 year of age is difficult. AFP typically nadirs at age 8 months. While teratomas can secrete AFP, levels rarely exceed 100 ng/mL in children >6 months of age harboring teratoma [8]. Lactate dehydrogenase (LDH) is used as a non-specific marker of disease burden. In the setting of a testis mass and precocious puberty, a hormonal panel consisting serum testosterone, estradiol, inhibin and 17-ketosteroid level can aid in establishing the diagnosis of a stromal tumor or congenital adrenal hyperplasia.

Further cross-sectional imaging consisting of CT chest, abdomen, and pelvis with oral and iv contrast for staging purposes is traditionally deferred until a histologic diagnosis is made, with the exception being patients presenting with markedly elevated AFP or symptomatic metastases. Sites of metastasis from most to least common are lung, retroperitoneal lymph nodes, liver, and bone [8]. If sedation for CT imaging is necessary in young children, this can commonly be coordinated with other procedures (orchiectomy, vascular access for chemotherapy, etc.). Additional considerations regarding fertility preservation include sperm banking for age-appropriate males, cryopreservation of testicular tissue, and early referral to an oncofertility specialist.

19.2.3 Diagnosis and Treatment

Considering the high incidence of benign lesions in children, there has been an evolution towards testis-sparring surgery (TSS), especially in prepubertal males. It is suggested that all patients undergo ultrasound-facilitated excisional biopsy and intra-operative frozen section analysis. However, in the largest series of prepubertal testes tumors, 75% of patients were managed with radical orchiectomy [9]. Completion radical orchiectomy is performed when malignancy is suggested on frozen section [8]. The exception is patients with pathologically elevated pre-operative AFP who are treated with radical orchiectomy for presumed YST. In post-pubertal patients, radical orchiectomy is the standard initial treatment. TSS in post-pubertal males is controversial and typically implemented in specialized circumstances (bilateral tumors, tumors in solitary testicle, when a benign tumor suspected, etc.). Pre-operatively, trans-scrotal biopsy is contraindicated and automatically portends stage II disease in the COG staging system. It also changes the lymphatic drainage of the testicle and can alter spread of disease, which usually occurs in a very predictable step-wise fashion. Histologic classification of prepubertal testes tumors, their incidence, histopathologic, and clinical characteristics are outlined in Table 19.5 [8, 10, 11].

Table 19.5 Histologic classification, incidence, and clinicopathologic characteristics of pediatric testis tumors

	Incidence	Pathologic characteristics	Clinical characteristics	Treatment	Surveillance
GCTs					
YST	• 15–62% • Most common malignant prepubertal tumor • Median age 1–2 years	• Schiller-Duval bodies are pathognomonic (papillary fibrovascular core lined by cuboidal or columnar cells) • May contain AFP, characterized as pink hyaline globules	• AFP elevated in 90% • 85% present as clinical stage I • Hematogenous spread (lung 20% of cases)	• Radical orchiectomy with stage-specific adjuvant therapy • Stage I: Observation • Recurrence of stage II–IV: Platinum-based chemotherapy • RPLND reserved only for residual RP mass or elevated AFP after surgery and chemotherapy	• AFP monthly, chest X-ray every 2 months, CT every 2–3 months for 2 years • After 2 years, increase surveillance interval
Teratoma	• 23–48% • Median age 1 year	• Composed of tissue from all 3 embryological germ cell layers • Lack cytological atypia and extensive mitoses	• Little or no AFP (<100 ng/ml) • Uniformly benign in prepubertal (in contrast to adults)	• TSS for prepubertal males • Radical orchiectomy for postpubertal males	• Pre-pubertal: No surveillance after TSS • Post-pubertal: Radical orchiectomy with surveillance protocols similar to adults
Epidermoid cyst	• 3–15%	• Cysts lined with keratin-producing epithelium	• Classic "onion skin" appearance on US • Normal AFP	• TSS	• No surveillance required
Seminoma	• Up to 10%			• Follow adult protocols	
Gonadal stromal tumors					
Juvenile Granulosa cell tumor	• 3–5% • Most common testicular tumor affecting neonates	• Granulosa-like cells lining cystic spaces with solid, nodular areas	• Associated with Y chromosome mutations and ambiguous genitalia • Benign	• TSS	• No surveillance required

Table 19.5 (continued)

	Incidence	Pathologic characteristics	Clinical characteristics	Treatment	Surveillance
Leydig cell	• 1–4% • Mean age 7 years	• Layers of polygonal cells • 40% contain Reinke crystals	• Associated with precocious puberty • Elevated testosterone and 17-ketosteroids, low gonadotropins • Benign	• TSS	• Virilization may persists despite testosterone normalization after excision
Sertoli cell	• 3% • Median age 6 months	• Well circumscribed, tan-gray • Contain hemorrhagic cysts	• 10% are hormonally active (virilization or feminization) • Mostly benign, malignant lesions limited to case reports	• TSS vs. radical orchiectomy • Full staging warranted if: Patient >5 years of age, tumor >5 cm, vascular invasion, necrosis, cellular atypia, high mitotic rate	
Other primary or secondary lesions					
Gonadoblastoma	• 1%	• Large germ cells with mesenchymal and stromal elements	• May occur bilaterally • Associated with DSD • Primarily in phenotypic female (46XY) with intraabdominal testis • Benign in neonatal period	• Radical orchiectomy	• 50% may undergo malignant transformation into dysgerminoma
Leukemia/ lymphoma	• 2–5% • Most common metastatic lesion to testes		• Represent majority of bilateral tumors • Testicular involvement portends poor prognosis • Testes are second-most common site for extramedullary leukemic relapse	• TSS if primary mass • If history of leukemia, open wedge biopsies through scrotal approach to establish diagnosis, followed by systemic treatment	

Staging of the primary tumor is completed with histologic evaluation of the completely excised tumor through an inguinal approach (Table 19.6). Pubertal status is critical in staging and treatment algorithms for pediatric testes tumors. Prepubertal boys are staged and treated using COG protocols (Table 19.7) while post-pubertal boys, adolescents and adults are more often staged and risk stratified per the adult AJCC TNMS and International Germ Cell Cancer Collaborative Group risk stratification systems (Tables 19.7 and 19.8) and therapeutic strategies commonly are derived from the adult National Comprehensive Cancer Network (NCCN) guidelines. Traditionally, application of pediatric chemotherapeutic regimens to older children has resulted in undertreatment and may have contributed to historically poorer outcomes in adolescents compared to prepubertal males [11]. Patients with localized disease that is completely resected with radical orchiectomy are typically managed with surveillance. High risk clinicopathologic features should not result in deviation from initial conservative management, as survival rates with salvage treatment are excellent and there is considerable morbidity associated with overtreatment and cumulative chemotherapeutic toxicity [11]. Chemotherapy is usually first-line in patients with metastatic disease, with radiotherapy reserved for seminoma. Retroperitoneal lymph node dissection plays a minor role in prepubertal tumors.

Population-based studies have suggested that teratoma is the most common benign and YST is the most common malignant testis tumor in a prepubertal boy, but discrepancy exists between the two in terms of which is truly the most prevalent [8, 10]. Up to 75% of prepubertal testis tumors in several series are benign. In a recent National Cancer Data Base study, nearly 10% of reported masses were seminomatous GCTs in patients <12 years of age, and in the absence of formal recommendations for prepubertal seminoma, it seems reasonable to apply adult treatment algorithms [9]. Leukemia and lymphoma are the most common metastatic lesions to the testes and, along with gonadoblastoma, should be considered with bilateral testicular lesions. Paratesticular tumors, including benign (leiomyoma, fibroma, lipoma, cystadenoma, adenomatoid hemangioma) as well as malignant (leiomyosarcoma, fibrosarcoma, liposarcoma, RMS) histologies are often managed similarly to intratesticular lesions, with complete excision via radical orchiectomy followed by histology-driven staging and treatment.

19.2.4 Prognosis and Surveillance

Malignant prepubertal tumors tend to be less aggressive than their post-pubertal counterparts. Prepubertal mature teratoma is typically localized and rarely metastasizes, with immature components conferring more malignant potential. Over 70% of prepubertal children with YST present with clinically localized disease, but approximately 20% experience relapse. Intratubular germ cell neoplasia (ITGCN) is a precursor of malignant germ cell tumors in adults, and it has been linked to pospubertal tumors but not prepubertal ones. Embryonal carcinoma is the most common pediatric postpubertal histology and commonly presents with metastasis at the time of diagnosis [8].

Table 19.6 American joint committee on cancer (AJCC) TNM staging system for testes cancer (seventh ed., 2010)

Stage	Extent of disease
Primary tumor (pT)	
pTX	Primary tumor cannot be assessed
pT0	No evidence of primary tumor
pTis	Intratubular germ cell neoplasia (ITGCN)
pT1	Tumor limited to testis and epididymis without lymphovascular invasion; tumor may invade into the tunica albuginea but not the tunica vaginalis
pT2	Tumor limited to the testis and epididymis with lymphovascular invasion or with involvement of the tunica vaginalis
pT3	Tumor invades the spermatic cord
pT4	Tumor invades the scrotum
Regional lymph nodes (N) clinical	
NX	Regional lymph nodes cannot be assessed
N0	No regional lymph node metastasis
N1	Metastasis with a lymph node mass 2 cm or less in greatest dimension and ≤5 nodes positive, none more than 2 cm
N2	Metastasis with a lymph node mass greater than 2 cm but not more than 5 cm in greatest dimension; or >5 nodes positive, none more than 5 cm; or evidence of extranodal extension
N3	Metastasis with a lymph node measuring >5 cm in greatest dimension
Distant metastasis (M)	
M0	No distal metastasis
M1a	Nonregional nodal or pulmonary metastasis
M1b	Distant metastasis other than M1a
Serum tumor markers (S)	
S1	AFP < 1000 ng/ml hCG < 5000 IU/l LDH < 1.5 times normal
S2	AFP 1000–10,000 ng/m hCG 5000–50,000 IU/l LDH 1.5–10 times normal
S3	AFP > 10,000 ng/ml hCG > 50,000 IU/l LDH > 10 times normal

Benign tumors are associated with a 100% survival with no reported cases of recurrence or metastasis. Malignant prepubertal tumors are associated with a 5 year overall survival between 94 and 100% [10]. There appears to be no difference in survival based upon surgical procedure (radical vs. partial orchiectomy) in any of the histologic subtypes, so long as the tumor is completely excised [9]. Prepubertal stromal tumors treated with TSS exhibit a local recurrence rate of just 3% and can be salvaged with completion radical orchiectomy. Patients with a diagnosis of malignant testicular tumor require lifelong follow-up consisting of imaging of the retroperitoneum, lungs, and physical examination of the contralateral testis (Table 19.5). The considerable late effects of chemotherapy and radiotherapy are

Table 19.7 Comparison of COG and AJCC staging systems for testicular tumors

Stage	AJCC	COG
I	pT1–4 N0 M0 S0 IA: pT1 N0 M0 S0 IB: pT2–4 N0 M0 S0 IS: pT1–4 N0 M0 S1–3	Tumor limited to testis completely resected by high inguinal orchiectomy No evidence of disease beyond testis STM negative after appropriate half-life decline If retroperitoneal LN >2 cm on imaging and normal/unknown STM, must have negative ipsilateral RPLN sampling
II	pT1–4 N1–3 M0 S0–1 IIA: pT1–4 N1 M0 S0–1 IIB: pT1–4 N2 M0 S0–1 IIC: pT1–4 N3 M0 S0–1	Microscopic residual disease present in scrotum or spermatic cord STM remain elevated after appropriate half-life interval Tumor rupture or scrotal biopsy prior to orchiectomy
III	pT1–4 N1–3 M1 S0–1 IIA: pT1–4 N1–3 M1A S0–1 IIB: pT1–4 N1–3 M0–1B S2 IIC: pT1–4 N1–3 M0–1B S3	RPLN involvement LN >4 cm by CT are considered metastases (biopsy-confirmation needed for LN > 2 cm and <4 cm)
IV		Distant metastasis

Adapted from Saltzman and Cost, 2018

Table 19.8 International Germ Cell Consensus Classification scheme for the assignment of prognostic category in patients with metastatic GCTs

Prognostic category	Nonseminoma	Seminoma
Good risk	• Testicular or primary retroperitoneal tumor • Absence of extrapulmonary visceral metastases • Low STM (TNMS stage S1)	• Any primary site • Any STM • Absence of extrapulmonary visceral metastases
Intermediate risk	• Testicular or primary retroperitoneal tumor • Absence of extrapulmonary visceral metastases • Intermediate STM (TNMS stage S2)	• Any primary site • Any STM Presence of extrapulmonary visceral metastases
Poor risk	• Testicular, primary retroperitoneal, or primary mediastinal tumor • Presence of extrapulmonary visceral metastases • High STM (TNMS stage S3)	None

increasingly evident with improved clinical outcomes. In addition to an increased risk of infertility, secondary malignancy, and psychosocial effects, cisplatin-based regimens are associated with nephrotoxicity (10% risk of stage III CKD), peripheral neuropathy (17%) and hearing loss (20–40%). Bleomycin has been associated with a 5% risk of developing pulmonary fibrosis, which is more common in older patients.

19.3 Part 3: Rhabdomyosarcoma

19.3.1 Introduction

Rhabdomyosarcoma (RMS) is a malignant soft tissue tumor of mesenchymal origin. Approximately 350 cases of RMS are diagnosed in the United States annually, making it the third most common solid tumor diagnosed in children. Up to 25% of cases arise in the genitourinary tract [12]. The incidence of RMS exhibits male predominance and a bimodal age distribution, commonly diagnosed from ages <2 years and again from 10 to 18 years [13]. While the bladder and prostate are commonly involved sites and both portend an unfavorable prognosis, RMS involvement of the testes (paratesticular masses), vagina, cervix, uterus and retroperitoneum are associated with a favorable prognosis (Table 19.9) [14].

The majority of genitourinary RMS is associated with a genetic mutation, with several well described predisposing conditions. These include Li-Fraumeni syndrome, pleuropulmonary blastoma, neurofibromatosis type I, Costello syndrome, Beckwith-Wiedemann syndrome, Noonan syndrome, multiple endocrine neoplasia type 2A (MEN 2A), and Gorlin syndrome (Table 19.10) [14].

19.3.2 Diagnosis and Evaluation

Genitourinary RMS typically presents with a palpable mass or symptoms related to mass effect, including upper urinary tract obstruction, urinary retention, vaginal bleeding, hematuria and irritative voiding symptoms [14]. Tumors are commonly localized at presentation. Nodal metastases are uncommon and typically involve pelvic and retroperitoneal lymph nodes. Paratesticular tumors commonly present as painless scrotal masses, and workup is similar to that of a primary testicular tumor. Serum tumor markers are indicated with paratesticular masses, especially in cases when the origin of the primary tumor is uncertain. Initial workup should include a thorough history and physical examination. The initial imaging of choice is pelvic ultrasound, which can confirm the presence and origin of solid masses, followed by complete staging with contrasted CT or MRI of the chest, abdomen, and pelvis to determine resectability (Fig. 19.3).

Table 19.9 Prognostic factors for RMS

	Favorable prognosis	Unfavorable prognosis
Location	Retroperitoneum, vagina, cervix, uterus, paratestis	Prostate and bladder
Age	1–9 years	<1 or ≥10 years
Histology	Embryonal (with variants)	Alveolar
Genetic alterations	None	Translocation of PAX3/PAX2 to FOXO1

Table 19.10 Genetic syndromes associated with pediatric RMS

Genetic predisposition syndrome (mode of transmission)	Mutated gene	Associated conditions	Cumulative incidence of RMS
Li-Fraumeni syndrome (AD)	*P53*	Sarcomas Breast cancer Brain tumors Adrenal carcinoma Leukemia	15–20%
Pleuropulmonary bastoma	*DICER1*	Carcinoid tumors Gonadal germ cell and stromal tumors Thyroid carcinomas Benign eye and nasal tumors	Unknown
Neurofibromatosis type I (AD)	*NF1*	Musculoskeletal disorders Neurofibromas Mental retardation Café au lait spots Lisch nodules of iris	10% (bladder/prostate predominance)
Costello syndrome (AD)	*HRAS*	Mental retardation Unusual facial features Heart abnormalities Short stature	7%
Beckwith-Wiedemann syndrome (variable)	*11p15*	Overgrowth features Abdominal wall defects Wilms tumor Hepatoblastoma Neuroblastoma	Unknown
Noonan syndrome (AD)	*PTPN11*	Facial abnormalities Short stature Cardiac abnormalities	Unknown
Multiple endocrine neoplasia (MEN) type 2A (AD)		Medullar thyroid carcinoma Pheochromocytoma Hyperparathyroidism	Unknown
Gorlin syndrome (nevoid-basal cell carcinoma syndrome; AD)	*PTCH*	Overgrowth features Skeletal abnormalities Benign and malignant tumors	Unknown

AD autosomal dominant

Definitive diagnosis is dependent on histologic evaluation. In cases of paratesticular tumors, a radical orchiectomy is indicated. While biopsy is contraindicated in testicular and paratesticular masses, endoscopic tissue sampling from other genitourinary organs may allow for diagnosis. It is often difficult to determine the site of origin, particularly in locally invasive masses. If adequate diagnostic tissue cannot be obtained endoscopically, it has been recommended that open transvesical biopsy with pelvic and para-aortic lymph node sampling (for staging) be performed. A portion of the biopsy should be reserved for genetic testing and not exposed to

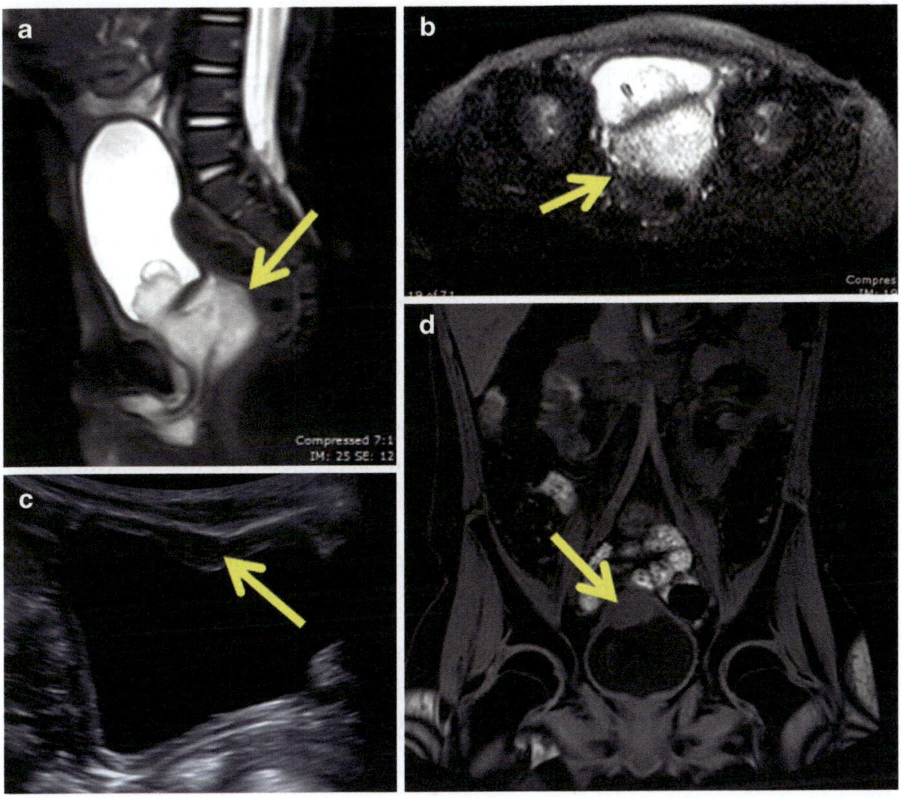

Fig. 19.3 Multiple rhabdomyosarcomas. T2-weighted MRI (A-sagital, B-axial) of a primary prostatic RMS extending posteriorly and into the bladder lumen. Primary bladder RMS depicting a large mass at the bladder dome (C-ultrasound, D-T1 MRI coronal section). (**a**) T2 weighted MRI, saggital, primary prostatic RMS extending posteriorly and into the bladder lumen (arrow). (**b**) T2 weighted MRI, axial, primary prostatic RMS extending posteriorly and into the bladder lumen (arrow). (**c**) US showing primary bladder RMS with lesion at dome (arrow). (**d**) MRI, coronal, primary bladder RMS with mass at bladder dome (arrow)

processing or preservatives. Prompt drainage of urinary tract obstruction is prudent to preserve renal function in anticipation of nephrotoxic adjuvant chemotherapy, if indicated. Percutaneous approaches to drainage (suprapubic catheter or nephrostomy tube placement) are discouraged.

The Intergroup Rhabdomyosarcoma Study Group (IRSG) recognizes two histologic subtypes of RMS: embryonal and alveolar [13]. Embryonal RMS is the most common form to involve the bladder and its incidence accounts for up to 90% of genitourinary cases [14]. Embryonal RMS is further subdivided into sarcoma botryoides (vagina) and spindle cell tumors which commonly involve hollow viscus organs (uterus, cervix, bladder) and paratesticular regions, respectively. Botryoid tumors have a characteristic polypoid appearance described as a "bunch of grapes." While botryoid RMS predominates in early childhood, alveolar RMS is most common in adolescents [13].

19.3.3 Treatment

Similar to advances in WT, protocol-driven multimodal treatment modalities have improved outcomes for RMS. Current COG recommendations will be outlined in this chapter. Recent focus has prioritized organ-preserving surgical approaches to limit morbidity from radical extirpative procedures, which historically, were associated with only modest outcomes [13].

Staging for RMS is complex and multifactorial, incorporating pre-operative COG soft tissue sarcoma committee (COG-STS) TNM classification, post-operative or post-biopsy clinical group designation (remaining tumor burden), as well as patient age and histologic subtype (Table 19.11). These designations culminate into a risk stratification system to guide subsequent treatment: low (localized disease), intermediate, and high risk (metastatic disease) (Table 19.12). The majority of bladder or prostate RMS are unresectable at initial presentation (at least intermediate risk). After adequate tissue sampling and diagnosis, patients are treated with appropriate risk-stratified definitive chemoradiation (Table 19.12). Upfront, complete surgical resection is the preferred local control strategy, however with many tumors and sites this is both impossible and considered to be overly mutilating. In situations where an entire tumor can be resected after biopsy but prior to chemotherapy initiation (common with paratestis or vagina, also possible with portions of bladder), complete excision is prudent to potentially avoid subsequent radiation for local control. While radiation is part of COG protocols as a local control strategy after chemotherapy, Europe utilizes surgery more often and there is continuous debate as to the best vs. least morbid local control strategy [15].

Radical cystectomy/cystoprostatectomy (anterior exenteration) with urinary diversion (e.g. neobladder, continent urinary diversion, or ileal/colon conduit) is typically reserved for patients who have persistent, biopsy-proven disease after chemotherapy and radiation. Notably, a persistent mass does not always represent

Table 19.11 TNM staging and clinical group designation for RMS

Pre-operative COG soft tissue sarcoma committee (COG-STS) TNM clinical staging	
Stage I	Favorable site, non-metastatic
Stage II	Unfavorable site, <5 cm, negative nodes, nonmetastatic
Stage III	Unfavorable site, >5 cm or positive nodes, nonmetastatic
Stage IV	Any site, metastatic
Intergroup rhabdomyosarcoma study (IRS) post-operative clinical group designation	
Group I	Localized disease, completely resected
Group II	(IIA) grossly resected tumor with microscopic residual disease; (IIB) regional disease with involved nodes, completely resected with no microscopic residual disease; (IIC) regional disease with involved nodes, grossly resected, but with evidence of microscopic residual and/or histologic involvement of the most distal regional node in the dissection
Group III	Incomplete resection or biopsy with gross residual mass
Group IV	Distant metastasis

Favorable site: GU sites *other than* bladder and prostate; Unfavorable site: GU sites *except* bladder and prostate

Table 19.12 Risk group stratification guiding treatment strategies for RMS

Risk group	Histology	Clinical group	Stage	Age	Treatment
Low	Embryonal with variants	I, II, III	I	All	VA or VAC (concomitant radiotherapy if residual disease)
	Embryonal with variants	I, II	II, III	All	
Intermediate	Embryonal with variants	III	II, III	All	VAC with radiotherapy
	Embryonal with variants	IV	IV	<10 years	
	Alveolar	I, II, III	I, II, III	All	
High	Embryonal with variants	IV	IV	≥10 years	Intensive regimen with VAC backbone
	Alveolar	IV	IV	All	

RMS risk stratification and treatment options, *V* vincristine, *A* Actinomycin D, *C* cyclophosphamide

viable tumor and close histologic evaluation should guide salvage therapy. While bladder preservation is possible in up to 40%, long term morbidity from limited bladder capacity and chemoradiation toxicity can be significant.

Non bladder/prostate genitourinary RMS is managed with biopsy/complete resection, followed by risk-stratified primary chemotherapy and radiotherapy, if indicated. Radiotherapy can be omitted in patients with embryonal histology and localized disease that is completely resected prior to chemotherapy initiation. Patients with paratesticular RMS are managed with radical inguinal orchiectomy. Because >40% of patients with paratesticular RMS present with metastatic disease primarily to the retroperitoneum, particularly in old children, all children ≥10 years of age with paratesticular RMS should undergo ipsilateral retroperitoneal lymph node dissection as they are often understaged by cross-sectional imaging [13].

19.3.4 Prognosis

The complexity of RMS group and stage classifications offer tailored treatment strategies and are highly prognostic. Histologic predictors of adverse clinical outcomes include local tumor invasion, tumor size, and histologic subtype. The 5-year failure-free survival for patients with localized tumors (low-risk) is approximately 75% with overall survival approaching 97% [12]. Intermediate-risk tumors historically confer up to 88% overall survival, while children in the high-risk group (metastatic disease) have poor prognosis with 5 year survival <50%. Age is an independent predictor of prognosis, with age <1 and >10 years significantly worse failure-free survival (Table 19.9) [13].

The discovery of oncogene fusions resulting from chromosomal translocation offers promising prognostic potential. Beyond histologic classification, RMS tumors can be subgrouped into fusion positive or fusion negative based on the presence of balanced translocations between *PAX3* (chromosome 2) or *PAX7* (chromosome 1) with *FOXO1* (chromosome 13). These oncogenes confer an aggressive phenotype and are evident in about 80% of alveolar RMS (Table 19.9). Recent studies suggest inferior oncologic outcomes in fusion positive patients, and it likely this classification will be incorporated into future risk group stratification [16].

Late effects of aggressive treatment strategies include bladder dysfunction as well as significant reproductive and sexual dysfunction [13]. With pelvic radiation to growing bones specifically, there is halt of pelvic growth resulting in disproportionate size and function for patients. Additionally, longitudinal studies suggest that survivors of pelvic RMS develop secondary malignancy at a rate six-times higher than normal children [17] and long-term surveillance in survivorship clinics has been recommended. Advances in proton therapy have resulted in more targeted therapy at lower maximum doses, resulting in decreased toxicity to surrounding tissues, but routine use has not yet been fully studied [15] (Fig. 19.3).

19.4 Part 4: Bladder Tumors

19.4.1 Urothelial Cell Carcinoma

19.4.1.1 Introduction

Urothelial cell carcinoma (UC) of the bladder is an uncommon pediatric malignancy. In a recent literature review and case series, there are <150 cases of UC of the bladder diagnosed in patients <20 years of age, with only 20 cases reported in children <10 years [18]. While several well-defined factors strongly predispose adults to UC, including smoking and environmental exposures, the etiology in children is less clear and the genetic and epigenetic changes regulating tumorigenesis in adults and children are different.

UC in children is typically low grade and low stage with infrequent recurrence [19]. Less than 7 cases of high grade UC have been reported in children <18 years [20]. Median age at diagnosis is around 12 years of age, with tumors in children <12 more likely representing bladder RMS.

19.4.1.2 Diagnosis and Evaluation

The most common presenting symptoms is hematuria. Unlike adults who are managed with a high index of suspicion and rigorous hematuria protocols, diagnosis if often delayed in children [18, 19]. Evaluation starts with a thorough history and physical exam, urinalysis, urine culture and renal and bladder ultrasound. Ultrasonography is highly sensitive in detecting bladder tumors in children as small as 5 mm (Fig. 19.4) [20, 21]. Cystoscopy is warranted for persistent symptoms and lack of identifiable cause of hematuria.

Tumors are typically solitary and roughly 75% are at the trigone [18, 20, 21]. No further staging imaging is indicated at the time of initial diagnosis. Nearly 75% of bladder UC in children is non-invasive or minimally invasive at index resection.

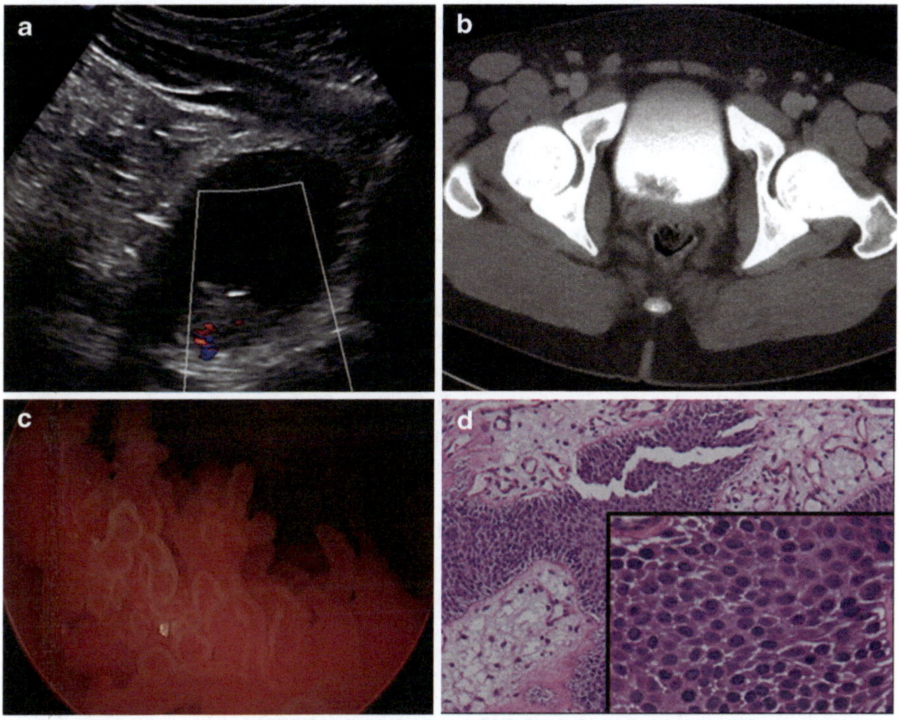

Fig. 19.4 Urothelial carcinoma in 15 year-old male who presented with painless gross hematuria. (**a**) Bladder ultrasonography revealed a 2.0 cm posterior wall bladder mass with internal blood flow. (**b**) Axial section from hematuria protocol CT confirming filling defect in posterior bladder wall. (**c**) Classic papillary appearance of posterior trigone tumor. (**d**) Histology section exhibiting low grade, non-invasive urothelial carcinoma (H&E section 200× magnification, insert 1000×)

19.4.1.3 Treatment and Surveillance

Complete visible transurethral resection is both diagnostic and therapeutic. There is no defined role for peri-operative or adjuvant intravesical therapy. Pathologic distinction of grade and depth of invasion is imperative, with stage and grading systems identical to that of adult UC of the bladder (Tables 19.13 and 19.14). Muscularis propria evaluation is mandatory to determine depth of invasion, and repeat resection is indicated in its absence from the initial specimen. No additional therapy beyond initial, complete resection is typically indicated. Repeat resection is performed with high grade or invasive lesions.

The 5-year survival rate for pediatric UC of the bladder is 98%. Deaths from high grade, muscle invasive disease are limited to a few case reports [19]. While recurrence rates in adults approach 70%, the recurrence rate for low grade Ta or PUNLMP lesions in children ranges from 14 to 60% in several studies [18]. Recurrences are commonly papilloma or PUNLMP, both of which have no metastatic potential.

Because of low recurrence rates in children, there are no guidelines regarding routine surveillance cystoscopy or imaging. Additionally, there are no definitive recommendations on upper tract surveillance as contrasted studies (pyelograms or CT) expose patients to radiation. Cytology also has a limited role in children with sensitivity <40% in low grade lesions [18]. Surveillance protocols should be guided by tumor stage and grade at the discretion of the treating urologist, and one may employ non-invasive strategies including ultrasonography.

19.4.2 Non-Urothelial Bladder Tumors

Longitudinal studies suggesting an increased risk of bladder malignancy in patients with history of bladder augmentation led to the general recommendation for annual endoscopic screening beginning 5–10 years after reconstruction. In one study of 153 patients, 7 developed cancer at a median time of 32 years from reconstruction. However, more recent reports suggest that it is the congenitally abnormal bladder itself, not the augmentation, that portends an increased risk of bladder cancer, and that perhaps augmentation is even protective [23]. Patients at greatest risk were those with history of tobacco abuse, end-stage renal disease, transplantation, or immunosuppression [24]. Given the low incidence of findings and relative invasiveness of surveillance cystoscopy, recent recommendations suggest that endoscopy of the augmented bladder should be limited to the following criteria: ≥4 symptomatic urinary tract infections per year, history of gross hematuria, chronic pain, abnormal radiographic studies, or patients 50 years of age with colon augmentations (consistent with current colonoscopy screening recommendations).

Table 19.13 World Health Organization classification of bladder tumors (2016)

WHO grading system for urothelial lesions of the bladder	
Non-invasive urothelial tumors	Urothelial carcinoma *in situ* (CIS) Papillary urothelial carcinoma, low grade Papillary urothelial carcinoma, high grade Papillary urothelial neoplasm of low malignant potential (PUNLMP) Urothelial papilloma Inverted urothelial papilloma Urothelial proliferation of uncertain malignant potential (hyperplasia) Urothelial dysplasia
Invasive urothelial tumors	Infiltrating urothelial carcinoma with divergent differentiation Nested Microcystic Micropapillary Lymphoepithelioma-lika Plasmacytoid Giant cell Poorly differentiated Lipid rich Clear cell tumors of Mullerian type Tumors arising in a bladder diverticulum

Table 19.14 American joint committee on cancer (AJCC) TNM Staging for urothelial carcinoma of the bladder (seventh Edition)

Primary tumor (pT)	
T0	Primary tumor cannot be assessed
T0	No evidence of primary tumor
Ta	Noninvasive papillary carcinoma
Tis	Carcinoma *in situ*
T1	Tumor invades subepithelial connective tissue
T2a	Tumor invades superficial muscularis propria (inner half)
T2b	Tumor invade deep muscularis propria (outer half)
T3a	Tumor invades perivesical tissue (microscopic)
T3b	Tumor invades perivesical tissue (macroscopic)
T4a	Tumor invades prostate, uterus, vagina
T4b	Tumor invades pelvic wall, abdominal wall
Nodal stage	
NX	Lymph nodes cannot be assessed
N0	No lymph node metastasis
N1	Single regional lymph node metastasis in true pelvis
N2	Multiple regional lymph node metastases in true pelvis
N3	Lymph node metastasis to common iliac lymph nodes
Metastasis stage	
M0	No distant metastases
M1	Distant metastases
Stage groupings	
Stage I	T1 N0 M0
Stage II	T2a/T2b N0 M0
Stage III	T3a/T3b/T4a N0 M0
Stage IV	T4b or N1–3 or M1

Adapted from Humphrey 2016 [22]

Primary non-urothelial bladder malignancies are uncommon in children. Patients with history of bladder exstrophy are at increased risk of primary bladder adenocarcinoma and squamous cell carcinoma. Primary bladder squamous cell carcinoma and urachal adenocarcinoma are exceedingly rare in children, limited to few case reports.

Benign bladder tumors are also uncommon, and their histologic distinction has important treatment and prognosis implications. Inflammatory myofibroblastic tumor (IMT) is a spindle cell tumor with myofibroblastic differentiation. IMT associated with specific genetic rearrangements have a high risk of recurrence and metastasis, but those without these alterations can be treated with a combination of NSAIDS and/or surgical excision. Bladder hemangiomas are vascular lesions which often present with gross hematuria and are indistinguishable from malignant lesions endoscopically. Treatments for hemangiomas include partial cystectomy and laser ablation. Nephrogenic adenoma is a benign papillary lesion of the bladder, commonly associated with prior bladder surgery, injury or recurrent infections. They are histologically characterized by papillary arrangement of cuboidal cells. Treatment focuses on limiting inflammatory stimuli, transurethral resection, or fulguration. Recurrence is common and follow up is warranted.

References

Kidney Tumors

1. Dénes FT, Duarte RJ, Cristófani LM, Lopes RI. Pediatric genitourinary oncology. Front Pediatr. 2013;1:48.
2. Saltzman AF, Cost NG. AUA update: childhood kidney tumors. 2018.
3. Craft AW, Parker L, Stiller C, Cole M. Screening for Wilms' tumour in patients with aniridia, Beckwith syndrome, or hemihypertrophy. Med Pediatr Oncol. 1995;24(4):231–4.
4. Saltzman AF, Carrasco A, Weinman J, Meyers ML, Cost NG. Initial imaging for pediatric renal tumors: an opportunity for improvement. J Urol. 2018;199(5):1330–6.
5. Geller JI, Ehrlich PF, Cost NG, Khanna G, Mullen EA, Gratias EJ, et al. Characterization of adolescent and pediatric renal cell carcinoma: a report from the Children's oncology group study AREN03B2. Cancer. 2015;121(14):2457–64.
6. Rialon KL, Gulack BC, Englum BR, Routh JC, Rice HE. Factors impacting survival in children with renal cell carcinoma. J Pediatr Surg. 2015;50(6):1014–8.
7. Seibel NL, Li S, Breslow NE, Beckwith JB, Green DM, Haase GM, et al. Effect of duration of treatment on treatment outcome for patients with clear-cell sarcoma of the kidney: a report from the National Wilms' tumor study group. J Clin Oncol. 2004;22(3):468–73.

Testes Tumors

8. Agarwal PK, Palmer JS. Testicular and paratesticular neoplasms in prepubertal males. J Urol. 2006;176(3):875–81.
9. Maizlin II, Dellinger M, Gow KW, Goldin AB, Goldfarb M, Nuchtern JG, et al. Testicular tumors in prepubescent patients. J Pediatr Surg. 2017;53(9):1748–52.
10. Ross JH, Rybicki L, Kay R. Clinical behavior and a contemporary management algorithm for prepubertal testis tumors: a summary of the Prepubertal testis tumor registry. J Urol. 2002;168(4 Pt 2):1675–8; discussion 1678–1679.
11. Saltzman AF, Cost NG. Adolescent and young adult testicular germ cell tumors: special considerations. Adv Urol. 2018;2018:2375176.

Rhabdomyosarcoma

12. Rodeberg DA, Anderson JR, Arndt CA, Ferrer FA, Raney RB, Jenney ME, et al. Comparison of outcomes based on treatment algorithms for rhabdomyosarcoma of the bladder/prostate: combined results from the Children's oncology group, German cooperative soft tissue sarcoma

study, Italian cooperative group, and International Society of Pediatric Oncology Malignant Mesenchymal Tumors Committee. Int J Cancer. 2011;128(5):1232–9.
13. Caldwell BT, Wilcox DT, Cost NG. Current Management for Pediatric Urologic Oncology. Adv Pediatr Infect Dis. 2017;64(1):191–223.
14. Kieran K, Shnorhavorian M. Current standards of care in bladder and prostate rhabdomyosarcoma. Urol Oncol. 2016;34(2):93–102.
15. Saltzman AF, Cost NG. Current treatment of pediatric bladder and prostate Rhabdomyosarcoma. Curr Urol Rep. 2018;19(1):11.
16. Skapek SX, Anderson J, Barr FG, Bridge JA, Gastier-Foster JM, Parham DM, et al. PAX-FOXO1 fusion status drives unfavorable outcome for children with rhabdomyosarcoma: a children's oncology group report. Pediatr Blood Cancer. 2013;60(9):1411–7.
17. Cohen RJ, Curtis RE, Inskip PD, Fraumeni JF. The risk of developing second cancers among survivors of childhood soft tissue sarcoma. Cancer. 2005;103(11):2391–6.

Bladder Tumors

18. Lerena J, Krauel L, García-Aparicio L, Vallasciani S, Suñol M, Rodó J. Transitional cell carcinoma of the bladder in children and adolescents: six-case series and review of the literature. J Pediatr Urol. 2010;6(5):481–5.
19. Paner GP, Zehnder P, Amin AM, Husain AN, Desai MM. Urothelial neoplasms of the urinary bladder occurring in young adult and pediatric patients: a comprehensive review of literature with implications for patient management. Adv Anat Pathol. 2011;18(1):79–89.
20. Berrettini A, Castagnetti M, Salerno A, Nappo SG, Manzoni G, Rigamonti W, et al. Bladder urothelial neoplasms in pediatric age: experience at three tertiary centers. J Pediatr Urol. 2015;11(1):26.e1–5.
21. Aguiar L, Danialan R, Kim C. A case of high-grade transitional cell carcinoma of the bladder in a pediatric patient with turner syndrome. Urology. 2015;85(6):1477–9.
22. Humphrey PA, Moch H, Cubilla AL, Ulbright TM, Reuter VE. The 2016 WHO classification of Tumours of the urinary system and male genital organs-part B: prostate and bladder Tumours. Eur Urol. 2016;70(1):106–19.
23. Rove KO, Husmann DA, Wilcox DT, Vricella GJ, Higuchi TT. Systematic review of bladder cancer outcomes in patients with spina bifida. J Pediatr Urol. 2017;13(5):456.e1–9.
24. Husmann DA, Rathbun SR. Long-term follow up of enteric bladder augmentations: the risk for malignancy. J Pediatr Urol. 2008;4(5):381–5; discussion 386.

Pediatric Urologic Trauma

20

Carter Boyd, Elena Gibson, and Pankaj P. Dangle

Learning Objectives

- Identify high grade renal injuries that potentially may need other surgical interventions.
- Proper imaging to grade the genitourinary trauma to prevent potential complications.
- Identify key elements of clinical and radiological findings to direct the treatment.
- Avoid immediate urethral surgery in posterior urethral distraction defect to prevent complications.
- Proper use of surgical instruments to prevent devastating complications such as circumcision.

20.1 Introduction

The following is a review of pertinent clinical information and surgical managements regarding pediatric urologic trauma. We review each of the organs of urologic trauma by presenting a case scenario, followed by several questions. There is a brief review after the questions addressing the answers and other relevant information in reference to the case or injury presented.

Genitourinary trauma is second only to central nervous system trauma in pediatric patient at an estimated rate of 3–10%. Most of these injuries are associated with other organ injuries; Death is uncommon following genitourinary trauma, though if

C. Boyd · E. Gibson
University of Alabama-Birmingham School of Medicine, Birmingham, AL, USA

P. P. Dangle (✉)
Department of Urology, University of Alabama-Birmingham, Birmingham, AL, USA

Pediatric Urology, Children's Hospital of Alabama, Birmingham, AL, USA
e-mail: Pankaj.Dangle@childrensal.org

P. Godbole et al. (eds.), *Practical Pediatric Urology*,
https://doi.org/10.1007/978-3-030-54020-3_20

missed delayed complications are more morbid and with complications. Herein we review each organ with pertinent clinical scenario, management (initial, intermediary and delayed) with supporting evidence of the current practice based on literature and guidelines.

20.2 Scenario 1

An 8-year-old healthy boy presented to the emergency department (ED) with unilateral flank pain after a fall from a treehouse 15 feet above the ground. The child had been resting with ice at home until he reported bright red urinary output to his mother who promptly brought him to the ED. Vital signs on admission are 98.6 °F, heart rate 79 beats per minute, respiratory rate 20 breaths per minute, and blood pressure 114/72. On physical exam, patient appears mildly distressed, left flank ecchymosis is visualized. Focused assessment with sonography in trauma (FAST) exam is unrevealing.

Question 1: What fact in this patient's presentation merits further radiological workup?

- A. Patient age
- **B. Fall from 15 feet or more**
- C. Hemodynamic stability
- D. Presence of gross hematuria
- E. Flank hematoma/ecchymosis

Triphasic CT with delayed imaging of abdomen and pelvis is ordered and image is below.

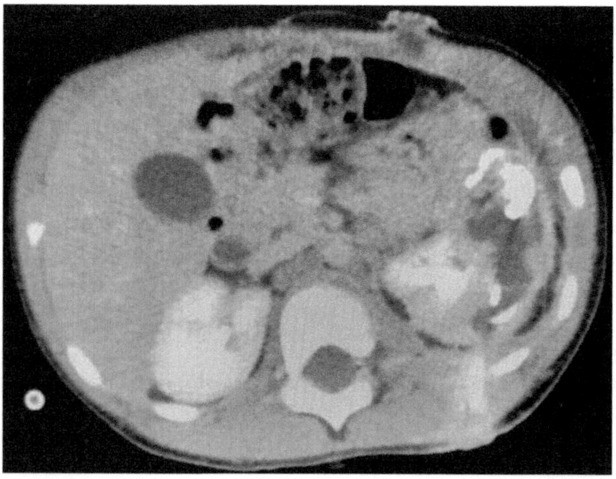

Patient is transported from the ED to the floor for conservative management. Patient is followed with serial hematocrit/hemoglobin and bed rest. Patient subsequently recovers and is discharged from the hospital. Two weeks later the patient presents again to the ED complaining of worsening flank pain and a distended abdomen. Vitals are now 101.2 °F, heart rate 94 beats per minute, respiratory rate 23 breaths per minute, and blood pressure 104/68. WBC is 7.2, hemoglobin is 12, and BMP is unremarkable.

Question 2: What is the most likely diagnosis?

- A. Sepsis
- **B. Urinoma**
- C. Renal Vein Thrombosis
- D. Retroperitoneal hematoma
- E. UTI

20.3 Discussion of Scenario 1

Pediatric renal trauma is most frequent site of urogenital trauma, the majority of which are secondary to blunt injury [1]. Children have been shown to be more susceptible to renal injury likely attributable to less protection from the pliable rib cage, lower positioning of the kidneys and a less developed abdominal wall and viscera for cushioning [2, 3].

The CT (Computed tomography) images shown demonstrate an example of Grade 4 Renal Trauma (AAST grading system). By definition, Grade 4 Renal Trauma involves a laceration which extends into the collecting system with evidence of urinary extravasation. Viability of the renal fragments is not considered in the definition. Grade 4 lesions also demonstrate injury to the principle renal vessels but demonstrate a confined hemorrhage. Grades 1–3 renal injuries are treated conservatively, whereas Grades 4–5 management depend more on the clinical picture.

While a conservative approach is the preferred initial modality for Grade 4–5 injury, however specific instances merit acute or subacute interventions. The goal of conservative management for renal trauma including high grade; has been demonstrated to avoid unnecessary surgery, decrease the rate of post-traumatic nephrectomies, and preserve renal function [4, 5]. Conservative management entails bed rest, continual hemodynamic assessment, serial hemoglobin monitoring, and prophylactic antibiotics.

Indications for imaging depend on the nature of the traumatic injury. All penetrating abdominal injuries merit advanced imaging workup most commonly accomplished with a triphasic CT scan of the abdomen and pelvis. Blunt abdominal trauma has relative indications for imaging which are similar in children and adults. Cases of gross hematuria require imaging as do cases presenting with microscopic hematuria (>50 RBC/hpf) in the context of low systolic blood pressures (<90 mm Hg) though AUA (American Urological Association) guidelines suggest that children typically do not present with hypovolemic shock [6]. Blunt abdominal trauma from high speed accidents, deceleration injuries, and falls from 10 feet or more also necessitate radiologic workup. Finally, traumatic injuries associated with ribs, spine, pelvic, or femur fractures pose high risk to the genitourinary tract and merit workup [6, 7].

With conservative management, it is essential to remain vigilant for potential complications that may develop. Urinary extravasation can lead to the development of a urinoma, with a classical triad of fever, worsening flank pain, and abdominal distension one to 2 weeks following the initial presentation. There is evidence to suggest that early stent placement may be merited in cases of blunt renal trauma that fail to demonstrate contrast material in the ipsilateral ureter. In cases where contrast is not visualized, these patients often go on to need stent placement and thus can be done prophylactically [8]. For diagnosis, repeat CT scan with delayed imaging is required, particularly to look for persistent urine extravasation. Treatment includes stenting or drainage [2, 8].

Patients requiring multiple blood transfusions are also a red flag and merit intervention either in the form of an open exploration or angioembolization [2]. Specific indications for endoscopic or angiographic intervention include hemodynamic instability, continued need for blood transfusions, persistent gross hematuria 72 h after initial presentation, non-resolving fever or ileus for greater than 72 h, or worsening flank pain.

Renal exploration has absolute indications. These include hemodynamic instability due to large volume renal bleeding, expanding or pulsatile retroperitoneal hematoma, in ability to stop persistent or delayed hemorrhage by selective vascular embolization. In each of these cases, the most frequent result is nephrectomy [6, 7].

Follow up should include blood pressure and urinalysis assessment at 6 and 12 weeks to assess for the development of hypertension and persistent microscopic hematuria. Grade 3 injuries and above merit follow-up with renal imaging 3 months after the trauma. For Grade 3 injuries that have viable fragments, ultrasound is sufficient. Grade 3 injuries with devitalized fragments, Grade 4, and Grade 5 injuries require either CT or MRI.

Special considerations for future activity should also be given to patients with renal trauma, particularly those who have a solitary kidney (either congenitally or secondary to a nephrectomy) or underlying renal malformation [9]. Special concern is given to children wanting to participate in contact sports as they are the third leading cause of renal trauma in the pediatric population [10].The American Association of Pediatrics states that children with only one kidney require special consideration for contact and collision sports, and in making their recommendations physicians should consider remaining kidney anatomy, position, and probable compliance with correct protective equipment [10, 11].

20.4 Scenario 2

A 12-year-old girl is brought to the nearest pediatric hospital following a pedestrian versus motor vehicle collision. Patient is stabilized in the trauma bay after initial Glasgow Coma Scale was 12. Imaging revealed lumbar vertebral ruptures at the L1–L3 levels, and CT nephrogram was normal though the ureters could not be visualized. Patient begins to complain of diffuse back and flank pain at this time. There is no evidence of gross or microscopic hematuria. Patient received proper neurologic and orthopedic surgical care 2 days after initial entry for vertebral injury and is recovering in the hospital.

On post-operative day 1 following back surgery, patient develops a fever peaking at 100.7 °F. No clear etiology is detected. On the subsequent day, the patient complains of worsening unilateral left sided flank pain and abdominal distention with fever spiking to 101.3 °F.

Question 1: What is the most appropriate next step?

- A. Blood culture followed by broad spectrum antibiotics
- B. Ultrasound
- C. Work for infection including Chest X-Ray, urine analysis
- D. Urgent exploration
- **E. Contrast CT Scan**

Repeat imaging is performed. The radiology report denotes changes consistent with post-operative orthopedic intervention in the lumbar region, inability to visualize the ureter on the left side, medial extravasation of contrast in the region of the left kidney. No other abnormalities are identified.

Question 2: What is the most likely diagnosis and next step in management?

- A. Grade 4 Renal Trauma
- B. Postoperative abscess
- **C. Ureteropelvic junction disruption**
- D. Obstructing ureteral calculi
- E. Ureteral stricture

20.5 Discussion

Ureteropelvic junction (UPJ) disruption is a rare complication of blunt abdominal trauma [12]. UPJ disruption most commonly occurs secondary to blunt abdominal trauma in deceleration injuries including falls from 10 feet or greater or due to pedestrian versus motor vehicles collisions creating excessive trunk hyperextension. These insults avulse or weaken the attachment of the ureter to the kidney [10, 13]. The most common injury is a complete avulsion of the UPJ where no attachment remains to the kidney. Partial UPJ disruptions are also possible and the management can be less invasive. Avulsion injuries necessitate surgical repair, while some incomplete UPJ disruptions can be managed with stenting [13].

UPJ disruption can be overlooked as it typically occurs in major trauma where there are other associated significant injuries warranting more timely attention [14]. Delay in diagnosis is reported to occur in more than 50% of patients and can be delayed more than 36 h [10]. Diagnosis may also be missed as hematuria is not always present to indicate a urologic workup [13]. Delays in diagnosis can occur for up to 12 weeks after the inciting trauma and have been demonstrated to increase the rate of nephrectomy [10, 15]. Thus, it is important to consider UPJ disruption as a diagnosis in pediatric blunt abdominal trauma [12].

When UPJ disruption is not actively pursued as a potential diagnosis, it is frequently discovered in the work up of other abnormalities with unclear etiology. Common symptoms precipitating work up and discovery of UPJ disruption include fever, sepsis, ileus, flank pain [10]. Radiographic findings described in these cases are classic for UPJ disruption and help distinguish it from other types of blunt renal trauma. Diagnosis of traumatic UPJ disruption can be established with atriphasic CT scan with delayed images [10, 13].Three findings commonly visualized in UPJ disruptions are maintained renal parenchyma with no evidence of laceration, medial extravasation of contrast in the perinephric area, and inability to locate the distal ureter on the side of the insult [10, 13].

Definitive treatment of UPJ disruption demands surgical repair. Ideally, surgical repair would be completed on the primary exploratory laparotomy performed after the presentation of the trauma. If identified immediately upon presentation or within the first 5 days of presentation, optimal anastomotic repair can be done with the use of a stent to achieve a patent anastomosis and placement of a nephrostomy tube for drainage [10, 15, 16]. In cases where the diagnosis is made later than 5 days, patients are given a temporizing nephrostomy tube and allowed to stabilize for several weeks before surgical repair is performed [10]. Delayed diagnosis may require more significant reconstruction and reimplantation of the ureter, and it may present more technical difficulties due to associated scarring from urine leak [10, 15, 16].

20.6 Scenario 3

A 9 year old girl a restrained passenger presents to the emergency department following a motor vehicle accident. Vitals on admission are 97.7 °F, heart rate 104 beats per minute, respiratory rate 22 breaths per minute, and blood pressure 104/56. Glasgow Coma Scale was 10 on arrival. Initial evaluation of patient identifies several right upper extremity abrasions and contusions, right rib fractures, and numerous lower extremity lacerations. Patient appears uncomfortable and complains of lower abdominal pain and distention. Patient has been unable to void since presentation. Further work up with cystography reveals imaging concerning for concomitant injury to the bladder. The patient is prepared for surgical exploration of the injury. Surgical exploration reveals an intraperitoneal injury at the dome of the bladder and the patient undergoes primary repair.

Question 1: What is management required in this child that would not be necessarily needed in an adult with a similar injury?

- A. Immediate post-operative voiding cystourethragram
- **B. Suprapubic catheter placement**
- C. Perivesical drain placement

- D. Cystogram 2 weeks after surgery
- E. Transurethral catheter drainage

Shortly after, a 10-year-old girl presents with a similar injury. Patient has a pelvic fracture and evidence of gross hematuria. Imaging reveals a tear drop sign and an extraperitoneal bladder injury at the bladder neck is diagnosed.

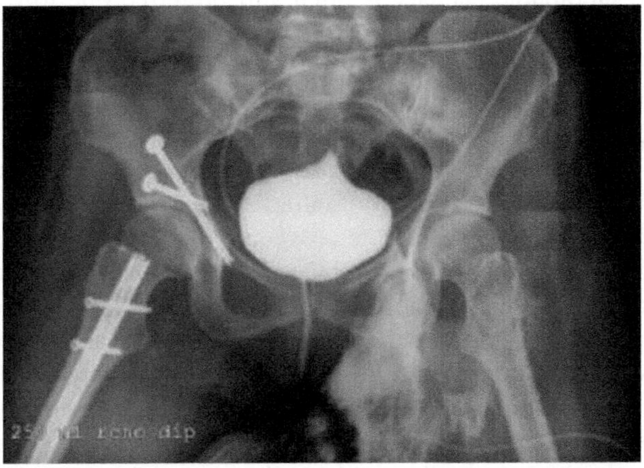

Image reprinted with permission from Elsevier from "Urinary-cutaneous Fistulae Following Conservative Management of Extraperitoneal Bladder Ruptures", by N. Johnsen et al., Urology, 109. Copyright November 2017 by Elsevier.

Question 2: Special consideration should be given to which of the following injuries in this particular case?

- A. Pelvic Hematoma
- B. Pelvic Urinoma
- **C. Concomitant Vaginal injury**
- D. Bladder neck injury
- E. Concomitant Rectal injury

Situated in the confines of the protective pelvis, bladder trauma requires high stress injury. While 80% of bladder trauma occurs in the setting of a pelvic fracture, bladder trauma occurs only in 10% of pelvic fractures [10, 17]. Because of this, bladder injuries are associated with approximately a 20% mortality rate and severe multi-organ trauma [18]. Extraperitoneal bladder injuries are about twice as common as intraperitoneal bladder injuries, though they can occur together [18]. The mechanism of extraperitoneal injury typically is due to osseous penetration of the bladder from fragments from fractured bones readily detected by the extravasation of contrast [10, 19]. Intraperitoneal injury is more commonly due to blunt abdominal trauma compressing a distended bladder and rupturing the weak dome of the bladder [19]. Intraperitoneal bladder injuries radiologically appear as fluid in the abdomen [10].

Clinical symptoms suspicious for bladder injury include abdominal pain, suprapubic pain, hematuria, and difficulty voiding [17]. Presence of these symptoms merit diagnostic workup with cystogram and close monitoring [17, 20].

Extraperitoneal injuries can be treated with simple large bore urethral catheter placement but suprapubic catheter is often still preferred due to risk of stricture particularly in pediatric males [10, 21]. However, surgical management is merited with the presence of a bony spicule or a fragment in the bladder, bladder neck involvement, or pelvic fracture [10]. Postoperatively continue 7–10 days of bladder drainage with a follow up cystogram to ensure adequate healing [10].

As distinguished in the first question of the case, according to guideline statements, following open surgical repair of intraperitoneal bladder injuries in the pediatric population, a suprapubic catheter is required [22]. A cystogram should be obtained after 7–10 days of catheter drainage prior to catheter removal [10].

The second case emphasizes the importance of investigating other complications of pelvic fractures and bladder neck injuries. Bladder neck involvement of bladder injuries is much more common in children than adults [10]. Any bladder neck injury necessitates rectal, vaginal, and urethral workup for coexisting trauma and may require immediate primary repair [23, 24]. Injuries to the bladder neck can be devastating and lead to high morbidity and incontinence requiring extensive future urologic workup [25].

While treatment depends on the classification of the injury, generally repair of the pediatric bladder has been demonstrated to improve survival [26] and has been shown to decrease immediate and long-term complication risks [10]. All patients should be placed on broad spectrum antibiotic upon presentation until the removal of catheters [10].

20.7 Urethral Injury

<u>Scenario 1</u>: A 10-year-old male is brought to the Emergency Department after being hit by a motor vehicle while riding a scooter. On presentation, he is alert, oriented and complains of abdominal pain. Blood pressure is 101/68, HR 154 beats per minute, pulse oximetry 100% on room air, and respiratory rate of 30 breaths per minute. Physical exam reveals an atraumatic head with no signs of cardiorespiratory distress. Abdominal exam reveals mild distention with tenderness in the lower quadrants. Imaging of his chest, head and spine do not reveal any acute injuries. CT Abdomen/pelvis reveals a stable fracture of his right pubic rami, left iliac wing, and sacrum. The fractures do not require fixation at this time. Patient is unable to void and retrograde urethrogram is completed.

1. What portion of the urethra would most likely be injured in this case?
   - a. Bulbous
   - **b. Membranous**
   - c. Prostatic

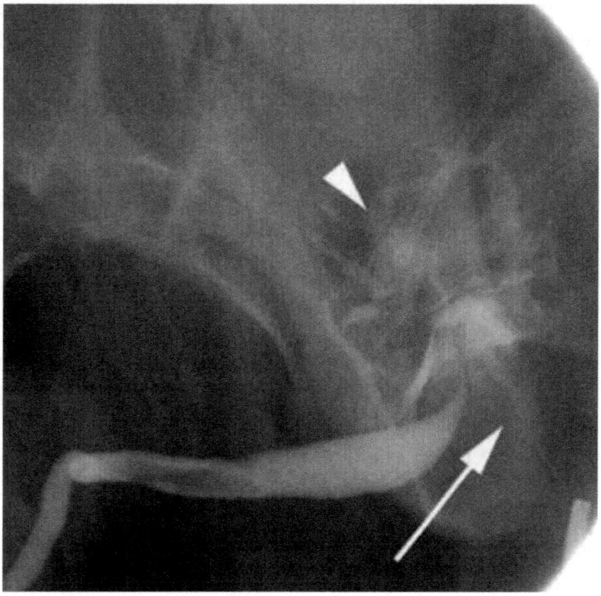

Fig. 20.1 Image from RUG with *white arrow* and *arrowhead* defining areas of contrast extravasation. (Reprinted with permission from Springer Nature from "Lower male genitourinary trauma: a pictorial review", by B. Lehnert et al., *Emergency Radiology, 21* [1], pp. 67–74. Copyright 2014 by Springer Nature)

- d. Penile
- e. Bladder neck

A retrograde urethrogram (RUG) is completed and the findings are demonstrated below an arrow and arrowhead defining the areas of contrast extravasation (Fig. 20.1):

2. Given these imaging findings, what would the Goldman classification for this injury be?
   - a. Grade I
   - b. Grade II
   - **c. Grade III**
   - d. Grade IV
   - e. Grade V
3. A complete transection of the posterior urethra is identified on imaging. What is the recommended management of this acute urethral injury?
   - a. Immediate anastomotic urethroplasty
   - b. Suprapubic catheterization and delayed anastomotic urethroplasty
   - c. Endoscopic realignment
   - d. Per urethral catheter placement
   - **e. B &C**

20.8 Discussion

Q1: Given this patient's mechanism of injury and pelvic fracture findings, he most likely injured his posterior urethra, and posterior injuries most commonly involve injuries to the membranous urethra [27]. Anatomically, the posterior urethra includes the prostatic and membranous portions of the urethra and the urogenital diaphragm while the anterior urethra includes the bulbous and penile portions of the urethra [6]. Urethral injuries are similarly categorized into anterior and posterior urethral injuries. Anterior urethral injuries most often result in damage to the bulbous urethra from straddle injuries such as direct trauma to the perineum from handlebars or kicks when anterior forces compress the bulbous urethra against the pubic symphysis [27, 28]. On the other hand, posterior urethral injuries are associated with blunt trauma and pelvic fractures. One study of posterior urethral disruptions in children found 71% were the result of a vehicle-pedestrian accident [29].

Q2: The image in this case reveals extravasation of contrast from the posterior urethra with extravasation of contrast above (*white arrowhead*) and below (*white arrow*) the urogenital diaphragm. By definition, this would be a Type III urethral injury, which is more likely to occur than type I and type II injuries [30]. Based on anatomic findings from retrograde urethrograms, the Goldman Classification [31] divides urethral, bladder neck and bladder injuries into five categories. The first three categories represent subtypes of posterior urethral injuries:

- **Type I**: Posterior urethra is intact but stretched resulting in superior movement of the prostate and the neck of the bladder. No contrast extravasation is visualized.
- **Type II**: Partial or complete urethral rupture above the urogenital diaphragm with extravasation of contrast-agent above an intact diaphragm.
- **Type III**: Partial or complete posterior urethral rupture with disruption of the urogenital diaphragm and bulbous urethra. Extravasation is seen within the extraperitoneal and intraperitoneal pelvis.

Anterior urethral, bladder neck, and bladder base, and anterior urethral injuries are classified as Type IV and Type V injuries [30].

- **Type IV**: Bladder neck injury extending into the urethra with extravasation of contrast surrounding the bladder neck.
- **Type IVa**: Bladder base injury with periurethral extravasation.
- **Type V:** Partial or complete anterior urethral injury.

Q3: Initial management of posterior urethral injuries remains controversial and options include primary endoscopic realignment, primary repair with end-to-end anastomosis, and suprapubic cystostomy (SC) placement with delayed anastomotic urethroplasty (DAU) [32]. However, primary anastomosis is only recommended in the setting of a concomitant bladder neck or rectal injury, as it has been associated with very high rates of incontinence and erectile dysfunction [6]. Ideally, management should divert urine immediately while reducing the development of potentially morbid long-term effects including stricture, incontinence and sexual dysfunction. DAU for posterior urethral injury has success rates of 75–92% reported in pediatric populations [27]. DAU can be performed using a perineal or perineal with partial pubectomy approach with similar success noted in the literature (Table 20.1). Although some studies describe worse outcomes with primary

Table 20.1 Delayed correction

Study	N	Primary Success N (%)
Posterior injury		
Voelzke [27]	18	16 (90)
Perineal	13	12
Perineal/partial Pubectomy	5	4
Koraitim [33]	65	60 (92)
Perineal	42	39
Transpubic	23	21
Podesta [29]	49	44 (90)
Perineal	28	23
Perineal/partial pubectomy	21	21
Anterior injury		
Voelzke [27]	8	7 (88)
Anastomotic	5	4
Ventral only Buccal mucosa graft	3	3

Table 20.2 Reported rates of complications in Pediatric Patients following Posterior Urethral Injury Management

Study	Stricture	Incontinence	Erectile Dysfunction
Podesta [29]			
SC then DAU (n = 35)	4	5	2
Primary realignment then DAU (n = 14)	1	4	1
Onen [35]			
Primary Realingment (n = 22)	5	4	5
Immediate repair (n = 8)	2	1	1
Delayed repair (n = 16)	4	3	3
Nerli [36]			
SC then DAU (n = 10)	10	0	NA
Primary realignment (n = 12) (endoscopic n = 7 and open n = 5)	6	0	NA

SC Suprapubic cystostomy, *DAU* Delayed anastomotic urethroplasty

realignment of a posterior urethral injury in adults [34], long-term research has identified similar rates of adverse outcomes such as stricture and incontinence when initial management options are compared among pediatric patients (Table 20.2). However, most of the research on this subject is observational and includes small numbers of patients. Therefore, depending on the injury, appropriate initial management of posterior urethral injuries may include initial placement of a suprapubic tube or primary realignment followed by a delayed repair 3–6 months after the initial injury [27].

<u>**Scenario 2**</u>: A 12-year-old boy is brought to the Emergency Department by his family. Two hours before presentation, he had a bicycle accident, resulting in a straddle-type blunt injury to his perineum from the handlebars. On presentation, his

vital signs are all within normal limits there is a small amount of bright red blood at the urethral meatus and a scrotal hematoma is present.

1. What is the most appropriate next step?
   - a. Placement of a urinary catheter
   - b. Suprapubic tube placement
   - **c. Retrograde urethrogram**
   - d. Urethroscopy
   - e. CT Abdomen/pelvis with contrast
2. A partial tear of the anterior urethra is identified (Grade V) is identified. What is the next best step for management?
   - a. Blind placement of a urinary catheter
   - b. Placement of suprapubic catheter with delayed anastomotic urethroplasty
   - **c. Guided placement of a urethral catheter with follow-up pericatheter study**
   - d. Surgical repair

20.9 Discussion

Q1: This patient presents blood at the urethral meatus and a scrotal hematoma, two findings highly suggestive of an acute urethral injury. The classic triad of an acute urethral injury includes (1) blood at the meatus/vaginal introitus (2) perineal/penile hematoma and (3) inability to void. If there is no evidence of blood at the meatus or a hematoma, a urethral injury is less likely; however, up to 20% of urethral injuries among male patients and 30% among females can be missed initially [37]. The diagnostic workup of urethral injuries frequently begins with a retrograde urethrogram. However, injuries in female patients are usually first suggested by findings on a CT such as perivesical hematoma, peri vesical hematoma around bladder neck,disruption at the level of the bladder neck, and given the short length of the female urethra, a cystoscopy/vaginoscopy can be used for diagnostic confirmation [37].

Q2: As this patient has a partial anterior urethral tear with no significant penile hematoma, management should include insertion of a urethral catheter with a follow-up pericatheter study in 2 weeks. Immediate repair is recommended in penetrating trauma to the anterior urethra [6], and among stable patients, it is recommended to avoid blind placement of a urinary catheter. However, blind placement may be attempted in critically ill patients with caution for any resistance and care to avoid balloon inflation until urine returns [37]. Unfortunately, there is limited data on outcomes following anterior urethral injuries in pediatric patients [27, 28].

<u>Scenario 3</u>: A 10-day-old male infant underwent circumcision completed with a Mogen clamp under anesthesia. After completing the procedure, partial amputation of the glans penis was noted with an oblique injury noted on examination.

1. What should be done with regard to the amputation at this time?
   - **a. Preserve amputated tissue by wrapping in saline soaked gauze and placing in bag immersed in cold water. Immediately take to OR for reimplantation**
   - b. Preserve amputated tissue and wrap penis in compressive bandage, wait for healing before reconstruction is attempted
   - c. Wrap in compressive bandage and attempt reconstruction with buccal mucosa in 1–3 months
   - d. Wrap in compressive bandage and attempt reconstruction with buccal mucosa immediately
2. What should be done to prevent urethral injury?
   - a. If patient is able to void, urethral injury is unlikely. No management is necessary
   - **b. Place a urethral stent for at least 1 week**
   - c. Place a urinary catheter for 48 h
   - d. Suprapubic catheter placement

Discussion: Although uncommon, glans amputation is a morbid potential complication of circumcision [38–40]. Circumcision clamp techniques, including the Mogen, Gomco and Plastibell clamps, have become popular given the convenience of the procedures [38, 41]. As most partial amputation injuries of the glans penis occur in an oblique pattern, the injury is believed to be the result of incomplete release of the balano-preputial adhesions around the frenulum [38, 40, 41]. To avoid this complication, providers should aim to ensure complete release of the mucosa from the glans before placing a circumcision clamp.

Q1: Successful reimplantation of a partially amputated glans penis has been successfully reported up to 8 h after removal [38].If immediate reimplantation is not possible or the original tissue is not available, reconstruction can be performed with a buccal mucosa graft after the initial injury has healed [38].

Q2*:* Circumcisions can lead to significant urethral injury leading to subsequent development of urethrocutaneous fistulas and urethral stenosis. Although meatal stenosis can occur as a complication of an uncomplicated circumcision [42], it is much more common in the setting of a partial glans amputation [38]. Therefore, a ureteral stent should be placed for at least 7 days to prevent significant stenosis.

20.9.1 Genital Trauma

Scenario 1: An 11-year-old male is brought to the Emergency Department following a high-speed bike injury. Patient sustained a "straddle injury" by striking his perineum and scrotum on bike frame during the crash. On presentation, he is alert, and complains of significant abdominal pain. Vital signs are within normal limits and no signs of cardiorespiratory distress or neurologic abnormalities are noted on exam. Genital exam reveals tenderness with mild swelling. Imaging reveals a left pubic rami fracture and patient is able to void without difficulty. A urinary catheter is placed without difficulty, and the patient is admitted to the hospital.

1. What is the next best step in management?
   - a. Retrograde urethrogram
   - **b. Doppler ultrasound of the testes**
   - c. CT Scan of Abdomen and Pelvis
   - d. Abdominal Ultrasound

24 h after admission, he began reporting increasing left scrotal pain and “dark” urine. A repeat ultrasound of the L testicle is seen below (Fig. 20.2):

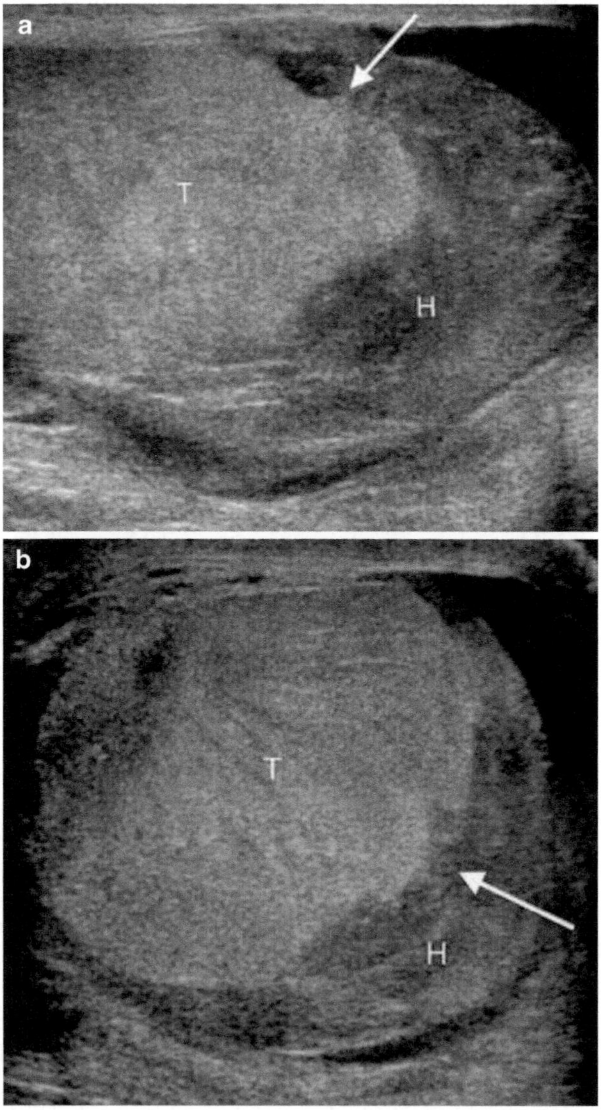

Fig. 20.2 Grey scale ultrasound with longitudinal (**a**) and transverse (**b**) left scrotum showing heterogeneous testicular echogenicity (T), irregular testicular contour (*arrows*) and hematocele (H). Tunica albuginea was not identified with certainty on imaging and doppler imaging is not shown but revealed absent flow. (Reprinted with permission from Springer Nature from “Sonography of pediatric blunt scrotal trauma: what the pediatric urologist wants to know”, by L. Fenton et al., *Pediatric Radiology*, 46 [7], p. 1054. Copyright 2016 by Springer Nature)

2. What is the next best step in the management of this patient?
   - **a. Immediate exploration**
   - b. Conservative Management
   - c. Repeat US in 48 h
   - d. Antibiotics

20.10 Discussion

Q1: Genital trauma accounts for a significant number of pediatric emergency care visits [43]. Direct blunt trauma to the scrotum often results in scrotal and testicular hematomas or concerningly, testicular rupture [44]. An ultrasound with doppler should be completed on both testes for comparison to identify complications requiring surgical intervention including testicular torsion, rupture and dislocation [45].

Q2: Ultrasound findings concerning for testicular rupture include loss of tunica continuity, testicular shape and heterogeneous testicular echotexture [6, 46].Given the ultrasound findings and the expanding hematoma in the L testis, this patient should be taken to the operating room for surgical exploration with debridement and tunica albuginea closure [6]. Early surgical intervention in the setting of scrotal trauma is associated with improved short- and long-term outcomes for patients [45].

References

1. Grimsby GM, Voelzke B, Hotaling J, Sorensen MD, Koyle M, Jacobs MA. Demographics of pediatric renal trauma. J Urol. 2014;192(5):1498–502.
2. Murphy GP, Gaither TW, Awad MA, et al. Management of Pediatric Grade IV renal trauma. Curr Urol Rep. 2017;18(3):23.
3. Brown SL, Elder JS, Spirnak JP. Are pediatric patients more susceptible to major renal injury from blunt trauma? A comparative study. J Urol. 1998;160(1):138–40.
4. Dangle PP, Fuller TW, Gaines B, et al. Evolving mechanisms of injury and Management of Pediatric Blunt Renal Trauma--20 years of experience. Urology. 2016;90:159–63.
5. Jacobs MA, Hotaling JM, Mueller BA, Koyle M, Rivara F, Voelzke BB. Conservative management vs early surgery for high grade pediatric renal trauma--do nephrectomy rates differ? J Urol. 2012;187(5):1817–22.
6. Morey AF, Brandes S, Dugi DD 3rd, et al. Urotrauma: AUA guideline. J Urol. 2014;192(2):327–35.
7. Serafetinides E, Kitrey ND, Djakovic N, et al. Review of the current management of upper urinary tract injuries by the EAU trauma guidelines panel. Eur Urol. 2015;67(5):930–6.
8. Cannon GM Jr, Polsky EG, Smaldone MC, et al. Computerized tomography findings in pediatric renal trauma--indications for early intervention? J Urol. 2008;179(4):1529–32; discussion 1532–1523.
9. Gerstenbluth RE, Spirnak JP, Elder JS. Sports participation and high grade renal injuries in children. J Urol. 2002;168(6):2575–8.
10. Hussman DA. Chapter 154: pediatric genitourinary trauma. In: Wein AJ, Kavoussi LR, Partin AW, Peters CA, editors. Campbell Walsh urology. 11th ed. Philadelphia, PA: Elsevier-Saunders. p. 3538.
11. Committee on Sports Medicine and Fitness. Medical conditions affected sports participation. Pediatrics. 2001;107:1205–9.

12. Pumberger W, Stoll E, Metz S. Ureteropelvic junction disruption following blunt abdominal trauma. Pediatr Emerg Care. 2002;18(5):364–6.
13. Kawashima A, Sandler CM, Corriere JN Jr, Rodgers BM, Goldman SM. Ureteropelvic junction injuries secondary to blunt abdominal trauma. Radiology. 1997;205(2):487–92.
14. Al-Qudah HS, Santucci RA. Complications of renal trauma. Urol Clin North Am. 2006;33(1):41–53, vi.
15. Kunkle DA, Kansas BT, Pathak A, Goldberg AJ, Mydlo JH. Delayed diagnosis of traumatic ureteral injuries. J Urol. 2006;176(6 Pt 1):2503–7.
16. Pereira BM, Ogilvie MP, Gomez-Rodriguez JC, et al. A review of ureteral injuries after external trauma. Scand J Trauma Resusc Emerg Med. 2010;18:6.
17. Guttmann I, Kerr HA. Blunt bladder injury. Clin Sports Med. 2013;32(2):239–46.
18. Carroll PR, McAninch JW. Major bladder trauma: mechanisms of injury and a unified method of diagnosis and repair. J Urol. 1984;132(2):254–7.
19. Zacharias C, Robinson JD, Linnau KF, Mannelli L. Blunt urinary bladder trauma. Curr Probl Diagn Radiol. 2012;41(4):140–1.
20. Bryk DJ, Zhao LC. Guideline of guidelines: a review of urological trauma guidelines. BJU Int. 2016;117(2):226–34.
21. Kotkin L, Koch MO. Morbidity associated with nonoperative management of extraperitoneal bladder injuries. J Trauma. 1995;38(6):895–8.
22. Summerton DJ, Djakovic N, Kitrey ND, et al. European association of urology. Guidelines on urological trauma. March 2015.
23. Kim S, Linden B, Cendron M, Puder M. Pediatric anorectal impalement with bladder rupture: case report and review of the literature. J Pediatr Surg. 2006;41(9):E1–3.
24. Routh JC, Graham DA, Nelson CP. Epidemiological trends in pediatric urolithiasis at United States freestanding pediatric hospitals. J Urol. 2010;184(3):1100–4.
25. Routh JC, Husmann DA. Long-term continence outcomes after immediate repair of pediatric bladder neck lacerations extending into the urethra. J Urol. 2007;178(4 Pt 2):1816–8; discussion 1818.
26. Deibert CM, Glassberg KI, Spencer BA. Repair of pediatric bladder rupture improves survival: results from the National Trauma Data Bank. J Pediatr Surg. 2012;47(9):1677–81.
27. Voelzke BB, Breyer BN, McAninch JW. Blunt pediatric anterior and posterior urethral trauma: 32-year experience and outcomes. J Pediatr Urol. 2012;8(3):258–63.
28. Holland AJ, Cohen RC, McKertich KM, Cass DT. Urethral trauma in children. Pediatr Surg Int. 2001;17(1):58–61.
29. Podesta M, Podesta M Jr. Delayed surgical repair of posttraumatic posterior urethral distraction defects in children and adolescents: long-term results. J Pediatr Urol. 2015;11(2):67.e61–66.
30. Lehnert BE, Sadro C, Monroe E, Moshiri M. Lower male genitourinary trauma: a pictorial review. Emerg Radiol. 2014;21(1):67–74.
31. Goldman SM, Sandler CM, Corriere JN Jr, McGuire EJ. Blunt urethral trauma: a unified, anatomical mechanical classification. J Urol. 1997;157(1):85–9.
32. Dixon AN, Webb JC, Wenzel JL, Wolf JS Jr, Osterberg EC. Current management of pelvic fracture urethral injuries: to realign or not? Translational andrology and urology. 2018;7(4):593–602.
33. Koraitim MM. Posttraumatic posterior urethral strictures in children: a 20-year experience. J Urol. 1997;157(2):641–5.
34. Barrett K, Braga LH, Farrokhyar F, Davies TO. Primary realignment vs suprapubic cystostomy for the management of pelvic fracture-associated urethral injuries: a systematic review and meta-analysis. Urology. 2014;83(4):924–9.
35. Onen A, Ozturk H, Kaya M, Otcu S. Long-term outcome of posterior urethral rupture in boys: a comparison of different surgical modalities. Urology. 2005;65(6):1202–7.
36. Nerli RB, Koura AC, Ravish IR, Amarkhed SS, Prabha V, Alur SB. Posterior urethral injury in male children: long-term follow up. J Pediatr Urol. 2008;4(2):154–9.

37. Meltzer JA, Reddy SH, Blumfield E, Alvayay C, Blumberg SM. Pelvic fracture urethral injuries in children: a case report and appraisal of their emergency management. Pediatr Emerg Care. 2016;32(9):627–9.
38. Pippi Salle JL, Jesus LE, Lorenzo AJ, et al. Glans amputation during routine neonatal circumcision: mechanism of injury and strategy for prevention. J Pediatr Urol. 2013;9(6 Pt A):763–8.
39. Baskin LS, Canning DA, Snyder HM 3rd, Duckett JW Jr. Surgical repair of urethral circumcision injuries. J Urol. 1997;158(6):2269–71.
40. Weiss HA, Larke N, Halperin D, Schenker I. Complications of circumcision in male neonates, infants and children: a systematic review. BMC Urol. 2010;10:2.
41. Mousavi SA, Salehifar E. Circumcision complications associated with the Plastibell device and conventional dissection surgery: a trial of 586 infants of ages up to 12 months. Adv Urol. 2008;606123.
42. Ozen MA, Gundogdu G, Tasdemir M, Eroglu E. Complication of newborn circumcision: Meatal stenosis or meatal web? J Pediatr Urol. 2017;13(6):617.e611–4.
43. Yang C Jr, Song B, Liu X, Wei GH, Lin T, He DW. Acute scrotum in children: an 18-year retrospective study. Pediatr Emerg Care. 2011;27(4):270–4.
44. Wang Z, Yang JR, Huang YM, et al. Diagnosis and management of testicular rupture after blunt scrotal trauma: a literature review. Int Urol Nephrol. 2016;48(12):1967–76.
45. Dalton DM, Davis NF, O'Neill DC, Brady CM, Kiely EA, O'Brien MF. Aetiology, epidemiology and management strategies for blunt scrotal trauma. The surgeon : journal of the Royal Colleges of Surgeons of Edinburgh and Ireland. 2016;14(1):18–21.
46. Fenton LZ, Karakas SP, Baskin L, Campbell JB. Sonography of pediatric blunt scrotal trauma: what the pediatric urologist wants to know. Pediatr Radiol. 2016;46(7):1049–58.

Functional Voiding Disorders 21

Anka Nieuwhof-Leppink and Prasad Godbole

Learning Objectives
- Understand the micturition cycle and the functions of the bladder
- Appropriate history taking and examination for functional voiding disorders
- Investigations for functional voiding disorders
- Understand the treatment for various functional voiding disorders

21.1 Case 1

Lisa an 8 years old girl presents to your outpatient clinic with a history of urinary incontinence during the day and recurrent lower urinary tract infections.

Situation at first intake:

- Incontinence during the day
- Urinary tract infections
- Nocturnal enuresis

Question 1: What other information would you like to know from the history?

Answer 1: Medical history

- Very wet during the day and night

A. Nieuwhof-Leppink
Wilhemina's Childrens Hospital, University Medical Center Utrecht, Utrecht, The Netherlands

P. Godbole (✉)
Department of Paediatric Surgery, Sheffield Children's NHS Foundation Trust, Sheffield, UK
e-mail: p.godbole@nhs.net

P. Godbole et al. (eds.), *Practical Pediatric Urology*,
https://doi.org/10.1007/978-3-030-54020-3_21

- Voiding frequency: 5 times a day
- Defecation 3 times a week
- BSC; 2–3
- Fecal incontinence; 1 times a week
- Urge complaints
- Fluid intake: 1 liter a day
- Wetting at night, uses diapers

Question 2; The frequency volume chart (bladder/bowel diary) is as shown as is the dysfunctional voiding scoring system. What further investigations would you like to consider?

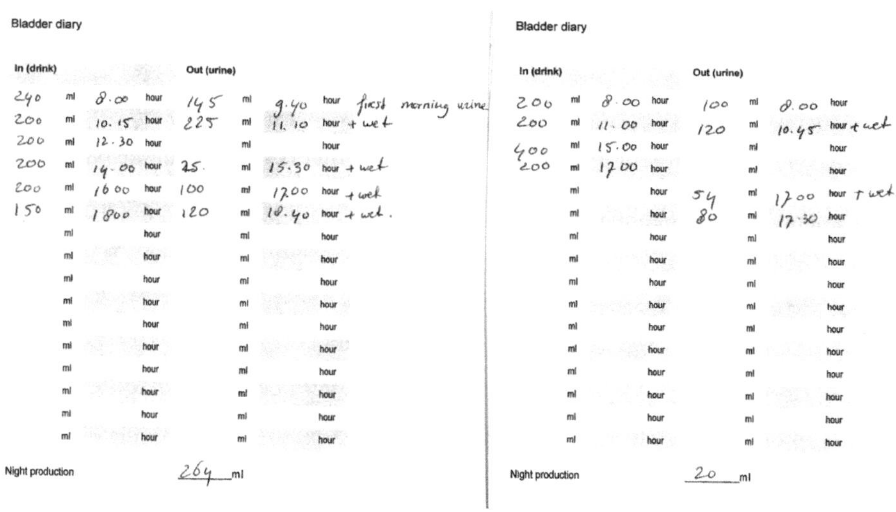

Dysfunctional Voiding Scoring System

Patient to answer if appropriate (Please circle best answer)

Patient Lisa)

Date _ Questionnaire

Reason for referral ____________________

Over the last month	Almost never	Less than half the time	About half the time	Almost every time	Not available or Not applicable
1. I have wet clothes or wet underwear during the day	0	1	2	3	N/A
2. When I wet myself my underwear is soaked.	0	1	2	3	N/A
3. I miss having a bowel movement every day.	0	1	2	3	N/A
4. I have to push for my bowel movements to come out	0	1	2	3	N/A
5. I only go to the bathroom to pee one or two times a day	0	1	2	3	N/A
6. I can hold onto my pee by crossing my legs, squatting or doing the "pee dance"	0	1	2	3	N/A
7. When I have to pee, I cannot wait	0	1	2	3	N/A
8. I have to push or strain to pee	0	1	2	3	N/A
9. When I pee it hurts	0	1	2	3	N/A
10. **Parents to answer:** Has your child experienced something stressful? For example: new baby, new home, divorce, death of someone close, abuse, school issues, injury, illness	NO = 0			YES = 3	
11. I leak pee when I play sports, cough, sneeze	0	1	2	3	N/A
12. I leak pee because I can not wait	0	1	2	3	N/A
13. I leak pee because I can not reach a bathroom in time	0	1	2	3	N/A
14. I leak pee at night while I am asleep	0	1	2	3	N/A
15. I leak pee without any warning or urge	0	1	2	3	N/A
16. I use protection (tissue, pads, pull-ups, goodnights) to protect against pee leaks during the day or night	0 Never	1 1 per day or less	2 2-3 per day	3 4 or more per day	N/A
17. I don't do sleepovers, other activities, or sports because I am afraid I will leak pee	0	1	2	3	N/A

Answer 2:
Uroflowmetry
Renal and bladder ultrasound with postvoid residual

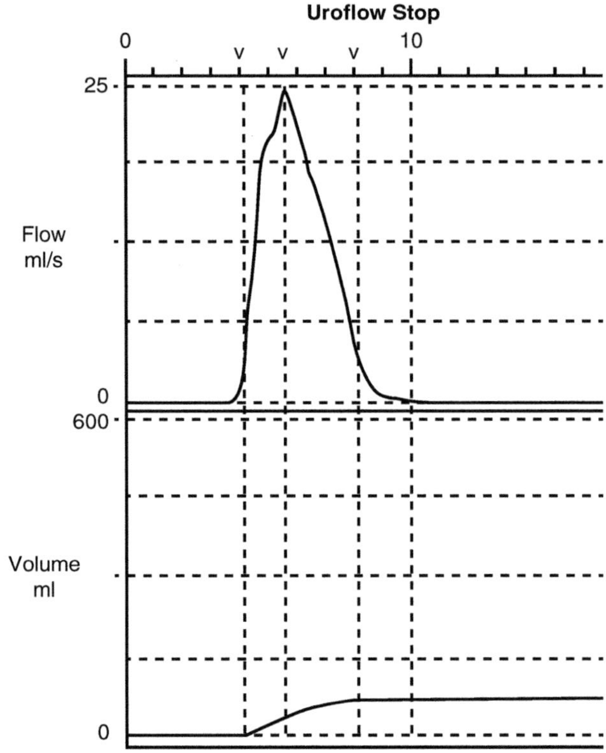

Uroflow Summary

Maximum flow:	24.1	ml/s
Average flow:	15.9	ml/s
Voiding time:	4.2	sec
Flow time:	4.2	sec
Time to peak flow:	1.6	sec
Voided volume:	66.9	ml
Flow at 2 seconds:	20.0	ml/s
Accelerations:	11.6	ml/s/s

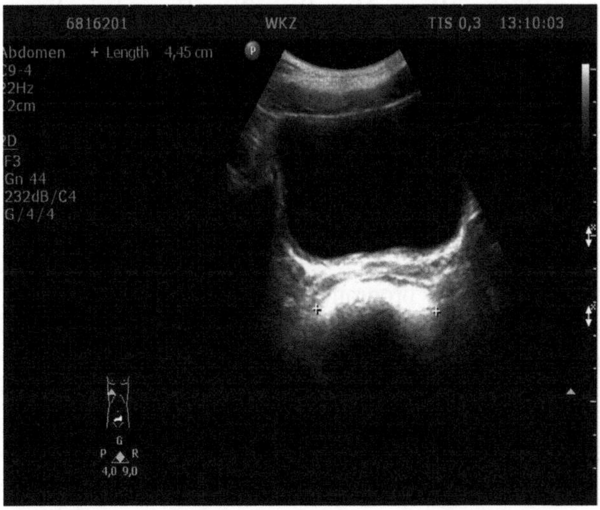

Postvoid Ultrasound (Normal kidneys)
Question 3
What is your impression of the uroflometry and renal ultrasound?
Answer

Lisa seems to have a functional small capacity bladder with urge incontinence based on the dysfunctional voiding scoring system. Ultrasound suggests faecal loading (constipation meets Rome IV criteria) and significant post void residual.

Question 4
What would be the next steps?
Answer 4

- Start standard urotherapy: explanation and instructions about normal bowel and bladder behavior
- Treat constipation; Laxatives (macrogol 2 × 2gr) and toilet sit for 3 months to guarantee daily bowel movement

Question 5:
After 3 months treatment of constipation the clinical situation is as follows:

- No fecal incontinence
- BSC 3–4
- Daily bowel movements.
- US: Rectum diameter 2.6 cm, PVR 10 ml
- Still daily wet accidents
- MF 6
- Still Urge complaints, holding maneuvers
- FI: 1000 ml

- Flow pattern: Tower shape, Max flow 26 ml/s and voiding time 11 s, volume 180 ml
- Enuresis

What would be the next steps?
Answer 5:

- Start anti cholinergic: Oxybutynin 2 × 2.5 mg
- Continuing laxatives,
- Start intensive urotherapy program;

bladder training program, focused on learning to react adequately on bladder signals (learns how to void, when to void and how often to void).

- Biofeedback session by real-time uroflowmetry and EMG,
- During 3 months, frequently contact/support provided by the nurse/urotherapists

21.2 Case 2

Lennart is an 8 year old boy with daytime urinary incontinence every day and voiding frequency of 6–7 times per day. He has urgency and does holding manoeuvres. He opens his bowels 5 times a week, Bristol Stool Chart 4. He has faecal incontinence up to twice a day. His fluid intake is 1500 ml/day. He also had nocturnal enuresis which has improved with enuresis alarm. He has never had any medication. Clinical examination is normal. His uroflometry and ultrasound are shown below:

Flowmetry

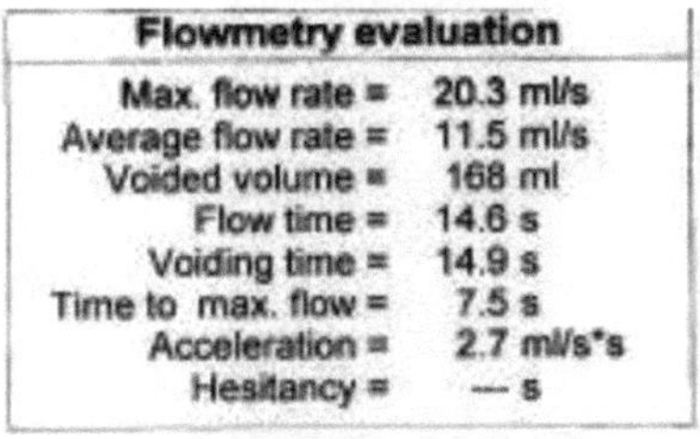

Flowmetry evaluation	
Max. flow rate =	20.3 ml/s
Average flow rate =	11.5 ml/s
Voided volume =	168 ml
Flow time =	14.6 s
Voiding time =	14.9 s
Time to max. flow =	7.5 s
Acceleration =	2.7 ml/s*s
Hesitancy =	--- s

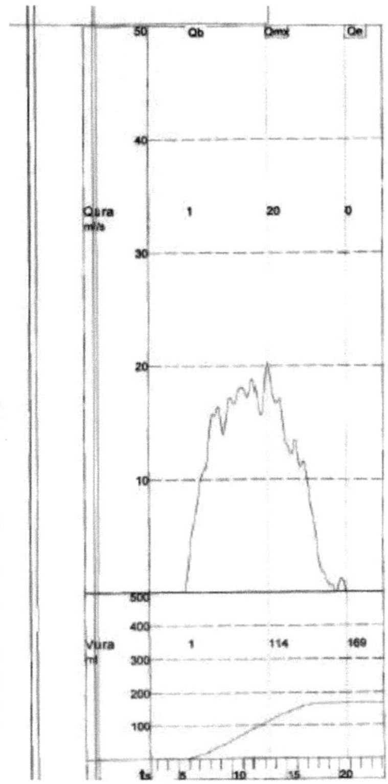

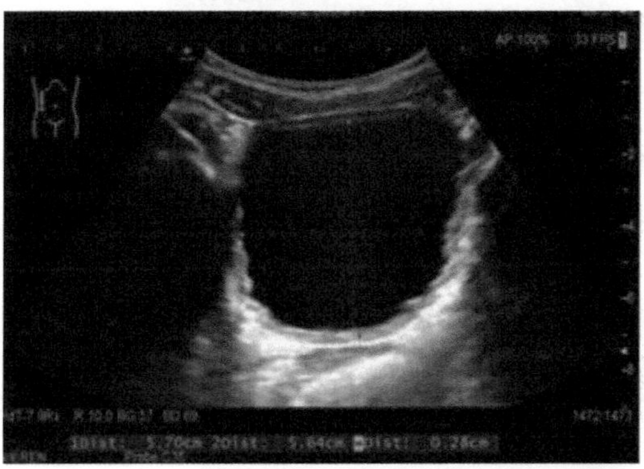

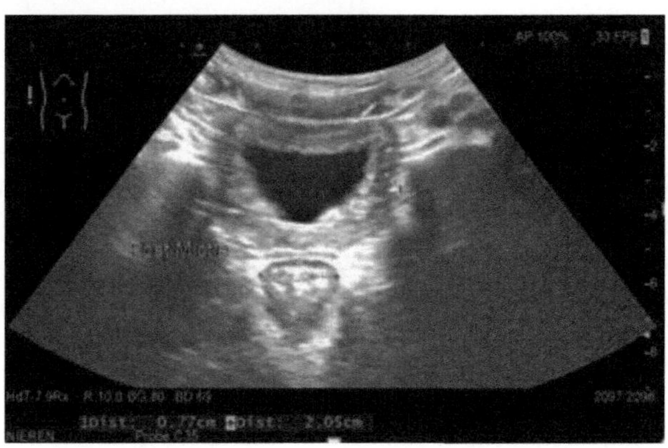

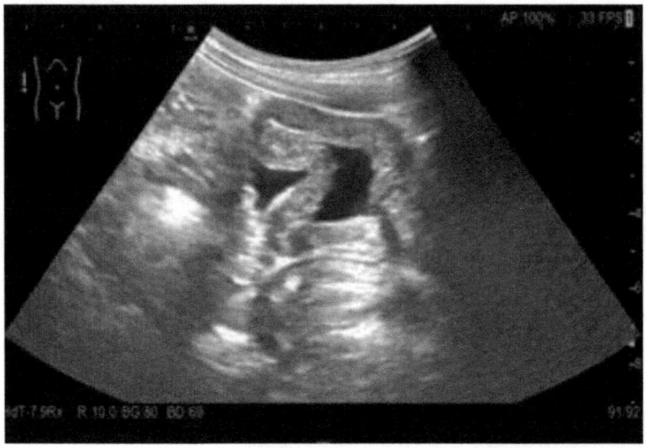

Question 1

What kind of incontinence is this? What is your interpretation of the ultrasound?

Answer 1:

- Daytime incontinence and enuresis based on OAB, **thick bladder-wall (>6 mm)**, constipation, No further anatomical or neurological issues.
- Attention: In light of the thick walled bladder, one must consider infravesical obstruction
- Constipation: meets Rome IV criteria

Question 2

What would be next step?

Answer 2:

- Start standard urotherapy: explanation and instructions about normal bowel and bladder behavior
- Treat constipation; Laxatives (macrogol 2 × 2gr) and regular toileting for 3 months to guarantee daily bowel movement
- Start anti cholinergics 2 × 2.5 mg oxybutinin

Treatment Results

After 3 months treatment of standard urotherapy. He puts a lot of efforts in his training and his clinical picture is as follows:

- No fecal incontinence, Bristol stool chart 3–4 and daily bowel movements
- US: Rectum diameter 1.5 cm, PVR 15 ml

- Still daily wetting accidents and urgency
- Voiding frequency 6/day
- Flow pattern: staccato bell-shaped, Max flow 35 ml/s and voiding time 25 s, volume 180 ml
- Nocturia

Question 3
What would the next investigation?
Answer 3:
Video urodynamics

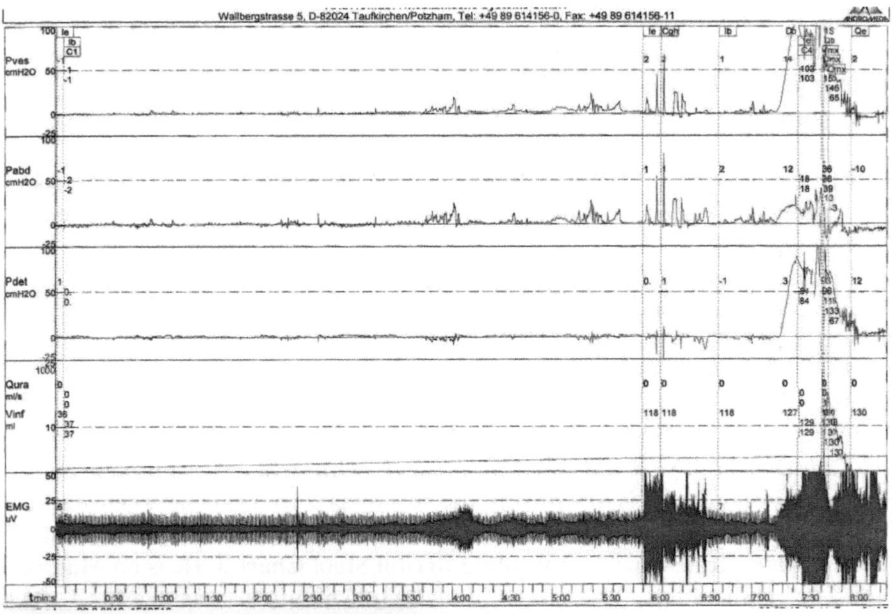

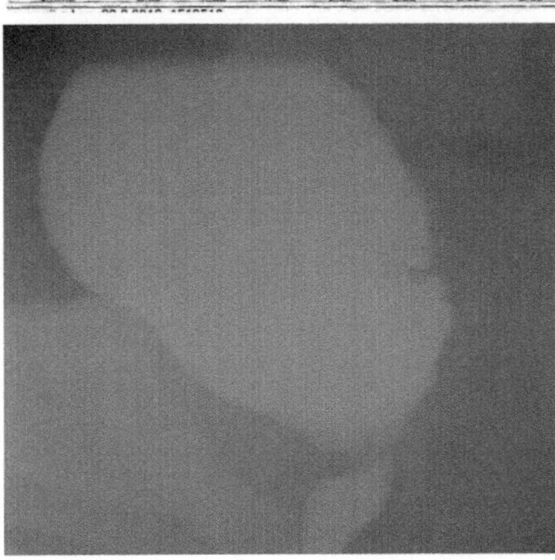

Question 4: What is your interpretation of the VUD?

Answer 4:

Bladder capacity +/– 180 cc, stable filling up to 150 cc (PQmax:67 cm H2 Qmax:17.6 ml/s with open bladder neck (without reaction of the detrusor), then terminal over activity, voiding without consent with high pressure and relatively low flow, relaxed pelvic floor during voiding, constriction proximal urethra.

Question 5

What surgical intervention would you consider?

Answer 5

Cystoscopy +/– relief of infravesical obstruction (if any)

Question 6

The boy went for cystoscopy and had resection of Posterior urethral valves (eponymously called Moorman's ring or Cobb's collar). 3 months following this, his symptoms improved. What further follow up is necessary?

Answer 6

- Regular urology follow up with renal ultrasound scans, uroflows and videourodynamics if evidence of bladder decompensation or if reconstructive surgery contemplated
- Functional radionuclide imaging for renal function
- Long term nephrological follow up

21.3 Case 3

Alexander is an 8 year old boy who presents with urinary incontinence every day with urgency. He is dry during the school day. He voids between 7 and 10 times a day with a maximum voided volume of 240 ml. His fluid intake is 1500 ml/day. He also has faecal soling Bristol Stool Chart 3. He is on Macrogol and Methylphenidate. After starting methylphenidate he was dry for 1 week. His ultrasound and uroflowmetry is shown below:

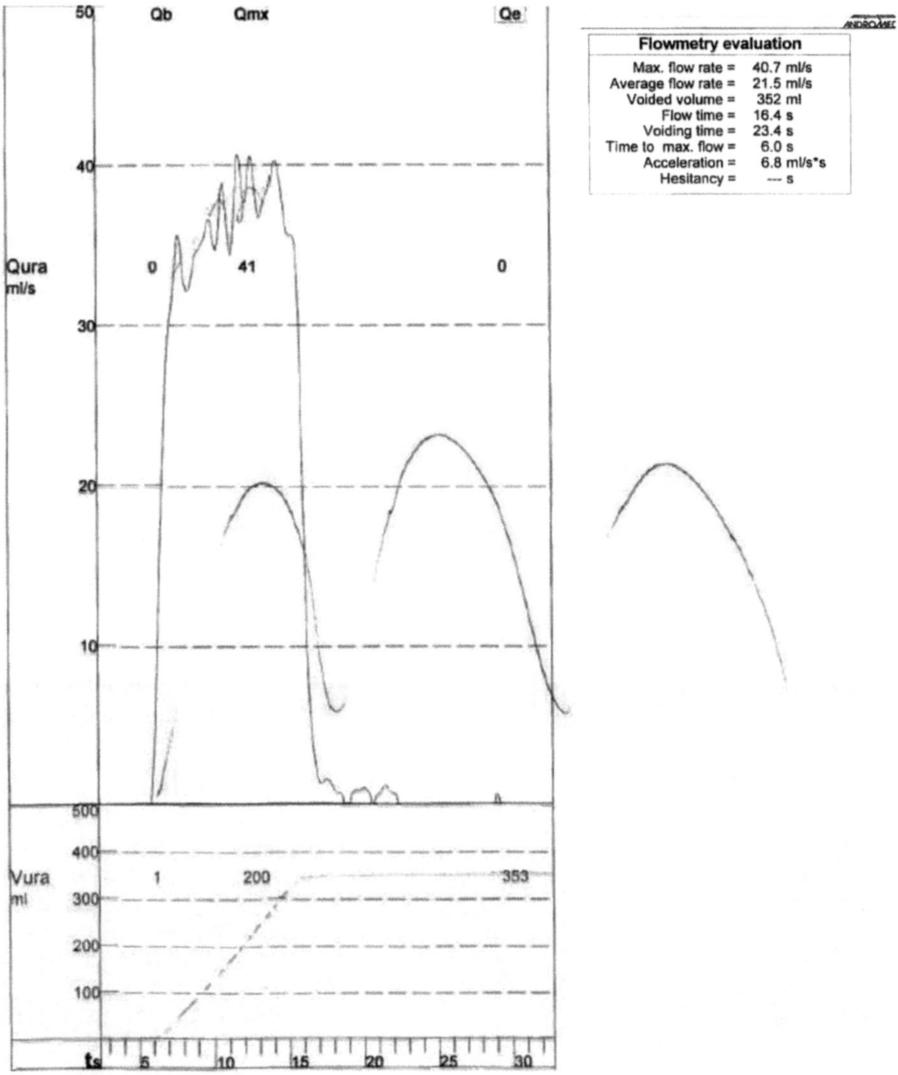

Qb
Qmx
Qe
Qura
ml/s
0
41
0
Vura
ml
1
200
353
ts
Flowmetry evaluation
Max. flow rate = 40.7 ml/s
Average flow rate = 21.5 ml/s
Voided volume = 352 ml
Flow time = 16.4 s
Voiding time = 23.4 s
Time to max. flow = 6.0 s
Acceleration = 6.8 ml/s*s
Hesitancy = --- s

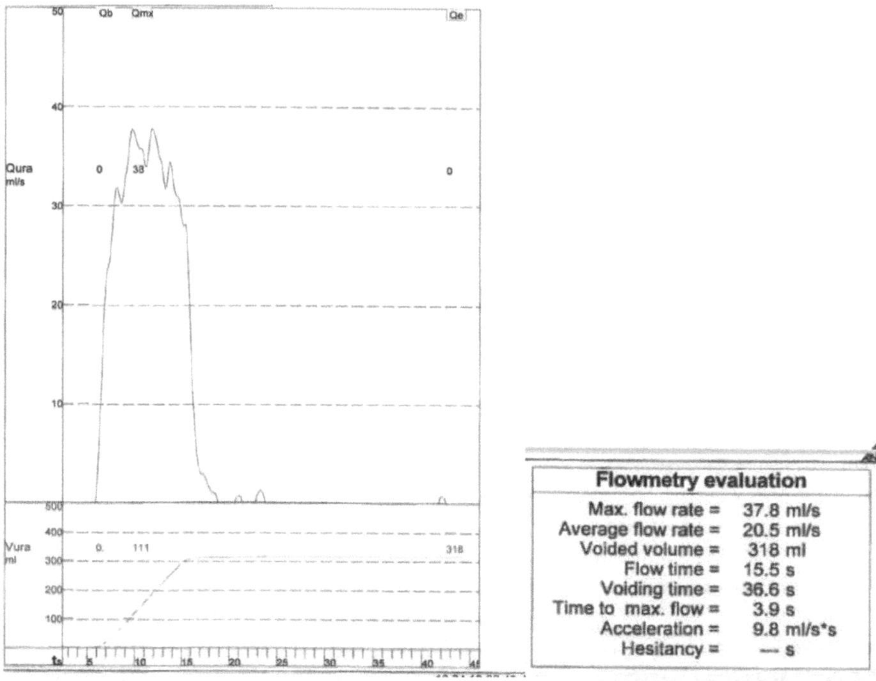
Qb
Qmx
Qe
Qura
ml/s
Vura
ml
Flowmetry evaluation
Max. flow rate = 37.8 ml/s
Average flow rate = 20.5 ml/s
Voided volume = 318 ml
Flow time = 15.5 s
Voiding time = 36.6 s
Time to max. flow = 3.9 s
Acceleration = 9.8 ml/s*s
Hesitancy = --- s

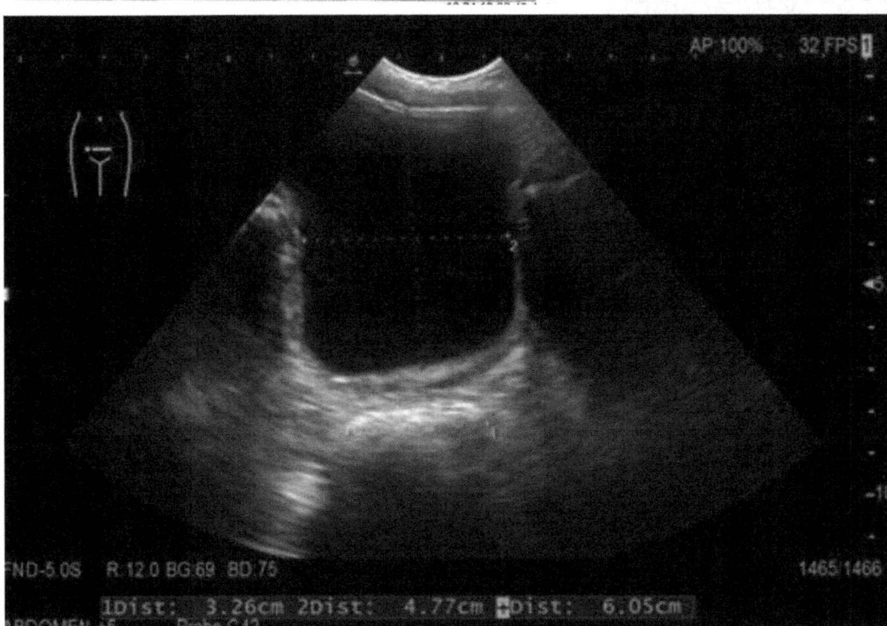
AP 100%
32 FPS
R 12.0 BG 69 BD 75
1465/1466
1Dist: 3.26cm 2Dist: 4.77cm
Dist: 6.05cm
Probe C42

Question 1: What further history would you like to know
Answer 1:
Psychological-social history
Dyslexia, IQ Verbal 118, performal 97
School results: concentration is low, results are fine
Brother is known with ADHD
Family: Father, mother, brother
Social: social contacts normal
Bullying and abuse: none
Question 2
What kind of incontinence is this?
Answer 2

- Daytime incontinence based on urgency and concentration problems. High flow rate, No further anatomical or neurological issues.

Question 3
How do you explain that he has been dry for 1 week after starting methylphenidate?
Answer 3

- Because of his concentration problems (ADHD) it is even more difficult to recognize the signals from his bladder. With methylphenidate his concentration improved and he is temporally able to react adequately on his bladder signals, but can't keep up. With therapy, he can learn to inhibit urgency complaints and to stay dry.

Question 4
What would be next steps?

- Start urotherapy: explanation and instructions about normal bowel and bladder behavior
- Start Intensive bladder training program, focused on learning to react adequately on bladder signals (learns how to void, when to void and how often to void).
- With biofeedback session by real-time uroflowmetry and EMG,
- During 3 months, frequently contact/support provided by the nurse/urotherapist
- Start anti cholinergics 2 × 2.5 mg oxybutynin and review in 3–4 months

21.4 Case 4

Charlotte 11 years old with daytime urge incontinence and giggle incontinence. She voids approximately 8 times a day with voided volumes varying between 50 and 200 ml per void. She has had recurrent cystitis and is on prophylactic antibiotics. Her bowels are open every 3 days, Bristol Stool Chart 1–3. Neurological examination is normal and the external genital examination shows a narrow meatus. Her urinary stream is deflected anteriorly with spraying. A perineal ultrasound demonstrates her inability to contract the pelvic floor muscle on coughing and a urethral length of 2 cm.

Her US and uroflowmetry with EMG is shown below

Charlotte US and flow

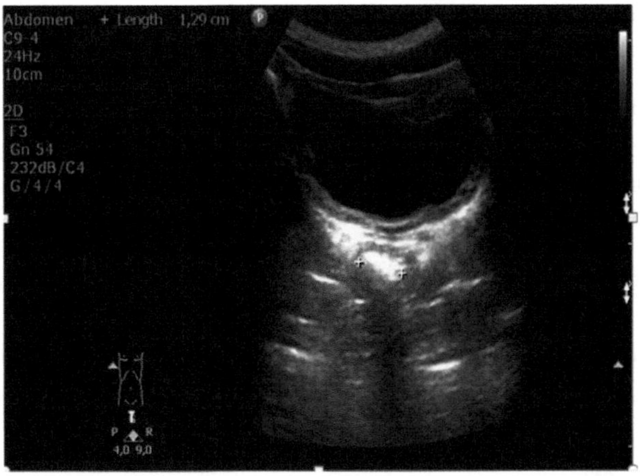

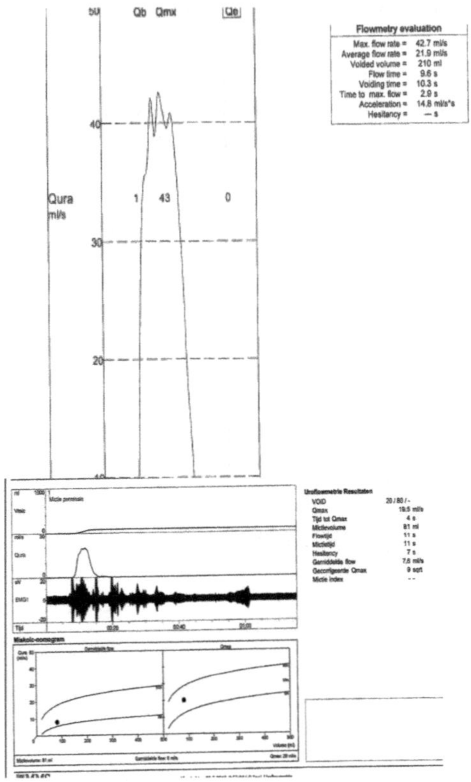

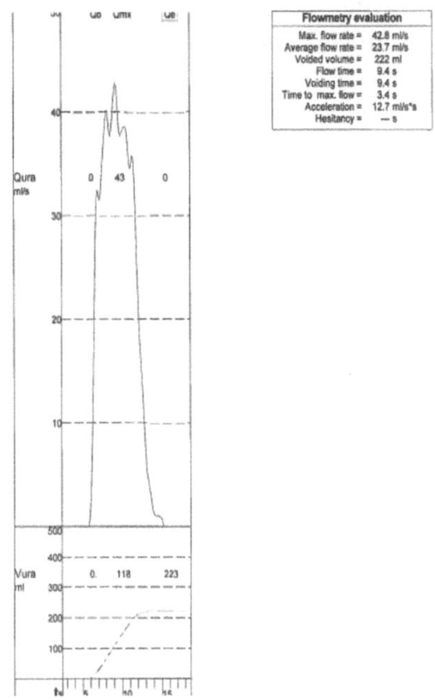

Question 1

What kind of incontinence is this?

Answer 1:

Daytime incontinence based on small bladder volume, UTI's and Anteriorly deflected urinary stream

Question 2

What would be next step?

Answer 2:

Cystoscopy and meatotomy to correct the direction of the urinary stream.

Question 3

Results after cystoscopy: She was able to relax during voiding, but still has daytime wetting once a day. What would your next treatment plan be?

Answer 3:

- bladder training program, focused on learning to react adequately on bladder signals (learns how to void, when to void and how often to void).
- With biofeedback session by real-time uroflowmetry and EMG,
- During 3 months, frequently contact/support provided by the nurse/urotherapist

Treatment Results urotherapy

After 4 months treatment with urotherapy. She was dry and happy

Author comment

Functioning voiding disorders are common and can be challenging to manage. Treatment strategies include a detailed history, clinical examination and appropriate investigations including bladder/bowel diary, uroflowmetry and renal ultrasound with post void residuals. For those children without organic pathology accounting for their symptoms, urotherapy, managing constipation, anticholinergics and most importantly psychological support from nurse specialists remains key. A checklist for evaluation is given below

Symptoms	Present?
Examination	Anatomical
	Neurological
UTI's	Yes/no
Urgency	Normal
	Imperative /urge
	Urge incontinence
	Urge on postponement
Bladder volume	Small (60% ebc)
	Normal
	Large (>150% ebc)
MF	<4
	5–7
	>7
Voiding behavior	Postponement
	Urgency
Incontinence	Yes/no
Wetting accidents	1/week.,
	2–5/week
	6–7/week
Wet during physical activity	Stress Y/N Giggle Y/N
Enuresis	Yes/no
Straining	Yes/no
PVR: >20 ml	Yes/no
Constipation	Yes/no
Rectum diameter	>3 cm
Fecal incontinence	Yes/no
Bristol stool score	1–7
Flow pattern	Bell shape
	Tower
	Staccato,
	Obstructive

21.5 Algorithm for Diagnostic Evaluation and Diagnosis of Children with Lower Urinary Tract Symptoms

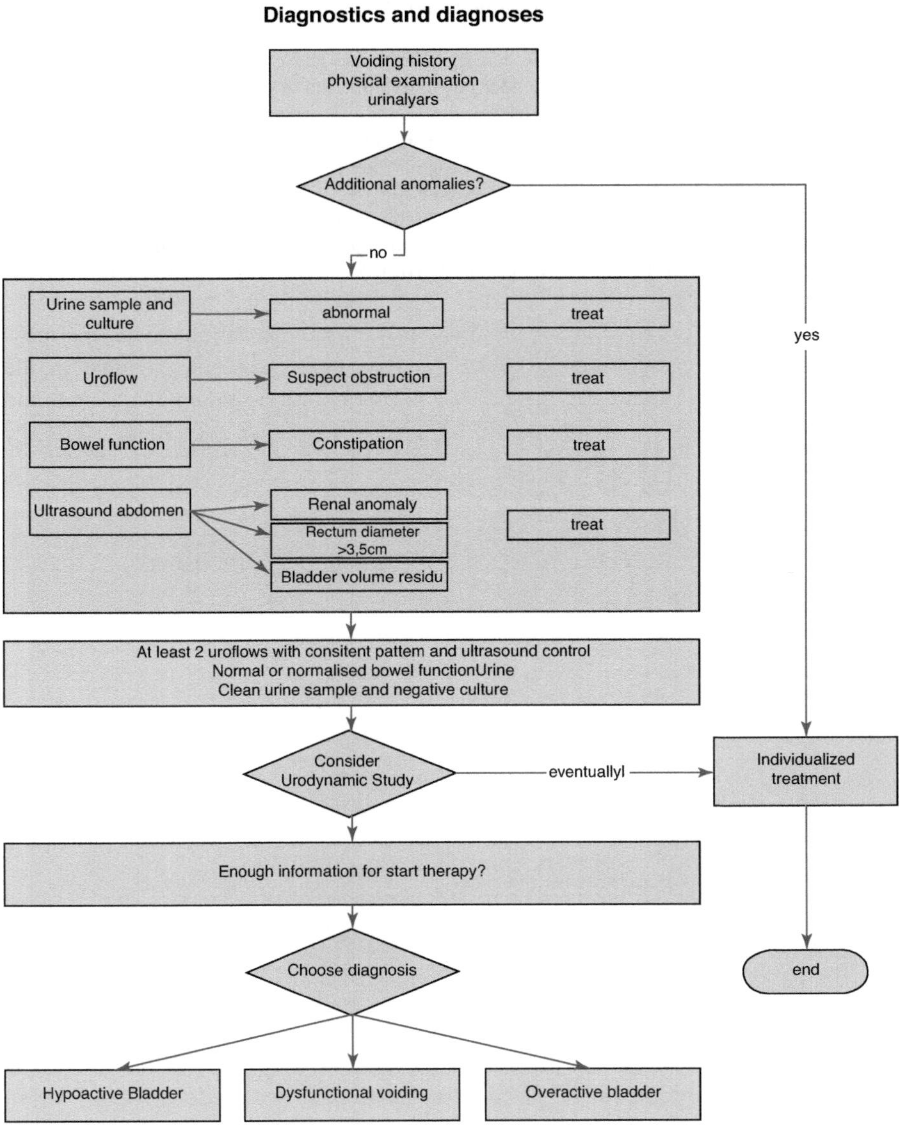

Suggested Further Reading

Fernandez-Ibieta M, Ayuso-Gonzalez L. Dysfunctional voiding in pediatrics: a review of pathophysiology and current treatment modalities. Curr Pediatr Rev. 2016;12(4):292–300.

Arlen AM. Dysfunctional Voiders-medication versus Urotherapy? Curr Urol Rep. 2017;18(2):14.

Tremback-Ball A, Gherghel E, Hegge A, Kindig K, Marsico H, Scanlon R. The effectiveness of biofeedback therapy in managing bladder bowel dysfunction in children: a systematic review. J Pediatr Rehabil Med. 2018;11(3):161–73.

Míguez-Fortes L, Somoza-Argibay I, Casal-Beloy I, García-González M, García-González M, Dargallo-Carbonell T. Analisys of non-neurogenic lower urinary tract dysfunction patterns controlled in a pediatric urodynamic unit. Arch Esp Urol. 2019;72(1):45–53.

Farhat W, Bägli DJ, Capolicchio G, O'Reilly S, Merguerian PA, Khoury A, McLorie GA. The dysfunctional voiding scoring system: quantitative standardization of dysfunctional voiding symptoms in children. J Urol. 2000;164(3 Pt 2):1011–5.

Neurogenic Bladder

22

Kyle O. Rove and Christopher S. Cooper

Learning Objectives

- Learn about the etiology of neurogenic bladder and common underlying disorders that gives rise to the condition.
- Understand the clinical management of a newborn with possible neurogenic bladder and differing strategies used by urologists.
- Discover nuances of formal urodynamic testing used in the assessment of patients with neurogenic bladder.
- Learn how surgery is used to reconstruct the urinary tract, aid with storage at low pressures, maintain adequate drainage and enhance continence.
- Understand the sexuality and reproductive health concerns of patients with neurogenic bladder and concomitant conditions that cause it.

22.1 Introduction and Definition

Neurogenic bladder non-specifically implies an abnormality of detrusor innervation causing dysfunction of the bladder. Nervous system injury may be congenital or acquired, peripheral or central, isolated or syndromic. The primary functions of the bladder are to store and empty urine through coordinated activity of the detrusor muscle and urinary sphincter, and dysregulation may result in leakage of urine, elevated pressures (storage or voiding), or inefficient emptying. Patients with

K. O. Rove (✉)
Department of Surgery, Division of Urology, Children's Hospital Colorado, University of Colorado, Aurora, CO, USA
e-mail: kyle.rove@childrenscolorado.org

C. S. Cooper
Division of Pediatric Urology, University of Iowa, Iowa City, IA, USA

P. Godbole et al. (eds.), *Practical Pediatric Urology*,
https://doi.org/10.1007/978-3-030-54020-3_22

neurogenic bladder are at risk for progressive injury to the urinary tract, including the kidneys. Appropriate attention and management are crucial to avoiding chronic kidney disease, achieving dryness, and improving quality of life.

22.2 Etiology

Case

A 41 year old grava-2-para-2 female presents to clinic at 30 weeks gestation with ultrasound findings of open myelomeningocele. What counseling would you provide regarding how common this diagnosis is and its underlying causes?

Spina bifida remains the most common cause of congenital neurogenic bladder in children. The worldwide incidence of spina bifida varies from 1.2 to 124.1 per 10,000 births [1]. The incidence has been decreasing over the last two decades owing to public health awareness of prenatal folic acid requirements [2–4]. The most severe form of neural tube defect is myelomeningocele and accounts for 90% of spina bifida cases, while lipomyelomeningocele or meningocele are less common. Other related causes of neurogenic bladder include closed and occult forms of neural tube defects such as tethered spinal cord, intradural lipoma, and intraspinal cysts. Spina bifida occulta represents the mildest form of spinal dysraphism, characterized by incomplete formation of the posterior spinous process and can be found in up to 15% of the population. It is not associated with neurologic dysfunction and is often an incidental finding.

One of the biggest risk factors for the development of neural tube defects is maternal low folate intake prenatally or dysregulated folate metabolic [5]. The first few weeks of gestation comprise the critical period of neuralation (closure of the neural tube from cephalad to caudad). Given this, adequate levels of folic acid are necessary, and supplementation of folic acid should start at least 2 months prior to planned pregnancies. In 1992, the United States recommended childbearing age women consume 400 mcg folic acid daily [6, 7]. Most developed countries now mandate folate supplementation in grain products, contributing to marked declines in the incidence of this disorder [8, 9]. Other risk factors that have been implicated in neural tube defects include maternal obesity, diabetes mellitus, and advanced maternal age (≥35 years old).

Other changes seen over the last 70 years include a marked improvement in survival of infants born with myelodysplasia [10, 11]. From 1956 to 1960, fewer than 20% of infants survived beyond 24 months of age. By the mid-1970s, survival rates increased to over 50%, and currently >90% of these infants will survive with the majority living into adulthood. Crucial advances over the years account for these dramatic changes. The ventriculoperitoneal (VP) shunt was introduced in the 1950s and changes how we care for those patients with Chiari malformation and hydrocephalus [12]. Lapides introduced the concept of clean intermittent catheterization in 1972, followed by the recognition of the need for proactively managing patients with an intravesical leak pressure over 40 cm of H_2O further improving outcomes [13, 14].

Prenatal recognition in now increasingly common with widespread use of screening ultrasounds. This has led to increased elective termination of the fetus with myelodysplasia [15, 16].

Although spina bifida is a common underlying cause of congentical forms of neurogenic bladder, other causes exist and include partial or complete sacral agenesis (caudal regression syndrome) and anorectal malformations. Acquired neurogenic bladder may occur after spinal cord trauma, tumors, extensive pelvic surgery, spinal cord infarction, transverse myelitis, and developmental syndromes such as cerebral palsy. Finally, idiopathic neurogenic bladder (non-neurogenic neurogenic bladder or Hinman's syndrome) is also encountered by urologists, and is characterized by long-standing dysfunction of the bladder, urinary retention and incontinence at presentation without neurological findings on exam or imaging studies.

22.3 Pathophysiology

Case

A 3 month old male with lumbosacral myelomeningocele present for initial urologic consultation with his parents. They are interested in knowing more about how the nerves in the spinal column have been disrupted and the implications for lower extremity, bowel, and bladder function.

Vertebral anomalies most commonly identified are in the lumbosacral spine, accounting for 50% of cases. Lumbar vertebral anomalies occur in 28% and thoracic anomalies account for the remaining 20%. Importantly, the bony level defect does not predict neurologic function or sensory level or bladder function.

The lower urinary tract functions to store and evacuate urine. The spine and brainstem coordinate these function. The hypogastric nerve fibers emanating from the lumbar region supply detrusor muscle sympathetics and urethral smooth muscle. Parasympathetic innervation of the detrusor occurs via pelvic nerves emanating out of the sacral spine. Pudendal nerve fibers travel from the sacral region and innervate the striated external urethral sphincter. The neural pathophysiology can be broken down into upper motor neuron and lower motor neuron lesions. The upper motor neuron lesions typically lead to an overactive bladder with no control of the sphincter. Contractions of an overactive bladder against a dyssynergic sphincter can lead to a thick-walled, hypertrophied bladder. Conversely a lower motor neuron lesion will lead to an acontractile, flaccid detrusor and some denervation of the external sphincter leading to urinary incontinence. Patients with these lesions usually have a small smooth-walled bladder. Because of spinal reflex pathways, lesions below the level of T6 may have some features of upper motor neuron lesion and some features of lower motor neuron lesions.

Arnold-Chiari malformation occurs in 85% of patients with meningomyelocele, in which the cerebellar tonsils herniate through the foramen magnum. Obstruction of the fourth ventricle then prevents the cerebrospinal fluid from entering the subarachnoid space around the brain and spinal cord leading to hydrocephalus. Ventricular peritoneal shunt has been key to prolonging survival in these patients.

22.4 Prenatal Intervention

Case

A G1P0 35 year old female presents at 20 weeks gestation with findings on prenatal ultrasound of open lumbar myelomeningocele of the fetus. She has read about prenatal intervention and seeks more information about the risks and benefits with regards to urinary function.

Surgical interventions on the growing fetus has become a reality in the last decade [17]. A prospective, randomized trial examined fetal intervention and repair of the meningomyelocele and subsequent clinical outcomes [18]. Called the MOMS trial, analysis of 158 randomized patients showed postnatal VP shunts were needed less often and suggested improvements in lower extremity function at 12 and 30 months age compared to patients who did not undergo fetal intervention. Bladder function, however, did not appear to be improved on urodynamics and need for intermittent catheterization did not change [19]. Fetal surgery interventions have been noted to increase the risk of preterm delivery and uterine dehiscence. More recent information suggests there might be a slight decrease in the need for clean intermittent catheterization and an increased ability to void spontaneously in children that had open neural tube defects closed prenatally although longer follow-up is needed.

22.5 Newborn Evaluation and Management

In order to minimize trauma to exposed neural tissues, cesarean section is recommended as the method of delivery for children with myelomeningocele. Initial management should involve a multidisciplinary team of neonatal intensivists, neurosurgery, urology, and orthopedic surgery. Spinal closure is recommended within the first 24 h of life to minimize the risk of meningitis.

No formal guidelines or recommendations currently exist for the urologic management of these patients. Many centers have transitioned from a reactionary approach to one motivated in trying to prevent any adverse changes in the upper and lower urinary tracts. This proactive strategy begins with placement of an indwelling bladder catheter after birth and initiation of clean intermittent catheterization in all children once they are cleared by the neurosurgery team to lay supine. Baseline postnatal renal and bladder ultrasound after 24–48 h and serum creatinine or cystatin c is also obtained. Once discharged, a voiding cystourethrogram or video urodynamic study is performed around 3 months to assess bladder capacity, filling pressures, compliance, presence of bladder overactivity, sphincteric function, and leak point pressures. Additionally the test will determine if there is vesicoureteral reflux and assess bladder neck configuration (open versus closed).

For patients with more subtle neural tube defects (spina bifida occulta), suggestive physical examination findings may include prominent sacral dimple, sacral mass, asymmetric gluteal cleft, posterior hair tuft, skin tag or hemangioma over the lower spine. These infants can be evaluated in the first 2–3 months of life with a spinal ultrasound to look for signs of tethered cord suggesting clinically important pathology. After this period, calcification of the spine makes ultrasound imaging less effective. The gold standard to rule out pathology is an MRI.

For patients who do not void spontaneously, intermittent catheterization is begun. For voiding patients, there are two strategies of clinical management. As noted above with the proactive approach, all children are started on intermittent catheterization and anticholinergics. The benefit of this approach is that parents and patients are accustomed to catheterization and avoids introduction at later ages. The other method of management after birth is close observation and with this approach the physician holds off on the initiation of anticholinergics and intermittent catheterization and follows these children frequently with renal and bladder ultrasounds as well as periodic urodynamic studies and only introduce catheterization and/or anticholinergics as needed. Patients eligible for this observation group should have safe bladder parameters on urodynamic studies. Patients with bladder parameters that would suggest the need to begin intermittent catheterization and possibly anticholinergics include a noncompliant high-pressure bladder or significant detrusor sphincter dyssynergia or high-grade of vesicoureteral reflux. In addition, indications to begin intermittent catheterization and anticholinergics include the development of hydronephrosis, worsening parameters on urodynamics, or recurrent urinary tract infections.

Proponents of early catheterization note that 80–90% of patients with meningomyelocele will have neurogenic bladder dysfunction and require catheterization at some point. The child and family incorporate intermittent catheterization into routine cares which may decrease problems with later acceptance of intermittent catheterization. While there is not great evidence at this time to support (or refute) proactive 'prophylactic' early intermittent catheterization and institution of anticholinergic therapy, it is hoped that it may prevent the need for subsequent bladder augmentation. Providers who select observation note that this decreases the burden on caregivers and introduces less bacteria into the urinary tract, avoiding some of the complexities of managing patients with asymptomatic bacteria and misidentification of urinary tract infections by other providers.

Asymptomatic bacteriuria is present in approximately 70% of patients who intermittently catheterize. Symptomatic urinary tract infections occur in <30%. Research has demonstrated that increasing the frequency of intermittent catheterization is associated with decreasing urinary tract infections. This may reduce stasis of urine, which can create an environment in which microorganisms have an increased chance to multiply and attach to the urothelium. Distinguishing between asymptomatic bacteruria and a urinary tract infection can be difficult to convey to caregivers and inexperienced providers. In general, providers ought to minimize the use of antibiotics wherever possible, as overuse leads to increased bacterial resistance and complicates future therapy.

22.6 Video Urodynamics

Case

A 6 year old male with history of resected sacrococcygeal teratoma is referred for urodynamics after recent issues with intermittent urinary retention and a urinary tract infection.

Urodynamics is a test of bladder and sphincteric function. It involves placement of a pressure-transducing catheter in the bladder and rectum [20]. If the patient has a vesicostomy, a balloon catheter should be used to occlude it during the test. For patients with colostomy or ileostomy, the rectal catheter can be placed in these structures to facilitate measuring abdominal pressures. Additionally, the vagina can be used to measure abdominal pressure. The bladder fill rate must be run at variable rates in pediatric patients because of different bladder capacities. The rate is typically 10% of the estimated bladder capacity per minute [21]. A patient's estimated bladder capacity is (age in years +2) × 30 ml [22]. During filling, the pressure in the bladder is recorded (P_{ves}). By subtracting abdominal pressure ($P_{ves} - P_{abd}$) from bladder pressure, the contribution of the detrusor muscle can be calculated (P_{det}). Sphincteric function is recorded with electromyography (typically patch electrodes). Fluoroscopic imaging can be used during the test to provide the video component which demonstrates bladder morphology, diverticulae, stones, trabeculations, vesicoureteral reflux, and bladder neck configuration (open versus closed) [23]. Recent studies have demonstrated that interpretation of urodynamics can be very subjective leading to significant intra- and inter-observer variations and interpretations [24, 25].

A healthy bladder should remain quiescent during filling with pressures less than 15 cm H_2O. During voiding, the detrusor muscle contracts after relaxation of the external sphincter allowing the bladder to empty. Post-void residual is routinely measured through urodynamic catheter drainage at the end of the study. During the filling, the following measurements are noted: maximum pressure (>40 cm H_2O is felt to be unsafe), presence of incontinence and associated pressure during the leakage (detrusor leak point pressures or DLPP > 40 cm H_2O are felt to be unsafe), compliance (volume over pressure, <20 ml/cm H_2O is abnormal) [13]. If the patient can void, providers look for evidence of detrusor-sphincter dyssynergia in addition to measuring voided volume, post-void residual, flow rate, flow curve appearance (bell-shaped, staccato, intermittent, flat) [26].

For patients with a dyssynergic sphincter, 70% will have subsequent urinary tract deterioration, including the development of hydronephrosis within 3 years. These patients with worrisome bladder parameters (detrusor sphincter dyssynergia, detrusor overactivity, elevated detrusor leak point pressures and elevated absolute filling pressures) should have escalation of bladder and urinary tract cares.

In 2016, a protocol was developed and published by the CDC National Spina Bifida Patient Registry establishing how often centers (21 total centers across the United States as of 2018) should perform various urologic testing and follow up in spina bifida patients [27]. At the moment, this is purely a research protocol to test thresholds and frequency for testing to detect clinically important changes. The protocol states that baseline studies be obtained around 3 months, and these are done again at ages 1, 2, and 3. In the presence of vesicoureteral reflux or a "hostile" bladder, formal urodynamics will be repeated every year up to age 5. In the future, this protocol will hopefully help clinicians determine appropriate testing frequencies.

Urodynamics can be used to guide patients in how often clean intermittent catheterization should be performed. For example, in patients who experience loss of compliance or increased absolute pressures near the end of filling, increasing the frequency of catheterization at home will help maintain filling pressures in the safe range, avoiding risk of upper tract changes like hydronephrosis or kidney injury. In general, patients are asked to adjust the frequency of catheterization so that the volume obtained is routinely held at a storage pressure <40 cm H2O.

As with early treatment options, there are two predominant schools of thought regarding how frequently to perform urodynamics on patients with spina bifida: annual testing or limited testing in response to changes in clinical status (e.g., new urinary tract infections, new or worsening urinary leakage, new or worsening upper tract dilation). Limited testing is not preferred by some because hydronephrosis is not a sensitive early indicator of changing lower tract function [28]. Proponents of this minimalist approach argue it is more cost effective and not solely predicated on hydronephrosis but all relevant clinical factors. Furthermore, annual testing itself may not provide great sensitivity and the number of studies required to be done to detect a meaningful change in one patient (that would result in a change in clinical management) may be cost prohibitive. Most agree regular follow up is key to ensuring safe upper tracts, avoiding long-term deleterious changes to the urinary tract, and minimizing risk of urinary tract infection. At the time of this writing, a simple hand-held device for home use that measures bladder pressure and attaches to the end of any catheter has been developed and is being tested at the University of Iowa (Cooper CS et al.). The hope is that this device will aid in monitoring the dynamic changes occurring in the neurogenic bladder and help improve management.

22.7 Tethered Spinal Cord

Case

A neurosurgeon refers a 5 year old male with concerns for tethered cord requesting a urologic evaluation prior to surgical intervention.

Tethered spinal cord is an evolving clinical entity that challenges neurosurgeons and urologists alike. In recent years, debate continues as to who should have surgery and who can be safely observed. Some of this complexity arises because 60% of the time, patients will have a normal urodynamic study as an infant. By 3 years of age, only 20% have a completely normal urodynamics result, however often, the abnormal findings are non-specific. Treatment in infancy with de-tethering of the spinal cord has improved outcome. In general children with a tethered spinal cord have a much better prognosis than those with meningomyelocele. Although deterioration is uncommon after surgery, 25% of children will have re-tethering of the spinal cord so these children also require continuous monitoring and follow-up. Studies have examined urodynamic outcomes before and after de-tethering for patients with tethered cord from occult spinal dysraphism and re-tethering after myelomeningocele closure [29–31]. Because of mixed results and the low intra- and inter-rater reliability of urodynamics testing, results should be interpreted with caution.

22.8 Appendicovesicostomy

Case

An 8 year old female with sacral agenesis performs clean intermittent catheterization. On urodynamics, her bladder capacity is 280 ml, she has minimal detrusor overactivity, no vesicoureteral reflux, and maximum detrusor pressure of 15 cm H_2O*. She and her parents are interested in increased independence with catheterization.*

Appendicovesicostomy has been a significant step forward for patients with neurogenic bladder who either cannot tolerate catheterization per urethra or who desire greater independence or continence. This technique or principle was first described by Paul Mitrofanoff, and requires the appendix (or other tubularized bowel) be disconnected from the gastrointestinal tract and connected to the bladder and skin allowing for intermittent catheterization to empty the bladder [32]. It permits increased independence by many patients. By itself, it is durable and allows patients to achieve continence in high numbers. About 15% of patients will develop stenosis over a 5-year time frame, which requires surgical revision typically at the skin stoma.

If an appendix is not available (removed in prior surgery, lumen is not patent, or it is planned to be used as another channel such as appendicocecostomy), alternatives include a straight, spiral, or double ileovesicostomy or colovesicostomy (also known as Monti or Yang-Monti channels named eponymously) [33, 34]. These channels involve selected a piece of ileum or sigmoid colon and reconfiguring them into a tube. False passages are less common with appendicovesicostomies than other techniques. Double ileovesicostomy (two independent tubularized segments of ileum sewn together end to end), for example, have the highest complications with catheterization (false passage, diverticulum, stenosis) [35].

22.9 Nocturnal Catheterization

Patients who perform intermittent catheterization do not usually catheterize at night, as this can be burdensome realizing that nighttime for most patients is the longest interval between catheterizations. In some patients, this can lead to high-pressure storage scenarios with poor downstream consequences for kidneys and bladder. Koff reported nighttime catheterization for children with a history of posterior urethral valves and borderline bladder pressures, and he demonstrated these patients subsequently had improved hydronephrosis, fewer urinary tract infections, less incontinence, and increased bladder capacity [36]. Similar improvements have been demonstrated in children with neurogenic bladder by either leaving an indwelling catheter overnight or having the patient undergo catheterization at night [37].

22.10 Vesicoureteral Reflux

As many as 20% of patients with neurogenic bladder will have vesicoureteral reflux [38]. About half resolve the reflux once they are started on intermittent catheterization and anticholinergic medication. In most patients, reflux in this setting is felt to represent secondary reflux from hostile bladder dynamics. By improving these dynamics, the reflux may improve or resolve. If reflux persists and the patient is having recurrent urinary tract infections, ureteral reimplantation does have a high success rate but can be challenging in patients with long-standing neurogenic bladder (thick-walled, fibrotic bladders). Endoscopic sub-ureteric bulking agents have a lower success rate of 60–70%. Ureteral obstruction is a risk following ureteral reimplantation into a poorly-compliant bladder, stressing how important medical (and surgical) management of the bladder is prior to treating reflux. In some cases, patients may require cutaneous vesicostomy or bladder augmentation to reduce pressures and aid with reflux resolution.

22.11 Continence

Although there is poor correlation between level of lesion and clinical outcomes, continence outcomes are better for children with certain types of lesions: tethered spinal cord, sacral myelomeningocele, or lipomeningocele. Continence may be achieved or improved with medical management options discussed above, including clean intermittent catheterization, anticholinergics, alpha sympathomimetics, intradetrusor botulinum toxin injection, or beta 3 agonists.

Oxybutynin, an anticholinergic medication used to treat detrusor overactivity and neurogenic bladder is the only FDA approved medication for children for this indication. It competitively binds the M2 and M3 acetylcholine receptors in the bladder. It can be dispensed in liquid, oral and transdermal forms. The oral form comes in both immediate-release tablets (dosing every 8 or 12 h) and extended-release capsules (once daily dosing with potentially fewer side effects from slow release pharmacokinetics). Common side effects of this class of medications include facial flushing, heat intolerance, dry mouth, confusion, and constipation. Of note, anticholinergic use has been associated with increased risk of dementia in the elderly, but has not been studied long-term in children [39].

Botulinum a toxin is produced by *Clostridium botulinum*, and when injected into the detrusor, the toxin cleaves SNAP-25, a SNARE protein required for fusion of vesicles in the presynaptic neuron which release acetylcholine into the neuromuscular junction. Without release of acetylcholine, no action potential is delivered to the postsynaptic membrane and the muscle does not contract. The common dosage used by pediatric urologists is 10 international units (IU) per kg up to 2–300 IU [40]. It is not currently FDA approved in children with neurogenic bladder, but it has been shown to be safe and efficacious in multiple studies of both children and adults with neurogenic bladder. Patients should be prepared to self-catheterize if they are not already because of risk of urinary retention. If efficacious for a patient, it can be re-dosed every as soon as every 3 months, but is typically re-injected every 6–12 months. Effects are monitored by clinical history or urodynamics. In one study of myelomeningocele patients, 73% of patients treated with botox were dry between catheterizations 4 months later, 88% had symptom improvement, and 73% improvement in reflux (if present) [41]. Systemic side effects are very rare. Urinary tract infections is a risk factor from instrumentation.

A number of surgical procedures have been described to reduce or eliminate leakage of urine in patients with neurogenic bladder. These operations are aimed at increasing resistance at the bladder outlet. When considering these surgeries, patients should be motivated to self-catheterize because access via the native urethra becomes more difficult. All patients should have preoperative evaluation that include upper tract imaging as well as video urodynamics to assess bladder capacity, ideally with the bladder outlet occluded. Surgeons should also consider bladder compliance and detrusor overactivity as these can continue to alter bladder dynamics in the future and should be planned for as necessary. To this end, increasing the outlet resistance should only be undertaking in a "safe" bladder otherwise bladder augmentation should be strongly considered at the time of bladder outlet procedure.

Surgical continence procedures can be grouped into those that increased the length of the urethra, narrow the opening of the bladder neck, compress the bladder neck or urethra with a bulking agent, placement of a urethral or bladder neck sling, implantation of an artificial urinary sphincter, or closure of the bladder neck. Bladder neck closure is considered a second line continence operation, and at least for these authors, is usually only considered and doneafter failure of other first line surgical options. One difficulty in interpreting the literature regarding success rates from these options is the significantly different definitions of continence used by authors, limiting comparisons. Furthermore, many studies suffer from small numbers, single center or single surgeon outcomes and render interpretation challenging. Bulking agents have been shown to have poor long-term outcomes. Bladder neck reconstructions or slings can increase the risk of bladder stones (as many as 40% in 5 years) with one third of these patients developing a recurrent stone.

In situations of persistent incontinence following an initial surgical procedure, the operation may be repeated or an injection of a bulking agent may be attempted. In these situations, success has been reported at a rate of 25% with 1 or 2 injections. As noted above the bladder neck closure is an alternative, second-line option to consider. Finally, a continent catheterizable reservoir or incontinent diversion (ileal conduit) are other long-term options that may deliver desired continence and long-term solution.

22.12 Bladder Augmentation

Case

A 7 year old, wheelchair-bound male with lumbar spina bifida has been followed with urodynamics and most recently noted to have markedly reduced compliance and increased filling pressures despite being on oxybutynin and having tried intra-detrusor botox.

Patients with small bladder capacity, high absolute filling pressures ($P_{ves} > 40$ cm H_2O), elevated detrusor leak point pressures (>35 cm H_2O), or poor compliance (< 10 ml/cm H_2O) may need to consider bladder augmentation. These patients often have upper tract changes like hydronephrosis, hydroureteronephrosis, or secondary vesicoureteral reflux. Bladder augmentation (also called cystoplasty, ileocystoplasty, or enterocystoplasty) is usually performed with a segment of ileum or sigmoid colon. The segment is detubularized and may be reconfigured. It is then attached to the bladder which is opened widely either with a transverse or longitudinal cystotomy. This results in an increase in bladder capacity and improved compliance. By lowering pressure, it may help with secondary vesicoureteral reflux as well. It is most frequently needed in those with thoracic and lumbar meningomyelocele. The rates are lower in those with sacral and lipomeningocele and is only rarely needed in those with a tethered spinal cord.

Most recently, there has been ongoing work to improve short-term patient outcomes after these surgeries, which typically leave patients in the hospital for 7–10 days on average [42, 43]. Colleagues at Children's Hospital Colorado adapted Enhanced Recovery After Surgery protocols from adult patients undergoing radical cystectomy for these patients to focus on consistently delivering care shown to improve outcomes throughout the pre-, intra- and postoperative phases of care [44]. The protocol focuses on minimizing *nil per os* times, omitting nasogastric tubes, minimizing opioids, favoring regional anesthetics [45] and scheduled non-opioid pain medications, and mobilization out of bed by the day after surgery. By consistently practicing in this manner, length of stay dropped from 8 to 5.4 days and complications per patient improved from 2.1 to 1.3 ($p = 0.035$). This pilot study demonstrated that this complex procedure could be made safer and allow patients to leave the hospital sooner without increasing the risk of visit to the emergency room, re-operation or re-admission. A larger multicenter trial is currently ongoing to determine if these results can be replicated at other centers [46].

The long-term complications of augmentation cystoplasty are not insignificant, and approximately one third of patients will require an additional operation at a mean of 13 years following the initial augmentation [47]. The metabolic complications that can occur include acid-base alterations and subsequent changes in bone metabolism. When ileum or colon is used, expect an increased risk of hyperchloremic hypokalemic metabolic acidosis. If terminal ileum is used as part of the reconstruction, patients are at risk of vitamin B_{12} deficiency, as this bowel segment contains essential receptors for intrinsic factor-bound B_{12}. Cystoplasty patients are at increased risk for asymptomatic bacteruria, recurrent urinary tract infections as well as bladder stone formation. Up to 5% of bladder augmentation patients may suffer a bladder perforation at some point during their life with significant risk of mortality. Clincians should have a high index of suspicion in bladder augmentation patients who present with abdominal pain and fever. A CT cystogram appears to be more sensitive than a standard fluoroscopic cystogram. If a fluoroscopic cystogram is performed, oblique and lateral views are key to ensure complete visualization of the bladder full of contrast. Posterior leaks may be missed with typical anterior-posterior views. Similarly, about 5% of augmenation patients will experience bowel obstruction within 15 years of their operation.

Bladder cancer risk after augmentation has been estimated to occur in between 1 and 4% of patients [48]. Higuchi et al. compared the rates of bladder cancer in a database of neurogenic bladder patients who were and were not augmented [49]. Of 153 ileal and colonic bladder augmentation patients matched to similarly aged controls without augmentation, there was no difference in the rates of bladder cancer (7 augmented patients [4.6%] vs. 4 controls [2.6%], $p = 0.54$). Similarly, the authors noted no differences between the groups in terms of age at diagnosis (51 vs. 49.5 years), stage (3.4 vs. 3.8), mortality rate (71 vs. 100%) or median survival (18 vs. 17 months). A follow up systematic review of the literature published in 2017 searched for publications that included patients with spina bifida and bladder cancer [50]. The authors found 28 articles with 50 patients, with an additional 2 patients from institutional databases. Median age of diagnosis was 41 years (ranging from 13 to 73 years), and 71% presented with stage III or IV bladder cancer. Overall survival was low at 1 and 2 years (48.5 and 31.5%, respectively). On analysis of overall survival, comparison of patients with and without bladder augmentation favored patients with bladder augmentation in those who develop bladder cancer (overall survival at 2 years was 61.4 vs. 14.5%, $p = 0.009$). Secondary analysis removed patients with gastric augmentation, and these differences disappeared. Importantly, these results do not reflect the risk of developing bladder cancer, but rather showed that bladder augmentation does not worsen cancer outcomes compared to other spina bifida patients with longstanding neurogenic bladder who also develop bladder cancer.

Bladder cancer in patients with neurogenic bladder often cause atypical or non-specific symptoms making early diagnoisis difficult. For a time, cystoscopy and cytology were advocated beginning 10 years after augmentation or urinary diversion. However, data from Higuchi and Husmann et al. demonstrated that of 250 cystoscopies, only 4 suspicious lesions were found and none identified cancer after biopsy [51]. Based on the rarity of bladder cancer in this population, routine screening was not cost effective. This same group published an algorithm that new pain, gross hematuria, 4 or more UTIs in a single year, or new onset of urinary incontinence should prompt further investigation with strong consideration of urine culture, cross-sectional imaging with and without contrast and endoscopy [52]. In the absence of these symptoms, patients should be seen annually and evaluated with serum creatinine or cystitis C, serum electrolytes, B_{12} levels, and urinalysis with microscopy. If there is gross hematuria ≥50 RBCs/HPF, patients should additionally be considered for renal bladder ultrasound. Often these patients with bladder cancer will have hematuria but it is be attributed to trauma from catheterization.

Because of the significant complications associated with bladder augmentation, work has been done to develop biological scaffolds that are purpose made for the individual [53]. At present there are no large clinical studies demonstrating efficacy of these techniques, but they hold promise for the future in eliminating some of the current described complications with bladder augmentation using intestine.

22.13 Transition to Puberty in Adulthood

Case

A 17 year old female with history of bladder augmentation, appendicovesicostomy for spina bifida presents with her parents and increasing concerns about non-compliance with intermittent catheterization.

Patients with congenital anomalies like neurogenic bladder with mental faculties and ability must be prepared to take charge of their own health care as they get older. There are studies of adolescents and young adults that show these patients are at risk for reduced compliance with self-cares [54]. 2/3 of adult neurogenic bladder patients do not seek regular urologic follow-up. 1/2 of those on intermittent catheterization stop intermittent catheterization in defiance of medical advice. Sometimes, we find young men using a catheter that is too small which can increase the risk of urethral injury, prolong drainage time and thus increase risk of noncompliance. Poor compliance increases risk of upper tract changes. Before the introduction of intermittent catheterization by Lapides, few would live into adulthood. Now, patients with neurogenic bladders are more likely to die from nonneurologic causes such as pulmonary embolism, infection or shunt failure [55]. Given the risks of these sequelae are not insignificant, these patients continue to require multispecialty healthcare throughout their lives.

22.14 Sexuality and Reproductive Health

In females with spina bifida, menarche has been reported to start earlier than the general population [56]. Early puberty in the general population has been estimated at 0.6% whereas it may occur as often as 12% in girls with spina bifida. These patients are at increased risk of uterine prolapse. Finally, these patients also report using less birth control when sexually active.

Female spina bifida patients who become pregnant have unique anatomic and surgical considerations, particularly if she has a history of prior urinary tract reconstructive operations. Each patient should be evaluated by a multidisciplinary team including obstetrician-gynecologist, urologist and other providers. In one recent case series, 17 women with spina bifida had 29 total pregnancies [57]. 23 (79%)

resulted in live offspring. No offspring had spina bifida, but 3 (13%) were born with other malformations. About 50% of patients required cesarean sections with postpartum complications that required prolonged hospitalization. Still, 37% of vaginal delivery mothers had postpartum complications. No problems were encountered specifically with ventriculoperitoneal shunts in patients who had them.

Males with spina bifida may experience erectile dysfunction to varying degrees. In one study of 40 male patients over 18 years age, each filled out the International Index of Erectile Function (IIEF) questionnaire [58]. Of the 16 patient who had had sexual intercourse during the previous month, 4 had no ED, 3 had mild, 4 mild to moderate, and 5 severe dysfunction. Another study of outcomes in men found the level of the spinal lesion (at least in patients with spina bifida) had no relation to erectile function, and testosterone levels were normally distributed in those tested [59].

One-quarter to one-third of meningomyelocele adolescent and young adults between 14 and 23 years age report having had sexual encounters [60]. This is more common in women than men. Most desired increased discussions of sexuality with providers. Providers have also expressed increased desire for better training in how to approach patients with these concerns [61]. Only 50% report satisfaction with sex life. Those male patients with neurologic lesions at S1 or lower are more likely to have normal sexual function.

It is important to note that a large fraction (up to 30%) of patients with spina bifida also report unwanted sexual attention. These patients may be vulnerable because they may depend on others for their urologic care, have few external relationships by which to report such activity [60].

22.15 Conclusions

Neurogenic bladder is a complex medical condition that is life-long and requires regular monitoring. Management can range from simple lifestyle changes to medicines to surgical reconstruction. Each patient should be evaluated and managed with the ultimate goals including kidney and bladder function preservation and continence as well as sexual and reproductive function as desired.

Funding No sources identified.

References

1. Zaganjor I, Sekkarie A, Tsang BL, et al. Describing the prevalence of neural tube defects worldwide: a systematic literature review. Edited by R Cruz-Martinez. PLoS One. 2016;11:e0151586.
2. Stein SC, Feldman JG, Friedlander M, et al. Is myelomeningocele a disappearing disease? Pediatrics. 1982;69:511–4.
3. Yen IH, Khoury MJ, Erickson JD, et al. The changing epidemiology of neural tube defects: United States, 1968-1989. Am J Dis Child. 1992;146:857–61.

4. Stevenson RE, Allen WP, Pai GS, et al. Decline in prevalence of neural tube defects in a high-risk region of the United States. Pediatrics. 2000;106:677–83.
5. Werler MM. Periconceptional folic acid exposure and risk of Occurrent neural tube defects. JAMA. 1993;269:1257–61.
6. Centers for Disease Control and Prevention: Recommendations for the Use of Folic Acid to Reduce the Number of Cases of Spina Bifida and Other Neural Tube Defects. CDC.gov 1992. https://www.cdc.gov/mmwr/preview/mmwrhtml/00019479.htm. Accessed 9 July 2019.
7. Bibbins-Domingo K, Grossman DC, Curry SJ, et al. Folic acid supplementation for the prevention of neural tube defects: US preventive services task force recommendation statement. JAMA. 2017;317:183–9.
8. Honein MA, Paulozzi LJ, Mathews TJ, et al. Impact of folic acid fortification of the US food supply on the occurrence of neural tube defects. JAMA. 2001;285:2981–6.
9. De Wals P, Tairou F, Van Allen MI, et al. Reduction in neural-tube defects after folic acid fortification in Canada. N Engl J Med. 2007;357:135–42.
10. Wong L-YC, Paulozzi LJ. Survival of infants with spina bifida: a population study, 1979–94. Paediatr Perinat Epidemiol. 2001;15:374–8.
11. Shin M, Kucik JE, Siffel C, et al. Improved survival among children with Spina bifida in the United States. J Pediatr. 2012;161:1132–1137.e3.
12. Jackson IJ, Snodgrass SR. Peritoneal shunts in the treatment of hydrocephalus and increased intracranial pressure; a 4-year survey of 62 patients. J Neurosurg. 1955;12:216–22.
13. McGuire EJ, Woodside JR, Borden TA, et al. Prognostic value of urodynamic testing in myelodysplastic patients. J Urol. 1981;126:205–9.
14. Bauer SB, Hallett M, Khoshbin S, et al. Predictive value of urodynamic evaluation in newborns with Myelodysplasia. JAMA. 1984;252:650–2.
15. Velie EM, Shaw GM. Impact of prenatal diagnosis and elective termination on prevalence and risk estimates of neural tube defects in California, 1989–1991. Am J Epidemiol. 1996;144:473–9.
16. Forrester MB, Merz RD, Yoon PW. Impact of prenatal diagnosis and elective termination on the prevalence of selected birth defects in Hawaii. Am J Epidemiol. 1998;148:1206–11.
17. Meller C, Aiello H, Otaño L. Sonographic detection of open spina bifida in the first trimester: review of the literature. Childs Nerv Syst. 2017;33:1101–6.
18. Adzick NS, Thom EA, Spong CY, et al. A randomized trial of prenatal versus postnatal repair of Myelomeningocele. N Engl J Med. 2011;364:993–1004.
19. Brock JW, Carr MC, Adzick NS, et al. Bladder function after fetal surgery for Myelomeningocele. Pediatrics. 2015;136:e906–13.
20. Schäfer W, Abrams P, Liao L, et al. Good urodynamic practices: uroflowmetry, filling cystometry, and pressure-flow studies**. Neurourol Urodyn. 2002;21:261–74.
21. Hjälmås K. Urodynamics in normal infants and children. Scand J Urol Nephrol Suppl. 1988;114:20–7.
22. Koff SA. Estimating bladder capacity in children. Urology. 1983;21:248.
23. Glazier DB, Murphy DP, Fleisher MH, et al. Evaluation of the utility of video-urodynamics in children with urinary tract infection and voiding dysfunction. J Urol. 1998;160:281–2.
24. Venhola M, Reunanen M, Taskinen S, et al. Interobserver and intra-observer agreement in interpreting urodynamic measurements in children. J Urol. 2003;169:2344–6.
25. Dudley AG, Casella DP, Lauderdale CJ, et al. Interrater reliability in pediatric urodynamic tracings: a pilot study. J Urol. 2017;197:865–70.
26. Austin PF, Bauer SB, Bower W, et al. The standardization of terminology of lower urinary tract function in children and adolescents: update report from the standardization Committee of the International Children's continence society. J Urol. 2014;191:1863–1865.e13.
27. Routh JC, CHENG EY, Austin JC, et al. Design and methodological considerations of the Centers for Disease Control and Prevention urologic and renal protocol for the newborn and young child with Spina bifida. J Urol. 2016;196:1728–34.
28. Kaufman AM, Ritchey ML, Roberts AC, et al. Decreased bladder compliance in patients with Myelomeningocele treated with radiological observation. J Urol. 1996;156:2031–3.

29. Fone PD, Vapnek JM, Litwiller SE, et al. Urodynamic findings in the tethered spinal cord syndrome: does surgical release improve bladder function? J Urol. 1997;157:604–9.
30. Nogueira M, Greenfield SP, Wan J, et al. Tethered cord in children: a clinical classification with urodynamic correlation. J Urol. 2004;172:1677–80. discussion 1680.
31. Hsieh MH, Perry V, Gupta N, et al. The effects of detethering on the urodynamics profile in children with a tethered cord. J Neurosurg Pediatr. 2006;105:391–5.
32. Mitrofanoff P. Trans-appendicular continent cystostomy in the management of the neurogenic bladder. Chir Pediatr. 1980;21:297–305.
33. Yang W-H. Yang needle tunneling technique in creating Antireflux and continent mechanisms. J Urol. 1993;150:830–4.
34. Monti PR, Lara RC, Dutra MA, et al. New techniques for construction of efferent conduits based on the mitrofanoff principle. Urology. 1997;49:112–5.
35. Narayanaswamy B, Wilcox DT, Cuckow PM, et al. The Yang–Monti ileovesicostomy: a problematic channel? Br J Urol. 2001;87:861–5.
36. Koff SA, Mutabagani KH, Jayanthi VR. The valve bladder syndrome: pathophysiology and treatment with nocturnal bladder emptying. J Urol. 2002;167:291–7.
37. Koff SA, Gigax MR, Jayanthi VR. Nocturnal bladder emptying: a simple technique for reversing urinary tract deterioration in children with neurogenic bladder. J Urol. 2005;174:1629–31. discussion 1632.
38. Wu CQ, Franco I. Management of vesicoureteral reflux in neurogenic bladder. Investig Clin Urol. 2017;58:S54–8.
39. Cooper CS. Fat, demented, and stupid: an unrecognized legacy of pediatric urology? J Pediatr Urol. 2017;13(4):341–4.
40. Dyer L, Franco I. Botulinum toxin-a therapy in pediatric urology: indications for the neurogenic and non-neurogenic neurogenic bladder. Sci World J. 2009;9:1300–5.
41. Kajbafzadeh A-M, Moosavi S, Tajik P, et al. Intravesical injection of botulinum toxin type a: management of neuropathic bladder and bowel dysfunction in children with myelomeningocele. Urology. 2006;68:1091–6.
42. Bowlin P, Siparsky G, Wilcox D. Nationwide review of bladder augmentation in pediatric hospitals. J Urol. 2011;185:e477.
43. Schlomer BJ, Saperston K, Baskin L. National Trends in augmentation Cystoplasty in the 2000s and factors associated with patient outcomes. J Urol. 2013;190:1352–8.
44. Rove KO, Brockel MA, Saltzman AF, et al. Prospective study of enhanced recovery after surgery protocol in children undergoing reconstructive operations. J Pediatr Urol. 2018;14:252.e1–9.
45. Chalmers DJ, Bielsky A, Wild TT, et al. Continuous local anesthetic infusion for children with spina bifida undergoing major reconstruction of the lower urinary tract. J Pediatr Urol. 2015;11:72.e1–5.
46. Clinical Trial NCT03245242: Pediatric Urology Recovery After Surgery Endeavor (PURSUE). U.S. National Institutes of Health 2017. https://clinicaltrials.gov/ct2/show/NCT03245242. Accessed 31 Aug 2017.
47. Schlomer BJ, Copp HL. Cumulative incidence of outcomes and urologic procedures after augmentation cystoplasty. J Pediatr Urol. 2014;10:1043–50.
48. Soergel TM, Cain MP, Misseri R, et al. Transitional cell carcinoma of the bladder following augmentation Cystoplasty for the neuropathic bladder. J Urol. 2004;172:1649–52.
49. Higuchi TT, Granberg CF, Fox JA, et al. Augmentation cystoplasty and risk of neoplasia: fact, fiction and controversy. J Urol. 2010;184:2492–6.
50. Rove KO, Husmann DA, Wilcox DT, et al. Systematic review of bladder cancer outcomes in patients with spina bifida. J Pediatr Urol. 2017;13:456.e1–9.
51. Higuchi TT, Fox JA, Husmann DA. Annual endoscopy and urine cytology for the surveillance of bladder tumors after Enterocystoplasty for congenital bladder anomalies. J Urol. 2011;186:1791–5.
52. Husmann DA, Fox JA, Higuchi TT. Malignancy following bladder augmentation: recommendations for long-term follow-up and cancer screening. AUA Update Ser. 2011;24:221–7.

53. Atala A, Bauer SB, Soker S, et al. Tissue-engineered autologous bladders for patients needing cystoplasty. Lancet. 2006;367:1241–6.
54. Husmann DA. Long-term complications following bladder augmentations in patients with spina bifida: bladder calculi, perforation of the augmented bladder and upper tract deterioration. Transl Androl Urol. 2016;5:3–11.
55. Oakeshott P, Hunt GM, Poulton A, et al. Expectation of life and unexpected death in open spina bifida: a 40-year complete, non-selective, longitudinal cohort study. Developmental medicine &amp. Child Neurology. 2010;52:749–53.
56. Jackson AB, Mott PK. Reproductive health care for women with spina bifida. Sci World J. 2007;7:1875–83.
57. Arata M, Grover S, Dunne K, et al. Pregnancy outcome and complications in women with spina bifida. J Reprod Med. 2000;45:743–8.
58. Gamé X, Moscovici J, Gamé L, et al. Evaluation of sexual function in young men with spina bifida and myelomeningocele using the international index of erectile function. Urology. 2006;67:566–70.
59. Decter RM, Furness PD, Nguyen TA, et al. Reproductive understanding, sexual functioning and testosterone levels in men with Spina bifida. J Urol. 1997;157:1466–8.
60. Sawyer SM, Roberts KV. Sexual and reproductive health in young people with spina bifida. Dev Med Child Neurol. 1999;41:671–5.
61. Streur CS, Schafer CL, Garcia VP, et al. "I Don't know what I'm doing… I Hope I'm not just an idiot": the need to train pediatric urologists to discuss sexual and reproductive health care with young women with Spina bifida. J Sexual Medicine. 2018;15:1403–13.

Disorders of Sex Development

23

Prasad Godbole and Neil Wright

Learning Objectives

- Understand the development of male and female internal and external genitalia
- Identify the different forms of disorders of sex development
- Understand the investigations of disorders of sex development
- Understand the principles of treatment of different forms of disorders of sex development including genital surgery

23.1 Scenario 1

You are called to the neonatal unit to see a newborn with appearances of the genitalia as shown below (Figs. 23.1 and 23.2):

23.1.1 Picture of CAH

23.1.1.1 Question 1

What specific points do you wish to address in the clinical examination in this case and of newborns with DSD in general?

23.1.1.2 Answer 1

The main question to be answered is if this is a overvirilised female (46XX DSD) or undervirilised male 46XY DSD).

P. Godbole (✉)
Department of Paediatric Surgery, Sheffield Children's NHS Foundation Trust, Sheffield, UK
e-mail: p.godbole@nhs.net

N. Wright
Department of Paediatric Endocrinology, Sheffield Children's NHS Foundation Trust, Sheffield, UK

P. Godbole et al. (eds.), *Practical Pediatric Urology*,
https://doi.org/10.1007/978-3-030-54020-3_23

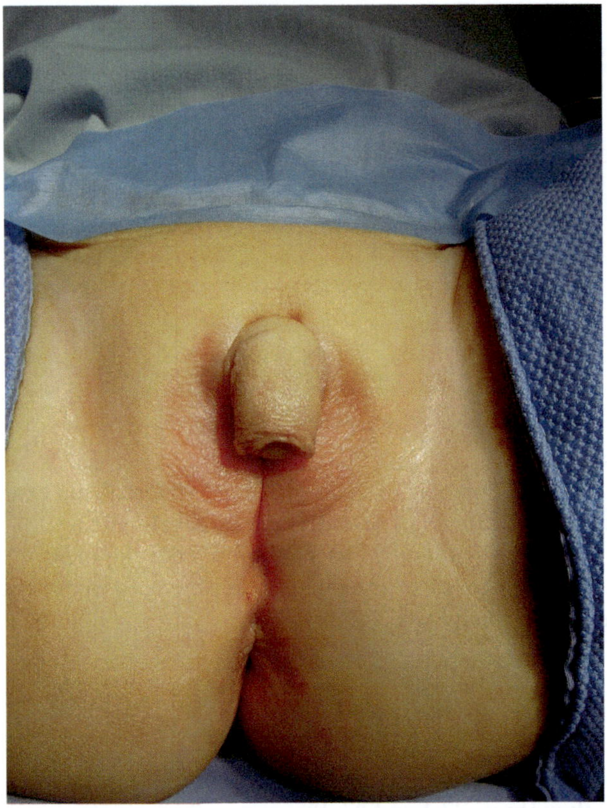

Fig. 23.1 External appearances of overvirilised 46XX female in CAH

Gonads: Documentation of palpable gonads is important; although ovotestes have been reported to descend completely into the bottom of labioscrotal folds, in most patients, only testicular material descends fully. If examination reveals palpable inguinal gonads, diagnoses of a gonadal female, and pure gonadal dysgenesis can be eliminated. Bilateral impalpable gonads, even in an apparently fully virilized infant, should raise the possibility of a severely virilized 46, XX DSD patient with for example CAH.

Phallus: Note the size and degree of differentiation of the phallus, since variations may represent clitoromegaly or hypospadias.

Labioscrotal folds: Labioscrotal folds may be separated or folds may be fused at the midline, giving an appearance of a scrotum. Labioscrotal folds with increased pigmentation suggest the possibility of increased corticotropin levels as part of CAH.

Urethral opening: Note the position of the urethral meatus and the number of openings on the perineum. This requires elevating the phallus to get a good view of the perineal openings.

In classical CAH in a virilzed female, no gonads will be palpable and there will be a single urogenital sinus. Depending on the degree of virilisation there will be

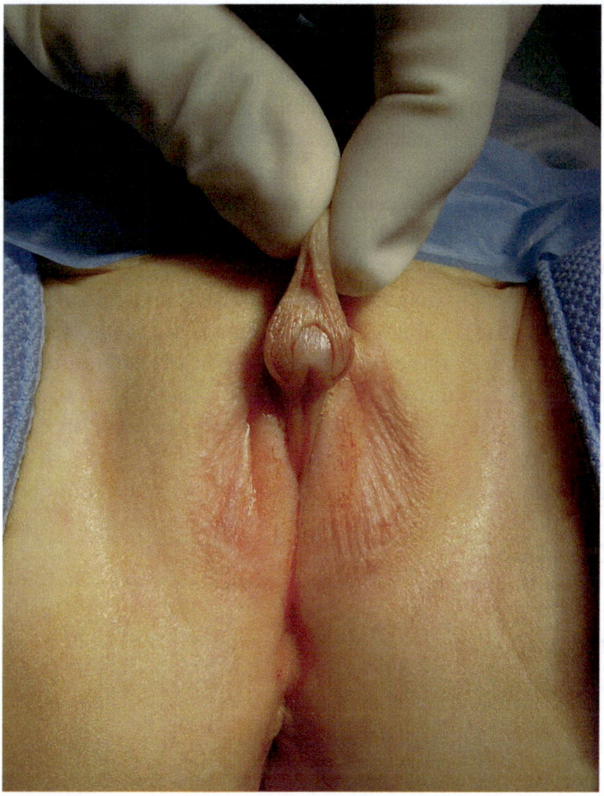

Fig. 23.2 External appearances of overvirilised 46XX female in CAH

hypertrophy and rugosity of the labioscrotal folds and hypertrophy of the phallus. If a gonad/s is palpable, this suggests a male karyotype with hypospadias which could be idiopathic, due to partial androgen insensitivity or a rarer testosterone biosynthetic defect. If a gonad is palpable on one side and impalpable on the contralateral side, one must consider a mixed gonadal dysgenesis.

As the classic type can be salt wasting, careful attention to the weight and state of hydration is important.

23.1.1.3 Question 2

Assuming neither gonads are palpable, what is the most likely diagnosis in the above case?

23.1.1.4 Answer 2

46XX DSD: Congenital adrenal hyperplasia.

23.1.1.5 Question 3

What investigations would assist in making the diagnosis?

23.1.1.6 Answer 3

Karyotype; The expected karyotype would be 46XX.

Endocrine investigations: The most common form (classic) is characterised by mutations in the 21-hydroxylase (21OH) enzyme, which normally converts 17-OHP to 11-dexoycortisol and progesterone to deoxycorticosterone. Loss of this enzyme activity results in the redirection of this pathway leading to an increase in androgens. To fully differentiate between the various enzymatic defects potentially causing CAH, clinicians should ideally send samples for measurement of 17-OHP, cortisol, 11-deoxycortisol, dehydroepiandrosterone, androstenedione and testosterone. Renin and aldosterone may be helpful to assess salt wasting. A urinary steroid profile if available is also a valuable investigation. Due to interference from placental and maternal hormones these investigations can't be sent until 48–72 h of age.

Pelvic ultrasound to identify presence of Mullerian structures.

A simple urine dip for protein and blood should be done in case of rare conditions like Denys-Drash.

Until the diagnosis is confirmed, the neonates' sex should not be registered.

23.1.1.7 Question 4

What would be your management of this baby with CAH?

23.1.1.8 Answer 4

Immediate

1. Resuscitation with attention to fluid and electrolyte balance and weight
2. Steroids; hydrocortisone and fludrocortisone and sodium chloride supplements under guidance of a paediatric endocrinologist once appropriate investions have been sent.
3. IV fluids as required in the newborn period.

Subsequent

1. Endocrine management: Treatment can include the use of hydrocortisone, fludrocortisone and sodium chloride replacement; however treatment will depend on the sex, age, duration (short, long term and stress dosing), pregnancy status and type of CAH. Care should also be taken to avoid under and over-replacement of steroids.
2. Surgical management: EUA, cystovaginoscopy at around 6–12 months of age with or without a genitogram. This will give a better understanding of the length of the common channel if early surgery is being considered, although this is controversial and is discussed below.

23.1.2 Further Surgical Management

23.1.2.1 Surgical Controversies in CAH Surgery and DSD Surgery in General

Increasingly there has become a reluctance for early surgical intervention to improve the external appearances of the genitalia in CAH. Previously this used to involve feminising genitoplasty with reduction in the size of the clitoris (reduction, recession or cavernous body sparing) and recreating the labioscrotal folds. The timing of vaginal reconstruction has been debated between reconstruction in early infancy to delayed vaginal reconstruction after puberty.

Increasingly, the principle of shared decision making (SDM) between parents and the clinicians has been advocated with a further extension of this shared decision making involving the child when they are old enough to participate in the decision making. Parents can make decisions under the SDM principle in the best interests of their child but opponents of this view cite the lack of autonomy of the child in making their own decisions. Certainly in some countries including the UK, widespread media attention to the topic of genital surgery in DSD has led to many healthcare providers putting a moratorium on such surgery.

Hence it is vitally important that parents receive full psychological support as part of an MDT while these issues are discussed and managed on a case by case basis.

23.1.2.2 Surgical Management for the Vagina

The timing of surgery for the vagina remains controversial. Opponents of early vaginal reconstruction consider this not to be required for functional reasons at this age along with the potential for complications requiring further surgical interventions. In the authors' practice, vaginal reconstruction is delayed until the peripubertal age. At this point a further evaluation of the common channel jointly with an adolescent gynaecologist by a cystovaginoscopy is carried out. Where there is no impedance to menstrual flow, depending on the length of the common channel and as per the wishes of the girl, the surgery can be differed to a later date. If there is impedance to menstrual flow, this will require earlier surgery. Any surgery should be undertaken by either a paediatric or adolescent urologist/urogynaecologist with experience in such surgery. The aim of the surgery for the vagina is for the entrance to the vagina to be on the perineum to enable intercourse and the use of tampons.

23.1.3 Scenario 2

A 6 month old infant girl presents with an irreducible right inguinal hernia. At surgical exploration a testicle like structure is seen within the hernia sac.

23.1.3.1 Question 1

What would be your surgical intervention?

23.1.3.2 Answer 1

As the child has been consented for a hernia repair, this would be the most appropriate course of action in the first instance. The gonad should be returned to the abdomen and after the procedure the parents should be counselled regarding the findings and the need for further investigations.

23.1.3.3 Question 2

What would be your subsequent investigations?

23.1.3.4 Answer 2

Endocrine: Karyotype. Depending on the age of the child, LH, FSH, DHEAS, Androstenedione and Testosterone. In some cases this may require an HCG test. Consider sending genetics for Androgen receptor mutations or a DSD gene panel as these are becoming more widely available.

Imaging: pelvic ultrasound to identify presence or absence of any Mullerian structures.

Surgery: laparoscopy to identify the nature of the gonads on either side and biopsy of the gonads to ascertain the gonadal sex. If the diagnosis is a complete androgen insensitivity, then a perineal examination will demonstrate a small vaginal pit as the distal vagina is not influenced by the secretion of AMH by the testis.

23.1.3.5 Question 3

What is the likely differential diagnosis?

23.1.3.6 Answer 3

Complete Androgen Insensitivity Syndrome.

Mixed Gonadal Dysgenesis.

Ovotesticular DSD.

23.1.3.7 Question 4

How would you manage this infant if the Karyotype is 46XY?

23.1.3.8 Answer 4

In this situation the phenotype is female. Attention should therefore be paid to the karyotype and the gonadal sex.

If the karyotype shows a Y chromosome, a full discussion needs to be undertaken with the family with psychological and genetic counselling as part of an MDT. The sex of rearing will be female in cases of CAIS and the future management would be for the child to function as a female both psychologically and anatomically. Managing the gonads and the timing thereof should also be discussed. It is generally agreed that the testes should be retained until puberty and then bilateral gonadectomy performed. The postponement of gonadectomy until at least puberty allows spontaneous pubertal development thanks to oestradiol deriving from the peripheral aromatization of testosterone produced by the retained testes. Input regarding vaginal reconstruction should be obtained from a urogynaecologist experienced in surgery for DSD and this can be delayed until the peripubertal age when the child can be part of the shared decision making process.

HRT is mandatory after bilateral gonadectomy and should be undertaken in consultation with an endocrinologist. This is to induce pubertal development or maintain secondary sexual characteristics. The classic HRT for CAIS patients is based on oestrogen therapy, and there are a number of consensus recommendations as to dose and route (oral or transdermal), for example the BSPED guidelines. As the child gets older, regular psychological counselling is essential.

23.1.4 Scenario 3

A 15 year old girl presents with primary amenorrhoea.

23.1.4.1 Question 1

What investigations would you do to make a diagnosis?

23.1.4.2 Answer 1

History: a good history of any coexistent disease or any weight changes.

Clinical examination: Height, weight, blood pressure, secondary sexual characteristics include any palpable gonads.

Endocrine investigations: Serum electrolytes, FSH, LH, TSH, T4, oestradiol, androstenedione, testosterone.

Imaging: Pelvic ultrasound looking for mullerian structures. Absent Mullerian structures along with raised gonadotrophins with or without breast bud development should prompt the need for a karyotype.

An algorithm for the management of primary amenorrhoea is shown below.

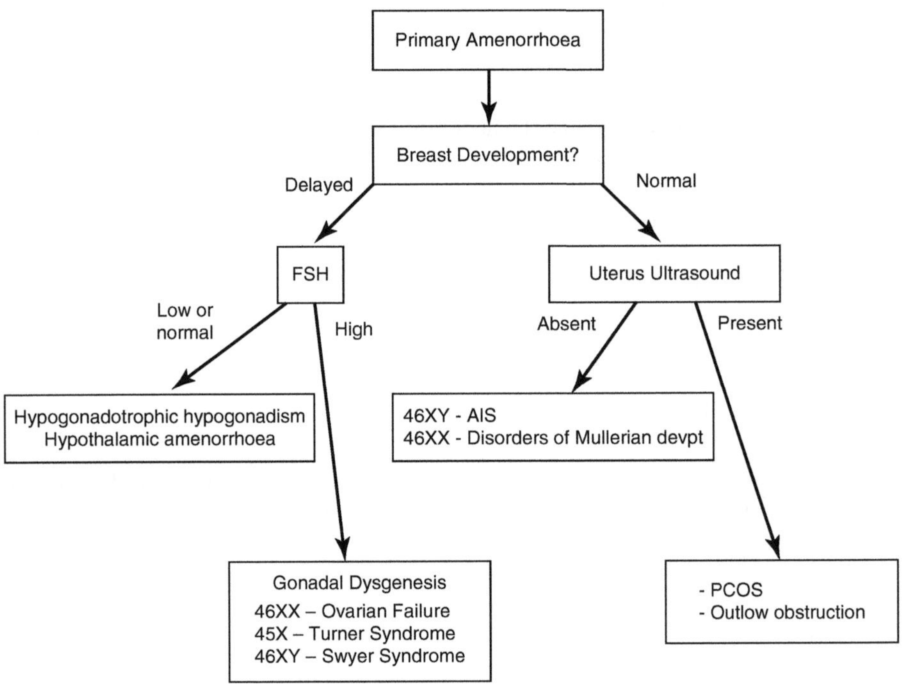

From: Society for Endocrinology UK guidance on the initial evaluation of an infant or an adolescent with a suspected disorder of sex development (Revised 2015).

LH to the measurement of FSH is advisable although FSH measurement alone can give the answer in the majority of cases. One has to also bear in mind that the primary amenorrhoea may be reflective of delayed pubertal development.

23.1.4.3 Question 2

The karyotype is 46XY with no Mullerian structures on US and palpable gonads bilaterally in the groin. Discuss current thoughts of management of the gonads and why?

In CAIS, the risk of Germ cell tumours (GCT) is considered low and related to age. The estimated risk of gonadal tumors (eg gonadoblastoma) in CAIS gonads is about 0.8–22%. The reports of malignant GCTs before puberty in CAIS are very rare. After puberty, the risk is low, but not negligible. Hence most clinicians would recommend gonadectromy after puberty after completion of breast development.

However some patients may wish to retain their gonads. In these patients regular monitoring with ultrasonography is recommended. If the gonads are intra-abdominal an MRI may be more helpful for monitoring.

23.1.4.4 Question 3

What are the options for vaginal reconstruction?

23.1.4.5 Answer 3

Non surgical dilatation only, may be accomplished in many cases, by self dilatation of the vaginal pit.

Surgical: McIndoe, Vechietti procedures.

Intestinal transplantation.

Any approach should be discussed with the patient, their families in an MDT setting along with an appropriately experienced urogynaecologist/adolescent urologist.

23.1.5 Scenario 4

A newborn male infant presents with a proximal hypospadias and a unilateral palpable descended testis and a contralateral impalpable testis. His karyotype is 46XY with normal urinary steroid profile. At 9 months of age he undergoes a laparoscopy for his impalpable testis and first stage hypospadias repair. At laparoscopy a streak gonad with appearances like an ovary and a hemiuterus with a rudimentary fallopian tube are seen on the side of the impalpable gonad.

23.1.5.1 Question 1

What is the most likely diagnosis?

23.1.5.2 Answer 1

This is most likely to be a sex chromosome DSD mixed gonadal dysgenesis. In most cases, this is due to a 45XO/46XY mosaicism. However if this is not a mosaicism, then this would come under the 46XY DSD category—partial gonadal dysgenesis or ovotesticular DSD.

23.1.5.3 Question 2

What investigations would you consider?

A karyotype should be undertaken with a microarray to ascertain mosaicism.

The endocrinological evaluation of 46, XY DSD infants includes assessment of testicular function by basal measurements of LH, FSH, inhibin B, anti-Mullerian hormone (AMH) and steroids.

23.1.5.4 Question 3

The karyotype is 46XY. What would be your management of the phallus?

23.1.5.5 Answer 3

In this case, either a single or 2 stage hypospadias repair would be the recommended option.

23.1.5.6 Question 4

What would be your management of the intraabdominal gonad and rudimentary mullerian structures?

23.1.5.7 Answer 4

Because of the high risk of gonadoblastoma (30%), one would recommend biopsy prior to gonadectomy unless frozen section could be examined in theatre to confirm the presence of ovarian stroma. If the Y chromosome is present in the gonadal biopsy, the option is to undertake an early gonadectomy. Removal of the Mullerian structures can be undertaken at the same time. In the absence of Y chromosome in the streak gonad, removal of the gonad and/or the mullerian structures is dependant on the parental/child wishes.

Because of the usually dysgenetic contralateral descended testicle, annual surveillance should be undertaken with the possibility of a testicular biopsy at puberty. Hormone replacement may be necessary in the run up to puberty.

Suggested Further Reading

1. Cools M, Nordenström A, Robeva R, Hall J, Westerveld P, Flück C, Köhler B, Berra M, Springer A, Schweizer K, Pasterski V, on behalf of the COST Action BM1303 working group. Expert consensus document caring for individuals with a difference of sex development (DSD): a consensus statement. Nat Rev Endocrinol. 2018;14:415–29.
2. Hughes IA., Houk C., Ahmed SF., Lee PA, LWPES Consensus Group, & ESPE Consensus Group. Consensus statement on management of intersex disorders. Arch Dis Child. 2006;91(7):554–63. https://doi.org/10.1136/adc.2006.098319.
3. Juliana Gabriel Ribeiro de Andrade, Antonia Paula Marques-de-Faria, Helena Campos Fabbri, Maricilda Palandi de Mello, Gil Guerra-Júnior, and Andréa Trevas Maciel-Guerra, "Long-term follow-up of patients with 46, XY partial gonadal Dysgenesis reared as males," International J Endocrinol, 2014, Article ID 480724, 8, 2014.

4. Gardner M, Sandberg DE. Navigating surgical decision making in disorders of sex development (DSD). Front Pediatr. 2018;6:339. https://doi.org/10.3389/fped.2018.00339.
5. Speiser PW, Arlt W, Auchus RJ, Baskin LS, Conway GS, Merke DP, et al. Congenital adrenal hyperplasia due to steroid 21-hydroxylase deficiency: an Endocrine Society clinical practice guideline. J Clin Endocrinol Metab. 2018;103(11):4043–88.
6. Lanciotti L, Cofini M, Leonardi A, Bertozzi M, Penta L, Esposito S. Different clinical presentations and Management in Complete Androgen Insensitivity Syndrome (CAIS). Int J Environ Res Public Health. 2019;16(7):1268.
7. Ahmed SF, Achermann JC, Arlt W, Balen A, Conway G, Edwards Z, Elford S, Hughes IA, Izatt L, Krone N, Miles H, O'Toole S, Perry L, Sanders C, Simmonds M, Watt A, Willis D. Society for Endocrinology UK guidance on the initial evaluation of an infant or an adolescent with a suspected disorder of sex development (revised 2015). Clin Endocrinol. 2016;84:771–88.
8. Batista RL, Frade Costa EM, de Santi Rodrigues A, et al. Androgen insensitivity syndrome: a review. Arch Endocrinol Metab. 2018;62(2):227–35.

Pediatric and Adolescent Gynecology 24

Veronica I. Alaniz

Learning Objectives

- Describe approaches for examination of the genitalia in a prepubertal female patient
- Identify etiologies and understand treatment options for pediatric vulvar conditions
- Discuss genital changes that occur at puberty and vulvovaginal concerns in adolescents
- Recognize hymenal and vaginal anomalies and describe surgical techniques for management

24.1 Pediatric Gynecology

The most common gynecological conditions in childhood involve the lower genital tract and are usually diagnosed with a careful history and examination of the external genitalia. The prepubertal genital exam can be challenging and the goal is to obtain information without causing trauma. Before starting the examination, it is important to discuss the nature of the exam and reassure both the patient and caregivers that the examination will only be visual inspection of the external genitalia. There are several positions that allow adequate visualization of the external genitalia. "Frog-leg" or "butterfly" is often used which can be done with the child on the exam table or a caregiver's lap. Alternate positions are prone or lateral decubitus with knees to chest. In either of these positions, visualization of the genitalia is enhanced with labial traction by grasping the bilateral labia majora with the thumb

V. I. Alaniz, MD, MPH (✉)
Division of Pediatric and Adolescent Gynecology, Children's Hospital Colorado, Aurora, CO, USA
e-mail: veronica.alaniz@cuanschutz.edu

P. Godbole et al. (eds.), *Practical Pediatric Urology*,
https://doi.org/10.1007/978-3-030-54020-3_24

and forefinger and gently pulling laterally and downward or alternatively, placing gentle downward traction on the buttocks [1].

Complete examination of the external genitalia includes evaluation of pubic hair, clitoris, prepuce, labia majora, labia minora, urethra, hymen, and anus. Due to the absence of estrogen, prepubertal labia majora are flat, labia minora are thin, hymen is thin, and the vagina is atrophic with a basic pH. The shape of the hymen should be noted and accurately describe [1, 2]. There are several hymenal configurations with the most common shapes being crescentic and annular in the prepubertal girl. Occasionally, a congenital anomaly of the hymen (septate, microperforate, imperforate) is detected on prepubertal exam which typically does not require surgical intervention until adolescence. See Fig. 24.1. Hymenal notches and bumps can be present and should not prompt evaluation of sexual abuse without associated history or parental concern. In a study of 147 prepubertal girls selected for non-abuse, 51% were noted to have hymenal irregularities [3]. The exception to this is the finding of

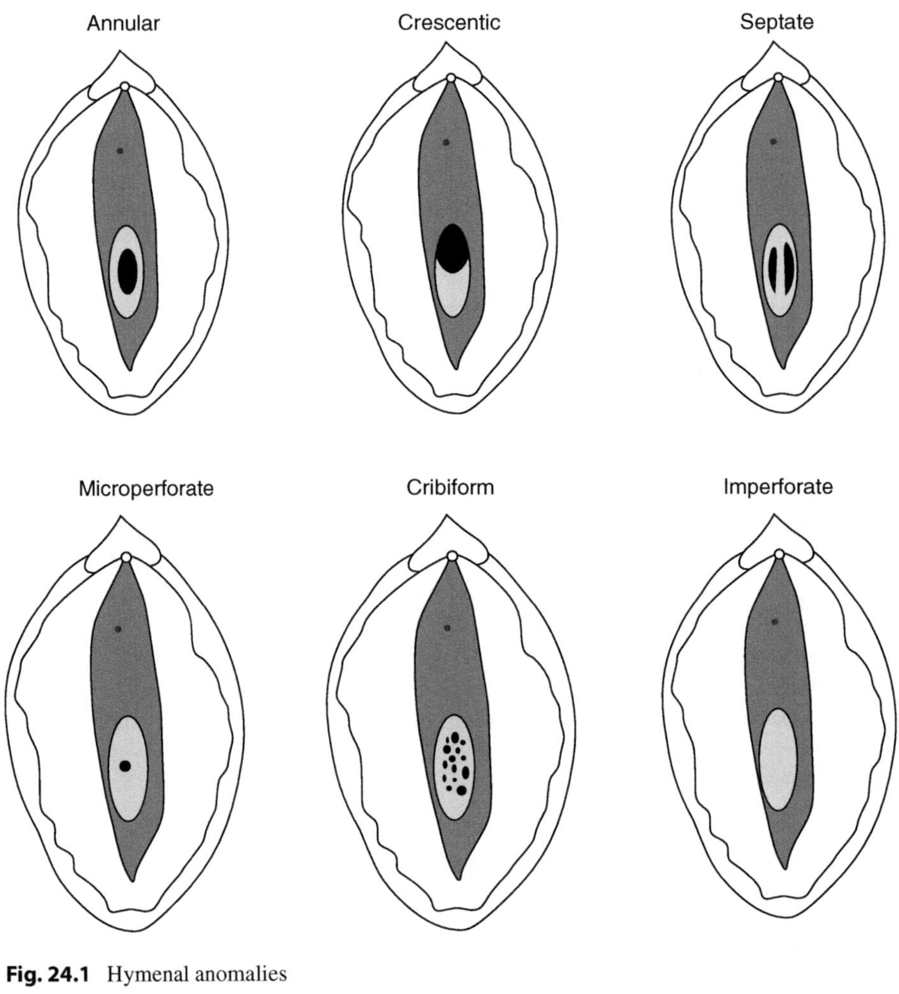

Fig. 24.1 Hymenal anomalies

deep notches or complete transection in the posterior portion of the hymen which is concerning for vaginal penetration [4].

Exam under anesthesia and vaginoscopy may be indicated when office examination in insufficient. In cooperative patients with narrow-caliber hysteroscopes, vaginoscopy can be done in the office setting. In most cases, vaginoscopy is done in the operating room with a pediatric cystoscope and saline as distending medium. To facilitate distension, the introitus should be occluded by gently pinching the labia majora closed [5].

24.2 Vulvovaginitis

Vulvovaginitis is one of the most common gynecological concerns in prepubertal girls and in most cases the etiology is non-specific [6]. Young girls are susceptible to vulvovaginal issues due to unestrogenized and alkaline vaginal mucosa, lack of labial fat pads and pubic hair that protect the vulva, poor hygiene, and proximity of the vulva to the rectum. Additionally, genital tissues are easily irritated by harsh soaps, chemicals, and clothing [7, 8]. Genital complaints in the prepubertal child include discomfort, vulvar redness, itching, vaginal discharge, dysuria and less commonly vaginal bleeding which occurs from mucosal irritation with skin breakdown. All patients with vulvovaginal complaints should be screened for abuse [6].

Prior studies have identified an infectious etiology in 20–36% of vulvovaginitis cases [6, 9]. Isolated bacteria are often enteric or respiratory in origin such as group A β-haemolytic streptococcus, *Haemopholius influenza, Klebsiella pneumoniae, Shigella flexnori, Staphylococcus aureus, Escherichia coli, Enterococcus faecalis* [8–10]. In toilet trained prepubertal girls without risk factors (diabetes, immunosuppressed state, or recent use of antibiotics), yeast is rarely the cause of vulvovaginitis. This is because a non-estrogenized atrophic vagina has a high vaginal pH which does not allow growth of Candida [6, 10, 11].

Vulvovaginitis can be diagnosed by history and examination of the external genitalia. Treatment for non-specific vulvovaginitis includes avoidance of any potential irritants and hygiene measures outlined in Box 24.1. Mild to moderate symptoms can be also be treated with cool compresses to the vulva and a non-medicated emollient such as Aquaphor (Beiersdorf Inc., Hamburg, Germany) and A&D (Schering-Plough Healthcare Products, Inc., Memphis, TN, USA). Patients that have failed conservative management may benefit from a course of topical steroids or oral antibiotics [12].

Those with bacterial vulvovaginitis tend to have marked vulvar erythema and more visible discharge [6]. If infection is suspected or discharge is visible at the introitus, an aerobic culture can be collected. In general, intravaginal specimens should not be obtained in the outpatient setting, unless a small moistened calgi swab is used. Amoxicillin is often used for bacterial vulvovaginitis since skin flora and respiratory pathogens are commonly implicated. Azithromycin or trimethroprim/sulfamethoxazole are options when gastrointestinal flora are isolated or suspected [12].

A vaginal foreign body can cause vulvovaginitis and typically presents with purulent, malodorous, and blood tinged discharge [8]. The most common item found is tissue paper but other items such as coins, beads, and small toys can also be recovered. In cooperative patients, vaginal irrigation can be used to expel tissue paper. Otherwise, vaginoscopy if often indicated to evaluate for and remove foreign bodies [13].

24.3 Labial Adhesions

Labial adhesions or agglutination occurs when the labia minora become adherent in the midline. This occurs most commonly between ages 3 months and 3 years in response to estrogen deficiency and local inflammation [14]. Inflammation from poor hygiene, infection, or vulvar trauma can cause agglutination by denuding of the mucosal surface of the labia which then stick together. Patients with labial adhesions are often asymptomatic, though can present discomfort, an abnormal urine stream, post void dribbling, and urinary tract infections. Diagnosis can be made with history and examination of the genitalia. The adhesion typically appears as a grey line (raphe) and can be the entire length of the labia or just a small portion [15]. See Fig. 24.2.

Many cases of labial adhesions resolve spontaneously. In patients that are asymptomatic, expectant management or use of a non-medicated emollient is a reasonable option. In cases where the adhesion is significant or causing symptoms, an estrogen based cream or steroid cream is often needed. When prescribed, a small (pea-sized) amount of estrogen cream is applied to the adhesion once to twice daily with gentle traction for at least 2 weeks and usually no more than 6 weeks [15]. Estrogen cream results in resolution of the adhesion in 50–90% of cases and is most successful when the adhesion is thin and translucent [16, 17]. The most common side effects include local irritation, vulvar pigmentation, and rarely pubertal changes. Patients should be assessed for breast budding with treatment and especially with repeat courses of topical estrogen [15]. Topical steroids, such as betamethasone 0.05% ointment, are an alternative to estrogen cream and are typically prescribed twice daily for 4–6 weeks [15, 18].

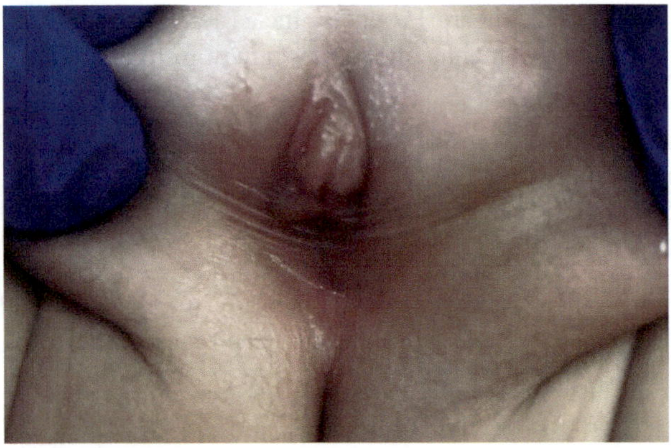

Fig. 24.2 Labial adhesions

Box 24.1 General Recommendations for Hygiene and Self-Care for the Vulva and Vagina

- Change diapers frequently and avoid irritants on the skin.
- If toilet trained, wear only plain white, cotton underpants.
- Use unscented detergent and avoid fabric softeners or any extra cleaning or "freshening" products.
- Wear a nightgown for sleeping. It's OK to sleep without underwear
- Avoid tights, one-piece leotards, tight jeans, or leggings.
- Take a bath every day and use clean, warm water only. No soap, vinegar or baking soda is needed.
- Gently pat the genital area dry.
- Don't use bubble bath or perfumed soap.
- Always wipe from front to back after bowel movements
- Change out of wet swimsuits and sweaty exercise clothes.

Manual separation of the labia without a topical anesthetic or sedation should be avoided due to associated pain and potential trauma caused to the child. Surgical separation in the operating room is only recommended in rare cases when the adhesion is very thick and topical treatment has failed. A lubricated Q-tip applied with tension to the raphe is usually sufficient to separate the adhesion. Occasionally, sharp dissection is needed.

Recurrence of labial adhesions is common. Regardless of treatment modality, a non-medicated emollient should be applied daily after separation to prevent recurrence. Good vulvar hygiene in an effort to prevent vulvar irritation should be reviewed with caregivers. See Box 24.1.

24.4 Lichen Sclerosus

Lichen sclerosus is a chronic inflammatory condition affecting the anogenital skin. Though it is most common in post-menopausal women, up to 15% of cases arise in childhood with a reported incidence of 1 in 900 girls [19, 20]. The pathogenesis of lichen sclerosus is likely multifactorial, but it is generally considered an autoimmune condition that peaks at times of low estrogen [20, 21]. Symptoms include intense vulvar itching, soreness, dysuria, pain with defecation, and sometimes genital bleeding. Examination findings are characteristic and most notable for thin and hypopigmented skin in a classic "figure of 8" distribution around the vulvar and anus. Subepithelial hemorrhages (blood blisters), ecchymosis, and fissures can also be present. In late stages, scarring can lead to loss of vulvar architecture including resorption of labia minora, buried clitoris, and introital narrowing [19, 21, 22]. See Fig. 24.3.

In prepubertal girls, vulvar biopsy is rarely indicated and the diagnosis of lichen sclerosus is made on history and physical exam only. On average, it takes 1–2 years after onset of symptoms before the correct diagnosis of LS is made, and infection, trauma, and/or sexual abuse are often first suspected [23]. For clinicians who are

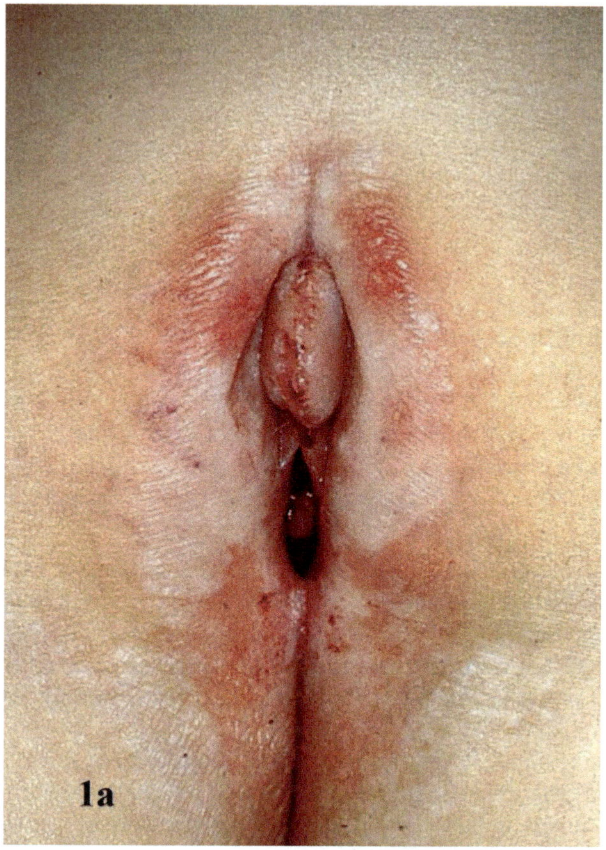

Fig. 24.3 Pediatric Lichen Sclerosus depicting vulvar hypopigementation, fissures, and subepithelial hemorrhages. (Reference: Boms, S., Gambichler, T., Freitag, M. et al. BMC Dermatol (2004) 4: 14. https://doi.org/10.1186/1471-5945-4-14)

unfamiliar with prepubertal lichen sclerosus, the clinical findings of genital bruising and bleeding can be confused with genital trauma and worrisome for abuse [20, 24]. The diagnosis of lichen sclerosus, as with any vulvar complaint in a prepubertal girl, should not prevent appropriate abuse screening.

The goals of treatment for lichen sclerosus are to provide symptom relief and prevent genital scarring. Acute symptoms are typically treated with high-potency steroids such as clobetasol propionate or betamethasone valerate [19]. A suggested regimen is topical clobetasol propionate 0.05% applied twice daily for two weeks, followed by daily application for two weeks, tapered to a lower-potency agent, such as triamcinolone acetonide 0.1% applied twice daily for two weeks followed by daily application for two weeks. Lichen sclerosus tends to be recurrent and often requires repeat courses of topical steroids. Physicians should monitor for thinning of the vulvar skin and superimposed bacterial or yeast infections, which can result from prolonged use of high-potency topical steroids [25]. Vulvar hygiene is important for symptom control and should be reviewed with the patient and caregivers. See Box 24.1.

24.5 Adolescent Gynecology

The anatomy and physiology of the reproductive system changes with endogenous estrogen production during puberty. Most adolescents follow up a predictable pubertal course that usually begins with breast budding around the age of 10. Pubic hair, body odor, and axillary hair results primarily from adrenal androgens and typically lags behind breast development. The major landmark of puberty is menarche which typically occurs 2–3 years after breast budding between 12 and 13 years of age [26]. Vaginal tissue changes in response to estrogen and becomes thickened and rugated. The hymen during puberty is redundant and in most cases can stretch without difficulty. Vaginal secretions are common and discharge that is clear or cloudy without an associated odor, itch, or burn is often physiologic. Changes to the external genitalia also occur during puberty and include thickening of the labia majora and enlargement of the labia minora to adult size. The labia minora are varied in size, shape, and color and asymmetry is not uncommon.

24.6 Labial Hypertrophy

There is no consensus for the definition of labial hypertrophy and few original studies attempt to define labia minora size. In the current literature, the typical width of the labia minora range from 3 to 50 mm in adult women [27]. When teen girls present with concerns about labial appearance, the provider should educate about normal variation and provide reassurance. Resources such as the *The Labia Library* (www.labialibrary.org.au) and *Great Wall of Vagina* (www.greatwallofvagina.co.uk) can be used to illustrate normal differences. Surgical intervention for cosmetic purposes should not be offered to patients <18 years old [27, 28].

In some cases, patients may present with functional concerns due to enlarged labia including irritation, pain, pulling with activity, difficulties with menstrual hygiene, and interference during sexual activity. Comfort measures and supportive care should be recommended first and include supportive garments, avoidance of soaps or gels to the vulva, a non-medicated emollient, and arrangement of labia minora during activity and sports [28].

Though there is an increasing awareness of external genitalia and request for labiaplasty, criteria for surgical intervention have not been established. Labiaplasty in patients less than 18 years of age should only be considered in girls with significant and persistent functional symptoms. Laws and regulations must also be considered prior to surgery; for example medically unnecessary genital surgery in minors is a violation of US federal law. In adolescents particularly, it is also important to assess the maturity of the teen and determine if she has ability to make a decision independent of peer and family pressures [25].

There are a variety of different surgical techniques described for labiaplasty including de-epitheliazation, excision or amputation of the free edge, central wedge excision, inferior wedge excision, W-shaped excision, and Z-plasty with excision and wedge techniques being the most commonly described [29]. See Fig. 24.4. With

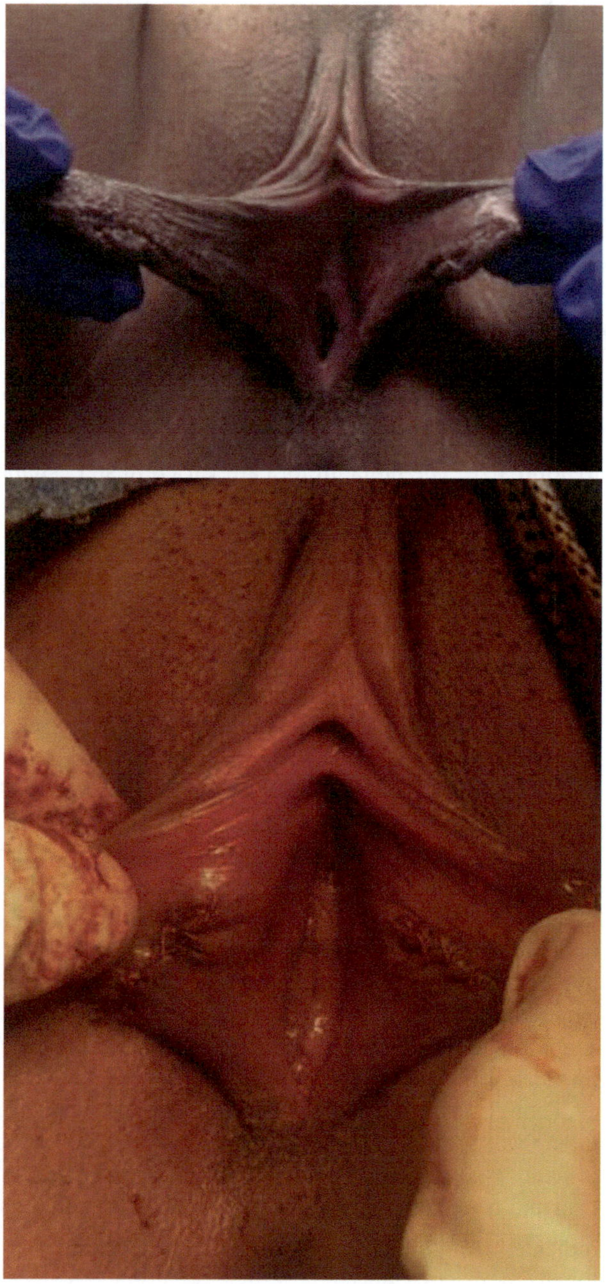

Fig. 24.4 Labial hypertrophy before and after wedge resection

any method, sensation may be altered due to removal of skin with many nerve endings. The most common complications are hematoma, wound dehiscence, discomfort, visible scarring, need for repeat surgery [27, 29].

24.7 Non Sexual Genital Ulcers

Acute genital ulcers in non-sexually active young girls have been attributed to a variety of causes including idiopathic aphthosis, post viral or infectious aphthosis, Bechet's disease, inflammatory bowel disease, drug reaction, and trauma. Patients typically present with intense vulvar pain from ulcerations on the inner mucosal surface of the labia minora which can be associated with difficulty urinating. Many patients have prodromal symptoms or report a recent history of febrile illness and symptoms typically last 10–14 days. Although Ebstein Barr Virus is commonly cited as an infectious etiology, the majority of cases are idiopathic [30, 31].

The goals of treatment are to provide pain relief and prevent super-imposed infection. Supportive care and comfort measures include sitz baths, topical anesthetics, oral analgesics, and efforts to minimize voiding discomfort such as voiding with legs apart or in the bathtub. Occasionally patients are admitted to the hospital for pain management and require placement of a foley catheter. Recurrence is common and seen in 30–35% of patients, although duration of symptoms is usually shorter and ulcers are smaller [30, 31]

24.8 Hymenal Anomalies

Congenital abnormalities of the hymen are either occlusive (imperforate hymen) or subocclusive (septate, microperforate, cribiform hymen). See Fig. 24.1. A septate hymen is the most common hymenal anomaly with an estimated prevalence of 0.7% [32]. This typically presents during adolescence with difficulty inserting or removing tampons. Diagnosis can be made with history and physical examination only. When evaluating the external genitalia, outward and lateral traction of the labia majora may be sufficient enough to open the vestibule and reveal hymenal anatomy. If not obvious with inspection, a lubricated Q tip can be used to delineate the borders of the hymen and identify a septum if present. Resection of the hymenal septum is usually performed in the operating room, however can also be offered in the outpatient setting with an injectable anesthetic. After removing the septum, mucosal edges should be reapproximated with 3-0 or 4-0 vicryl. Removal of the septum allows use of tampons for menstrual hygiene and penetrative vaginal intercourse.

An imperforate hymen is less common occurring in 1/2000 girls. This is an obstructive anomaly that presents with primary amenorrhea and cyclic pelvic pain, increasing in severity due to worsening hematometrocolpos. If the vagina is very distended, the patient may also complain of urinary retention and constipation. On

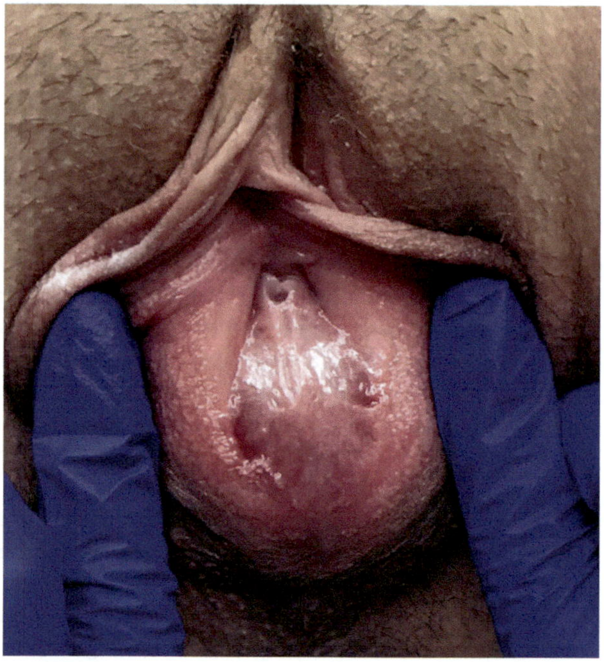

Fig. 24.5 Imperforate hymen

examination of the vulva, no hymenal opening is present and a flesh colored or bluish bulge is seen at the introitus. See Fig. 24.5. If the obstruction has been present for some time, an abdominal mass from the hematometrocolpos will be present. A rectal exam is generally well tolerated and can aid in diagnosis. With an imperforate hymen, a vaginal bulge is palpated throughout the rectum. If the diagnosis is unclear or a more complex anomaly like vaginal agenesis or transverse vaginal septum is suspected, MRI should be performed for further evaluation. An imperforate hymen is treated surgically with hymenectomy. Hymenal tissue is excised in a cruciate or circular fashion to create a patent vaginal opening and obstructed menstrual blood is evacuated with suction. The mucosal edges are then reapproximated with 3-0 or 4-0 vicryl using interrupted stitches. Post operative dilation is not necessary since the risk of reobstruction is minimal [33]. If surgical services are not available, then menstrual suppression should be initiated with a combined estrogen and progestin hormonal contraception (pill or patch used continuously) or a progestin only pill such as Norethindrone Acetate.

24.9 Longitudinal Vaginal Septum

A longitudinal vaginal septum or duplicated vagina results from failed fusion of the distal mullerian ducts. Patients can be asymptomatic or present with painful intercourse and difficulty using tampons, specifically continued menstrual bleeding because the tampon is placed in only one of the hemi-vaginas. A longitudinal

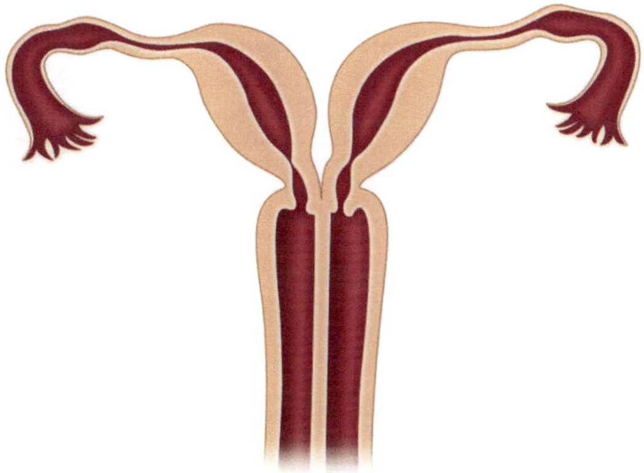

Fig. 24.6 Didelphys uterus with complete longitudinal vaginal septum

vaginal septum may be complete from the level of the cervix to the introitus or partial. See Fig. 24.6. It is typically diagnosed with pelvic exam and palpated on bimanual exam. A uterine anomaly is present in up 87% of cases, which should be evaluated with pelvic imaging [34]. Septum resection should be considered in patients that are symptomatic or those considering pregnancy. Although there are reports of successful vaginal delivery with a longitudinal vaginal septum, there is also risk of laceration or vaginal dystocia [35]. During surgical resection, the midline septum is removed completely with care to avoid injury to the cervix. The vaginal mucosa on either end of the septum is then reapproximated with a delayed absorbable suture [34]. Alternatively, a bipolar cutting forceps can be used to remove the septum [36].

24.10 Obstructed Hemi-Vagina and Ipsilateral Renal Anomalies (OHVIRA)

An obstructed hemi-vagina occurs with a partially formed vaginal septum and may be associated with ipsilateral renal agenesis or renal anomalies. See Fig. 24.7. Most patients with OHVIRA have complete uterine duplication. Patients typically present with worsening dysmenorrhea not responsive to oral pain medications or hormonal suppression of periods. With a chronic obstruction, an abdominal mass may be palpated from a large hematometrocolpos. If digital vaginal exam is performed, then a lateral bulge is often palpated in the vagina. Pelvic imaging with MRI confirms the diagnosis OHVIRA [37].

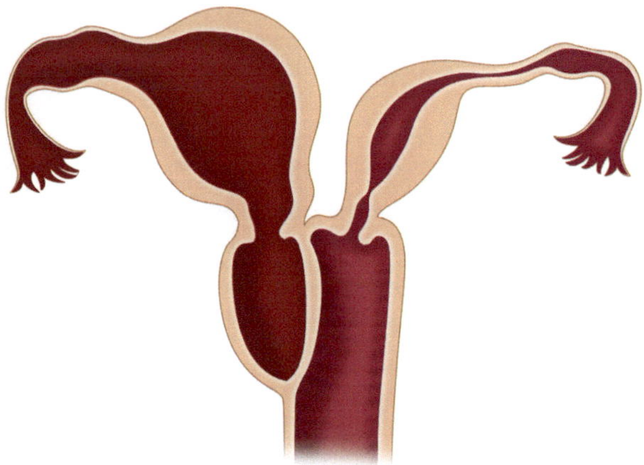

Fig. 24.7 Didelphys uterus with obstructed hemi vagina and hematocolpos

Resection of the obstructing vaginal septum provides definitive surgical treatment. Typically the septum is incised at a low point and old menstrual blood is evacuated. If the septum is thick or margins are unclear, a spinal needle can be inserted to help locate the obstructed vagina and guide the excision. All septal tissue should be excised with care not to injury nearby structures. Often times, the obstructed cervix is dilated making edges difficult to delineate. The vaginal mucosa is then re-approximated circumferentially with interrupted stitches [38]. With a thick septum, risk of stenosis and re-obstruction increases and surgical techniques such as a “Z-plasty” in conjunction with a vaginal stent or post-operative dilation might be considered. Occasionally, hemi-hysterectomy may be indicated [39].

24.11 Vaginal Agenesis

Mullerian agenesis, also referred to as Mayer-Rokitansky-Kuster-Hauser Syndrome (MRKH) or vaginal agenesis results from incomplete development of the mullerian ducts and occurs in approximately 1 in 4,500–5,000 females [40]. Patients typically present with normal pubertal development and primary amenorrhea. External genitalia appear typical with normal hymenal fringe. If a single digit exam is tolerated, the distal vagina will palpate short without any identifiable cervix. If digital exam is not tolerated, a lubricated Q-tip can be used to confirm an underdeveloped vagina [34]. Pelvic imaging with ultrasound or MRI will confirm mullerian agenesis and rule out obstructive anomalies which can present similarly. Some patients with mullerian agenesis have rudimentary mullerian remnants and laparoscopic removal of these remnants may be indicated if active endometrium is present or if the patient has cyclic abdominal pain. Work up should include a testosterone and karyotype to differentiate mullerian agenesis from Androgen Insensitivity Syndrome (AIS). Evaluation for associated congenital anomalies, especially skeletal and urologic, is necessary [41].

The diagnosis of mullerian agenesis and loss of fertility is difficult for patients and families. Emotions range from fear, isolation, depression and all patients should be offered counseling and connected to support groups. Fertility options should be discussed with patients and generally include adoption and assisted reproduction with use of a gestational carrier [34]. Live births have been reported from uterine transplantation, however this is only available on a research protocol at few centers. Vaginal creation should only be considered when the patient is emotionally ready and expresses a desire for treatment [41]. Dilation is an appropriate first line approach and is successful in creating a functional vagina in 90–95% of motivated patients [42, 43]. Depending on the frequency and duration of treatment, it usually takes 4–11 months to create a functional vagina. Surgical vaginoplasty is alternative for some patients, especially those that fail dilation. Various techniques exist including surgically assisted dilation and vaginoplasty with bowel, skin, oral mucosa, or peritoneum grafts. With any procedure, post operative dilation or penetrative intercourse is needed to maintain length and prevent stenosis [34]

References

1. Jacobs AM, Alderman EM. Gynecologic examination of the Prepubertal girl. Pediatr Rev. 2014;35(3):227–35.
2. Kass-Wolff JH, Wilson EE. Pediatric gynecology: assessment strategies and common problems. Semin Reprod Med. 2003;21(4):329–38.
3. Heger AH, Ticson L, Guerra L, Lister J, Zaragoza T, McConnell G, et al. Appearance of the genitalia in girls selected for nonabuse: review of hymenal morphology and nonspecific findings. J Pediatr Adolesc Gynecol. 2002;15(1):27–35.
4. Pillai M. Genital findings in prepubertal girls: what can be concluded from an examination? J Pediatr Adolesc Gynecol. 2008;21(4):177–85.
5. Simms-Cendan J. Examination of the pediatric adolescent patient. Best Pract Res Clin Obstet Gynaecol. 2018;48:3–13.
6. Jaquiery A, Stylianopoulos A, Hogg G, Grover S. Vulvovaginitis: clinical features, aetiology, and microbiology of the genital tract. Arch Dis Child. 1999;81(1):64–7.
7. Kives S. Pediatric Vulvovaginitis. Practical pediatric and adolescent gynecology. Hoboken, NJ: Blackwell Publishing Ltd.; 2013. p. 33–7.
8. Kokotos F. Vulvovaginitis. Pediatr Rev. 2006;27(3):116–7.
9. Stricker T, Navratil F, Sennhauser FH. Vulvovaginitis in prepubertal girls. Arch Dis Child. 2003;88(4):324–6.
10. Bumbuliene Z, Venclaviciute K, Ramasauskaite D, Arlauskiene A, Bumbul E, Drasutiene G. Microbiological findings of vulvovaginitis in prepubertal girls. Postgrad Med J. 2014;90(1059):8–12.
11. Banerjee K, Curtis E, de San LC, Graham JC. Low prevalence of genital candidiasis in children. Eur J Clin Microbiol Infect Dis. 2004;23(9):696–8.

12. Zuckerman A, Romano M. Clinical Recommendation: Vulvovaginitis. J Pediatr Adolesc Gynecol. 2016;29(6):673–9.
13. Smith YR, Berman DR, Quint EH. Premenarchal vaginal discharge: findings of procedures to rule out foreign bodies. J Pediatr Adolesc Gynecol. 2002;15(4):227–30.
14. Leung AK, Robson WL, Tay-Uyboco J. The incidence of labial fusion in children. J Paediatr Child Health. 1993;29(3):235–6.
15. Bacon JL, Romano ME, Quint EH. Clinical recommendation: labial adhesions. J Pediatr Adolesc Gynecol. 2015;28(5):405–9.
16. Muram D. Treatment of prepubertal girls with labial adhesions. J Pediatr Adolesc Gynecol. 1999;12(2):67–70.
17. Aribarg A. Topical oestrogen therapy for labial adhesions in children. Br J Obstet Gynaecol. 1975;82(5):424–5.
18. Mayoglou L, Dulabon L, Martin-Alguacil N, Pfaff D, Schober J. Success of treatment modalities for labial fusion: a retrospective evaluation of topical and surgical treatments. J Pediatr Adolesc Gynecol. 2009;22(4):247–50.
19. Bercaw-Pratt JL, Boardman LA, Simms-Cendan JS. Clinical recommendation: pediatric lichen sclerosus. J Pediatr Adolesc Gynecol. 2014;27(2):111–6.
20. Powell J, Wojnarowska F. Childhood vulvar lichen sclerosus: an increasingly common problem. J Am Acad Dermatol. 2001;44(5):803–6.
21. Murphy R. Lichen sclerosus. Dermatol Clin. 2010;28(4):707–15.
22. Val I, Almeida G. An overview of lichen sclerosus. Clin Obstet Gynecol. 2005;48(4):808–17.
23. Lagerstedt M, Karvinen K, Joki-Erkkila M, Huotari-Orava R, Snellman E, Laasanen SL. Childhood lichen sclerosus—a challenge for clinicians. Pediatr Dermatol. 2013;30(4):444–50.
24. Jenny C, Kirby P, Fuquay D. Genital lichen sclerosus mistaken for child sexual abuse. Pediatrics. 1989;83(4):597–9.
25. Smith YR, Quint EH. Clobetasol propionate in the treatment of premenarchal vulvar lichen sclerosus. Obstet Gynecol. 2001;98(4):588–91.
26. Chulani VL, Gordon LP. Adolescent growth and development. Prim Care. 2014;41(3):465–87.
27. Runacres SA, Wood PL. Cosmetic Labiaplasty in an adolescent population. J Pediatr Adolesc Gynecol. 2016;29(3):218–22.
28. Committee Opinion No. 662: breast and labial surgery in adolescents. Obstet Gynecol. 2016;127(5):e138–40.
29. Motakef S, Rodriguez-Feliz J, Chung MT, Ingargiola MJ, Wong VW, Patel A. Vaginal labiaplasty: current practices and a simplified classification system for labial protrusion. Plast Reconstr Surg. 2015;135(3):774–88.
30. Huppert JS, Gerber MA, Deitch HR, Mortensen JE, Staat MA, Adams Hillard PJ. Vulvar ulcers in young females: a manifestation of aphthosis. J Pediatr Adolesc Gynecol. 2006;19(3):195–204.
31. Rosman IS, Berk DR, Bayliss SJ, White AJ, Merritt DF. Acute genital ulcers in nonsexually active young girls: case series, review of the literature, and evaluation and management recommendations. Pediatr Dermatol. 2012;29(2):147–53.
32. Watrowski R, Jager C, Gerber M, Klein C. Hymenal anomalies in twins—review of the literature and case report. Eur J Pediatr. 2014;173(11):1407–12.
33. Breech LL, Laufer MR. Obstructive anomalies of the female reproductive tract. J Reprod Med. 1999;44(3):233–40.
34. Dietrich JE, Millar DM, Quint EH. Non-obstructive mullerian anomalies. J Pediatr Adolesc Gynecol. 2014;27(6):386–95.
35. Haddad B, Louis-Sylvestre C, Poitout P, Paniel BJ. Longitudinal vaginal septum: a retrospective study of 202 cases. Eur J Obstet Gynecol Reprod Biol. 1997;74(2):197–9.
36. Chatzipapas I, Zacharakis D, Michala L, Grigoriadis T, Antsaklis P, Protopapas A. Complete longitudinal vaginal septum resection. Description of a bloodless new technique. Clin Exp Obstet Gynecol. 2016;43(2):209–11.
37. Santos XM, Dietrich JE. Obstructed Hemivagina with Ipsilateral renal anomaly. J Pediatr Adolesc Gynecol. 2016;29(1):7–10.

38. Dietrich JE, Millar DM, Quint EH. Obstructive reproductive tract anomalies. J Pediatr Adolesc Gynecol. 2014;27(6):396–402.
39. Rieger MM, Santos XM, Sangi-Haghpeykar H, Bercaw JL, Dietrich JE. Laparoscopic outcomes for pelvic pathology in children and adolescents among patients presenting to the pediatric and adolescent gynecology service. J Pediatr Adolesc Gynecol. 2015;28(3):157–62.
40. Fontana L, Gentilin B, Fedele L, Gervasini C, Miozzo M. Genetics of Mayer-Rokitansky-Kuster-Hauser (MRKH) syndrome. Clin Genet. 2017;91(2):233–46.
41. Committee Opinion No ACOG. 728: Mullerian Agenesis: Diagnosis, Management. And Treatment Obstetrics and gynecology. 2018;131(1):e35–42.
42. Roberts CP, Haber MJ, Rock JA. Vaginal creation for mullerian agenesis. Am J Obstet Gynecol. 2001;185(6):1349–52; discussion 52–3.
43. Edmonds DK, Rose GL, Lipton MG, Quek J. Mayer-Rokitansky-Kuster-Hauser syndrome: a review of 245 consecutive cases managed by a multidisciplinary approach with vaginal dilators. Fertil Steril. 2012;97(3):686–90.

Index

P. Godbole et al. (eds.), *Practical Pediatric Urology*,
https://doi.org/10.1007/978-3-030-54020-3

W

<u>GPSR Compliance</u>

The European Union's (EU) General Product Safety Regulation (GPSR) is a set of rules that requires consumer products to be safe and our obligations to ensure this.

If you have any concerns about our products, you can contact us on ProductSafety@springernature.com

In case Publisher is established outside the EU, the EU authorized representative is:

Springer Nature Customer Service Center GmbH
Europaplatz 3
69115 Heidelberg, Germany

Batch number: 10732076

Printed by Printforce, the Netherlands